Copyright 2020 by Darryl Parker -All rights reserved.

No part of this book may be reproduced or transmitted in any form or by any means, electronic or mechanical, including photocopying and recording, or by any information storage and retrieval system, without permission in writing from the publisher. This is a work of fiction. Names, places, characters and incidents are either the product of the author's imagination or are used fictitiously, and any resemblance to any actual persons, living or dead, organizations, events or locales is entirely coincidental. The unauthorized reproduction or distribution of this copyrighted work is ilegal.

Disclaimer Notice:

Please note the information contained within this document is for educational and entertainment purposes only. All effort has been executed to present accurate, up to date, reliable, complete information. No warranties of any kind are declared or implied. Readers acknowledge that the author is not engaged in the rendering of legal, financial, medical, or professional advice. The content within this book has been derived from various sources. Please consult a licensed professional before attempting any techniques outlined in this book.

By reading this document, the reader agrees that under no circumstances is the author responsible for any losses, direct or indirect, that are incurred as a result of the use of the information contained within this document, including, but not limited to, errors, omissions, or inaccuracies.

CONTENTS

Chapter 1: Appetizer Slow Cooker Recipes 11
1. Amazing Buffalo Dip 11
2. Anne's Hot Ham And Swiss Dip 11
3. Awesome Slow Cooker Buffalo Wings 11
4. BBQ Bison Phyllo Bites 11
5. Bacon Wrapped Smokies 11
6. Bavarian Style Meatballs 12
7. Beef Enchilada Dip 12
8. Big Game Salsa Dip 12
9. Big Game Sunday Chili Dip 12
10. Black Eyed Pea Sausage Dip 12
11. Cajun Boiled Peanuts 13
12. Candied Bacon Pigs 13
13. Candied Kielbasa 13
14. Carolina Pulled Pork Slow Cooker Dip 13
15. Carrie's Southern Queso 13
16. Cheese Dip II 13
17. Cheesy Taco Dip 14
18. Chicken Nachos From Reynolds Wrap® 14
19. Chorizo Queso Dip 14
20. Cocktail Wieners 14
21. Crab Rangoon Dip For The Slow Cooker 14
22. Cranberry Chipotle Meatballs 14
23. Crock Pot® Party Meatballs 15
24. Currant Jelly Wiener Sauce 15
25. Dog Food Dip 15
26. Drunken Sailors 15
27. Easy Beer And Ketchup Meatballs 15
28. Easy Cheesy Crawfish Dip 15
29. Easy Marinated Mushrooms 16
30. Easy Slow Cooker Chicken Wings 16
31. Famous Meatballs 16
32. Guinness® Beer Cheese Dip 16
33. Healthier Buffalo Chicken Dip 16
34. Hot Mexican Dip 17
35. Hot Roasted Red Pepper And Artichoke Dip 17
36. Kansas City BBQ Chicken Dip 17
37. Kevin's Sausage Dip 17
38. Kielbasa Appetizer 17
39. Krista's Queso 18
40. Laurie's Creamy Slow Cooker Queso 18
41. Little Smokies 18
42. Marinated Mushrooms 18
43. Meatballs And Kraut 18
44. Mexican Cheese And Hamburger Dip 18
45. Outrageous Warm Chicken Nacho Dip 19
46. Party Kielbasa 19
47. Pupu Balls 19
48. Queso (Cheese) Dip 19
49. Queso Blanco And Black Bean Slow Cooker Dip 20
50. Rachael's Superheated Cajun Boiled Peanuts 20
51. Rachel's Crockpot Seafood Cheese Dip 20
52. Ranch Taco Chicken Dip 20
53. Shannon's White Cheese Dip 20
54. Slim's Bad Attitude Nacho Sauce 21
55. Slow Cooker BBQ Meatballs And Polish Sausage 21
56. Slow Cooker Bar B Q Party Mix 21
57. Slow Cooker Buffalo Chicken Lettuce Wraps 21
58. Slow Cooker Cocktail Smokies 21
59. Slow Cooker Cocktail Wieners 22
60. Slow Cooker Jalapeno Popper Taquitos 22
61. Slow Cooker Philly Cheesesteak Dip 22
62. Slow Cooker Reuben Dip 22
63. Spicy Hot Chicken Legs 22
64. Sweet 'N Sour Meatballs 23
65. Sweet And Sour Meatballs 23
66. Sweet And Sour Meatballs I 23
67. Taco Bean Dip 23
68. Tangy Barbecued Wings 23
69. Vegetarian Buffalo Chicken Dip 24
70. Warm Chili Cheese Dip 24
71. Warm Mexican Corn Dip 24

Chapter 2: Side Dish Slow Cooker Recipes 25
72. Alfredo Green Bean Casserole 25
73. Baked Beans With Beef 25
74. Bandito Beans 25
75. Becca's Barbequed Beans 25
76. Betty's 3 Bean Hot Dish (a La Minnesota) ... 25
77. Bourbon Barbecue Slow Cooker Beans 26
78. Cajun Red Beans 26
79. Cola Beans 26
80. Deborah's Slow Cooker Spicy Black Eyed Peas 26
81. Deborah's Slow Cooker Collard Greens 27
82. Easy Slow Cooker Cheesy Potatoes 27
83. Easy Slow Cooker Spanish Rice 27
84. Easy Slow Cooker Squash 27
85. Garlic Mashed Potatoes In The Slow Cooker 27
86. Grandpa's Classic Coney Sauce 28
87. Hash Brown Casserole For The Slow Cooker 28
88. Hobo Beans 28
89. Hot As Hell Hickory Beans 28
90. Hungarian Noodle Side Dish 28
91. Maple And Ginger Baked Beans 29
92. Minnesota Real Wild Rice Stuffing 29
93. Mother Earth's Baked Beans 29
94. Pammy's Slow Cooker Beans 30
95. Rebellion Sauerkraut 30
96. Risi Bisi 30
97. Sandy's Sweet Slow Cooker Sauerkraut 30
98. Sauerkraut With Pigtails 30
99. Slow Cooker Barbecue Beans 30
100. Slow Cooker Black Eyed Peas 31
101. Slow Cooker Cheesy Mushroom Potatoes 31
102. Slow Cooker Chicken Dressing 31
103. Slow Cooker Chinese Carrots 31
104. Slow Cooker Collard Greens 32
105. Slow Cooker Cranberry Apple Stuffing 32
106. Slow Cooker Creamed Corn 32
107. Slow Cooker Creamed Spinach 32
108. Slow Cooker Garlic Mashed Potatoes 32
109. Slow Cooker Green Bean Casserole 32
110. Slow Cooker Ham And Scalloped Potatoes 33
111. Slow Cooker Mashed Potatoes 33
112. Slow Cooker Mashed Potatoes And Cauliflower 33
113. Slow Cooker Northern White Bean 33
114. Slow Cooker Pizza Potatoes 33
115. Slow Cooker Refried Beans With Bacon 34
116. Slow Cooker Sausage 'n' Grits Meatloaf 34

117. Slow Cooker Scalloped Potatoes With Chicken 34
118. Slow Cooker Scalloped Potatoes With Ham 34
119. Slow Cooker Southern Collard Greens 35
120. Slow Cooker Spaghetti Squash 35
121. Slow Cooker Sweet Potato Casserole 35
122. Slow Cooker Sweet Potatoes (Yams) And Marshmallows 35
123. Slow Cooker Western Omelet 35
124. Spicy Chipotle Black Eyed Peas 35
125. Spicy Slow Cooker Potatoes 36
126. Spinach Noodle Casserole 36
127. Stuffing For Slow Cooker 36
128. Sweet Barbeque Beans 36
129. Sweet And Sour Beans 37
130. Swiss Corn Slow Cooker Casserole 37
131. Tender Taters 37
132. Texas Style Baked Beans 37
133. The Best Slow Cooker Baked Beans (Dad's Recipe) 37
134. The Best Slow Cooker Cream Corn 38
135. Tomato And Bacon Creamed Corn Casserole 38
136. Western Style Baked Beans 38
137. Wild Rice Casserole I 38

Chapter 3: Main Dish Slow Cooker Recipes 39
138. Amazing Ribs 39
139. Anna's Amazing Easy Pleasy Meatballs Over Buttered Noodles 39
140. Apple Breakfast (Easy Slow Cooker Oatmeal) 39
141. Apple And Brown Sugar Corned Beef 39
142. Asian Bison Short Ribs 39
143. Authentic Cochinita Pibil (Spicy Mexican Pulled Pork) 40
144. Awesome Pulled Pork BBQ 40
145. Bandito Slow Cooker Chili Dogs 40
146. Barbecued Pulled Pork With Sweet Sour Slaw 41
147. Barbeque Pork Two Ways 41
148. Barbeque Shredded Beef 41
149. Beef Roast In Red Wine (Carni Arrosto Al Vino Rosso) 42
150. Big V's Slow Cooker Pulled Pork 42
151. Busy Mom Lasagna 42
152. Cabbage Rolls II 42
153. Cajun Roast Beef 43
154. Carnitas With Pico De Gallo 43
155. Charley's Slow Cooker Mexican Style Pork 43
156. Cheesy Italian Tortellini 43
157. Chicken Delicious 44
158. Chicken Livers Fandango 44
159. Christmas Morning Oatmeal 44
160. Classic Beef Stroganoff In A Slow Cooker. 44
161. Classic Chulent 45
162. Corny Ham And Potato Scallop 45
163. Country Cooking Slow Cooker Neck Bones 45
164. Cream Of Mushroom And Soy Sauce Pork Chops 45
165. Creamy Slow Cooker Chicken And Vegetables 45
166. Creole Pork Shanks With Sweet Potato Gravy 46
167. Crock Pot Cheesy Mushroom Chicken 46
168. Crock Pot Portobello Chicken 46
169. Cuban Style Pork And Sweet Potatoes 46
170. Cyndee's Best Slow Cooker Italian Pot Roast 47
171. Dad's Home With The Kids Slow Cooker Roast 47
172. Delicious Beef Tongue Tacos 47
173. Easy Corned Beef And Cabbage 47
174. Easy Ground Beef Stroganoff 48
175. Easy Overnight Oatmeal 48
176. Easy Slow Cooker Carne Guisada 48
177. Easy Slow Cooker Chicken Curry With Potatoes And Coconut Milk 48
178. Easy Slow Cooker Chicken Thighs With Honey 48
179. Easy Slow Cooker Swiss Steak 49
180. Easy Sweet And Spicy Meatballs 49
181. Eaton's Easy Pulled Pork 49
182. Egg, Spinach, And Mushroom Slow Cooker Casserole 49
183. Havana Slow Cooker Pork Tenderloin 49
184. Honey Ribs 50
185. Honey Baked Spiral Ham In The Slow Cooker 50
186. IPA Corned Beef 50
187. Italian Beef In A Bucket 50
188. Jennie's Heavenly Slow Cooker Chicken ... 50
189. Jenny's Cuban Style Slow Cooker Chicken Fricassee 51
190. Julia's Easy Slow Cooker Chicken 51
191. Kalua Pig In A Slow Cooker 51
192. Kathy's Roast And Vegetables 51
193. Kay Kay's Pulled Pork 51
194. Low Fat Slow Cooker Glazed Meatloaf 52
195. Melt In Your Mouth Meat Loaf 52
196. Melt In Your Mouth Beef Cacciatore 52
197. Monterey Spaghetti 52
198. Mother's Pot Roast 53
199. No Fuss Shredded Beef Tacos 53
200. Not Barbecued Short Ribs 53
201. O'Kee's Healthy Gray Corned Beef Brisket From Scratch 53
202. Our Favorite Olive Beef 54
203. PHILLY Slow Cooker Beef Stroganoff 54
204. Parmesan Chicken I 54
205. Pot Roast With Balsamic Onions 54
206. Pulled BBQ Pork Poutine 54
207. Ropa Vieja In A Slow Cooker 55
208. Salsa Verde Pork 55
209. Sarge's EZ Pulled Pork BBQ 55
210. Shredded Tri Tip For Tacos In The Slow Cooker 55
211. Simple Slow Cooker Pulled Pork 56
212. Slow Cooker 5 Ingredient Ham 56
213. Slow Cooker Adobo Chicken 56
214. Slow Cooker Barbecue Goose Sandwich ... 56
215. Slow Cooker Barbecued Ribs 56
216. Slow Cooker Beef Enchiladas 56
217. Slow Cooker Beef Tinga 57
218. Slow Cooker Blackberry Pork Tenderloin 57
219. Slow Cooker Breakfast Casserole 57
220. Slow Cooker Chicken Curry 58

221. Slow Cooker Chicken Curry With Coconut Milk 58
222. Slow Cooker Chicken Marsala 58
223. Slow Cooker Chicken And Dumplings 58
224. Slow Cooker Corned Beef Style Brisket 58
225. Slow Cooker Country Style Spareribs 59
226. Slow Cooker Cranberry Chicken 59
227. Slow Cooker Cranberry And Muscadine Pork Roast 59
228. Slow Cooker Dump And Go Cheesy Chicken 59
229. Slow Cooker Ham 59
230. Slow Cooker Honey Garlic Chicken 59
231. Slow Cooker Kielbasa And Beer 60
232. Slow Cooker Lancaster County Pork And Sauerkraut 60
233. Slow Cooker Lasagna II 60
234. Slow Cooker Lengua (Beef Tongue) 60
235. Slow Cooker London Broil 60
236. Slow Cooker Mexican Chicken And Rice ... 61
237. Slow Cooker Orange Chicken 61
238. Slow Cooker Overnight Breakfast Casserole 61
239. Slow Cooker Pepper Steak II 61
240. Slow Cooker Philly Steak Sandwich Meat 61
241. Slow Cooker Pork Loin Roast With Apple Cranberry Rice 62
242. Slow Cooker Pork And Sauerkraut With Apples 62
243. Slow Cooker Pork With Mushrooms And Barley 62
244. Slow Cooker Pulled Pork 62
245. Slow Cooker Pulled Pork Roast 62
246. Slow Cooker Red Curry Beef Pot Roast 63
247. Slow Cooker Roast Beef 63
248. Slow Cooker Sauerkraut And Sausage 63
249. Slow Cooker Shoyu Pork 64
250. Slow Cooker Shredded Venison For Tacos 64
251. Slow Cooker Sloppy Swiss Steak 64
252. Slow Cooker Spanish Rice 64
253. Slow Cooker Tender And Yummy Round Steak 64
254. Slow Cooker Texas Pulled Pork 65
255. Slow Cooker Texas Smoked Beef Brisket . 65
256. Slow Cooker Tropical Chicken 65
257. Slow Cooker Venison Burritos 65
258. Slow Cooker Venison Sloppy Joes 66
259. Slow Cooker Wieners In Wiener BBQ Sauce 66
260. Slow Cooked Turkey Legs 66
261. Slow Cooker Posole 66
262. Sour Cream Pork Chops 66
263. Southern Barbeque Pulled Beef Sandwiches 67
264. Spanish Chicken 67
265. Sunday Sticky Chicken 67
266. Sweet Ham Recipe 67
267. Sweet And Savory Brisket 67
268. Sweet And Savory Slow Cooker Pulled Pork 68
269. Sweet And Sour Beef 68
270. Tangy Slow Cooker Pork Roast 68
271. Two Corn Chicken Posole 68
272. Vegetarian Slow Cooker Meal 69
273. Verenike Casserole For The Slow Cooker 69
274. Waikiki Style Meatballs 69
275. Zesty Pulled Pork Sandwiches 69
Chapter 4: Dessert Slow Cooker Recipes 70
276. Alexander's Chocolate Covered Peanuts ... 70
277. Amazing Slow Cooker Chocolate Cake 70
278. Ashley And Whitney's Apple Cherry Cobbler 70
279. Bread Pudding In The Slow Cooker 70
280. Chocolate Cherry Slow Cooker Cake 70
281. Chocolate Pudding Cake IV 71
282. Gluten Free Slow Cooker Chocolate Lava Cake 71
283. Heaven In A Slow Cooker 71
284. Meadowwood Tapioca Pudding 71
285. Pumpkin Pie Pudding 71
286. Reindeer Poop 72
287. Rice Pudding In A Slow Cooker 72
288. Slow Cooked Apple Brown Betty 72
289. Slow Cooker Apple Cinnamon Bread Pudding 72
290. Slow Cooker Apple Crisp 72
291. Slow Cooker Apples With Cinnamon And Brown Sugar 73
292. Slow Cooker Bananas Foster 73
293. Slow Cooker Cherry Cobbler 73
294. Slow Cooker Cherry Delight 73
295. Slow Cooker Chocolate Candy 73
296. Slow Cooker Fruit Cobbler 73
297. Slow Cooker Peach Cobbler 74
298. Slow Cooker Peach Upside Down Cake 74
299. Slow Cooker Peanut Butter Fudge Cake 74
300. Slow Cooker Tapioca Pudding 74
301. Slow Cooker Vanilla Tapioca Pudding 75
302. Slow Cooker Peanut Butter Fudge Cake 75
303. Stef's Slow Cooker Creme Brulee 75
304. Triple Coconut Cake 75
305. Unbelievably Easy Slow Cooker Black Forest Cake 76
306. Warm Berry Compote 76
307. Warm Chocolate Peanut Butter Pudding Cake 76
Chapter 5: Soup And Stew Slow Cooker Recipes 77
308. African Sweet Potato Stew 77
309. Alison's Slow Cooker Vegetable Beef Soup 77
310. Amelia's Slow Cooker Brunswick Stew 77
311. Award Winning White Chicken Chili 77
312. Babushka's Slow Cooker Root Vegetable And Chicken Stew 77
313. Bachelor's Stew 78
314. Beef And Barley Soup I 78
315. Beer Beef Stew II 78
316. Beer Baked Irish Beef 78
317. Beezie's Black Bean Soup 79
318. Best Italian Sausage Soup 79
319. Best No Bean Chili 79
320. Black Lentil Veggie Soup 80
321. Black Eyed Pea Bratwurst Stew 80
322. Bull Riders All Beef Chili 80
323. Busy Day Slow Cooker Chili 80
324. Cabbage Beef Soup 81
325. Cabbage Patch Stew 81
326. Cabbage Soup 81
327. Campbell's® Slow Cooker Chicken And Dumplings 81
328. Cauliflower Potato Soup 82

329. Caveman Chili 82
330. Chad's Slow Cooker Taco Soup 82
331. Chane's Beer And Rye Beef Stew 82
332. Cheddar Bratwurst Stew 83
333. Cheesy Brat Stew For The Slow Cooker 83
334. Chicken Broth In A Slow Cooker 83
335. Chicken Gumbo Over Rice 83
336. Chicken Soup With Drop In Noodles 84
337. Chicken Stew With Pepper And Pineapple 84
338. Chicken Tortilla Soup In The Slow Cooker 84
339. Chicken And Pumpkin Goulash 84
340. Chorizo Chili 85
341. Christina's Slow Cooker Chili 85
342. Classic Slow Cooker Corn Chowder 85
343. Coconut Chicken Curry Stew 85
344. Collard Kielbasa Soup 86
345. Colleen's Slow Cooker Jambalaya 86
346. Colorado Buffalo Chili 86
347. Cozy Cottage Beef Stew Soup 86
348. Crabmeat And Asparagus Soup 87
349. Creamy Slow Cooker Beef Stroganoff 87
350. Creamy Slow Cooker Potato Cheese Soup 87
351. Creamy Vegetable Soup 87
352. Crock Pot® Chicken Chili 88
353. Crocked Tater Tot® Soup 88
354. Dan's Slow Cooker Ham And White Bean Soup 88
355. Diego's Special Beef Stew 88
356. Different Ham And Potato Soup 89
357. Easy Slow Cooker Butternut Squash Soup 89
358. Easy Slow Cooker Cauliflower Soup With Cheese 89
359. Easy Slow Cooker Chicken Soup 89
360. Easy Slow Cooker Chicken And Dumplings 89
361. Easy Slow Cooker White Chicken Chili 90
362. Easy Sweet Chili 90
363. Easy Venison Stew 90
364. Eggplant Stew 90
365. Emily's Broccoli Cheese Soup 91
366. Emma's Slow Cooker Clam Chowder 91
367. Ez's Slow Cooker Hot Chili 91
368. Fall French Onion Soup 91
369. Fisherman's Catch Chowder 92
370. Five Star Venison Stew 92
371. German Texas Chili 92
372. Gram's Irish Stew 92
373. Grandma B's Bean Soup 93
374. Great Aunt Nina's Noodles And Chicken .. 93
375. Greek Style Beef Stew 93
376. Gringo Posole 94
377. Ham Bone Chowder 94
378. Ham Bone Soup 94
379. Ham Bone And Vegetable Soup 94
380. Hamburger Corn Soup 95
381. Hamburger Soup II 95
382. Harvest Pork Stew 95
383. Hearty Beef Stew 95
384. Hearty Ham Bone Black Bean Soup 96
385. Hearty Lentil And Sausage Soup 96
386. Hearty Slow Cooked Beef Stew 96
387. Hearty Vegan Slow Cooker Chili 96
388. Hobo Ground Beef And Vegetable Soup ... 97
389. Homemade Chili 97
390. Homemade Potato Soup 97
391. Hungarian Goulash II 97
392. It's Chili By George!! 98
393. Jamie's Pulled Pork Chili 98
394. Jay's Spicy Slow Cooker Turkey Chili 98
395. Jerre's Black Bean And Pork Tenderloin Slow Cooker Chili 98
396. Kale Soup With Portuguese Sausage 99
397. Kas' Chili 99
398. Kathy's Perfect Turkey Bisque 99
399. Kelly's Slow Cooker Beef, Mushroom, And Barley Soup 99
400. Kyera's Hearty Beef Borscht 100
401. Leek And Potato Chowder 100
402. Leftover Ham And Shrimp Slow Cooker Gumbo 100
403. Leftover Turkey Soup (Slow Cooker) 100
404. Lemon Salmon Soup 101
405. Lentil Soup With Garlicky Vinaigrette 101
406. Low Carb Cream Of Broccoli Soup........... 101
407. Luscious Lima Bean Soup II 101
408. Main Line Chicken Chili 102
409. Maine Venison Stew 102
410. Make Ahead Slow Cooker Beef Stew 102
411. Maverick Moose Chili 102
412. Meat Lovers' Vegetarian Chili 103
413. Mexican Chocolate Chili 103
414. Mile High Green Chili 103
415. Miner's Chili 104
416. Mixed Beans And More 104
417. Mo's Spicy Beef Stew 104
418. Mom's Chicken And Dumplings (Slow Cooker Version) 104
419. Mom's Italian Beef Barley Soup 105
420. Nikki's Creamy Crock Pot Potato Soup ... 105
421. No Peek Beef Stew 105
422. Old Fashioned Beef Stew 105
423. Old Fashioned Onion Soup 106
424. Old School Bean Soup With Wheat Berries 106
425. Paleo Chili You Won't Miss The Beans 106
426. Pareve Cholent 106
427. Potato And Corn Chowder (Freezer Dump Meal) 107
428. Pozole In A Slow Cooker 107
429. Pretty Easy Chili 107
430. Pulled Pork Chili 107
431. Pumpkin Pulled Pork Chili 108
432. Quick And Easy Clam Chowder 108
433. Red Chicken Chili 108
434. Rustic Slow Cooker Stew 108
435. Sauerkraut Soup II 109
436. Sausage Barley Soup 109
437. Savory Pork Stew 109
438. Scallop And Shrimp Chowder 109
439. Shipwreck Stew 110
440. Short Rib Tsimmes 110
441. Simple Slow Cooker Jambalaya 110
442. Slow Cooked Beef Stew 110
443. Slow Cooked Chicken Stew 111
444. Slow Cooked Ham And Potato Chowder 111
445. Slow Cooker 5 Mushroom Barley Soup .. 111
446. Slow Cooker BBQ Chicken Pizza Soup ... 111
447. Slow Cooker Beef Barley Soup 112
448. Slow Cooker Beef Neck Bones And Gravy 112

449. Slow Cooker Beef Stew..................................112
450. Slow Cooker Beef Stew Al La Catherine..112
451. Slow Cooker Beef Stew I 113
452. Slow Cooker Beef Stew III 113
453. Slow Cooker Beef Stew IV 113
454. Slow Cooker Beef Vegetable Soup 113
455. Slow Cooker Belgian Chicken Booyah.......113
456. Slow Cooker Black Eyed Pea And Sausage Soup 114
457. Slow Cooker Bone Broth................................114
458. Slow Cooker Borscht......................................114
459. Slow Cooker Buffalo Chicken Wing Soup115
460. Slow Cooker Butternut Squash Soup With Sausage..115
461. Slow Cooker Cactus Chili 115
462. Slow Cooker Cassoulet 115
463. Slow Cooker Chicken Chili With Greens And Beans 115
464. Slow Cooker Chicken Enchilada Soup.......116
465. Slow Cooker Chicken Gumbo With Shrimp 116
466. Slow Cooker Chicken Pot Pie Stew.............116
467. Slow Cooker Chicken Pozole Blanco..........116
468. Slow Cooker Chicken Thai Ramen Noodles 117
469. Slow Cooker Chicken And Corn Congee..117
470. Slow Cooker Chicken And Mushroom Stew 117
471. Slow Cooker Chicken And Sausage Gumbo 117
472. Slow Cooker Chili..118
473. Slow Cooker Chili II..118
474. Slow Cooker Chipotle Chili 118
475. Slow Cooker Clam Chowder.........................118
476. Slow Cooker Corn Chowder 119
477. Slow Cooker Cream Of Broccoli Soup 119
478. Slow Cooker Cream Of Potato Soup..........119
479. Slow Cooker Creamy Chicken And Dumplings..119
480. Slow Cooker Creamy Potato Soup 119
481. Slow Cooker French Onion Soup................120
482. Slow Cooker Fresh Vegetable Beef Barley Soup 120
483. Slow Cooker Game Day Chili.......................120
484. Slow Cooker Ground Beef Stew 121
485. Slow Cooker Ham And Bean Soup 121
486. Slow Cooker Ham And Bean Stew 121
487. Slow Cooker Hearty Mixed Bean Stew With Sausage..121
488. Slow Cooker Hoppin John 122
489. Slow Cooker Hoppin' John Chowder 122
490. Slow Cooker Island Beef 122
491. Slow Cooker Italian Beef Stew 122
492. Slow Cooker Jambalaya..................................123
493. Slow Cooker Jambalaya (Vegan) 123
494. Slow Cooker Kielbasa Stew 123
495. Slow Cooker Lentil Rice Soup 123
496. Slow Cooker Lentil And Ham Soup...........123
497. Slow Cooker Low Carb Santa Fe Chicken124
498. Slow Cooker Manly Stew 124
499. Slow Cooker Mexican Beef Stew.................124
500. Slow Cooker Mexican Chili Bowls From Del Monte®...124
501. Slow Cooker Northern White Bean Bacon Chowder..125
502. Slow Cooker Onion Soup 125
503. Slow Cooker Oxtail Soup 125
504. Slow Cooker Potato Broccoli Soup 125
505. Slow Cooker Pumpkin Soup 126
506. Slow Cooker Pumpkin Turkey Chili 126
507. Slow Cooker Quinoa Sweet Potato Chicken.. 126
508. Slow Cooker Salmon Chowder 126
509. Slow Cooker Spanish Beef Stew................. 127
510. Slow Cooker Spanish Rice Chili................. 127
511. Slow Cooker Split Pea Sausage Soup 127
512. Slow Cooker Split Pea Soup With Bacon And Hash Browns 127
513. Slow Cooker Squirrel And Veggies 127
514. Slow Cooker Stout Stew 128
515. Slow Cooker Sweet Chicken Chili.............. 128
516. Slow Cooker Sweet Potato Soup................. 128
517. Slow Cooker Taco Bean Soup...................... 128
518. Slow Cooker Tofu Chili 128
519. Slow Cooker Tomato Soup........................... 129
520. Slow Cooker Tortellini................................... 129
521. Slow Cooker Turkey Soup With Dumplings.. 129
522. Slow Cooker Turkey Stew 129
523. Slow Cooker Turkey And Dumplings 130
524. Slow Cooker Turkey And White Bean Chili 130
525. Slow Cooker Vegan Sweet Potato Chili... 130
526. Slow Cooker Vegetable Soup With Ground Beef 130
527. Slow Cooker Vegetarian Minestrone 131
528. Slow Cooker Veggie Beef Soup With Okra 131
529. Slow Cooker Venison Stew 131
530. Slow Cooker White Chili 131
531. Slow Cooker White Chili With Chicken... 131
532. Slow Cooker Zucchini Soup 132
533. Slow Cooker Zuppa Toscana 132
534. Slow Cooker, Easy Baked Potato Soup.... 132
535. Slow Cooked Chicken And Sausage Gumbo 132
536. Slow Cooked Chili 133
537. Slow Cooked White Chili.............................. 133
538. Slow Cooker Baked Bean Stew................... 133
539. Slow Cooker Fish Chowder.......................... 133
540. Smashed Potato Soup.................................... 134
541. Smashing Pumpkin Soup.............................. 134
542. Snert (Split Pea Soup).................................... 134
543. Sonte's Slow Cooker Potato Soup 135
544. Southwest Style Creamy Corn Chowder 135
545. Spaghetti Squash And Polish Sausage Slow Cooker Soup 135
546. Spicy Beef Curry Stew For The Slow Cooker.. 135
547. Spicy Beef Vegetable Stew 136
548. Spicy Black And Red Bean Soup 136
549. Spicy Pumpkin Chili 136
550. Spicy And Savory Slow Cooker Beef Ragout.. 136
551. Split Pea Smoked Turkey Soup 137
552. Split Pea Soup With Homemade Ham Bone Stock... 137
553. Spooky Slow Cooker Turkey Lentil Chili 137
554. Sunday Brunswick Stew 138
555. Sweet Pork Slow Cooker Chili 138

556. Sweet Potato Chili 138
557. Swink's Chili 138
558. Swiss Steak Stew 139
559. Taco Chili From Publix® 139
560. Taiwanese Spicy Beef Noodle Soup 139
561. Tangy Vegan Crockpot Corn Chowder 139
562. Teddy's Duck Gumbo 140
563. Ten Bean Soup II 140
564. Teriyaki Beef Bean Rice Bowls From Del Monte® 140
565. Texas Beef Soup 140
566. The Big Game Barbeque Meat Chili 141
567. The Ultimate Chili 141
568. The Ultimate Slow Cooked Chili 141
569. Thunderbird Stew 142
570. Traditional Irish Stew 142
571. Turkey And Okra Soup With Barley And Bacon 142
572. V Eight Vegetable Beef Soup 142
573. Vegetarian Bacon Chili 142
574. Vegetarian Pumpkin Spinach Chili 143
575. White Chicken Chili With Salsa Verde 143
576. White Chili V 143
577. White Chili VI 143
578. White Chili VII 144
579. White Chili With Chicken Corn 144
580. Wild Turkey Gumbo 144
581. Winter Lentil Vegetable Soup 144
Chapter 6: Steak Slow Cooker Recipes 146
582. All Day Soup 146
583. Asian Style Round Steak 146
584. Barbecues For The Bunch 146
585. Beef Braciole 146
586. Beef And Beans 147
587. Beef Wrapped Stuffed Peppers 147
588. Burgundy Beef Stew 147
589. Chipotle Beef Chili 147
590. Colony Mountain Chili 148
591. Cuban Ropa Vieja 148
592. Easy Ham With Cherry Sauce 148
593. Easy Slow Cooked Swiss Steak 148
594. Fabulous Fajitas 149
595. Fiesta Beef Bowls 149
596. Flank Steak Fajitas 149
597. Game Stopper Chili 149
598. Garlic Beef Stroganoff 150
599. Gone All Day Casserole 150
600. Grandma Schwartz's Rouladen 150
601. Herbed Beef With Noodles 150
602. Hunter's Delight 151
603. Louisiana Round Steak 151
604. Mushroom 'n' Steak Stroganoff 151
605. Mushroom Round Steak 151
606. Mushroom Steak 152
607. No Fuss Swiss Steak 152
608. Pepper Steaks 152
609. Portobello Beef Burgundy 152
610. Pumpkin Harvest Beef Stew 153
611. Round Steak Italiano 153
612. Round Steak Roll Ups 153
613. Round Steak Sauerbraten 154
614. Roundup Chili 154
615. Sausage Stuffed Flank Steak 154
616. Savory Beef Fajitas 154
617. Shredded Steak Sandwiches 155
618. Skillet Steak Fajitas 155
619. Slow Cook Beef Stew 155
620. Slow Cooker Beef Stroganoff 155
621. Slow Cooker Beef Tostadas 156
622. Slow Cooker Burgundy Beef 156
623. Slow Cooker Fajitas 156
624. Slow Cooker Flank Steak Fajitas 157
625. Slow Cooker Mushroom Beef Stroganoff 157
626. Slow Cooker Steak 'n' Gravy 157
627. Slow Cooker Swiss Steak 157
628. Slow Cooker Swiss Steak Supper 158
629. Slow Cooker Vegetable Beef Soup 158
630. Slow Cooker Vegetable Soup 158
631. Slow Cooked Beef 'n' Veggies 158
632. Slow Cooked Mushroom Swiss Steak 159
633. Slow Cooked Round Steak 159
634. Slow Cooked Sirloin 159
635. Slow Cooked Steak Fajitas 159
636. Slow Cooked Stroganoff 160
637. Slow Cooked Stuffed Flank Steak 160
638. Slow Cooked Swiss Steak 160
639. Smothered Round Steak 160
640. Steak 'n' Gravy 161
641. Steak Strips With Dumplings 161
642. Steak Stroganoff 161
643. Steak And Mushroom Sauce 161
644. Stuffed Flank Steak 161
645. Sweet Sour Beef 162
646. Tangy Venison Stroganoff 162
647. Tomato Basil Steak 162
648. Veggie Topped Swiss Steak 162
649. Zesty Orange Beef 163
650. Zippy Beef Fajitas 163
651. Zippy Steak Chili 163
Chapter 7: Bean Slow Cooker Recipes 164
652. Apple Sausage Beans 164
653. Bacon Lima Beans 164
654. Baked Beans With Bacon 164
655. Barbecued Beans 164
656. Black Eyed Peas Ham 164
657. Boston Baked Beans 165
658. Chuck Wagon Beans With Sausage 165
659. Cowboy Calico Beans 165
660. Fiesta Corn And Beans 165
661. Four Bean Medley 166
662. Georgian Bay Baked Beans 166
663. Hawaiian Barbecue Beans 166
664. Hearty Pork N Beans 166
665. Partytime Beans 167
666. Pineapple Baked Beans 167
667. Root Beer Apple Baked Beans 167
668. Simple Vegetarian Slow Cooked Beans .. 167
669. Slow Cooker BBQ Baked Beans 168
670. Slow Cooker Calico Beans 168
671. Slow Cooker Potluck Beans 168
672. Slow Cooker Baked Beans 168
673. Slow Cooked Bean Medley 168
674. Slow Cooked Calico Beans 169
675. Slow Cooked Pork Beans 169
676. Smoky Baked Beans 169
677. Sweet Hot Baked Beans 170
678. Sweet Spicy Beans 170
679. Sweet N Sour Beans 170
680. Sweet And Tangy Ranch Beans 170
681. Tangy Cranberry Beans 170

Chapter 8: Rib Slow Cooker Recipes ... 171
- 682. "Secret's In The Sauce" BBQ Ribs ... 171
- 683. 4Switch And Go Ribs ... 171
- 684. 5 Ingredient Chinese Pork Ribs ... 171
- 685. BBQ Country Style Ribs ... 171
- 686. Baby Back Ribs ... 171
- 687. Barbecue Country Ribs ... 171
- 688. Barbecued Beef Ribs ... 172
- 689. Beef Short Ribs Vindaloo ... 172
- 690. Braised Beef Short Ribs ... 172
- 691. Brazilian Pork Black Bean Stew ... 172
- 692. Busy Day Barbecued Ribs ... 173
- 693. Caribbean Beef Short Ribs ... 173
- 694. Chinese Pork Ribs ... 173
- 695. Chinese Style Ribs ... 173
- 696. Coffee Braised Short Ribs ... 174
- 697. Cola Barbecue Ribs ... 174
- 698. Contest Winning Braised Short Ribs ... 174
- 699. Country Ribs Dinner ... 174
- 700. Country Style Ribs ... 175
- 701. Country Style Barbecue Ribs ... 175
- 702. Cranberry Ginger Pork Ribs ... 175
- 703. Crazy Delicious Baby Back Ribs ... 175
- 704. Farm Style BBQ Ribs ... 176
- 705. German Style Short Ribs ... 176
- 706. Ginger Country Style Pork Ribs ... 176
- 707. Gingered Short Ribs ... 176
- 708. Gingered Short Ribs With Green Rice ... 177
- 709. Green Chili Ribs ... 177
- 710. Hearty Short Ribs ... 177
- 711. Home Style Ribs ... 178
- 712. Lazy Man's Ribs ... 178
- 713. Lip Smackin' Ribs ... 178
- 714. Maple Pork Ribs ... 178
- 715. My Brazilian Feijoada ... 178
- 716. Peachy Baby Back Ribs ... 179
- 717. Pork Baby Back Ribs ... 179
- 718. Pork Ribs Lo Mein ... 179
- 719. Pork Ribs With Apple Mustard Glaze ... 179
- 720. Pork Spareribs ... 180
- 721. Root Beer BBQ Ribs ... 180
- 722. Seasoned Short Ribs ... 180
- 723. Sesame Pork Ribs ... 180
- 724. Short Rib Poutine ... 181
- 725. Simple Sparerib Sauerkraut Supper ... 181
- 726. Slow Easy Baby Back Ribs ... 181
- 727. Slow Cooked BBQ Pork Ribs ... 181
- 728. Slow Cooker Jerked Short Ribs ... 182
- 729. Slow Cooker Memphis Style Ribs ... 182
- 730. Slow Cooker Peach BBQ Ribs ... 182
- 731. Slow Cooker Ribs ... 182
- 732. Slow Cooker Short Ribs ... 183
- 733. Slow And Easy BBQ Ribs ... 183
- 734. Slow Cooked Country Ribs In Gravy ... 183
- 735. Slow Cooked Mesquite Ribs ... 183
- 736. Slow Cooked Peachy Spareribs ... 183
- 737. Slow Cooked Ribs ... 184
- 738. Slow Cooked Short Ribs ... 184
- 739. Slow Cooked Short Ribs With Salt Skin Potatoes ... 184
- 740. Stack Of Bones ... 184
- 741. Super Easy Country Style Ribs ... 185
- 742. Super Short Ribs ... 185
- 743. Sweet 'n' Sour Ribs ... 185
- 744. Sweet Chili Short Ribs ... 185
- 745. Sweet And Savory Ribs ... 186
- 746. Sweet And Spicy Jerk Ribs ... 186
- 747. Tasty Pork Ribs ... 186
- 748. Tender 'n' Tangy Ribs ... 186
- 749. Tender Spareribs ... 186

Chapter 9: Mexican Slow Cooker Recipes ... 187
- 750. Barbacoa Style Shredded Beef ... 187
- 751. Bean And Beef Shaloupias ... 187
- 752. Big Ben's Beef Machaca ... 187
- 753. Birria De Chivo ... 187
- 754. Cabbage Tamales ... 188
- 755. Carne Adovada ... 188
- 756. Charley's Slow Cooker Mexican Style Meat ... 188
- 757. Chicken Butternut Squash Posole ... 188
- 758. Chicken Enchilada Slow Cooker Soup ... 189
- 759. Chicken Taco Filling ... 189
- 760. Chicken Verde Sandwiches ... 189
- 761. Chile Chicken Chili ... 189
- 762. Chili Cumin Stuffed Chicken Breasts ... 189
- 763. Chipotle Barbacoa ... 190
- 764. Cowboy Mexican Dip ... 190
- 765. Easy Slow Cooker Chicken Fajitas ... 190
- 766. Easy Slow Cooker Enchiladas ... 190
- 767. Frijoles II ... 190
- 768. Frijoles A La Charra ... 191
- 769. Green Chile Beef Tacos ... 191
- 770. Ground Turkey Enchilada Stew With Quinoa ... 191
- 771. Kris' Amazing Shredded Mexican Beef ... 191
- 772. Latin Inspired Spicy Cream Chicken Stew ... 191
- 773. Mexican Pintos With Cactus ... 192
- 774. Mexican Pot Roast ... 192
- 775. Mexican Style Shredded Pork ... 192
- 776. Mijo's Slow Cooker Shredded Beef ... 192
- 777. Paddy's Chile Verde ... 193
- 778. Paleo Mexican Pulled Pork ... 193
- 779. Pork Chalupas ... 193
- 780. Pork Chile Rojo (Pulled Pork With Red Chile Sauce) ... 194
- 781. Queso Con Carne ... 194
- 782. Simple Slow Cooked Korean Beef Soft Tacos ... 194
- 783. Slow Cooker Beef Barbacoa ... 194
- 784. Slow Cooker Carnitas ... 195
- 785. Slow Cooker Cheesy Chicken And Tortillas ... 195
- 786. Slow Cooker Chicken Taco Soup ... 195
- 787. Slow Cooker Chicken Tacos With Chipotle Cream Sauce ... 195
- 788. Slow Cooker Chicken Tinga ... 196
- 789. Slow Cooker Chicken Tinga Tacos ... 196
- 790. Slow Cooker Chile Verde ... 196
- 791. Slow Cooker Chile Verde (Green Chile) ... 196
- 792. Slow Cooker Cilantro Lime Chicken ... 197
- 793. Slow Cooker Enchiladas ... 197
- 794. Slow Cooker Guisado Verde ... 197
- 795. Slow Cooker Mexican Style Chicken ... 197
- 796. Slow Cooker Posole With Pork And Chicken ... 197
- 797. Slow Cooker Salsa Chicken ... 198
- 798. Slow Cooker Shredded Beef For Tacos And Burritos ... 198
- 799. Slow Cooker Spicy Chicken ... 198

800. Slow Cooker Taco Soup 198
801. Slow Cooker Tacos Al Pastor 198
802. South Of The Border Mac And Cheese 199
803. Southwest Black Bean Chicken Soup 199
804. Southwestern Style Chalupas 199
805. Southwestern Style Fifteen Bean Soup 199
806. Spicy Turkey Tacos 200
807. Super Easy Slow Cooker Chicken Enchilada Meat 200
808. Sweet Pork For Burritos 200
809. Tex Mex Pork 200
810. Texas Venison 200
811. Turkey Burrito 201
812. White Chicken Enchilada Slow Cooker Casserole 201
813. Zesty White Chicken Chili 201

Chapter 10: Family Slow Cooker Recipes 202
814. Apple Cinnamon Slow Cooker Oatmeal ... 202
815. Brunswick Stew 202
816. Cajun Style Pork And Shrimp Pasta 202
817. Carnitas Tacos 202
818. Chicken Pho 203
819. Chicken Ragout 203
820. Chicken And Vegetables With Herbs 203
821. Cider Pork Stew 204
822. Corn Bread Topped Chicken Enchilada Casserole 204
823. Creamy Turkey Soup 204
824. Hearty Beef Chili 205
825. Hearty Vegetable Beef Stew 205
826. Mushroom Sauced Pork Chops 205
827. Pork Chops With Herb Tomato Sauce 205
828. Pork Zuppa 206
829. Pot Roast Rigatoni Stew 206
830. Provencal Vegetable Stew 206
831. Pulled Pork Tenderloin With Vidalia Onion BBQ Sauce 207
832. Rosemary Chicken 207
833. Savory Barbecue Chicken 207
834. Seeded Pork Roast 207
835. Slow Cooked Ranch Chicken And Vegetables 208
836. Slow Cooker Baby Back Ribs 208
837. Slow Cooker Beef Stew 208
838. Slow Cooker Braised Beef With Carrots Turnips 209
839. Slow Cooker Brisket Sandwiches With Quick Pickles 209
840. Slow Cooker Cassoulet 210
841. Slow Cooker Chicken Noodle Soup Meal Prep Freezer Pack 210
842. Slow Cooker Chicken Parmesan Meatballs 210
843. Slow Cooker Picadillo 211
844. Slow Cooker Sausage Apple Stuffing 211
845. Slow Cooker Vegetarian Lasagna 211
846. Spanish Chicken Stew 212
847. Sweet And Sour Pork With Cabbage 212
848. Tried And True Chili Mac 212
849. Vegetarian Pinto Bean Sloppy Joes 212
850. Zesty Sloppy Joes 213

Chapter 11: Healthy Slow Cooker Recipes 214
851. A Crock Of Curried Pork Soup 214
852. Amazing Apple Butter 214
853. Amazing Pork Tenderloin In The Slow Cooker 214
854. Apple Tapioca Pudding 214
855. Ashley's African Peanut Soup 215
856. Balsamic Pear, Chicken, And Asparagus 215
857. Beer Chops I 215
858. Better Slow Cooker Robust Chicken 215
859. Bloody Mary Chicken 215
860. Blueberry And Banana Steel Cut Oats 216
861. Blueberry And Chia Quinoa 216
862. Bone Broth 216
863. CB's Black Eyed Peas 216
864. Chicken Tagine With Couscous 216
865. Chicken Wild Rice Soup III 217
866. Chicken And Corn Chili 217
867. Chicken And Fresh Tomato Slow Cooker Stew 217
868. Chicken With Sausage And Dried Fruit .. 217
869. Cindy's Snappy Sensational Superfood Soup 217
870. Clean Eating Refried Beans 218
871. Dee's Special Chicken 218
872. Deer Chop Hurry 218
873. Easy Peasy Venison Stew 218
874. Easy Slow Cooker Thai Chicken With Basil 218
875. Easy And Quick Swiss Steak 219
876. Gluten Free Vegan Stock For The Slow Cooker 219
877. Grandma's Slow Cooker Vegetarian Chili 219
878. Greek Slow Cooker Chicken 219
879. Ham And Chickpea Slow Cooker Soup ... 220
880. Healthier (but Still Awesome) Awesome Slow Cooker Pot Roast 220
881. Healthier Amazing Pork Tenderloin In The Slow Cooker 220
882. Healthier BBQ Pork For Sandwiches 220
883. Healthier Baked Slow Cooker Chicken ... 220
884. Healthier Marie's Easy Slow Cooker Pot Roast 221
885. Healthier Slow Cooker Beef Stew I 221
886. Healthier Slow Cooker Chicken Stroganoff 221
887. Healthier Slow Cooker Chicken Taco Soup 221
888. Healthier Slow Cooker Chicken And Dumplings 222
889. Healthier Slow Cooker Chicken Tortilla Soup 222
890. Hearty Cabbage Rutabaga Slow Cooker Soup 222
891. Honey Wheat Bread IV 222
892. Hunter's Roast 223
893. Karen's Slow Cooker Pizza Chicken 223
894. Laura's Quick Slow Cooker Turkey Chili 223
895. Lorene's Slow Cooker Potato Soup 223
896. Lower Sugar Spicy All Day Apple Butter . 223
897. Middle Eastern White Beans 223
898. Momma OB's Chicken Chili 224
899. Montigott 224
900. Moroccan Tagine 224
901. Mushroom Lentil Barley Stew 224
902. NO YOLKS® Easy Slow Cooker Beef Noodle Stew 225
903. Old Fashioned Baked Beans 225

904. Paleo Chicken With Apple And Sweet Potato 225
905. Pinto Beans Muy Facil 225
906. Pork Chops With Apples, Sweet Potatoes, And Sauerkraut 225
907. Quick Chick! 226
908. Refried Beans Without The Refry 226
909. Savory Slow Cooker Squash And Apple Dish 226
910. Shrimp Jambalaya 226
911. Sleeper Heater Lentil Soup 226
912. Slow Cook 3 Bean Chili (Vegetarian And Gluten Free) 227
913. Slow Cooked Apple Peach Sauce 227
914. Slow Cooked Baked Beans 227
915. Slow Cooker Apple Butter 227
916. Slow Cooker Apple Cider Pot Roast .. 227
917. Slow Cooker Baked Beans 228
918. Slow Cooker Baked Potatoes 228
919. Slow Cooker Balsamic Chicken 228
920. Slow Cooker Butternut Squash Soup . 228
921. Slow Cooker Calico Bean Soup 228
922. Slow Cooker Caribou Stew 229
923. Slow Cooker Carrot Cake Steel Cut Oats . 229
924. Slow Cooker Chicken Creole 229
925. Slow Cooker Chicken Curry With Quinoa 229
926. Slow Cooker Chicken Marrakesh 229
927. Slow Cooker Chicken Mole 230
928. Slow Cooker Chicken And Noodles .. 230
929. Slow Cooker Chocolate Banana Steel Cut Oats 230
930. Slow Cooker Cider Applesauce (No Sugar Added) 230
931. Slow Cooker Cilantro Lime Chicken Tacos 230
932. Slow Cooker Cinnamon Apple Steel Cut Oats 231
933. Slow Cooker Garlic And Herb Pork Tenderloin 231
934. Slow Cooker Ham And Beans 231
935. Slow Cooker Homemade Beans 231
936. Slow Cooker Mediterranean Lentil Soup 231
937. Slow Cooker Mediterranean Stew 232
938. Slow Cooker Mock Roast 232
939. Slow Cooker Moroccan Chicken 232
940. Slow Cooker Oats 232
941. Slow Cooker Potato Soup 233
942. Slow Cooker Pozole 233
943. Slow Cooker Pumpkin Steel Cut Oats 233
944. Slow Cooker Ratatouille From RED GOLD® 233
945. Slow Cooker Root Vegetable Tagine . 233
946. Slow Cooker Root Veggie Winter Soup 234
947. Slow Cooker Rosemary And Red Pepper Chicken 234
948. Slow Cooker Southern Lima Beans And Ham 234
949. Slow Cooker Spaghetti Sauce I 234
950. Slow Cooker Spicy Black Eyed Peas 235
951. Slow Cooker Turkey Chili With Kidney Beans 235
952. Slow Cooker White Chicken Chili 235
953. Slow Cooked Habanero Chili 235
954. Spiced Slow Cooker Applesauce 236
955. Spicy Chicken Thai Noodle Soup 236
956. Spicy Slow Cooker Black Bean Soup 236
957. Spicy Turkey Chili 236
958. Sweet And Simple Pork Roast 236
959. Tunisian Slow Cooked Turkey Breast 236
960. Tykvenitsa Millet Breakfast Cereal 237
961. Vegetarian Cassoulet 237
Chapter 12: Easy Slow Cooker Recipes 238
962. Bacon Cheese Breakfast Casserole .. 238
963. Barbecue Pulled Chicken 238
964. Beef And Red Bean Chili 238
965. Buffalo Chicken Salads 239
966. Cheese Fondue With Fennel Tomatoes 239
967. Chile, Cheese, And Scrambled Egg Grits 239
968. Creamy Chicken Noodle Soup 239
969. Easy Chicken Enchiladas 240
970. Eggplant Chickpea Stew 240
971. Ethiopian Spiced Chicken Stew 240
972. Fennel Pork Stew 241
973. Fireside Beef Stew 241
974. Flemish Beef Stew 241
975. Fork Tender Pot Roast 242
976. Greek Chicken Vegetable Ragout 242
977. Pasta With Marinara Sauce 242
978. Pulled Pork With Caramelized Onions 243
979. Sausage And Sweet Pepper Hash 243
980. Slow Cooked Beans 243
981. Slow Cooked Brisket In Onion Gravy 244
982. Slow Cooker Beef Stroganoff 244
983. Slow Cooker Beef Tacos With Rhubarb Salsa 244
984. Slow Cooker Chicken Tortilla Soup ... 245
985. Slow Cooker Garlic Mashed Potatoes 245
986. Slow Cooker Lamb Stew With Artichokes White Beans 245
987. Slow Cooker Moroccan Lentil Soup .. 245
988. Slow Cooker Pasta E Fagioli Soup Freezer Pack 246
989. Slow Cooker Shredded Beef Tacos With Pico De Gallo 246
990. Slow Cooker Southwestern Bean Soup 246
991. Slow Cooker Sweet Potato Casserole With Marshmallows 247
992. Slow Cooker Turkish Lamb Vegetable Stew 247
993. Slow Cooker Vegetable Soup 247
994. Slow Cooker Yankee Bean Pot 247
995. Southwestern Three Bean Barley Soup 248
996. Spanish Potato Omelet 248
997. Sweet Ginger Root Vegetables 248
998. Tangy Cherry Barbecue Sausage 249
999. Vegetable And Pasta Soup 249
1000. Veggies, Turkey, And Pasta 249
1001. Wine Tomato Braised Chicken 249

Chapter 1: Appetizer Slow Cooker Recipes

1. Amazing Buffalo Dip

Serving: 10 | Prep: 10mins | Cook: 20mins | Ready in:

Ingredients
2 cups diced cooked chicken
1 (8 ounce) package cream cheese, softened
1/2 cup blue cheese salad dressing
1/2 cup hot pepper sauce (such as Frank's RedHot®)
1/2 cup crumbled blue cheese
1/4 cup ranch dressing, or to taste

Direction
Prepare a slow cooker and put in the blue cheese dressing, ranch dressing, cream cheese, hot pepper sauce, chicken and crumbled blue cheese then mix together.
Turn on the slow cooker to high temperature for about 20 minutes until cooked and heated through.

Nutrition Information
Calories: 246 calories;Protein: 11.5;Total Fat: 21.4;Sodium: 665;Total Carbohydrate: 2.1;Cholesterol: 54

2. Anne's Hot Ham And Swiss Dip

Serving: 8 | Prep: 10mins | Cook: 2hours | Ready in:

Ingredients
1 pound thinly sliced deli ham, sliced into thin strips
1 (8 ounce) package cream cheese, cut into cubes
1 (10.75 ounce) can condensed cream of mushroom soup, undiluted
1 (10.75 ounce) can condensed cream of celery soup, undiluted
2 cups shredded Swiss cheese
2 (1 pound) loaves cocktail rye bread

Direction
Mix cream of celery soup, cream of mushroom soup, cream cheese and ham in a slow cooker; mix in Swiss cheese. Cover; cook for approximately 2 hours till cheese is melted on Low while occasionally mixing. Serve over cocktail rye slices.

Nutrition Information
Calories: 483 calories;;Total Carbohydrate: 11.6;Cholesterol: 123;Protein: 29.1;Total Fat: 35.6;Sodium: 1476

3. Awesome Slow Cooker Buffalo Wings

Serving: 8 | Prep: | Cook: 4hours30mins | Ready in:

Ingredients
1 (12 ounce) bottle hot pepper sauce (such as Frank's RedHot®)
1/2 cup butter
2 tablespoons Worcestershire sauce
2 teaspoons dried oregano
2 teaspoons onion powder
2 teaspoons garlic powder
1 (4 pound) frozen chicken wing sections, thawed
1/2 cup butter
1 (12 ounce) bottle hot pepper sauce (such as Frank's RedHot®)

Direction
In a saucepan, mix together garlic powder, onion powder, oregano, Worcestershire sauce, 1/2 cup butter, and 1 bottle hot pepper sauce over medium heat. Heat the mixture to a boil then decrease to low heat and simmer for 5 minutes.
In the slow cooker, put chicken wings then spread sauce mixture over the wings.
Choose High setting and cook for 2 hours. Switch to Low then cook for 2 more hours.
Set oven to 200° C (400° F) and start preheating. Oil some baking trays.
Arrange wings on the prepared baking trays then put them into the oven; bake for 30 minutes until wings are browned and crisp.
In a small saucepan, melt 1/2 cup butter together with 1 bottle hot sauce; simmer 20 minutes until thickened. Brush wings with the sauce just prior to serving.

Nutrition Information
Calories: 385 calories;;Total Fat: 34.4;Sodium: 2472;Total Carbohydrate: 3.5;Cholesterol: 109;Protein: 16.1

4. BBQ Bison Phyllo Bites

Serving: 30 | Prep: 40mins | Cook: 12hours10mins | Ready in:

Ingredients
1 (4.5 pound) bison brisket
1 1/2 cups beef broth
1/4 cup Worcestershire sauce
3 tablespoons cider vinegar
4 teaspoons chili powder
1/4 teaspoon cayenne pepper
3 cloves garlic, minced
1/2 cup bottled barbecue sauce
2 (1.9 ounce) packages baked miniature phyllo dough shells
1/2 cup shredded Cheddar cheese
Sour cream
Chopped fresh cilantro

Direction
Slice bison brisket into 2-inch slices. In a 4- 5-quart slow cooker, put the bison brisket slices. In a medium-sized bowl, mix together garlic, cayenne pepper, chili powder, vinegar, Worcestershire sauce, and broth. Put on the bison slices in the slow cooker. Put a cover on and cook on low for 12 hours. Take the bison brisket slices out of the cooker and put in a big bowl, dispose of the cooking juices. Shred the bison brisket slices with 2 forks. In a bowl, save enough shredded bison brisket to measure 2 cups. Keep the rest of the shredded bison brisket in 2-cup portions in airtight containers. Refrigerate a maximum of 3 days or freeze a maximum of 3 months.
Start preheating the oven to 375°F. In a 15x10x1-inch baking pan, put phyllo dough shells. In the bowl, mix barbecue sauce into the saved 2 cups of shredded bison. Split the shredded bison evenly between phyllo shells. Put an equal amount of shredded cheese on top each.
Put in the preheated oven and bake without a cover until cooked through, about 10 minutes. Put cilantro and sour cream on top.

Nutrition Information
Calories: 119 calories;;Total Carbohydrate: 6.4;Cholesterol: 20;Protein: 13.9;Total Fat: 3.5;Sodium: 807

5. Bacon Wrapped Smokies

Serving: 16 | Prep: 45mins | Cook: 45mins | Ready in:

Ingredients
1 pound sliced bacon, cut into thirds
1 (14 ounce) package beef cocktail wieners
3/4 cup brown sugar, or to taste

Direction

Set the oven to 325°F (165°C) to preheat.
Chill two-third of the bacon until required. Easily wrap each wiener with a cold bacon and poke with a toothpick. Wrap each cocktail wiener with a piece of bacon. Position on a big baking sheet. Sprinkle sufficiently with brown sugar over all.
Bake in the preheated oven until the sugar is bubbly, for 40 minutes. Set the slow cooker to low, and place the wieners in it to serve.

Nutrition Information
Calories: 163 calories;;Total Fat: 10.5;Sodium: 458;Total Carbohydrate: 10.7;Cholesterol: 26;Protein: 6.5

6. Bavarian Style Meatballs

Serving: 7 | Prep: 5mins | Cook: 4hours | Ready in:

Ingredients
12 fluid ounces tomato-based chili sauce
1 (16 ounce) can whole cranberry sauce
27 ounces Bavarian-style sauerkraut, undrained
1 cup water
1 cup packed brown sugar
1 (16 ounce) package frozen meatballs

Direction
Combine brown sugar, water, sauerkraut, cranberry sauce, and chili sauce in a medium-size mixing bowl. Mix well. Next, in a slow cooker, put the meatballs and the sauce, stir well.
Cover and cook for 4 hours at a medium temperature. Stir infrequently to coat the meatballs.

Nutrition Information
Calories: 494 calories;Protein: 11.5;Total Fat: 17.1;Sodium: 1954;Total Carbohydrate: 76.7;Cholesterol: 50

7. Beef Enchilada Dip

Serving: 10 | Prep: 20mins | Cook: 25mins | Ready in:

Ingredients
1/2 pound ground beef
1/4 onion, chopped, or more to taste
2/3 cup water
1 (1 ounce) packet taco seasoning mix
1 (28 ounce) can mild red enchilada sauce
2 (10.75 ounce) cans cream of mushroom soup
1/2 cup shredded Cheddar cheese, or to taste

Direction
Over medium-high heat, heat large skillet. In hot skillet, cook while stirring onion and beef for 5-7 mins or until crumbly and browned; drain, then remove any grease. Put in taco seasoning and water; cook while stirring for 5 mins or until water has been evaporated.
In a slow cooker, mix together Cheddar cheese, enchilada sauce and cream of mushroom soup; turn the cooker on High. Put the ground beef mixture into the enchilada sauce mixture. Cook for 15-20 mins, until the sauce starts to bubble, stirring occasionally. Set on 'Keep Warm' mode or lower the heat to Low. Serve!

Nutrition Information
Calories: 178 calories;;Sodium: 859;Total Carbohydrate: 11.9;Cholesterol: 21;Protein: 7.6;Total Fat: 11

8. Big Game Salsa Dip

Serving: 80 | Prep: 30mins | Cook: 1hours30mins | Ready in:

Ingredients
1 (2 pound) loaf processed cheese, cubed
1 cup milk
1 (12 ounce) package ground pork sausage
1 white onion, chopped
1 (24 ounce) jar medium salsa
1/2 (15 ounce) can black beans, drained and rinsed
1 bunch green onions, chopped
1 (12 ounce) package tortilla chips

Direction
Set a slow cooker on high heat, put in the milk and processed cheese. Cook with a cover while stirring from time to time till the cheese is melted and blended well with milk.
In a medium skillet, put the ground pork sausage. Cook it over medium high heat till evenly browned. Add white onion. Cook while stirring till the onion becomes translucent. Take it away from the heat and strain.
Mix the sausage mixture into the cheese mixture. Turn the heat down to low. Put in black beans and salsa. Keep cooking while stirring from time to time for about 1 hour.
Use green onions for garnish. Serve with tortilla chips.

Nutrition Information
Calories: 83 calories;;Sodium: 252;Total Carbohydrate: 5.1;Cholesterol: 12;Protein: 3.4;Total Fat: 5.6

9. Big Game Sunday Chili Dip

Serving: 8 | Prep: | Cook: 1hours5mins | Ready in:

Ingredients
1 (14 ounce) can black beans, drained
1 (8 ounce) jar salsa
1 pound ground turkey
salt and ground black pepper to taste
1 (8 ounce) package shredded Mexican cheese blend

Direction
In slow cooker set on low, mix salsa and black beans. In skillet, break ground turkey on medium heat; season with pepper and salt. Mix and cook turkey for 5-7 minutes till browned completely. Mix turkey into black bean mixture. Sprinkle the cheese on bean and turkey mixture.
Cook mixture for 1 hour on high. Lower to low setting while serving to keep dip hot.

Nutrition Information
Calories: 246 calories;;Total Fat: 13.6;Sodium: 630;Total Carbohydrate: 10.9;Cholesterol: 69;Protein: 21

10. Black Eyed Pea Sausage Dip

Serving: 14 | Prep: 10mins | Cook: 16hours10mins | Ready in:

Ingredients
3 tablespoons unsalted butter
1 large onion, chopped
4 stalks celery, chopped
salt and ground black pepper to taste
1 (12 ounce) package reduced fat pork sausage
3 (15.5 ounce) cans black-eyed peas, undrained
2 (10 ounce) cans diced tomatoes with green chiles (such as Rotel®)

Direction
Melt butter in a big skillet on medium high heat. Add celery and onion; mix and cook for 5 minutes till translucent. Season with pepper and salt. Put vegetables in a slow cooker.
Put sausage in the same skillet; cook, using a wooden spoon to break apart, for 5-6 minutes till browned.

Put in the slow cooker; put diced tomatoes with green chiles and black-eyed peas in.
Cook for 16 hours on low till black-eyed peas are tender.
Nutrition Information
Calories: 170 calories;;Cholesterol: 20;Protein: 8.3;Total Fat: 8.2;Sodium: 521;Total Carbohydrate: 16

11. Cajun Boiled Peanuts
Serving: 32 | Prep: 5mins | Cook: 8hours | Ready in:
Ingredients
5 pounds raw peanuts, in shells
1 (6 ounce) package dry crab boil
1 (4 ounce) can sliced jalapeno peppers, with liquid
Direction
In a slow cooker, place peanuts. Sprinkle dry crab boil over; pour in water to cover. Mix in in sliced jalapeno peppers and the liquid accompanied with them. Put cover on the slow cooker and cook peanuts 8 hours or all night on low setting, till peanuts float to the surface of the water.
Nutrition Information
Calories: 403 calories;;Sodium: 71;Total Carbohydrate: 11.6;Cholesterol: 0;Protein: 18.3;Total Fat: 35

12. Candied Bacon Pigs
Serving: 10 | Prep: 20mins | Cook: 4hours40mins | Ready in:
Ingredients
1 (14 ounce) package little smokie sausages
1 pound bacon slices, cut into thirds crosswise
1 1/2 cups brown sugar, divided
1/2 (12 fluid ounce) can cola-flavored carbonated beverage
1/2 teaspoon Chinese five-spice powder
1 dash hot pepper sauce, or to taste (optional)
Direction
Let your oven heat to 165°C (325°F).
Wrap sausage in a third of the slice of bacon and pin with toothpicks.
Spread the appetizers on a big baking sheet then top it with about 3/4 cup brown sugar.
Let it bake for 40 minutes until the sugar is bubbling and melted; turn after 20 minutes.
Transfer appetizers, using a slotted spoon, from the pan to a slow cooker. Sprinkle with the leftover 3/4 cup brown sugar. Also, sprinkle the Smokies with five-spice powder. Dribble with cola. You can also add hot sauce to add flavor if you want.
For up to 4 hours, heat on High. Serve while hot.
Nutrition Information
Calories: 291 calories;;Cholesterol: 41;Protein: 10.5;Total Fat: 17.1;Sodium: 752;Total Carbohydrate: 24.3

13. Candied Kielbasa
Serving: 8 | Prep: 5mins | Cook: 1hours | Ready in:
Ingredients
1 cup packed brown sugar
1/2 cup ketchup
1/4 cup prepared horseradish
2 pounds kielbasa sausage, sliced thin
Direction
Mix horseradish, ketchup and sugar in a slow cooker. Put in the sausage, then stir well. Cook on High until it begins boiling. Lower heat to Low and cook for about 45 minutes to 1 hour, until sauce thickens.

Nutrition Information
Calories: 473 calories;;Total Carbohydrate: 34.8;Cholesterol: 75;Protein: 14.3;Total Fat: 31.1;Sodium: 1224

14. Carolina Pulled Pork Slow Cooker Dip
Serving: 32 | Prep: 15mins | Cook: 4hours | Ready in:
Ingredients
1 pound pork tenderloin, cut into 1-inch chunks
1 (1.6 oz) package McCormick® Slow Cookers BBQ Pulled Pork Seasoning Mix
1 cup cider vinegar
1/2 cup firmly packed brown sugar
1/4 cup chopped dill pickles
8 ounces processed cheese product, such as Velveeta®, cubed
2 tablespoons chopped green onions
Direction
In medium bowl, put pork. Sprinkle two tablespoons of Seasoning Mix over; coat by tossing. Put aside.
In slow cooker, mix the remaining Seasoning Mix, pickles, vinegar and brown sugar. Put seasoned pork into the slow cooker.
Cook on HIGH or until the pork becomes tender, about 3 1/2-4 hours. Discard pork from the slow cooker.
Using 2 forks, shred pork. Put the pork back to the slow cooker. Put in cheese; allow to stand with a cover until cheese melts, about 10 mins. Stir well. Sprinkle green onions over. If desired, top with coleslaw.
Nutrition Information
Calories: 58 calories;;Total Fat: 2.5;Sodium: 261;Total Carbohydrate: 4.2;Cholesterol: 13;Protein: 3.8

15. Carrie's Southern Queso
Serving: 10 | Prep: 5mins | Cook: 1hours | Ready in:
Ingredients
2 (14.5 ounce) cans diced tomatoes with mild green chiles
1 pound processed cheese food, cubed
Direction
In a slow cooker, mix cheese food, chiles and tomatoes together; cook while stirring occasionally on high setting for around 1 hour, till melted.
Nutrition Information
Calories: 170 calories;;Total Fat: 11.1;Sodium: 679;Total Carbohydrate: 7.8;Cholesterol: 29;Protein: 10.3

16. Cheese Dip II
Serving: 48 | Prep: 5mins | Cook: 25mins | Ready in:
Ingredients
1 (2 pound) loaf processed cheese, cubed
1 1/2 pounds ground beef
2/3 cup water
1 (1.25 ounce) package taco seasoning mix
1 (16 ounce) jar picante sauce
Direction
Let processed cheese melt over high heat in a slow cooker. Stir occasionally to prevent the cheese from burning.
In a large skillet, add ground beef. Over medium high heat, cook to brown evenly. Drain and mix the beef with taco seasoning mix and water. Cook for 2-4 minutes, stirring.

Add seasoned beef into the melted processed cheese and stir. Add salsa and mix. Cook to blend well, stirring. Serve warm.
Nutrition Information
Calories: 109 calories;;Total Fat: 8.5;Sodium: 307;Total Carbohydrate: 2;Cholesterol: 27;Protein: 5.8

17. Cheesy Taco Dip

Serving: 9 | Prep: 5mins | Cook: 1hours5mins | Ready in:
Ingredients
1 pound lean ground beef
3/4 cup water
1 (1.25 ounce) package taco seasoning mix
1 (16 ounce) can crushed tomatoes
1 (1 pound) loaf processed cheese, shredded
Direction
Browning ground beef in a large skillet. Strain fat. Mix in water and seasoning packet. Bring to a boil, lower heat to simmer. Allow to cook for 5 minutes, occasionally stirring.
In a slow cooker, lay ground beef. Add into the slow cooker with cheese and tomatoes.
Allow to cook for an hour on low.
Nutrition Information
Calories: 327 calories;;Cholesterol: 78;Protein: 18.9;Total Fat: 23.1;Sodium: 1018;Total Carbohydrate: 10.2

18. Chicken Nachos From Reynolds Wrap®

Serving: 6 | Prep: 20mins | Cook: 4hours | Ready in:
Ingredients
4 boneless, skinless chicken breasts
1 (14 ounce) can enchilada sauce
1 (12 ounce) package tortilla chips
1 (14 ounce) can black beans, rinsed and drained
Shredded Mexican blend cheese
Sliced black olives
Salsa
Avocados
Banana peppers
1 Reynolds® Slow Cooker Liner
Reynolds Wrap® Non Stick Aluminum Foil
Direction
Using a Reynolds(R) Slow Cooker Liner, line a 5-6-qt. slow cooker. Open the slow cooker liner; cover it inside a cooker bowl. Keep the sides and bottom of the bowl fit closely with the liner; pull the top of the liner over the rim of the bowl.
Put chicken into the slow cooker. Place 1 can of enchilada sauce on top.
Cook on low with a cover for 4-6 hours.
Remove the lid to let the steam out. Take the chicken out; put on a cutting board. Shred with two forks; or speed up the process with a stand mixer. Transfer the chicken into the mixer; process for about 30 seconds on low. Allow the slow cooker to cool completely; take away the liner and toss.
Set the oven to 350°F (175°C) and start preheating. Using non-stick foil of Reynolds Wrap, line a cookie sheet; dull side up.
Arrange tortilla chips on the foil; put shredded cheese, black beans and the chicken on top. Bake until the cheese is melted, around 10 minutes. Take the nachos out of oven, cover the top with banana peppers, avocados, salsa, sliced olives and any other toppings of your choice.
Nutrition Information
Calories: 631 calories;;Sodium: 1339;Total Carbohydrate: 60.2;Cholesterol: 62;Protein: 31.2;Total Fat: 31.4

19. Chorizo Queso Dip

Serving: 16 | Prep: 5mins | Cook: 1hours30mins | Ready in:
Ingredients
10 ounces bulk chorizo sausage
1 (10 ounce) can diced tomatoes with green chile peppers (such as RO*TEL®), drained
1 (8 ounce) package cream cheese, cubed
1 (8 ounce) package processed cheese (such as Velveeta®), cubed
Direction
In a skillet, stir and cook chorizo sausage on medium heat for 5-7 minutes until completely cooked. Drain. Put into a slow cooker.
Mix processed cheese, cream cheese and diced tomatoes in with chorizo.
Cook on low for 1 1/2-2 hours, occasionally stirring, until cheese melts.
Nutrition Information
Calories: 178 calories;;Total Fat: 15.2;Sodium: 508;Total Carbohydrate: 2.4;Cholesterol: 42;Protein: 8

20. Cocktail Wieners

Serving: 10 | Prep: 10mins | Cook: 2hours | Ready in:
Ingredients
1 cup barbeque sauce
3/4 cup grape jelly
2 (16 ounce) packages cocktail sausages (such as Lit'l Smokies®)
Direction
In a slow cooker, stir grape jelly and barbeque sauce together; put in cocktail sausages and mix.
Cook for 2 - 3 hours on Low.
Nutrition Information
Calories: 389 calories;;Total Fat: 27.1;Sodium: 1159;Total Carbohydrate: 27.3;Cholesterol: 59;Protein: 11.8

21. Crab Rangoon Dip For The Slow Cooker

Serving: 6 | Prep: 5mins | Cook: 2hours | Ready in:
Ingredients
2 (8 ounce) packages cream cheese, softened
1 (12 ounce) package crabmeat, flaked and cartilage removed
1/2 cup sour cream
4 green onions, chopped
2 tablespoons confectioners' sugar
1 1/2 teaspoons Worcestershire sauce
1/2 teaspoon garlic powder
Direction
In the crock of a slow cooker, stir together garlic powder, Worcestershire sauce, confectioners' sugar, green onions, sour cream, crabmeat and cream cheese.
Cook on Low for 2 hours, mixing at least once.
Nutrition Information
Calories: 353 calories;Protein: 14;Total Fat: 30.5;Sodium: 374;Total Carbohydrate: 6.8;Cholesterol: 116

22. Cranberry Chipotle Meatballs

Serving: 16 | Prep: 10mins | Cook: 4hours | Ready in:
Ingredients

1 (16 ounce) package frozen cooked meatballs, thawed
1 (16 ounce) can jellied cranberry sauce
1 (15 ounce) can pineapple chunks, drained
1/4 cup packed brown sugar
1 canned chipotle chile in adobo sauce, chopped - or more to taste
Direction
Into a slow cooker, put the meatballs. Mash cranberry sauce coarsely in a bowl, and combine with chipotle chili, brown sugar and pineapple chunks. Put the sauce on top of meatballs, and mix to incorporate. Put the cooker cover, turn to Low setting, and allow to cook for 4 to 5 hours till meatballs have soaked in the sauce flavors and sauce is thickened. Serve together with toothpicks.
Nutrition Information
Calories: 132 calories;;Total Carbohydrate: 20.2;Cholesterol: 24;Protein: 4.9;Total Fat: 3.7;Sodium: 48

23. Crock Pot® Party Meatballs
Serving: 8 | Prep: 5mins | Cook: 3hours | Ready in:
Ingredients
1 (2 pound) bag frozen cooked meatballs
1 (14.5 ounce) can whole berry cranberry sauce
1 (12 ounce) bottle tomato-based chili sauce
1/2 lemon, juiced
2 drops hot sauce (such as Tabasco®), or more to taste
Direction
In a slow cooker, put frozen meatballs. Add the hot sauce, lemon juice, chili sauce, and cranberry sauce. Stir to evenly distribute the sauce over meatballs. Cook on High for about 3 hours, or until the meatballs are completely defrosted and hot.
Nutrition Information
Calories: 320 calories;;Sodium: 210;Total Carbohydrate: 27.3;Cholesterol: 94;Protein: 19.1;Total Fat: 14.6

24. Currant Jelly Wiener Sauce
Serving: 24 | Prep: 10mins | Cook: 2hours | Ready in:
Ingredients
1 cup red currant jelly
1 cup prepared Dijon-style mustard
1/4 cup ketchup
3/4 cup brown sugar
4 (16 ounce) packages little smokie sausages
Direction
In a slow cooker, combine brown sugar, ketchup, Dijon-style mustard and red currant jelly together over medium low heat. Add little smokie sausages into the mixture, let it simmer for at least 2 hours. Serve with toothpicks.
Nutrition Information
Calories: 300 calories;Protein: 9.3;Total Fat: 20.4;Sodium: 1032;Total Carbohydrate: 19.9;Cholesterol: 47

25. Dog Food Dip
Serving: 48 | Prep: 15mins | Cook: 20mins | Ready in:
Ingredients
2 pounds lean ground beef
1 onion, chopped
1 (10.75 ounce) can condensed cream of mushroom soup
1 pound processed cheese food, cubed
pickled jalapeno pepper slices, to taste (optional)

Direction
Place a large, deep skillet pan on the stove and turn on to medium high heat, then put the ground beef and onion together. Stir and cook until onion becomes soft beef is equally brown. Turn the stove to medium low heat then let the liquid dry out.
Add in the condensed cream of mushroom soup. Then stir in your wish amount of jalapeno pepper and processed cheese food. Mix and let it cook for about 10 minutes until all are well combined.
Place the mixture in medium size bowl. Use a plastic wrapper to cover the bowl and let it chill in the refrigerator for 8 hour or overnight.
Using a slow cooker to reheat the mixture, you can 1 tablespoon of water to make it thin if needed, then serve.
Nutrition Information
Calories: 88 calories;;Total Carbohydrate: 1.5;Cholesterol: 20;Protein: 5.3;Total Fat: 6.6;Sodium: 166

26. Drunken Sailors
Serving: 6 | Prep: 15mins | Cook: 6hours | Ready in:
Ingredients
1 (14 ounce) bottle ketchup
1 (12 ounce) bottle barbeque sauce
1/2 cup brown sugar
1/2 cup whiskey
1 (16 ounce) package kielbasa sausage, sliced into 1/2 inch pieces
1 box toothpicks
Direction
Pour the barbecue sauce and ketchup into a slow cooker. Then stir in the sausage, whiskey, and brown sugar. Cook for about 6 hours on Low. Serve hot using toothpicks.
Nutrition Information
Calories: 499 calories;;Sodium: 2054;Total Carbohydrate: 57.1;Cholesterol: 50;Protein: 10.4;Total Fat: 21

27. Easy Beer And Ketchup Meatballs
Serving: 8 | Prep: 40mins | Cook: 3hours | Ready in:
Ingredients
1 (28 ounce) bottle ketchup
24 fluid ounces beer
1 1/2 pounds ground beef
2 teaspoons garlic powder
1 onion, chopped
Direction
Set an oven to 200°C (400°F) and start preheating.
In a slow cooker on a high setting, arrange the ketchup and beer and bring to a simmer.
At the same time, blend the onion, garlic powder, and ground beef in a large bowl and mix thoroughly. Shape the mixture into meatballs with a diameter of about 3/4 inch. In a 9x13-inch baking dish, arrange meatballs.
Bake for 20 minutes at 200°C (400°F).
Place the meatballs into the slow cooker with the ketchup and beer and bring to a simmer for 3 hours; the sauce will become thickened.
Nutrition Information
Calories: 405 calories;;Total Fat: 22.9;Sodium: 1154;Total Carbohydrate: 29.6;Cholesterol: 72;Protein: 16.5

28. Easy Cheesy Crawfish Dip
Serving: 25 | Prep: 35mins | Cook: 1hours | Ready in:

Ingredients
2 pounds processed cheese food (such as Velveeta®), cubed
1 teaspoon condensed cream of mushroom soup
1/2 cup butter, divided
2 onions, chopped
1 green bell pepper, chopped
1 tablespoon minced garlic
3 pounds peeled crawfish tails
1 teaspoon cayenne pepper, or to taste
salt and ground black pepper to taste
1 (10 ounce) can diced tomatoes with green chile peppers (such as RO*TEL®)
Direction
Put 1 tsp cream of mushroom soup and processed cheese in a slow cooker. Set to High. Set aside.
In a pan, melt half of the butter over medium heat. Sauté and stir green pepper and onion for 10 minutes, until the onion is translucent and tender. Scrape the onion mix and transfer to a bowl. Set aside. Take the rest of the butter and melt it in the pan with the garlic. When the garlic becomes fragrant and sizzling, add the crawfish tails. Sprinkle with salt, pepper, and cayenne pepper to taste. Stir and cook until the tails are hot, then mix them into the pepper and onion mixture.
Put the crawfish mix in a blender or food processor. Blend until it's finely ground, or to your preferred texture. Add the crawfish mix to the slow cooker. Add the diced tomatoes too.
Put the lid on. Cook for 45 minutes. Stir frequently. Turn the heat to Low once it is hot, until you're about to serve.
Nutrition Information
Calories: 199 calories;;Total Fat: 13.4;Sodium: 566;Total Carbohydrate: 4.5;Cholesterol: 97;Protein: 15.1

29. Easy Marinated Mushrooms
Serving: 16 | Prep: 15mins | Cook: 8hours | Ready in:
Ingredients
2 cups soy sauce
2 cups water
1 cup butter
2 cups white sugar
4 (8 ounce) packages fresh mushrooms, stems removed
Direction
On low heat, mix butter, water and soy sauce in a medium saucepan. Mix till melted butter, then slowly stir in the sugar till sugar totally dissolved.
In a slow cooker on Low setting, put mushrooms and coat mushrooms with the soy sauce mixture. Cook 8 to 10 hours while mixing roughly every hour. Keep chilled in the fridge till serving.
Nutrition Information
Calories: 228 calories;;Sodium: 1889;Total Carbohydrate: 29.3;Cholesterol: 31;Protein: 3.9;Total Fat: 11.7

30. Easy Slow Cooker Chicken Wings
Serving: 8 | Prep: 5mins | Cook: 5hours | Ready in:
Ingredients
5 1/2 pounds chicken wings, split and tips discarded
1 (12 fluid ounce) can or bottle chile sauce
1/4 cup fresh lemon juice
1/4 cup molasses
2 tablespoons Worcestershire sauce
3 drops hot pepper sauce
1 tablespoon salsa
2 1/2 teaspoons chili powder
1 teaspoon garlic powder
2 teaspoons salt
Direction
Put chicken into a slow cooker. Combine salt, garlic powder, chili powder, salsa, hot pepper sauce, Worcestershire sauce, molasses, lemon juice and chile sauce in a medium bowl. Mix together then spread over the chicken.
In slow cooker, cook for 5 hours on Medium Low setting.
Nutrition Information
Calories: 284 calories;;Total Fat: 15.3;Sodium: 720;Total Carbohydrate: 13.7;Cholesterol: 66;Protein: 22.4

31. Famous Meatballs
Serving: 6 | Prep: 10mins | Cook: 2hours10mins | Ready in:
Ingredients
1 (13.25 ounce) can pineapple chunks in juice
1 green bell pepper, sliced
1/2 cup brown sugar
2 tablespoons cornstarch
2 tablespoons soy sauce
2 tablespoons lemon juice
1 (3 pound) bag frozen cooked meatballs, thawed
Direction
Pour pineapple chunks with juice into a saucepan. Stir lemon juice, soy sauce, cornstarch, brown sugar, and green bell pepper through the pineapple chunks until the cornstarch and sugar dissolve.
Next, bring the mixture to a boil; then cook and stir for about 10 minutes, until thickened.
Put the meatballs into slow cooker crock; pour over the meatballs with the pineapple mixture.
Cook for 2 hours on medium, stirring every half an hour.
Nutrition Information
Calories: 611 calories;;Total Fat: 29.2;Sodium: 587;Total Carbohydrate: 46.4;Cholesterol: 189;Protein: 38.9

32. Guinness® Beer Cheese Dip
Serving: 16 | Prep: 10mins | Cook: 30mins | Ready in:
Ingredients
32 ounces processed cheese food (such as Velveeta®), cut into 1/2-inch cubes
1 cup Irish stout beer (such as Guinness®)
1/2 cup salsa
2 tablespoons Worcestershire sauce
1 teaspoon chili powder
1/2 teaspoon onion powder
1/4 teaspoon cayenne pepper (optional)
Direction
In a slow cooker, heat cheese on high for 20 minutes until it melts.
Mix salsa, beer, chili powder, Worcestershire sauce, cayenne pepper and onion powder into the cheese. Stir frequently for 10 minutes until it's heated through and smooth.
Nutrition Information
Calories: 224 calories;;Cholesterol: 53;Protein: 12.8;Total Fat: 17.8;Sodium: 916;Total Carbohydrate: 2.5

33. Healthier Buffalo Chicken Dip
Serving: 20 | Prep: 5mins | Cook: 40mins | Ready in:

Ingredients
2 (10 ounce) cans natural chunk chicken, drained
3/4 cup hot pepper sauce (such as Frank's RedHot®)
2 (8 ounce) packages Neufchatel cheese, softened
1 cup light ranch dressing
1 cup shredded reduced-fat Cheddar cheese, divided
1 bunch celery, cleaned and cut into 4 inch pieces
8 ounces multi-grain crackers
Direction
Place a skillet on the stove and turn on to medium heat then put in the hot pepper sauce and chicken, let it heat for about 5 minutes. Add in the ranch dressing and Neufchatel cheese. Continue to cook for 5 to 7 minutes until mixed well and heat enough. Stir in half of the shredded cheddar cheese and place the mixture to a slow cooker.
Dash the left cheddar cheese on top, cover, and let it cook on low heat for about 30 minutes until becomes bubbly and hot. Pair with crackers and celery when served.
Nutrition Information
Calories: 177 calories;;Total Fat: 10.1;Sodium: 664;Total Carbohydrate: 9.9;Cholesterol: 39;Protein: 11

34. Hot Mexican Dip

Serving: 32 | Prep: 10mins | Cook: 20mins | Ready in:
Ingredients
1 (15 ounce) can chili without beans
1 (8 ounce) jar salsa
1 (8 ounce) jar taco sauce
2 chopped green chile peppers
crushed red pepper to taste
2 pounds processed cheese, cubed
Direction
Put processed cheese, crushed red pepper, green chile peppers, taco sauce and chili without beans in slow cooker set on low heat. Occasionally mixing, heat till all ingredients are blended well and processed cheese melts.
Nutrition Information
Calories: 110 calories;;Cholesterol: 25;Protein: 6.3;Total Fat: 7.5;Sodium: 497;Total Carbohydrate: 4.4

35. Hot Roasted Red Pepper And Artichoke Dip

Serving: 20 | Prep: 15mins | Cook: 2hours | Ready in:
Ingredients
2 (8 ounce) packages cream cheese, softened
1 1/2 cups sour cream
1/2 cup mayonnaise
2 cups shredded mozzarella cheese, divided
1 (12 ounce) jar roasted red peppers in oil with garlic, drained and chopped
1 (6 ounce) jar artichoke hearts, drained and chopped
1 loaf Italian bread, sliced
Direction
In a big bowl, use an electric mixer to beat mayonnaise, cream cheese, and sour cream together until smooth.
Add about half of the mozzarella cheese, artichoke hearts, and roasted red peppers.
Transfer mixture into a slow cooker.
Sprinkle the top with remaining mozzarella cheese.
Use low heat to cook cheese for about 2 to 3 hours until cheese is melted and the dip is bubbly. Serve with sliced Italian bread.

Nutrition Information
Calories: 316 calories;;Total Carbohydrate: 21.1;Cholesterol: 42;Protein: 8.5;Total Fat: 19.9;Sodium: 431

36. Kansas City BBQ Chicken Dip

Serving: 34 | Prep: 10mins | Cook: 2hours | Ready in:
Ingredients
1/2 cup ketchup
1/2 cup molasses
1/2 cup water
1 (1.25 ounce) package McCormick® Slow Cookers Sweet Smoky Pulled Chicken Seasoning Mix
1 pound boneless, skinless chicken thighs
1 (8 ounce) container whipped cream cheese
1 cup shredded Cheddar cheese
2 tablespoons finely chopped red onion
Direction
In a 4-quart slow cooker, combine together the seasoning mix, water, molasses and ketchup and mix. Add in the chicken; mix to coat.
Let it cook for 2 hours on high temperature or until chicken is cooked well. Use an instant-read thermometer and insert it in the middle and should read 165 degrees F (174 degrees C). Get the chicken from slow cooker.
Use 2 forks to shred the chicken. Put it back to slow cooker. Mix in the shredded cheese and cream cheese. Dust with onion and serve.
Nutrition Information
Calories: 71 calories;Protein: 3.4;Total Fat: 3.9;Sodium: 154;Total Carbohydrate: 5.6;Cholesterol: 18

37. Kevin's Sausage Dip

Serving: 24 | Prep: 10mins | Cook: 25mins | Ready in:
Ingredients
1 pound fresh, ground pork sausage
1/2 pound fresh, ground spicy pork sausage
1 (8 ounce) package cream cheese
1 (14.5 ounce) can diced tomatoes with green chile peppers
Direction
Brown sausage in a big skillet, then drain excess fat. Cube the cream cheese blocks into small portion; put sausage, tomatoes and cream cheese into a slow cooker. Heat on medium heat and stir constantly. Serve right away once cream cheese is melted thoroughly.
Nutrition Information
Calories: 153 calories;;Total Carbohydrate: 1.2;Cholesterol: 30;Protein: 4.1;Total Fat: 14.7;Sodium: 285

38. Kielbasa Appetizer

Serving: 6 | Prep: 10mins | Cook: 30mins | Ready in:
Ingredients
1 pound kielbasa, cut into 1/4-inch slices
1 onion, chopped
1/2 cup mustard
1 (10 ounce) jar prepared jalapeno pepper jelly
Direction
In a slow cooker, combine jalapeno jelly, mustard, onion and kielbasa; stir.
Set the slow cooker on high. Cook for half an hour or until heated completely.
Nutrition Information

Calories: 373 calories;Protein: 10.4;Total Fat: 21.5;Sodium: 945;Total Carbohydrate: 35.6;Cholesterol: 50

39. Krista's Queso

Serving: 24 | Prep: 10mins | Cook: 40mins | Ready in:
Ingredients
1 (16 ounce) package bulk pork breakfast sausage
1 (16 ounce) package processed cheese food, cubed
1 (4 ounce) jar mushrooms, drained
1 (14 ounce) can diced tomatoes with green chile peppers, drained
Direction
Place a large skillet on medium heat; cook in sausage till browned completely; strain.
In a slow cooker, mix green chile peppers, diced tomatoes, mushrooms, cheese and the cooked sausage. Set the slow cooker on low. Cook while stirring occasionally till the cheese is completely melted, 30-40 minutes.
Nutrition Information
Calories: 153 calories;;Total Fat: 13.5;Sodium: 491;Total Carbohydrate: 1.3;Cholesterol: 30;Protein: 6.6

40. Laurie's Creamy Slow Cooker Queso

Serving: 16 | Prep: 30mins | Cook: 1hours30mins | Ready in:
Ingredients
cooking spray
1 pound processed cheese (such as Velveeta®), cubed
1 (10.75 ounce) can condensed cream of mushroom soup
1 (10 ounce) can diced tomatoes with green chiles (such as Rotel®)
1 (5 ounce) can evaporated milk
1/2 cup sour cream
1/3 cup 2% milk
1/3 (8 ounce) package cold cream cheese, cubed
1 tablespoon vegetable oil
1 poblano pepper, seeded and chopped
1/2 yellow onion, chopped
2 small jalapeno peppers, seeded and chopped
1/3 cup canned chopped green chiles
2 teaspoons garlic, minced
2 tablespoons chopped fresh cilantro
1/2 cup Mexican-style shredded four-cheese blend
Direction
Set a slow cooker (such as Crock Pot(R)) on High; gently cover with cooking spray. Fill with cream cheese, milk, sour cream, evaporated milk, diced tomatoes with green chiles, mushroom soup, and processed cheese. Use a lid to cover. Cook for 1 hour until mostly melted.
In a skillet, heat oil over medium-high heat. Sauté jalapeno peppers, yellow onion, and poblano peppers for 5 minutes until tendered. Bring vegetables to the slow cooker; put in cilantro, garlic, and green chiles. Continue to cook with a cover for 20 minutes until cheese melts completely. Put in the Mexican cheese blend; mix until cooked through, about 10 more minutes.
Nutrition Information
Calories: 188 calories;;Total Carbohydrate: 6.9;Cholesterol: 38;Protein: 8.2;Total Fat: 14.4;Sodium: 580

41. Little Smokies

Serving: 16 | Prep: 10mins | Cook: 2hours | Ready in:
Ingredients
1 (18 ounce) bottle barbeque sauce
1 cup packed brown sugar
1/2 cup ketchup
1 tablespoon Worcestershire sauce
1/3 cup chopped onion
2 (16 ounce) packages little wieners
Direction
In the bowl of a slow cooker, combine wieners, onion, Worcestershire sauce, ketchup, brown sugar, and barbecue sauce. Cook on low until ready to enjoy, about 2 hours.
Nutrition Information
Calories: 285 calories;;Cholesterol: 31;Protein: 6.4;Total Fat: 16.4;Sodium: 1040;Total Carbohydrate: 28.6

42. Marinated Mushrooms

Serving: 8 | Prep: 15mins | Cook: 10mins | Ready in:
Ingredients
1 cup red wine
1/2 cup red wine vinegar
1/3 cup olive oil
2 tablespoons brown sugar
2 cloves garlic, minced
1 teaspoon crushed red pepper flakes
1/4 cup red bell pepper, diced
1 pound small fresh mushrooms, washed and trimmed
1/4 cup chopped green onions
1/4 teaspoon dried oregano
1/2 teaspoon salt
1/4 teaspoon ground black pepper
Direction
Mix together the mushrooms, red pepper flakes, bell pepper, garlic, sugar, oil, vinegar and wine in a saucepan on medium heat, then boil. Put cover and put aside to let it cool.
Mix in pepper, salt, oregano and green onions once cooled. Serve it at room temperature or chilled.
Nutrition Information
Calories: 139 calories;;Sodium: 151;Total Carbohydrate: 8.1;Cholesterol: 0;Protein: 2;Total Fat: 9.3

43. Meatballs And Kraut

Serving: 8 | Prep: 10mins | Cook: 1hours | Ready in:
Ingredients
1 (16 ounce) package frozen cooked meatballs, thawed
1 (14 ounce) can sauerkraut, drained
1 (12 ounce) bottle ketchup-style chili sauce (such as Heinz®)
1 cup white sugar
1 cup brown sugar
1/4 cup hot water
2 tablespoons vinegar
Direction
In a slow cooker, combine vinegar, hot water, brown sugar, white sugar, chili sauce, sauerkraut, and meatballs and stir them to dissolve the sugar. Cook for an hour on High.
Nutrition Information
Calories: 336 calories;;Total Fat: 7.4;Sodium: 459;Total Carbohydrate: 58.7;Cholesterol: 47;Protein: 10.1

44. Mexican Cheese And Hamburger Dip

Serving: 16 | Prep: 10mins | Cook: 1hours | Ready in:
Ingredients
1 pound ground beef
1 onion, diced
1 (1 ounce) package taco seasoning
1/4 cup water
1 (2 pound) loaf processed cheese food (such as Velveeta®), cut into cubes
2 (8 ounce) cans chopped green chilies
1 (8 ounce) can tomato sauce
1 tablespoon diced jalapeno peppers
Direction
In a skillet, cook and stir onion and hamburger over medium heat for 7 to 10 minutes until hamburger is entirely browned.
Scatter with taco seasoning. Pour water over the hamburger mixture; heat to a simmer and cook for 5 minutes.
Place cheese cubes in the crock of a slow cooker; add jalapeno peppers, tomato sauce, green chiles, and hamburger mixture.
Cook for about 45 minutes on low setting, stirring sometimes, until cheese melts and mixture is smooth.
Nutrition Information
Calories: 260 calories;;Sodium: 1275;Total Carbohydrate: 9.2;Cholesterol: 63;Protein: 15.8;Total Fat: 17.8

45. Outrageous Warm Chicken Nacho Dip
Serving: 12 | Prep: 20mins | Cook: 1hours15mins | Ready in:
Ingredients
1 (14 ounce) can diced tomatoes with green chile peppers (such as RO*TEL®), drained
1 (1 pound) loaf processed cheese food (such as Velveeta®), cubed
2 large cooked skinless, boneless chicken breast halves, shredded
1/3 cup sour cream
1/4 cup diced green onion
1 1/2 tablespoons taco seasoning mix
2 tablespoons minced jalapeno pepper, or to taste (optional)
1 cup black beans, rinsed and drained
Direction
In a slow cooker, place jalapeno pepper, taco seasoning, green onion, sour cream, chicken meat, processed cheese and diced tomatoes. Cook and stir occasionally for 1-2 hours on High till the dip is hot and cheese melts. Add black beans, stir and cook for 15 minutes longer to reheat.
Nutrition Information
Calories: 232 calories;;Total Fat: 13.6;Sodium: 790;Total Carbohydrate: 8.7;Cholesterol: 60;Protein: 18.6

46. Party Kielbasa
Serving: 15 | Prep: 5mins | Cook: 30mins | Ready in:
Ingredients
2 pounds kielbasa sausage
2 cups ketchup
2 cups grape jelly
Direction
Cut kielbasa into circles or strips.
In a slow cooker, put jelly and ketchup. Set the heat to medium, whisk from time to time while the ketchup and jelly melt together. Once the mixture turns into a thin glaze, add kielbasa and cook until the kielbasa is hot.
Nutrition Information
Calories: 331 calories;;Total Carbohydrate: 39.2;Cholesterol: 40;Protein: 8;Total Fat: 16.6;Sodium: 904

47. Pupu Balls
Serving: 10 | Prep: 10mins | Cook: 30mins | Ready in:
Ingredients
1 pound ground beef
1 small onion, chopped
1/2 cup seasoned bread crumbs
1/2 cup water
1/2 cup soy sauce
2 cloves garlic, crushed
1 (1.5 fluid ounce) jigger whiskey
Direction
Combine seasoned bread crumbs, onion, and ground beef in a medium bowl. Shape the mixture to bite-size balls.
Place the balls and cook in a big skillet set on medium-high heat until equally brown throughout.
Stir whiskey, garlic, soy sauce, and water in a big bowl. Put the balls in the mixture. Keep in the refrigerator to chill for a minimum of 1 hour, covered. Place the sauce mixture and the balls in a slow cooker over low heat. Then cook for a minimum of 30 minutes prior to serving.
Nutrition Information
Calories: 185 calories;;Sodium: 859;Total Carbohydrate: 5.9;Cholesterol: 39;Protein: 9.3;Total Fat: 12.4

48. Queso (Cheese) Dip
Serving: 12 | Prep: 20mins | Cook: 35mins | Ready in:
Ingredients
2 poblano peppers, halved lengthwise and seeded
2 Anaheim peppers, halved lengthwise and seeded
1 fresh jalapeno pepper, halved lengthwise and seeded
2 pounds processed cheese food (such as Velveeta ®), cut into cubes
3 large roma (plum) tomatoes, diced
1 large white onion, diced
1 tablespoon butter
2 teaspoons ground cumin
1/4 cup heavy whipping cream
Direction
The oven rack should be at least 6 inches from heat. Heat the broiler of the oven then line the baking sheet with foil.
Put the jalapeno pepper, Anaheim peppers and poblano peppers into the baking sheet with the cut facing down.
Let the peppers cook under broiler 5-8 minutes until the skin turns into black and blistered. Put the cooked peppers in a bowl then cover it with plastic wrap tightly. Let it steam for 20 minutes then peel off the skins of the peppers and dices.
Mix together the tomatoes, butter, onion, diced peppers, cheese food cubes and cumin in slow cooker. Let it cook on low while slowly adding the cream for half an hour until dip is heated and cheese has melted.
Nutrition Information
Calories: 293 calories;;Sodium: 744;Total Carbohydrate: 9.9;Cholesterol: 58;Protein: 15.7;Total Fat: 21.5

49. Queso Blanco And Black Bean Slow Cooker Dip

Serving: 8 | Prep: 15mins | Cook: 2hours30mins | Ready in:
Ingredients
1 (14 ounce) package Johnsonville® Jalapeno and Cheese Smoked Sausage, finely diced
1 (8 ounce) package cream cheese, softened
1/2 cup sour cream
1 (15 ounce) can BUSH'S® Black Beans, drained and rinsed
1 cup shredded Monterey Jack cheese
1 cup salsa verde
1 clove garlic, minced
Tortilla chips
Optional Garnish:
jalapeno peppers, sliced
tomatoes, chopped
chopped fresh cilantro
lime
Direction
Mix sour cream and softened cream cheese in a big bowl until smooth.
Put in garlic, salsa, shredded cheese, black beans and diced sausage; gently stir to mix.
Move to a 2-quarts slow cooker. Cover and cook until heated through, about 2 1/2 hours on Low, mixing every 30 minutes. To serve, lower heat to warm to hold.
Enjoy with tortilla chips. Top with a squeeze of fresh lime juice or cilantro, tomatoes and jalapenos, if desired.
Nutrition Information
Calories: 555 calories;;Total Fat: 36.3;Sodium: 882;Total Carbohydrate: 42.3;Cholesterol: 70;Protein: 16.6

50. Rachael's Superheated Cajun Boiled Peanuts

Serving: 8 | Prep: 20mins | Cook: 1Day | Ready in:
Ingredients
1 pound raw peanuts, in shells
1 (3 ounce) package dry crab boil (such as Zatarain's® Crab and Shrimp Boil)
1/2 cup chopped jalapeno peppers
1 tablespoon garlic powder
1/2 cup salt
2 tablespoons Cajun seasoning
1/2 cup red pepper flakes
Direction
In a slow cooker, combine the peanuts, jalapenos, Crab boil, salt, Cajun seasoning, garlic powder and red pepper flakes. Add water until covered and stir to mix well. Cook the mixture with cover on Low until the peanuts are soft for atleast24 hours. Stir frequently while cooking and add more water if needed so that the peanuts are covered. Drain the water and serve warm or cooled.
Nutrition Information
Calories: 360 calories;;Total Fat: 29.6;Sodium: 369;Total Carbohydrate: 16.2;Cholesterol: 0;Protein: 16.1

51. Rachel's Crockpot Seafood Cheese Dip

Serving: 10 | Prep: 5mins | Cook: 1hours | Ready in:
Ingredients
1 (8 ounce) package processed cheese food (such as Velveeta®)
2 tablespoons reduced-fat cream cheese
1 1/2 cups sour cream
1/2 cup cooked small shrimp
1/2 cup cooked crabmeat, flaked
1/2 cup cooked lobster, flaked
2 teaspoons seafood seasoning (such as Old Bay®)
1 teaspoon Worcestershire sauce
1 loaf (1/2-inch-thick) slices French bread, lightly toasted
Direction
In a crockpot, mix together the lobster, crab, shrimp, sour cream, cream cheese and processed cheese food. Cover with a lid and let it cook for about 1 hour on low heat until cheese melts, regularly stir to smash up chunks. When the cheese melted, mix in the Worcestershire sauce and seafood seasoning. Pair with French bread then serve.
Nutrition Information
Calories: 308 calories;;Total Fat: 14.5;Sodium: 777;Total Carbohydrate: 29.3;Cholesterol: 61;Protein: 15.3

52. Ranch Taco Chicken Dip

Serving: 8 | Prep: 5mins | Cook: 30mins | Ready in:
Ingredients
2 (12.5 fl oz) cans white meat chicken
1 cup sharp Cheddar cheese
1 cup plain Greek yogurt
1/4 cup taco sauce
1 (1.25 ounce) package taco seasoning mix
1/2 (1 ounce) package ranch dressing mix
Direction
In a slow cooker, mix together ranch dressing mix, taco seasoning mix, taco sauce, Greek yogurt, and chicken.
Cook for about 30 minutes on low heat until warmed through.
Nutrition Information
Calories: 268 calories;;Total Fat: 15.2;Sodium: 1054;Total Carbohydrate: 5.6;Cholesterol: 78;Protein: 24.8

53. Shannon's White Cheese Dip

Serving: 20 | Prep: 10mins | Cook: 2hours | Ready in:
Ingredients
2 (10 ounce) cans diced tomatoes with green chile peppers (such as RO*TEL®)
2 (8 ounce) packages cream cheese, cut into cubes
1 cup heavy whipping cream
1 (8 ounce) package processed cheese food (such as Velveeta®), cut into cubes
1 (8 ounce) package frozen chopped spinach, thawed and drained
1/2 cup milk
1/2 onion, finely diced
1/4 cup chopped jalapeno pepper, or to taste
4 cubes chicken bouillon
Direction
In the crock of a slow cooker, mix together chicken bouillon, jalapeno pepper, onion, milk, spinach, cheese food, cream, cream cheese, green chile peppers and diced tomatoes.
Cook on low for 2 hours while stirring often, until smooth.
Nutrition Information
Calories: 171 calories;Protein: 5;Total Fat: 15.3;Sodium: 566;Total Carbohydrate: 4.4;Cholesterol: 51

54. Slim's Bad Attitude Nacho Sauce

Serving: 20 | Prep: 15mins | Cook: 10mins | Ready in:
Ingredients
7 (15 ounce) jars nacho cheese dip
3 pounds ground beef
3 (1.25 ounce) packages dry Mexican or taco seasoning
1 yellow onion, diced
1 teaspoon chili powder
4 (10 ounce) cans diced tomatoes with green chilies, drained
water (optional)
Direction
Put the cheese sauce into a large slow cooker. Put a cover on and set it to High.
Arrange a large skillet on medium heat. Cook the ground beef until it is browned completely; add in the taco seasoning and stir. Retain the fat in the skillet, place the beef into the slow cooker with a slotted spoon and stir it into the cheese.
Place the skillet back on medium heat. In the skillet, blend chili powder and onion; cook the blend until the onion gets soft. Stir in green chiles with tomatoes. Put into the cheese mixture and stir thoroughly. Stir in half a cup of water if the sauce becomes too thick.
Nutrition Information
Calories: 478 calories;;Total Fat: 34.8;Sodium: 1797;Total Carbohydrate: 23;Cholesterol: 70;Protein: 14.2

55. Slow Cooker BBQ Meatballs And Polish Sausage

Serving: 16 | Prep: 20mins | Cook: 1hours10mins | Ready in:
Ingredients
1 (16 ounce) package kielbasa sausage
1 (16 ounce) jar salsa
1 (10 ounce) jar grape jelly
1 cup water
1 tablespoon lemon juice
2 eggs
1 small onion, chopped
2 pounds ground beef
1 teaspoon salt
1 teaspoon ground black pepper
1/2 cup cornflakes cereal, crushed
Direction
Bring lightly salted water in a large pot to a rolling boil over high heat. Mix in kielbasa and bring back to a boil. Cook for 8 to 10 minutes or until heated through; drain kielbasa; cut into bite-sized portion. Put cut kielbasa into a slow cooker; mix in lemon juice, water, grape jelly, and salsa. In the meantime, whisk eggs in a mixing bowl; whisk in crushed cornflakes, pepper, salt, ground beef, and onion. Combine everything using your hands until well distributed. Shape mixture into large walnut-sized balls; put into the slow cooker.
Cook meatballs on high setting in the slow cooker until no longer pink in the center, about 60 minutes.
Nutrition Information
Calories: 330 calories;;Total Fat: 23.5;Sodium: 624;Total Carbohydrate: 15.5;Cholesterol: 90;Protein: 14.2

56. Slow Cooker Bar B Q Party Mix

Serving: 16 | Prep: 10mins | Cook: 1hours5mins | Ready in:
Ingredients
2 cups crispy corn cereal squares (such as Corn Chex®)
2 cups crispy wheat cereal squares (such as Wheat Chex®)
2 cups crispy rice cereal squares (such as Rice Chex®)
1 cup cheese-flavored crackers (such as Cheez-It®)
1 cup mini pretzels
1/4 cup melted butter
2 tablespoons barbeque sauce
2 tablespoons Worcestershire sauce
1 teaspoon onion powder
1 teaspoon garlic powder
1/2 teaspoon hickory bacon-flavored salt
Direction
In a gallon-sized resealable bag, combine together pretzels, cheese-flavored crackers, rice cereal, wheat cereal and corn cereal, then seal bag and toss together to mix.
In a bowl, stir together salt, garlic powder, onion powder, Worcestershire sauce, barbecue sauce and butter. Pour over cereal mixture with a half of the butter mixture, then seal bag and shake until mixed entirely. Put into cereal mixture with leftover liquid mixture, seal bag to shake until cereal mixture is coated thoroughly. Put into the slow cooker with coated cereal mixture.
Cook on low setting about a half hour, while stirring after each 15 minutes. Increase heat to high and cook about 15 minutes. Stir and cook without a cover for 20-25 minutes longer, or until the coating has cooked into cereal mixture. Spread onto a baking sheet with the party mixture to let it cool and dry.
Nutrition Information
Calories: 102 calories;;Sodium: 244;Total Carbohydrate: 14.3;Cholesterol: 8;Protein: 1.9;Total Fat: 4.7

57. Slow Cooker Buffalo Chicken Lettuce Wraps

Serving: 10 | Prep: 10mins | Cook: 6hours | Ready in:
Ingredients
2 pounds skinless, boneless chicken breasts
1 (12 ounce) bottle cayenne pepper sauce (such as Frank's® RedHot®)
1 (1 ounce) package ranch dressing mix
1 head Boston lettuce leaves
Direction
Into crock of slow cooker, place the chicken.
In a bowl, mix ranch dressing mix and cayenne pepper sauce together till smooth; add on top of chicken.
Allow to cook for 6 to 7 hours on Low.
Turn chicken onto a big bowl and shred chicken into strands with 2 forks.
Into a bowl, strain the liquid from slow cooker crock to serve alongside.
Into the lettuce leaves, scoop the chicken and roll lettuce around chicken.
Nutrition Information
Calories: 105 calories;Protein: 18;Total Fat: 2;Sodium: 1123;Total Carbohydrate: 2.4;Cholesterol: 47

58. Slow Cooker Cocktail Smokies

Serving: 10 | Prep: 5mins | Cook: 2hours | Ready in:
Ingredients
2 (16 ounce) packages miniature smoked sausage links
1 (8 ounce) jar grape jelly

1 (12 ounce) bottle barbeque sauce
Direction
Mix together the barbeque sauce and grape jelly in a slow cooker. Add in the miniature smoked sausage links and give it a stir. Set on High for roughly 2 to 3 hours until heated completely.
Nutrition Information
Calories: 377 calories;Protein: 11.1;Total Fat: 24.6;Sodium: 1278;Total Carbohydrate: 28.3;Cholesterol: 56

59. Slow Cooker Cocktail Wieners
Serving: 8 | Prep: 10mins | Cook: 2hours | Ready in:
Ingredients
1 (16 ounce) package weiners, cut into bite-size pieces
3/4 cup ketchup
3/4 cup brown sugar
2 teaspoons liquid smoke flavoring
1 teaspoon Worcestershire sauce
1/4 teaspoon garlic powder
Direction
Mix together garlic powder, Worcestershire sauce, liquid smoke, brown sugar, ketchup, and wieners into a slow cooker.
Cook on low setting for around 2-4 hours.
Nutrition Information
Calories: 269 calories;;Sodium: 900;Total Carbohydrate: 21.5;Cholesterol: 30;Protein: 6.7;Total Fat: 17.8

60. Slow Cooker Jalapeno Popper Taquitos
Serving: 4 | Prep: 15mins | Cook: 3hours15mins | Ready in:
Ingredients
8 skinless, boneless chicken thighs
1 (8 ounce) package cream cheese, softened
1 (4 ounce) can diced jalapeno peppers with juice
1/4 cup green enchilada sauce
1 pinch salt and ground black pepper to taste
16 (6 inch) flour tortillas
2 cups shredded pepperjack cheese
2 tablespoons vegetable oil
Direction
In a slow cooker, mix black pepper, green enchilada sauce, salt, jalapeno peppers with juice, cream cheese and chicken thighs together.
Allow to cook for 3 to 4 hours on High. Pull chicken apart using 2 forks and in the slow cooker, mix with sauce to incorporate.
Preheat the oven to 220 °C or 425 °F. With cooking spray, coat a baking sheet.
On a flat work area, lay tortillas out and scatter pepper jack cheese equally in the middle of every tortilla. Scatter approximately 2 tablespoons of chicken mixture on top of cheese on every tortilla. Securely roll every tortilla and arrange on prepped baking sheet, seam-side facing down. Brush vegetable oil on surface and sides of every rolled tortilla.
In the prepped oven, let bake for 10 to 15 minutes till tortillas begin to brown and cheese melts. Position oven rack approximately 6-inch away from heat source and preheat an oven's broiler. Let taquitos cook below the broiler for 2 to 3 minutes longer till crisped.
Nutrition Information
Calories: 1207 calories;;Total Fat: 67.6;Sodium: 2087;Total Carbohydrate: 71.7;Cholesterol: 326;Protein: 74.7

61. Slow Cooker Philly Cheesesteak Dip
Serving: 16 | Prep: 20mins | Cook: 58mins | Ready in:
Ingredients
1 pound cream cheese, softened and cut into 2-inch pieces
1 (8 ounce) package processed cheese (such as Velveeta®), cut into 1-inch pieces, or more to taste
3 tablespoons olive oil
1 large yellow onion, chopped
1 large green bell pepper, chopped (optional)
1 tablespoon Worcestershire sauce
1 pound thinly sliced rib-eye steak, cut into 1-inch pieces
salt and ground black pepper to taste
1 (15 ounce) jar pasteurized process cheese spread (such as Cheez Whiz®)
Direction
In a slow cooker, mix the processed cheese and cream cheese on low.
In a big pan, heat the olive oil on medium heat. Cook and stir the green bell pepper and onion for about 8 minutes, until it becomes soft. Put Worcestershire sauce and simmer. Stir the pepper, salt and rib-eye steak into the onion mixture, then cook and stir for about 5 minutes until the steak turns brown. Drain off the excess grease. Mix the process cheese spread into the steak mixture until it melts. Put the steak-cheese mixture in the slow cooker.
Cook for 45 minutes on low.
Nutrition Information
Calories: 285 calories;;Sodium: 726;Total Carbohydrate: 5.9;Cholesterol: 73;Protein: 11.2;Total Fat: 24.2

62. Slow Cooker Reuben Dip
Serving: 12 | Prep: 4mins | Cook: 45mins | Ready in:
Ingredients
1 (16 ounce) jar sauerkraut, drained
1 (8 ounce) package cream cheese, softened
2 cups shredded Swiss cheese
2 cups shredded cooked corned beef
1/4 cup thousand island dressing
Direction
Mix thousand island dressing, corned beef, Swiss cheese, cream cheese and sauerkraut in slow cooker. Cover; cook for 45 minutes on high if you're hungry/low if you're not till cheese melts and it's hot. Occasionally mix while cooking. Use crackers or cocktail rye to serve
Nutrition Information
Calories: 298 calories;Protein: 17.9;Total Fat: 22.9;Sodium: 636;Total Carbohydrate: 5.5;Cholesterol: 76

63. Spicy Hot Chicken Legs
Serving: 6 | Prep: 5mins | Cook: 3hours | Ready in:
Ingredients
12 chicken drumsticks
1 (5 ounce) bottle hot red pepper sauce
1/4 cup butter, cubed
1/2 teaspoon garlic powder
1/2 teaspoon onion powder
salt and pepper to taste
1 1/2 cups blue cheese salad dressing
Direction

In slow cooker, put drumsticks. Evenly sprinkle with butter pieces. Put hot sauce on chicken. Season with pepper, salt, onion powder and garlic powder; cover. Cook for 3 hours on high till tender. Serve chicken legs alongside with blue cheese dressing.
Nutrition Information
Calories: 685 calories;;Sodium: 1025;Total Carbohydrate: 5;Cholesterol: 159;Protein: 41.4;Total Fat: 55.6

64. Sweet 'N Sour Meatballs
Serving: 4 | Prep: 20mins | Cook: 30mins | Ready in:
Ingredients
4 (12 ounce) bottles chili sauce
1 (18 ounce) jar grape jelly
1 pound ground beef
1/2 cup plain bread crumbs
1 small onion, chopped
2 eggs
1/4 teaspoon salt
1/4 teaspoon ground black pepper
Direction
Combine grape jelly and chili sauce on medium heat in a slow cooker.
Turn oven to 350°F (175°C) to preheat.
In a bowl, combine ground beef with black pepper, salt, eggs, onion, and breadcrumbs; shape mixture into golf ball-sized balls. Place meatballs on an ungreased baking sheet.
Bake for about 10 minutes in the preheated oven until thoroughly cooked and browned.
Transfer cooked meatballs to the slow cooker and let simmer for 20 minutes.
Nutrition Information
Calories: 669 calories;Protein: 24;Total Fat: 19.7;Sodium: 756;Total Carbohydrate: 101.5;Cholesterol: 161

65. Sweet And Sour Meatballs
Serving: 12 | Prep: 20mins | Cook: 1hours30mins | Ready in:
Ingredients
1 (12 fluid ounce) can or bottle chile sauce
2 teaspoons lemon juice
9 ounces grape jelly
1 pound lean ground beef
1 egg, beaten
1 large onion, grated
salt to taste
Direction
Mix grape jelly, lemon juice, and chili sauce. Pour into the slow cooker and simmer on low heat until warm. Mix salt, onion, egg, and ground beef. Stir well and roll into 1 inch balls. Put into the sauce and simmer for 1 1/2 hours.
Nutrition Information
Calories: 152 calories;;Total Carbohydrate: 17.4;Cholesterol: 38;Protein: 8.3;Total Fat: 5.6;Sodium: 22

66. Sweet And Sour Meatballs I
Serving: 7 | Prep: 10mins | Cook: 5hours | Ready in:
Ingredients
2 pounds ground beef
1 egg
1 onion, chopped
1 pinch salt
1 (12 fluid ounce) can or bottle chili sauce
2 teaspoons lemon juice

1 cup grape jelly
Direction
Place the salt, onion, egg, and beef in a large bowl. Combine them together, form into little balls. Blend the grape jelly, lemon juice, and chili sauce in a slow cooker. Add in the meatballs and stir, cook for 4-5 hours on high.
Nutrition Information
Calories: 562 calories;;Sodium: 99;Total Carbohydrate: 37.5;Cholesterol: 137;Protein: 24;Total Fat: 35.2

67. Taco Bean Dip
Serving: 12 | Prep: 5mins | Cook: 1hours | Ready in:
Ingredients
2 (11.5 ounce) cans condensed bean with bacon soup
1 (1 ounce) package taco seasoning mix
8 ounces sour cream
1/4 cup salsa
1/2 cup shredded Cheddar cheese
Direction
Mix salsa, sour cream, seasoning mix and soup in a slow cooker. Put cheese on top; heat on low for 1 hour till cheese melts.
Nutrition Information
Calories: 132 calories;;Sodium: 639;Total Carbohydrate: 12.5;Cholesterol: 15;Protein: 5.3;Total Fat: 6.7

68. Tangy Barbecued Wings
Serving: 15 | Prep: 15mins | Cook: 3hours50mins | Ready in:
Ingredients
5 pounds whole chicken wings, cut into 3 sections and tips discarded
2 1/2 cups hot and spicy ketchup
2/3 cup white vinegar
1/2 cup honey
2 tablespoons honey
1/2 cup molasses
1 teaspoon salt
1 teaspoon Worcestershire sauce
1/2 teaspoon onion powder
1/2 teaspoon chili powder
1/2 teaspoon liquid smoke, or more to taste
Direction
Set the oven to 190 degrees C or 375 degrees F. Grease 2 baking pans (15x10x1 inches).
Place the chicken onto the baking pans.
Bake them for 30 minutes, then drain and turn the wings over. Continue to bake until the center is no longer pink and the juices run clear, around 20-25 minutes. If you insert an instant-read thermometer near the bone, it should read 74 degrees C or 165 degrees F; drain.
In a big saucepan, combine liquid smoke, chili powder, onion powder, Worcestershire sauce, salt, molasses, 1/2 cup plus 2 tablespoons of honey, vinegar, and ketchup, then boil. Turn the heat down and simmer until the flavors blend and the sauce thickens, roughly 25-30 minutes.
Move 1/3 of the chicken into a slow cooker and top with about 1 cup of sauce. Repeat the layers with the leftover sauce and chicken.
Cook them on a low setting for around 3-4 hours, then stir before you serve.
Nutrition Information

Calories: 225 calories;;Total Fat: 7.7;Sodium: 641;Total Carbohydrate: 30;Cholesterol: 32;Protein: 10.9

69. Vegetarian Buffalo Chicken Dip

Serving: 16 | Prep: 10mins | Cook: 1hours | Ready in:
Ingredients
1 (8 ounce) package seasoned chicken-style vegetarian strips (such as Morningstar Farms® Chik'n Strips), diced
2 (8 ounce) packages reduced fat cream cheese, softened
1 (16 ounce) bottle reduced-fat ranch salad dressing
1 (12 fluid ounce) bottle hot buffalo wing sauce (such as Frank's® REDHOT Buffalo Wing Sauce)
1 cup Colby-Monterey Jack cheese blend
Direction
In a slow cooker, place buffalo wing sauce, ranch dressing, cream cheese and diced vegetarian chicken strips. Cook and stir occasionally on Low for 1-2 hours till the dip is hot and cheese is melted. Add shredded cheese, stir to serve.
Nutrition Information
Calories: 186 calories;;Total Fat: 11.4;Sodium: 1024;Total Carbohydrate: 11.7;Cholesterol: 24;Protein: 8.9

70. Warm Chili Cheese Dip

Serving: 20 | Prep: 10mins | Cook: 30mins | Ready in:
Ingredients
1 (2 pound) loaf processed cheese (such as Velveeta®), cubed
2 (15 ounce) cans chili without beans (such as Hormel®)
2 (8 ounce) packages cream cheese, cubed
1 (16 ounce) jar picante sauce (such as Pace®)
Direction
Put picante sauce, cream cheese, chili and processed cheese in a slow cooker, set to Low, then allow processed cheese to melt for 30 minutes. Mix until blended thoroughly; serve warm.
Nutrition Information
Calories: 269 calories;;Total Fat: 20.5;Sodium: 958;Total Carbohydrate: 8.5;Cholesterol: 67;Protein: 13.4

71. Warm Mexican Corn Dip

Serving: 28 | Prep: 5mins | Cook: 1hours | Ready in:
Ingredients
2 (8 ounce) packages cream cheese, softened
1 cup butter, softened
2 (15.25 ounce) cans white corn, drained
2 (14 ounce) cans diced tomatoes with green chile peppers
Direction
In a slow cooker, mix together green chile peppers, tomatoes, corn, butter and cream cheese. Set the slow cooker to low and cook for an hour, until the butter as well as cream cheese are melted thoroughly.
Nutrition Information
Calories: 138 calories;;Total Carbohydrate: 6.2;Cholesterol: 35;Protein: 2.1;Total Fat: 12.3;Sodium: 273

Chapter 2: Side Dish Slow Cooker Recipes

72. Alfredo Green Bean Casserole
Serving: 12 | Prep: 10mins | Cook: 3hours | Ready in:
Ingredients
1 (28 ounce) package frozen cut green beans
1 (28 ounce) package French-fried onions
1 (10 ounce) container Alfredo sauce
1 (8 ounce) can sliced water chestnuts, drained
1 (2.25 ounce) can sliced ripe olives, drained
1/2 cup roasted red bell peppers, cut into strips
1 tablespoon dried parsley (optional)
1/4 teaspoon salt
ground black pepper (optional)
Direction
In a 4-6-qt. slow cooker, mix together black pepper, salt, parsley, roasted red bell peppers, olives, water chestnuts, Alfredo sauce, onions, and green beans. Put the lid on and cook on High for 3-4 hours until the flavors blend.
Nutrition Information
Calories: 528 calories;Protein: 2.3;Total Fat: 40.1;Sodium: 914;Total Carbohydrate: 36.6;Cholesterol: 9

73. Baked Beans With Beef
Serving: 20 | Prep: 15mins | Cook: 4hours15mins | Ready in:
Ingredients
1 pound ground beef
1 large onion, finely chopped
1 pound peppered bacon
7 (28 ounce) cans baked beans (such as Bush's® Original)
1 (15 ounce) can black beans, drained
1 (15 ounce) can light red kidney beans, drained
1 (15 ounce) can dark red kidney beans, drained
1 (15 ounce) can great northern beans, drained
1/2 cup brown sugar
1/4 cup prepared yellow mustard
1/4 cup soy sauce
Direction
Heat your large skillet over medium-high heat. Stir in onion and ground beef, and then let it cook for 5-7 minutes until the beef is crumbly and all browned. Drain and remove the grease. Leave it for a while. Brown the bacon in a large skillet over medium-high heat for 10 minutes. Flip the bacon to brown all of its sides by turning occasionally. Use paper towels to drain bacon slices. Grind them into small pieces. Mix the bacon and the beef-onion mixture together in a slow cooker. Stir in mustard, soy sauce, sugar, and beans. Allow it to cook on Medium setting for 4 hours until the flavors are well-blended.
Nutrition Information
Calories: 500 calories;Protein: 26.8;Total Fat: 10.3;Sodium: 1514;Total Carbohydrate: 79.9;Cholesterol: 42

74. Bandito Beans
Serving: 24 | Prep: 15mins | Cook: 5hours | Ready in:
Ingredients
1 pound mild pork sausage
1 (15 ounce) can wax beans, drained
1 (15 ounce) can cut green beans, drained
1 (15 ounce) can lima beans, drained
1 (15 ounce) can black beans, drained
1/2 (28 ounce) can barbeque baked beans, with liquid
1 (15 ounce) can chili beans, with liquid
1 (6 ounce) can tomato paste
1 cup packed light brown sugar
1/4 cup barbeque sauce
1 small green bell pepper, diced
1 small yellow onion, diced
1 teaspoon fennel seed
Direction
Cook sausage till evenly brown in skillet on medium heat; drain grease. Put sausage in slow cooker. Mix black beans, lima beans, green beans and wax beans into slow cooker with sausage; mix chili beans with liquid and baked beans with liquid in. Mix fennel seed, onion, green bell pepper, barbeque sauce, brown sugar and tomato paste in.
Cover slow cooker; cook for a minimum of 5 hours on Low.
Nutrition Information
Calories: 169 calories;;Total Fat: 4.4;Sodium: 591;Total Carbohydrate: 26.5;Cholesterol: 11;Protein: 7.1

75. Becca's Barbequed Beans
Serving: 10 | Prep: 20mins | Cook: 40mins | Ready in:
Ingredients
1 1/2 pounds lean ground beef
1/4 cup chopped onion
1/4 teaspoon ground black pepper
2/3 cup barbeque sauce
1/4 cup diced dill pickles
1 teaspoon Worcestershire sauce
2 (15 ounce) cans pork and beans
Direction
Set oven to 350°F (175°C) to preheat.
Cook onion and ground beef together with pepper in a saucepan or large skillet until browned; drain. Combine beans, pork, Worcestershire sauce, pickles, barbeque sauce, and beef mixture in a large casserole dish. Cover with foil or lid; bake for 40 to 45 minutes in the preheated oven until bubbly and thoroughly heated. Another way, simmer on high setting in a slow cooker until heated through, 1 hour.
Nutrition Information
Calories: 247 calories;;Total Fat: 9.7;Sodium: 627;Total Carbohydrate: 23.5;Cholesterol: 50;Protein: 17.4

76. Betty's 3 Bean Hot Dish (a La Minnesota)
Serving: 8 | Prep: 10mins | Cook: 1hours20mins | Ready in:
Ingredients
1/4 pound bacon
1 pound ground beef
1 onion, diced
1 (15 ounce) can pork and beans, drained
1 (15 ounce) can kidney beans, drained
1 (15 ounce) can butter beans, drained
1/2 cup ketchup
1/2 cup brown sugar
2 tablespoons white vinegar
1 tablespoon yellow mustard
Direction
In a big skillet, cook bacon over medium high heat for about 10 minutes with occasional turning until completely brown. Put bacon slices on a paper towels.

When cool enough, crumble. Use paper towel to wipe out the skillet.
In the heated skillet, cook and stir ground beef for 5 to 7 minutes; until it turns brown and crumbly. Drain and remove grease. Add and cook onion for about 5 minutes until it becomes transparent.
In a slow cooker, mix in vinegar, brown sugar, mustard, cooked beef, butter beans, pork and beans, kidney beans, cooked bacon and ketchup. Stir the mixture until completely combine. Let it cook completely over high heat for 60 minutes until heated through.

Nutrition Information
Calories: 360 calories;;Total Fat: 11.9;Sodium: 810;Total Carbohydrate: 44.7;Cholesterol: 44;Protein: 19.7.

77. Bourbon Barbecue Slow Cooker Beans

Serving: 14 | Prep: 30mins | Cook: 10hours | Ready in:

Ingredients
1 (16 ounce) package dry 15 bean mix for soup
1 bay leaf
1 pound bacon
1 pound ground beef
1 pound kielbasa sausage, sliced
1 onion, chopped
1 green bell pepper, chopped
1 red bell pepper, chopped
2 (10.5 ounce) cans chicken broth
1 (16 ounce) bottle hickory flavored barbeque sauce (such as Open Pit®)
1 1/2 teaspoons Worcestershire sauce
1/3 cup honey
1/4 cup real maple syrup
2/3 cup bourbon whiskey
3 tablespoons coarse-grain mustard

Direction
Wash beans, and put in a very large pot. Pour water over beans to cover, add bay leaf, and bring to boiling. Simmer for 45 to 60 minutes until all liquid is absorbed. Discard bay leaf.
Cook chopped bacon over medium-high heat in a large, deep skillet for about 5 minutes, stirring well, until browned on all sides. Transfer bacon to a plate lined with paper towel to drain. Reheat the skillet; add ground beef, and cook for about 5 minutes until browned and thoroughly cooked. Drain drippings.
Combine mustard, bourbon, maple syrup, honey, Worcestershire sauce, barbeque sauce, chicken broth, red pepper, green pepper, onion, sliced kielbasa, ground beef, bacon, and beans in the crock of a slow cooker; stir well. Cook mixture for 8 to 10 minutes on low setting until beans are softened.

Nutrition Information
Calories: 466 calories;;Total Carbohydrate: 44.2;Cholesterol: 54;Protein: 21.1;Total Fat: 19.1;Sodium: 1237

78. Cajun Red Beans

Serving: 8 | Prep: 20mins | Cook: 7hours10mins | Ready in:

Ingredients
1 pound dried pinto beans
3 tablespoons bacon grease
1/4 cup chopped salt pork
1 1/2 cups chopped yellow onion
3/4 cup chopped celery
3/4 cup chopped green bell pepper
1/2 teaspoon freshly ground black pepper
1 pinch chipotle chile powder
1/2 pound smoked sausage, split in half and cut into 1-inch pieces
3 bay leaves
2 tablespoons chopped fresh parsley
2 teaspoons chopped fresh thyme
3 tablespoons chopped garlic
water as needed

Direction
In a large container, put pinto beans; pour in several inches of cool water to cover. Soak beans for 10 mins; then drain and rinse.
In a large pot, heat bacon grease over medium high heat. Cook while stirring salt pork for 1 min in hot grease. Put in chipotle, black pepper, bell pepper, celery, and onion; cook while stirring for 4 mins, until vegetables are soft.
Mix thyme, parsley, bay leaves, and smoked sausage into salt pork mixture; cook while stirring for 4 mins, until sausage is browned. Put in garlic, cook for 1 minute more, until fragrant.
Mix beans in sausage mixture, cover the beans with enough water. Boil, remove from heat, then remove beans mixture to slow cooker.
Cook for 1 hour on High. Lower to low heat and continue to cook for about 6 hours more, until tender; if needed, add water.
Using the back of a heavy spoon, mash 1/4 beans against sides of slow cooker crock. Continue to cook for 15-20 mins more on Low, until creamy and tender. Discard bay leaves.

Nutrition Information
Calories: 430 calories;;Sodium: 555;Total Carbohydrate: 41.2;Cholesterol: 30;Protein: 19.6;Total Fat: 20.7

79. Cola Beans

Serving: 24 | Prep: 15mins | Cook: 10hours | Ready in:

Ingredients
4 (28 ounce) cans baked beans, drained
1/2 pound bacon
1 cup brown sugar
1 (12 fluid ounce) can cola soft drink (such as Coke®)

Direction
Layer alternately the brown sugar, bacon, and baked beans in a slow cooker. Pour in some cola to fill each layer until all has run out.
Allow to cook, covered, on High for 4-6 hours or on Low for 8-10 hours (Check the oven instructions in Cook's Note).
Set an oven to 175°C (350°F) and start preheating.

Nutrition Information
Calories: 207 calories;;Total Carbohydrate: 38.3;Cholesterol: 6;Protein: 7.3;Total Fat: 4.7;Sodium: 530

80. Deborah's Slow Cooker Spicy Black Eyed Peas

Serving: 12 | Prep: 10mins | Cook: 4hours | Ready in:

Ingredients
4 (14 ounce) cans black-eyed peas, rinsed and drained
1/4 cup butter
1 cup chopped onion
1 cup diced cooked ham
1 1/2 cups chopped green bell pepper
1 (14.5 ounce) can diced tomatoes with green chile peppers, drained
2 cloves garlic, minced

1 tablespoon seasoned salt
Direction
In a slow cooker, combine seasoned salt, garlic, diced tomatoes with green chile peppers, bell pepper, ham, onion, butter, and black-eyed peas.
Cook on Low mode for 4 hours.
Nutrition Information
Calories: 179 calories;;Sodium: 933;Total Carbohydrate: 21.8;Cholesterol: 16;Protein: 9;Total Fat: 6.7

81. Deborah's Slow Cooker Collard Greens

Serving: 8 | Prep: 20mins | Cook: 4hours | Ready in:
Ingredients
2 (10.75 ounce) cans beef stock
1 (10 ounce) can diced tomatoes with green chiles
1 cup chopped onion
1 cup diced fully cooked ham
2 teaspoons red wine vinegar
1 teaspoon white sugar
1 teaspoon garlic powder
1 teaspoon seasoned salt
1/2 teaspoon red pepper flakes
1 bay leaf
2 bunches collard greens, thinly sliced
2 bunches mustard greens, thinly sliced
2 bunches turnip greens, thinly sliced
Direction
In a slow cooker, put the diced tomatoes, beef stock with bay leaf, red pepper flakes, seasoned salt, garlic powder, sugar, vinegar, ham, onion and green chiles.
Put the collard greens, the mustard greens, and turnip greens in order listed into slow cooker.
Cook for 4-6 hours on Low or until greens are very tender.
Nutrition Information
Calories: 131 calories;;Total Carbohydrate: 16.7;Cholesterol: 9;Protein: 9.6;Total Fat: 4.2;Sodium: 560

82. Easy Slow Cooker Cheesy Potatoes

Serving: 10 | Prep: 20mins | Cook: 2hours | Ready in:
Ingredients
1 (2 pound) package frozen Southern-style hash brown potatoes, thawed
4 cups shredded Cheddar cheese
2 (10.75 ounce) cans condensed cream of chicken soup
1 (8 ounce) container sour cream
1 cup chopped yellow onion (optional)
1 cup milk
1 pinch seasoned salt, or to taste
1 teaspoon minced garlic
1 cup crushed cheese-flavored crackers (such as Cheez-It®), divided
Direction
In a slow cooker, combine 1/2 cup cheese-flavored crackers, garlic, seasoned salt, milk, onion, sour cream, cream of chicken soup, Cheddar cheese, and hash brown potatoes.
Cook for about 2 hours on low, stirring sometimes, until thoroughly cooked. Mix and sprinkle with the remaining 1/2 cup cheese-flavored cracker.
Nutrition Information
Calories: 413 calories;;Cholesterol: 65;Protein: 17;Total Fat: 31.1;Sodium: 826;Total Carbohydrate: 28.8

83. Easy Slow Cooker Spanish Rice

Serving: 8 | Prep: 10mins | Cook: 3hours5mins | Ready in:
Ingredients
2 pounds ground beef
1 (28 ounce) can whole peeled tomatoes
2 (8 ounce) cans tomato sauce
2 green bell peppers, chopped
1 cup water
2 yellow onions, chopped
1 cup converted raw rice
2 tablespoons Worcestershire sauce
2 tablespoons chili powder
hot sauce, or to taste (optional)
1 cup shredded Cheddar cheese, or to taste
Direction
Turn a large skillet to medium-high heat on the stove. Sauté beef in the heated skillet for 5 to 7 minutes until lightly browned and crumbly. Drain beef and discard drippings.
Pour beef into a slow cooker. Add hot sauce, chili powder, Worcestershire sauce, rice, onions, water, green bell peppers, tomato sauce, and tomatoes.
Cook for 3 hours on high setting until rice is tender.
Ladle into bowls to serve, sprinkle with Cheddar cheese on top.
Nutrition Information
Calories: 403 calories;;Sodium: 660;Total Carbohydrate: 31.5;Cholesterol: 86;Protein: 26.6;Total Fat: 19.1

84. Easy Slow Cooker Squash

Serving: 6 | Prep: 10mins | Cook: 1hours10mins | Ready in:
Ingredients
4 pounds yellow summer squash, sliced
1 small onion, chopped
1/4 cup butter, cubed
1/4 pound processed cheese food (such as Velveeta®), cubed
Direction
Cover onion and squash with enough water in a pot. Boil; cover. Simmer veggies for 10 minutes till tender; don't mix. Drain onion and squash in colander in sink. Layer cheese food cubes, butter cubes, cooked onions and squash gently in slow cooker. Put cooker on low; cook for 1 hour till cheese and butter makes creamy sauce and squash is very tender. Don't mix.
Nutrition Information
Calories: 183 calories;Protein: 7.4;Total Fat: 13;Sodium: 300;Total Carbohydrate: 12.7;Cholesterol: 35

85. Garlic Mashed Potatoes In The Slow Cooker

Serving: 8 | Prep: 30mins | Cook: 3hours20mins | Ready in:
Ingredients
5 pounds red potatoes, peeled and cut into chunks
1 (8 ounce) package cream cheese
1 (8 ounce) container sour cream
1 1/2 cups chicken broth
2 teaspoons garlic powder
salt to taste
1/2 cup butter, melted
Direction
In a big pot with potatoes, pour salted water to cover potatoes; heat to a boil. Decrease to medium-low heat and allow to simmer for 20 minutes until tender. Drain.

Remove potatoes to a big bowl, mash with sour cream and cream cheese until entirely blended. Gradually mash in the chicken broth then blend in salt and garlic powder.
With an electric mixer, beat potatoes for 2 minutes on high speed until whipped. Remove to a slow cooker, cook 3 hours on Low. Mix melted butter into potatoes just prior to serving.

Nutrition Information
Calories: 464 calories;;Sodium: 396;Total Carbohydrate: 47.8;Cholesterol: 75;Protein: 8.8;Total Fat: 27.7

86. Grandpa's Classic Coney Sauce

Serving: 12 | Prep: 10mins | Cook: 2hours | Ready in:

Ingredients
2 pounds ground beef
1/2 cup chopped onion
1 1/2 cups ketchup
1/4 cup white sugar
1/4 cup white vinegar
1/4 cup prepared yellow mustard
1/2 teaspoon celery seed
3/4 teaspoon Worcestershire sauce
1/2 teaspoon ground black pepper
3/4 teaspoon salt

Direction
In a large skillet, put onion and ground beef over medium-high heat. Cook while stirring to crumble, until the beef is browned. Then drain. Put onion and beef into a slow cooker. Stir in mustard, vinegar, sugar and ketchup. Add salt, pepper, Worcestershire sauce and celery seed to season. Simmer, covered, for a few hours on Low setting before enjoying.

Nutrition Information
Calories: 186 calories;;Total Carbohydrate: 12.8;Cholesterol: 46;Protein: 13.5;Total Fat: 9.2;Sodium: 586

87. Hash Brown Casserole For The Slow Cooker

Serving: 16 | Prep: 15mins | Cook: 4hours | Ready in:

Ingredients
2 cups sour cream
1 (10.75 ounce) can condensed cream of mushroom soup, undiluted
2 cups shredded processed cheese
1/2 cup chopped onion
1/4 teaspoon salt
1/4 teaspoon pepper
1 (32 ounce) package frozen hash brown potatoes, thawed

Direction
Combine pepper, salt, onion, cheese, cream of mushroom soup, and sour cream in a large bowl. Slowly stir in hash browns until well coated. Grease the inside of a slow cooker with butter or cooking spray. Ladle the hash brown mixture into the slow cooker. Cook, covered for 1 hour and 30 minutes on high setting; turn heat to low, and cook for 2 hours and 30 minutes longer.

Nutrition Information
Calories: 198 calories;;Total Fat: 16.2;Sodium: 472;Total Carbohydrate: 14.8;Cholesterol: 30;Protein: 6.5

88. Hobo Beans

Serving: 8 | Prep: 10mins | Cook: 3hours10mins | Ready in:

Ingredients
1 pound hamburger
1/2 pound bacon
1 (28 ounce) can baked beans with pork
1 (15 ounce) can kidney beans, rinsed and drained
1 (15 ounce) can lima beans, rinsed and drained
2 onions, chopped
1 cup ketchup
1 cup brown sugar
1 teaspoon prepared mustard

Direction
Warm your large skillet over medium-high heat. Stir in bacon and hamburger together in a hot skillet, and then let it cook for 7-10 minutes until the hamburger is crumbly and browned.
In the crock of your slow cooker, combine the cooked hamburger and bacon together with lima beans, ketchup, baked beans with pork, brown sugar, onions, mustard, and kidney beans.
Set the cooker into Low setting and cook for at least 3 hours until thickened and hot.

Nutrition Information
Calories: 471 calories;;Total Fat: 12.6;Sodium: 1217;Total Carbohydrate: 67.7;Cholesterol: 53;Protein: 24.8

89. Hot As Hell Hickory Beans

Serving: 8 | Prep: 10mins | Cook: 8hours | Ready in:

Ingredients
1 pound dried pinto beans
4 cups water
1 (7 ounce) can sliced jalapeno peppers, drained
1 (14.5 ounce) can diced tomatoes
1 1/2 teaspoons salt
1/2 teaspoon ground black pepper
1/4 teaspoon onion powder
1/4 teaspoon garlic powder
1/4 teaspoon liquid smoke flavoring
1/4 cup barbeque sauce

Direction
In a big container, put pinto beans and fill with a few inches of cool water. Let sit overnight to soak.
Strain and rinse the next day, and then put the beans in a slow cooker together with barbeque sauce, liquid smoke, garlic powder, onion powder, pepper, salt, tomatoes, jalapenos, and 4 cups of water; mix thoroughly.
Cook in the slow cooker for 4 hours on High. Mix the beans again, and set the slow cooker to Low, and keep cooking for another 3 hours until the beans are soft and the sauce thickens.

Nutrition Information
Calories: 218 calories;;Sodium: 1018;Total Carbohydrate: 40.1;Cholesterol: 0;Protein: 12.4;Total Fat: 1.2

90. Hungarian Noodle Side Dish

Serving: 10 | Prep: | Cook: | Ready in:

Ingredients
1 (16 ounce) package wide egg noodles
3 cubes chicken bouillon
1/4 cup water
1 (10.75 ounce) can condensed cream of mushroom soup
1/2 cup chopped onion
2 tablespoons Worcestershire sauce
1 tablespoon poppy seeds
1/4 teaspoon garlic powder
1/4 teaspoon hot pepper sauce

2 cups cottage cheese
2 cups sour cream
1/4 cup grated Parmesan cheese
1 pinch paprika
Direction
Boil a big pot of salted water, cook in egg noodles; drain.
Dissolve chicken bouillon cube in a big bowl of boiling water. Stir in hot pepper sauce, cream of mushroom soup, garlic powder, chopped onion, poppy seeds, and Worcestershire sauce. Fold in cooked egg noodles, sour cream, and cheese.
Place in a lightly oiled slow cooker; add paprika and parmesan cheese on top.
Cook for 3-4 hours, covered, on high. Serve right away.
Nutrition Information
Calories: 365 calories;;Total Carbohydrate: 39.3;Cholesterol: 67;Protein: 15.2;Total Fat: 16.5;Sodium: 826

91. Maple And Ginger Baked Beans
Serving: 10 | Prep: 1hours | Cook: 10hours | Ready in:
Ingredients
1 1/2 pounds dry great Northern beans
1 large onion, cut into wedges
4 ounces salt pork, diced
3/4 cup real maple syrup
1/4 cup molasses
1/4 cup brown sugar
1 teaspoon ground ginger
1 teaspoon mustard powder
1/2 teaspoon salt
1/4 teaspoon ground black pepper
2 cups boiling water
Direction
Steep dried beans overnight in a large pot of water; drain. Pour clean water into the pot, and bring to a boil. Simmer for about 1 hour until beans are really soft.
Meanwhile, combine water, pepper, salt, mustard powder, ginger, brown sugar, molasses, and maple syrup. Put to one side.
Arrange onion wedges in the bottom of a 3-qt. slow cooker or a larger one. Add salt pork cubes over the onion. Drain beans and put into the cooker. Drizzle maple syrup mixture over the beans. Add little more hot water (if needed) just enough to cover the beans.
Cook, covered for 5 to 6 hours on high or 10 to 12 hours on low. Occasionally check if the mixture needs more water if you cook the beans on high setting. If the mixture looks too watery, uncover the cooker to allow liquid to vaporize for the last 30 minutes.
Nutrition Information
Calories: 384 calories;;Cholesterol: 10;Protein: 13.9;Total Fat: 10;Sodium: 290;Total Carbohydrate: 62

92. Minnesota Real Wild Rice Stuffing
Serving: 20 | Prep: 30mins | Cook: 1hours10mins | Ready in:
Ingredients
8 cups chicken broth
4 cups wild rice
3 cups cubed, stale cranberry-walnut bread
1 cup chicken broth
1 1/2 cups finely chopped celery
1 (8 ounce) can sliced water chestnuts, drained
3/4 cup chopped pecans
3/4 cup pine nuts
1 onion, diced
1 Granny Smith apple, diced
1/2 cup finely chopped dried apricots
4 cloves garlic, pressed
Direction
In a saucepan, heat wild rice and eight cups of chicken broth to a boil. Decrease the heat and let to simmer for half an hour until the rice becomes partially tender.
In a slow cooker, combine the partially-cooked wild rice together with garlic, water chestnuts, chicken broth, cranberry-walnut bread, pecans, one cup of chicken broth, onion, celery, pine nuts, apple, and apricots.
Cook for at least 40 minutes on Low heat until the wild rice has split and softened.
Nutrition Information
Calories: 246 calories;;Sodium: 515;Total Carbohydrate: 38.5;Cholesterol: 8;Protein: 7.9;Total Fat: 7.7

93. Mother Earth's Baked Beans
Serving: 16 | Prep: 15mins | Cook: 7hours20mins | Ready in:
Ingredients
1 pound thick-cut bacon
1 pound ground beef
1 large onion, chopped
1 1/3 cups brown sugar
1/2 cup barbeque sauce (such as Sweet Baby Ray's® Honey)
1/2 cup ketchup
2 tablespoons prepared mustard
1 tablespoon molasses
1 teaspoon liquid smoke flavoring
1 teaspoon ground black pepper
1 teaspoon chili powder
1 (28 ounce) can baked beans (such as Bush's Original®)
2 (16 ounce) cans kidney beans, drained and rinsed
2 (16 ounce) cans Great Northern beans, drained and rinsed
2 (16 ounce) cans pinto beans, drained and rinsed
Direction
In a big skillet, cook bacon over medium-high heat for about 10 minutes until evenly brown, turning it occasionally. On the paper towels place the bacon slices to drain; in the skillet, spare about 2 tablespoons bacon drippings. In a slow cooker, transfer crumbled bacon.
In a skillet, cook and stir onion and ground beef in bacon drippings over medium heat for 5 to 10 minutes until beef crumbles and becomes brown. In a slow cooker, transfer ground beef mixture.
In a bowl, combine chili powder, mustard, barbeque sauce, ketchup, black pepper, brown sugar, liquid smoke flavoring, and molasses.. Mix well and pour over ground beef bacon mixture. Combine pinto beans, kidney beans, baked beans and Great Northern beans then stir well.
Let it cook in low for 6 hours then place in the refrigerator for 8 hours overnight. Heat again in a slow cooker until hot for at least 60 minutes.
Nutrition Information
Calories: 394 calories;;Total Fat: 9.8;Sodium: 888;Total Carbohydrate: 58.4;Cholesterol: 28;Protein: 20.8

94. Pammy's Slow Cooker Beans

Serving: 10 | Prep: 15mins | Cook: 8hours | Ready in:
Ingredients
2 pounds dried pinto beans
8 cups water, or more if needed
1 small onion, chopped
2 teaspoons garlic powder
1/2 teaspoon onion powder
1 teaspoon ground black pepper
2 bay leaves
1 smoked turkey leg
1/3 cup olive oil
Direction
Rinse and pick on the beans, then put in a big bowl. With cold water, fill the bowl, and let the beans submerge for 6 to 8 hours.
Let drain and wash the beans, then put into slow cooker. Add in 8 cups water. Mix in bay leaves, black pepper, onion powder, garlic powder and onion. Into the cooker, put the turkey leg, place the cover, and allow to cook for 6 hours on Low setting. Mix in olive oil, and put additional water in case beans are starting to dry out; let cook for 2 hours longer till beans are really soft.
Nutrition Information
Calories: 415 calories;;Sodium: 728;Total Carbohydrate: 56;Cholesterol: 19;Protein: 25.3;Total Fat: 10.8

95. Rebellion Sauerkraut

Serving: 4 | Prep: 5mins | Cook: 3hours | Ready in:
Ingredients
1 (16 ounce) jar sauerkraut
1 cup hard apple cider
Direction
In small slow cooker, mix hard cider and sauerkraut. Cook for 3 hours till very tender on high.
Nutrition Information
Calories: 56 calories;Protein: 1;Total Fat: 0.2;Sodium: 755;Total Carbohydrate: 8.7;Cholesterol: 0

96. Risi Bisi

Serving: 6 | Prep: 30mins | Cook: 3hours40mins | Ready in:
Ingredients
1 1/2 cups converted long-grain white rice
1/3 cup chopped onion
2 cloves garlic, chopped
2 (14 ounce) cans chicken broth
1/3 cup water
3/4 teaspoon Italian seasoning
1/2 teaspoon dried basil
1/2 cup frozen green peas, thawed
1/4 cup grated Parmesan cheese
1/4 cup pine nuts, toasted
Direction
In a bowl of a slow cooker, mix together garlic, onion and rice. Add into a small saucepan with water and chicken broth, then bring mixture to a boil on high heat.
Stir into the rice mixture with basil, Italian seasoning and boiling liquid. Cook, covered, on low setting until liquid has been absorbed, about 2-3 hours. Stir in peas, then cook for an hour with a cover. Stir in cheese, then spoon mixture into a serving dish. Use pine nuts to sprinkle over top.
Nutrition Information
Calories: 271 calories;;Total Fat: 4.8;Sodium: 721;Total Carbohydrate: 46.8;Cholesterol: 6;Protein: 8.9

97. Sandy's Sweet Slow Cooker Sauerkraut

Serving: 8 | Prep: 20mins | Cook: 8hours | Ready in:
Ingredients
1 quart sauerkraut, drained and rinsed
1 1/2 cups water
3/4 cup diced carrot
3/4 cup brown sugar
2/3 cup chopped apple
1/2 sweet onion, minced
1 teaspoon caraway seeds
salt and ground black pepper to taste
1 pound fully cooked kielbasa, cut into 1-inch pieces (optional)
Direction
Add the black pepper, salt, caraway seeds, sweet onion, apple, brown sugar, carrot, water and sauerkraut into the slow cooker. Cook over Low heat for roughly 7 hours; put in the kielbasa. Cook for 60 minutes longer.
Nutrition Information
Calories: 264 calories;;Total Fat: 15.7;Sodium: 1302;Total Carbohydrate: 23.5;Cholesterol: 37;Protein: 8.3

98. Sauerkraut With Pigtails

Serving: 8 | Prep: 30mins | Cook: 2hours | Ready in:
Ingredients
4 pounds sauerkraut - rinsed and drained
5 (14 ounce) cans chicken broth
1 tablespoon caraway seeds
2 1/4 cups water
1 cup milk
1 tablespoon (1 stick) margarine, melted
2 1/4 cups instant mashed potato flakes
2 eggs
1 tablespoon baking powder
3 cups all-purpose flour, or as needed
salt and pepper to taste
Direction
In a slow cooker, combine caraway seeds, one can of chicken broth and sauerkraut. Cook, covered, on low for 120 minutes.
In a big pot, pour remaining cans of chicken broth, bring to a rapid boil.
In another saucepan, combine margarine, milk and water, bring to a boil. Mix in instant potato flakes until well incorporated, remove from heat and stir in baking powder, eggs and just enough amount of flour to form a firm but not sticky dough.
In a large pot, pour remaining cans of chicken broth, bring to a rapid boil. Shape dough into long thin dumplings (like pigtails) by rolling small pieces of potato dough. Add tails to boiling chicken broth, cook for 15 to 20 minutes.
Strain dumplings, add to the slow cooker with sauerkraut. Add salt and pepper to season.
Nutrition Information
Calories: 328 calories;Protein: 12;Total Fat: 4.7;Sodium: 2860;Total Carbohydrate: 60;Cholesterol: 55

99. Slow Cooker Barbecue Beans

Serving: 8 | Prep: 15mins | Cook: 6hours | Ready in:
Ingredients
1 pound lean ground beef

3/4 cup chopped raw bacon
1 small onion, finely chopped
2 (16 ounce) cans baked beans with pork
1 (15.25 ounce) can red kidney beans, with liquid
1 (15 ounce) can lima beans, partially drained
1 cup ketchup
1 tablespoon liquid smoke flavoring
1 tablespoon salt
1 tablespoon hot sauce
1/4 tablespoon garlic powder

Direction
In a big and deep skillet, cook beef over medium-high heat until completely brown. Discard then put aside. In a big and deep skillet, cook bacon over medium-high heat until completely brown, Discard then put aside. Mix onion, salt, ketchup, kidney beans, lima beans, baked beans, hot sauce, liquid smoke, garlic powder, bacon and ground beef. Let it cook in low fire for 4 to 6 hours,

Nutrition Information
Calories: 472 calories;;Total Fat: 18.4;Sodium: 2150;Total Carbohydrate: 53.2;Cholesterol: 60;Protein: 25

100. Slow Cooker Black Eyed Peas

Serving: 4 | Prep: 10mins | Cook: 15hours30mins | Ready in:

Ingredients
1 pound dried black-eyed peas
3 smoked ham hocks, or more to taste
6 cups water, plus more as needed
1 onion, chopped small
1 large clove garlic, crushed
1/4 teaspoon red pepper flakes
1/8 teaspoon white sugar
salt to taste

Direction
In a large container, put black-eyed peas with enough cool water to cover by several inches; soak for 8 hours to overnight.
Put ham hocks together with 6 cups of water into a stockpot; boil. Reduce heat to low, cover pot, and simmer for about 90 minutes until meat is falling off bone. Eliminate ham hocks and reserve for another use. Cool ham hock in refrigerator for 8 hours to overnight.
Drain and rinse thoroughly black-eyed peas; transfer to a slow cooker. Bury in the peas one of the cooked ham hocks; add red pepper flakes, sugar, garlic, and onion.
Skim congealed fat of ham stock from surface; discard. In slow cooker, pour stock. Add water enough to cover the peas by 1 and a half inches. Cook for 14 hours on Low setting. Add salt for seasoning.

Nutrition Information
Calories: 802 calories;;Total Fat: 33.1;Sodium: 114;Total Carbohydrate: 74.1;Cholesterol: 102;Protein: 53

101. Slow Cooker Cheesy Mushroom Potatoes

Serving: 10 | Prep: 20mins | Cook: 4hours10mins | Ready in:

Ingredients
2 tablespoons olive oil
1 teaspoon butter
1/2 pound white mushrooms, sliced
5 large Yukon Gold potatoes, quartered and sliced
4 cups shredded Cheddar cheese
1/2 cup milk
1/4 cup minced onion
2 tablespoons butter
1 tablespoon garlic salt
1/4 teaspoon ground black pepper

Direction
Heat 1 tsp. of the butter and olive oil on medium heat in the skillet. Cook and whisk the mushrooms in the butter for 10 minutes till becoming brown and soft.
In the slow cooker, whisk together black pepper, garlic salt, 2 tbsp. of the butter, onion, milk, Cheddar cheese, potatoes and cooked mushrooms.
Cook over High heat for 4 hours till the Cheddar cheese melts and the potatoes soften.

Nutrition Information
Calories: 386 calories;Protein: 16.2;Total Fat: 20.9;Sodium: 861;Total Carbohydrate: 34.7;Cholesterol: 56

102. Slow Cooker Chicken Dressing

Serving: 16 | Prep: 30mins | Cook: 4hours30mins | Ready in:

Ingredients
5 skinless, boneless chicken breast halves
1 (9x9 inch) pan cornbread, cooled and crumbled
8 slices day-old bread, torn into small pieces
4 eggs, beaten
1 onion, chopped
1 teaspoon salt
1 teaspoon ground black pepper
2 teaspoons dried sage
2 (14.5 ounce) cans chicken broth
2 (10.75 ounce) cans condensed cream of chicken soup
2 tablespoons margarine

Direction
Cover chicken in water in a pot; boil on medium heat. Boil till cooked through for 20 minutes. Cool; cut to pieces.
Mix chicken soup, chicken broth, sage, pepper, salt, onion, eggs, bread, cornbread and chicken in a slow cooker. Dot using margarine.
Cover; cook for 3-4 hours on low. Remove lid; fluff using fork. Allow to rest 15 minutes before serving.

Nutrition Information
Calories: 246 calories;;Cholesterol: 85;Protein: 13.7;Total Fat: 9.5;Sodium: 991;Total Carbohydrate: 25.8

103. Slow Cooker Chinese Carrots

Serving: 6 | Prep: 10mins | Cook: 8hours30mins | Ready in:

Ingredients
2 pounds baby carrots
1/2 cup orange juice concentrate
1/4 cup tamari sauce
2 cloves garlic, minced
1 teaspoon minced fresh ginger
1 teaspoon grated orange zest
1 tablespoon Asian (toasted) sesame oil
1 tablespoon honey

Direction
In a slow cooker, put honey, toasted sesame oil, orange zest, ginger, garlic, tamari sauce, orange juice concentrate, and baby carrots, and stir thoroughly. Turn the cooker on low, close the lid and cook for 8 hours. Set the cooker to high, and cook for 30 minutes.

104. Slow Cooker Collard Greens

Serving: 16 | Prep: 30mins | Cook: 8hours | Ready in:
Ingredients
4 bunches collard greens - rinsed, trimmed and chopped
1 pound ham shanks
4 pickled jalapeno peppers, chopped
1/2 teaspoon baking soda
1 teaspoon olive oil
ground black pepper to taste
garlic powder to taste
Direction
Pour water in a large pot until 1/2 full. Put the ham shanks in the water and as many of the greens as you can fit. Heat to a gentle boil.
When the greens start to wilt, remove the greens to the slow cooker. Alternate layers of greens with the jalapeno and ham shanks until the slow cooker is full. Mix in garlic powder, pepper, olive oil, and baking soda. Cover and heat to a boil on high. Lower the heat to low and cook for about 8 to 10 hours.
Nutrition Information
Calories: 99 calories;;Total Fat: 6.6;Sodium: 82;Total Carbohydrate: 4.2;Cholesterol: 19;Protein: 6.6

105. Slow Cooker Cranberry Apple Stuffing

Serving: 15 | Prep: 20mins | Cook: 3hours | Ready in:
Ingredients
1/4 cup butter
2 cups chopped celery
1 cup chopped onion
2 medium apples, cored and chopped
1 cup dried cranberries
2 cups Kitchen Basics® Original Chicken Stock
2 teaspoons McCormick® Sage, Rubbed
2 teaspoons McCormick® Parsley Flakes
1 teaspoon McCormick® Garlic Salt
1/2 teaspoon McCormick® Black Pepper, Coarse Grind
8 cups cubed day-old Italian or French bread
Direction
Put butter in a large skillet and melt it over medium heat. Add the onion and celery. Cook and stir the mixture for 5 minutes until softened. Mix in cranberries and apples.
Coat the inside of the slow cooker with nonstick cooking spray. Add the seasonings and the stock, stirring well until blended. Mix in vegetable mixture and bread cubes. Cover the slow cooker.
Cook it on a low setting for 3 hours until reached the desired texture.
Nutrition Information
Calories: 122 calories;;Sodium: 330;Total Carbohydrate: 20.2;Cholesterol: 8;Protein: 2.7;Total Fat: 3.8

106. Slow Cooker Creamed Corn

Serving: 12 | Prep: 10mins | Cook: 4hours | Ready in:
Ingredients
1 1/4 (16 ounce) packages frozen corn kernels
1 (8 ounce) package cream cheese
1/2 cup butter
1/2 cup milk
1 tablespoon white sugar
salt and pepper to taste
Direction
Mix together the sugar, milk, butter, cream cheese and corn in a slow cooker. Sprinkle pepper and salt to season.
Let it cook for 4-6 hours on Low or 2-4 hours on High.
Nutrition Information
Calories: 192 calories;;Total Carbohydrate: 13.7;Cholesterol: 42;Protein: 3.4;Total Fat: 15;Sodium: 114

107. Slow Cooker Creamed Spinach

Serving: 8 | Prep: 20mins | Cook: 5hours | Ready in:
Ingredients
2 (10 ounce) packages frozen chopped spinach, thawed, drained and squeezed dry
2 cups cottage cheese
1/2 cup butter, cubed
3 eggs, beaten
1 1/2 cups cubed process American cheese
1/4 cup all-purpose flour
1 teaspoon salt
Direction
Oil lightly a 4 1/2-quart slow cooker. Combine the salt, flour, eggs, American cheese, butter, cottage cheese and spinach in a big bowl till all are evenly distributed. Turn out onto the lightly oiled slow cooker.
Cook for an hour on high, then lower the heat to low, and keep cooking for 4 hours to 5 hours.
Nutrition Information
Calories: 320 calories;Protein: 18.3;Total Fat: 24.6;Sodium: 1070;Total Carbohydrate: 8.1;Cholesterol: 133

108. Slow Cooker Garlic Mashed Potatoes

Serving: 6 | Prep: 10mins | Cook: 4hours | Ready in:
Ingredients
2 pounds red potatoes, diced with peel
1/4 cup water
1/4 cup butter
1 1/4 teaspoons salt
1/2 teaspoon garlic powder
1/4 teaspoon ground black pepper
1/2 cup milk, or as needed
Direction
In a slow cooker, place butter, water, and potatoes. Season with pepper, garlic powder, and salt. Cook, covered for 4 hours on high setting or 7 hours on low setting.
Mash potatoes using an electric beater or masher, pouring in your preferred amount of milk until a creamy consistency is reached. Keep the mashed potatoes warm on low until serving.
Nutrition Information
Calories: 197 calories;;Total Fat: 8.2;Sodium: 553;Total Carbohydrate: 28.6;Cholesterol: 22;Protein: 3.3

109. Slow Cooker Green Bean Casserole

Serving: 8 | Prep: 10mins | Cook: 5hours | Ready in:
Ingredients
2 (16 ounce) packages frozen cut green beans
2 (10.75 ounce) cans cream of chicken soup
2/3 cup milk
1/2 cup grated Parmesan cheese
1/4 teaspoon salt
1/4 teaspoon ground black pepper

1 (6 ounce) can French-fried onions, divided
Direction
In a slow cooker, combine 1/2 can of French-fried onions, black pepper, salt, Parmesan cheese, milk, cream of chicken soup, and green beans.
Cook, with cover for 5 to 6 hours on Low setting. Put the remainder of French-fried onions on top of casserole and serve.
Nutrition Information
Calories: 272 calories;;Total Carbohydrate: 22.9;Cholesterol: 12;Protein: 5.9;Total Fat: 16.7;Sodium: 837

110. Slow Cooker Ham And Scalloped Potatoes

Serving: 6 | Prep: 15mins | Cook: 9hours | Ready in:
Ingredients
1 cup water
1/2 teaspoon cream of tartar
5 potatoes, thinly sliced
1 cup chopped onion
salt and ground black pepper to taste
2 cups milk
1/4 cup all-purpose flour
1 cup shredded Cheddar cheese
2 cups cubed smoke ham
Direction
In the big bowl, combine the cream of tartar and water.
Whisk the potatoes to the water mixture till the potatoes become well-coated; strain.
Layer the potatoes and onion in the slow cooker; use the black pepper and salt to season.
Heat the flour and milk on medium heat in the sauce pan, whisking frequently, for 5 minutes till boiling; use the black pepper and salt to season.
Add 1/2 milk sauce on top of potato mixture.
Scatter the ham and Cheddar cheese to slow cooker; cover with the rest of the milk sauce.
Cook over High heat setting for 4.5 to 5 hours or over Low heat setting for 9-10 hours.
Nutrition Information
Calories: 394 calories;;Total Fat: 16.4;Sodium: 741;Total Carbohydrate: 41.7;Cholesterol: 51;Protein: 20.1

111. Slow Cooker Mashed Potatoes

Serving: 8 | Prep: 15mins | Cook: 3hours15mins | Ready in:
Ingredients
5 pounds red potatoes, cut into chunks
1 tablespoon minced garlic, or to taste
3 cubes chicken bouillon
1 (8 ounce) container sour cream
1 (8 ounce) package cream cheese, softened
1/2 cup butter
salt and pepper to taste
Direction
Cook bouillon, garlic, and potatoes in a big pot of lightly salted boiling water for 15 minutes until the potatoes are softened but firm. Drain, putting the water aside. Mash potatoes with cream cheese and sour cream in a bowl, pouring in reserved water if needed to reach the wanted consistency.
Bring the potato mixture into a slow cooker, put the lid on and cook for 2-3 hours on low. Mix in butter right before eating, then add pepper and salt to taste.
Nutrition Information
Calories: 470 calories;;Total Fat: 27.7;Sodium: 703;Total Carbohydrate: 47.9;Cholesterol: 74;Protein: 8.8

112. Slow Cooker Mashed Potatoes And Cauliflower

Serving: 12 | Prep: 15mins | Cook: 6hours10mins | Ready in:
Ingredients
2 1/2 pounds potatoes, peeled and cubed
1 cup chicken broth
1 head cauliflower, chopped
1/4 cup milk
1/4 cup butter, softened
1/4 cup sour cream
1 tablespoon ground black pepper, or to taste
1 teaspoon garlic powder
1/4 teaspoon paprika
salt to taste
Direction
In a slow cooker, combine chicken broth and potatoes.
Cook potatoes for 3 hours on low setting. Add cauliflower and keep cooking for 3 more hours on low setting.
Mix salt, paprika, garlic powder, black pepper, sour cream, butter, and milk. Stir mixture into potatoes and mash until a desired consistency is reached using an immersion blender or potato masher.
Keep cooking the mashed potato mixture in the slow cooker for about 10 minutes longer until heated through.
Nutrition Information
Calories: 134 calories;;Sodium: 52;Total Carbohydrate: 20;Cholesterol: 13;Protein: 3.3;Total Fat: 5.1

113. Slow Cooker Northern White Bean

Serving: 6 | Prep: 15mins | Cook: 3hours | Ready in:
Ingredients
1 1/2 cups dried great Northern beans, rinsed
2 large smoked neck bones
2 (14 ounce) cans chicken broth
1/2 teaspoon soul seasoning
1/2 onion, finely chopped
1/2 teaspoon white vinegar, or to taste (optional)
1 pinch white sugar, or to taste (optional)
1 dash hot sauce, or to taste (optional)
Direction
In a big container, put beans; pour in some inches of cold water to cover, let sit 8 hours to all night. Drain and wash.
In a slow cooker, place neck bones, arrange chicken broth over top; mix in soul seasoning.
Cook on High for 1 hour until meat falls off from the bones. Remove meat and bones to a plate, tear meat from bones, take out bones.
Mix hot sauce, sugar, vinegar, onion, and beans into the slow cooker. Arrange shredded meat over beans.
Cook on Low 4-6 hours (or 2-4 hours on High)
Nutrition Information
Calories: 252 calories;;Cholesterol: 34;Protein: 21.7;Total Fat: 4.5;Sodium: 1149;Total Carbohydrate: 31.1

114. Slow Cooker Pizza Potatoes

Serving: 6 | Prep: 15mins | Cook: 6hours10mins | Ready in:
Ingredients

1 tablespoon olive oil
6 potatoes, peeled and thinly sliced
1 large onion, thinly sliced
1/4 pound grated mozzarella cheese
1 ounce sliced pepperoni
1 (8 ounce) can pizza sauce
Direction
Heat oil over medium-high heat in a big skillet. Cook and toss onion and potatoes in oil for 7 to 10 minutes, until the onion is semitransparent; drain. In a slow cooker, put the potato mixture and then the pepperoni and mozzarella cheese. Drizzle pizza sauce over the blend.
Cook for 6 to 10 hours on Low.
Nutrition Information
Calories: 248 calories;Protein: 9.2;Total Fat: 7.5;Sodium: 406;Total Carbohydrate: 36.3;Cholesterol: 17

115. Slow Cooker Refried Beans With Bacon

Serving: 6 | Prep: 10mins | Cook: 8hours17mins | Ready in:
Ingredients
1 cup dried pinto beans
1 ham hock
2 teaspoons salt
1/2 (16 ounce) package bacon, chopped
1/2 onion, finely chopped
2 teaspoons finely chopped garlic
1 teaspoon chili powder
Direction
Fill a bowl with water to cover beans. Soak the beans from 8 hours to overnight.
Drain beans and put in slow cooker with salt and ham hock. Cover using water. Cook for 8 hours on low until the beans are soft.
Put bacon in a big pot. Cook on medium-high heat while turning occasionally for 6 minutes until it starts to crisp. Place in onion; stir and cook for 5-7 minutes or until soft. Place in garlic; stir and cook for 3 minutes or until it starts to brown.
Move beans into the bacon mix with a slotted spoon. Mash mixture with a potato masher and add the liquid as needed from the slow cooker. Place in chili powder. Stir and cook for 3-5 minutes until combined.
Nutrition Information
Calories: 276 calories;;Total Fat: 12.7;Sodium: 1088;Total Carbohydrate: 22.6;Cholesterol: 36;Protein: 17.5

116. Slow Cooker Sausage 'n' Grits Meatloaf

Serving: 6 | Prep: 10mins | Cook: 5hours | Ready in:
Ingredients
2 16-inch square sheets of heavy duty aluminum foil
1 pound ground beef
1/2 pound bulk pork sausage
1/3 cup liquid egg whites
1/3 cup dry grits
1 tablespoon onion powder
1 tablespoon garlic powder
1/2 cup ketchup
2 dashes liquid smoke flavoring, or to taste (optional)
Direction
Fold the sheets of foil lengthwise in half and fold it again in half lengthwise to make 2 foil strips at 4x16 inches. Place the strips in the bottom of a slow cooker making a cross with the long ends coming partway up the insides of the cooker to make into lifting handles. Use cooking spray to spray the foil strips and the inside of the slow cooker.
Mix liquid smoke flavoring, ketchup, garlic powder, onion powder, grits, egg whites, pork sausage, and ground beef until combined thoroughly, then form into a round loaf. Place the loaf gently into the slow cooker over the crossed foil strips.
Cover and set the cooker on a low and cook for around 5-6 hours. To serve, hold the foil ends carefully and lift the meatloaf gently from the cooker by the foil handles to place onto a serving platter to slice.
Nutrition Information
Calories: 302 calories;;Sodium: 626;Total Carbohydrate: 14.2;Cholesterol: 69;Protein: 20.8;Total Fat: 17.7

117. Slow Cooker Scalloped Potatoes With Chicken

Serving: 5 | Prep: 30mins | Cook: 10hours | Ready in:
Ingredients
1/2 onion, chopped
1/2 green bell pepper, chopped
1 (10.75 ounce) can reduced fat condensed cream of mushroom soup
1 (10.75 ounce) can skim milk
1 1/4 cups cubed mozzarella cheese
2 tablespoons pressurized canned cheese spread (such as Cheez Whiz®)
1/2 teaspoon celery seed
1/2 teaspoon paprika
1 teaspoon dried parsley
5 (4 ounce) skinless, boneless chicken breast halves
7 large russet potatoes, peeled and thinly sliced
sea salt to taste
1 tablespoon cornstarch
2 tablespoons water
Direction
Combine parsley, paprika, celery seed, cheese spread, mozzarella cheese, milk, mushroom soup, green pepper, and onion together in a large mixing bowl until thoroughly incorporated. Add 1/4 of the sauce into the bottom of a slow cooker. Spread potatoes all over the sauce; add the remaining sauce atop the potatoes. Put chicken breasts into the slow cooker and season with a pinch or 2 of sea salt; press the chicken down into the sauce mixture.
Cook for 6 hours on low setting; adjust the cooker to high and cook for 4 hours longer until potatoes and chicken are very tender. Stir cornstarch and water, pour into the sauce, stir well to thicken, during the last 60 minutes of cooking time.
Nutrition Information
Calories: 686 calories;;Total Fat: 9.7;Sodium: 672;Total Carbohydrate: 107;Cholesterol: 85;Protein: 44.1

118. Slow Cooker Scalloped Potatoes With Ham

Serving: 8 | Prep: 20mins | Cook: 4hours | Ready in:
Ingredients
3 pounds potatoes, peeled and thinly sliced
1 cup shredded Cheddar cheese
1/2 cup chopped onion
1 cup chopped cooked ham
1 (10.75 ounce) can condensed cream of mushroom soup
1/2 cup water
1/2 teaspoon garlic powder
1/4 teaspoon salt
1/4 teaspoon black pepper
Direction

Put the sliced potatoes into the slow cooker. In the medium-sized bowl, combine the ham, onion and shredded cheese. Combine with the potatoes in the slow cooker. Using that bowl, combine the water and condensed soup. Use pepper, salt and garlic powder to season to taste. Add evenly on top of potato mixture.
Keep covered and cook over High heat for 4 hours.
Nutrition Information
Calories: 265 calories;Protein: 10.8;Total Fat: 10.2;Sodium: 634;Total Carbohydrate: 33.3;Cholesterol: 24

119. Slow Cooker Southern Collard Greens

Serving: 12 | Prep: 15mins | Cook: 12hours2mins | Ready in:
Ingredients
3 tablespoons olive oil
2 tablespoons minced garlic
5 cups chicken stock
3 ham hocks
1/2 cup olive oil
4 bunches collard greens - rinsed, trimmed, and chopped
1 (16 ounce) package cubed fully cooked ham
4 teaspoons red pepper flakes
salt and ground black pepper to taste
Direction
On medium heat, heat 3 tablespoons olive oil in a pan. Cook and stir garlic in hot oil for 2 minutes until pale brown. Move to a slow cooker. Put in ham hocks and chicken stock; cover. Cook for 8 hours to overnight on Low.
Take two cups of liquid in the slow cooker; reserve. On medium heat, heat 2 tablespoons olive oil in a pan. Add a teaspoon of red pepper, a quarter of the cubed ham, and a quarter of the collard greens; sprinkle black pepper and salt to season. Pour in half a cup of the reserved liquid. Cook for 4 minutes while mixing from time to time until the greens are a bit wilted and bright green; move to the slow cooker. Repeat three times more with the rest of the slow cooker liquid, greens, red pepper, and ham.
Cook for 4-6 hours on Low until the flavors combine.
Nutrition Information
Calories: 332 calories;;Cholesterol: 45;Protein: 15.7;Total Fat: 27.6;Sodium: 823;Total Carbohydrate: 6.8

120. Slow Cooker Spaghetti Squash

Serving: 4 | Prep: 5mins | Cook: 4hours | Ready in:
Ingredients
1 whole spaghetti squash, washed thoroughly
1 1/2 cups water
Direction
For 10 to 15 times, puncture outer of squash and put in slow cooker crock. Add water into the crock.
Allow to cook on Low for 4 to 6 hours. Take off squash to a chopping board till cool to handle, for 15 minutes to half an hour.
Slice squash in half lengthwise. Scrape out seeds and throw. Using a fork, shred flesh from skin to create strands.
Nutrition Information
Calories: 54 calories;;Sodium: 32;Total Carbohydrate: 12.1;Cholesterol: 0;Protein: 1.1;Total Fat: 1

121. Slow Cooker Sweet Potato Casserole

Serving: 8 | Prep: 30mins | Cook: 4hours | Ready in:
Ingredients
2 (29 ounce) cans sweet potatoes, drained and mashed
1/3 cup butter, melted
2 tablespoons white sugar
2 tablespoons brown sugar
1 tablespoon orange juice
2 eggs, beaten
1/2 cup milk
1/3 cup chopped pecans
1/3 cup brown sugar
2 tablespoons all-purpose flour
2 teaspoons butter, melted
Direction
Briefly oil a slow cooker.
Combine 2 tablespoons brown sugar, white sugar, 1/3 cup butter, and sweet potatoes in a big bowl. Stir in milk, eggs, and orange juice. Remove this mixture into the prepared casserole dish.
Mix together 2 tablespoons butter, flour, 1/3 cup brown sugar, and pecans in a small bowl. Spread on the sweet potatoes with the mixture. Put the lid on the slow cooker and cook for 3-4 hours on high.
Nutrition Information
Calories: 406 calories;;Total Fat: 13.8;Sodium: 103;Total Carbohydrate: 66.1;Cholesterol: 77;Protein: 6.3

122. Slow Cooker Sweet Potatoes (Yams) And Marshmallows

Serving: 8 | Prep: 5mins | Cook: 3hours15mins | Ready in:
Ingredients
cooking spray
2 (29 ounce) cans sweet potatoes, drained
1/3 cup butter, cut into 1/4-inch pieces
3/4 cup light brown sugar
1 (16 ounce) package miniature marshmallows
Direction
Spray cooking spray inside a slow cooker.
Put sweet potatoes in the slow cooker; put butter over sweet potatoes. Sprinkle sweet potatoes with brown sugar.
Cook for 3-3 1/2 hours on high. Add marshmallows; cook for 15 minutes till somewhat puffy and soft.
Nutrition Information
Calories: 531 calories;;Sodium: 238;Total Carbohydrate: 109.1;Cholesterol: 20;Protein: 3.5;Total Fat: 8.1

123. Slow Cooker Western Omelet

Serving: 12 | Prep: 20mins | Cook: 12hours | Ready in:
Ingredients
1 (2 pound) package frozen shredded hash brown potatoes
1 pound diced cooked ham
1 onion, diced
1 green bell pepper, seeded and diced
1 1/2 cups shredded Cheddar cheese
12 eggs
1 cup milk
salt and pepper to taste
Direction
Grease 4-qt. or bigger slow cooker lightly. In 1 layer, put 1/3 hash brown potatoes on the bottom. Layer 1/3 of ham, onion, green pepper and Cheddar cheese. Repeat layers twice. Whisk milk and eggs in big bowl; season with pepper and salt. Put over the contents in slow cooker.
Cover. Cook for 10-12 hours on low.
Nutrition Information
Calories: 310 calories;;Cholesterol: 227;Protein: 19.9;Total Fat: 22.7;Sodium: 696;Total Carbohydrate: 16.1

124. Spicy Chipotle Black Eyed Peas

Serving: 20 | Prep: 20mins | Cook: 8hours | Ready in:

Ingredients
- 2 tablespoons olive oil
- 1 tablespoon balsamic vinegar
- 1 cup chopped orange bell pepper
- 1 cup chopped celery
- 1 cup chopped carrot
- 1 cup chopped onion
- 1 teaspoon minced garlic
- 2 (16 ounce) packages dry black-eyed peas
- 4 cups water
- 4 teaspoons vegetable bouillon base (such as Better Than Bouillon® Vegetable Base)
- 1 (7 ounce) can chipotle peppers in adobo sauce, chopped, sauce reserved
- 2 teaspoons liquid mesquite smoke flavoring
- 2 teaspoons ground cumin
- 1/2 teaspoon ground black pepper

Direction
In a skillet, heat balsamic vinegar and olive oil. Cook while stirring garlic, onion, carrot, orange bell pepper, and celery in the hot oil for 5 to 8 minutes until the onion becomes translucent. Pour the mixture into a slow cooker and add in vegetable base, water and black-eyed peas, while stirring to dissolve the vegetable base. Mix in black pepper, liquid smoke, chipotle peppers, cumin and about one tablespoon of the reserved adobo sauce (or to taste).
Cook for about 8 minutes in the slow cooker on Low until the flavors are blended and the black-eyed peas become very tender.

Nutrition Information
Calories: 165 calories;;Sodium: 170;Total Carbohydrate: 26.9;Cholesterol: 0;Protein: 9.2;Total Fat: 2.7

125. Spicy Slow Cooker Potatoes

Serving: 8 | Prep: 25mins | Cook: 3hours30mins | Ready in:

Ingredients
- 2 tablespoons olive oil
- 1 large onion, thinly sliced
- 2 green chile peppers, thinly sliced (optional)
- 1 tablespoon mustard seeds
- 1 tablespoon cumin seeds
- 1 teaspoon white sugar
- 1 clove garlic, minced
- salt and ground black pepper to taste
- 8 potatoes, peeled and cubed
- 2 tablespoons red pepper flakes

Direction
Add olive oil to the bottom of a slow cooker. Place onion slices in layer over the oil. Add pepper, salt, garlic, sugar, cumin seeds, mustard seeds, and green chile peppers. Place a layer of potatoes on top, sprinkle on top of each layer with salt and red pepper flakes to season.
Cook for 3-1/2 to 4 hours on high until potatoes are softened. Stir gradually and serve.

Nutrition Information
Calories: 225 calories;;Total Carbohydrate: 42.8;Cholesterol: 0;Protein: 5.5;Total Fat: 4.6;Sodium: 36

126. Spinach Noodle Casserole

Serving: 8 | Prep: 45mins | Cook: 2hours30mins | Ready in:

Ingredients
- 8 ounces dry spinach noodles
- 2 tablespoons vegetable oil
- 1 1/2 cups sour cream
- 1/3 cup all-purpose flour
- 1 1/2 cups cottage cheese
- 4 green onions, minced
- 2 teaspoons Worcestershire sauce
- 1 dash hot pepper sauce
- 2 teaspoons garlic salt

Direction
In a large pot, cook noodles in the salted boiling water until they are barely tender. Drain, then rinse under the cold water. Toss with the vegetable oil.
In large bowl, combine flour and sour cream while the noodles are cooking. Mix well. Stir in garlic salt, hot pepper sauce, Worcestershire sauce, green onions and cottage cheese. Stir the noodles into the mixture. Grease inside of the slow cooker generously. Pour in the noodle mixture. Cook, covered, for 90-120 mins on high.

Nutrition Information
Calories: 226 calories;;Total Fat: 14.9;Sodium: 669;Total Carbohydrate: 14.7;Cholesterol: 35;Protein: 8.8

127. Stuffing For Slow Cooker

Serving: 11 | Prep: | Cook: | Ready in:

Ingredients
- 1 cup butter
- 2 cups chopped celery
- 2 cups chopped onion
- 1/4 cup chopped parsley
- 2 (8 ounce) cans mushrooms, drained
- 12 cups white bread, cut into cubes
- 1 teaspoon poultry seasoning
- 1 teaspoon dried thyme
- 1 1/2 teaspoons sage
- 1/2 teaspoon ground black pepper
- 1 1/2 teaspoons salt
- 1/2 teaspoon dried marjoram (optional)
- 2 eggs, beaten
- 4 cups chicken broth

Direction
Melt the butter in a large skillet that is set over medium heat. Sauté the mushrooms, onion, celery, and parsley until the onions softened.
Mix the vegetables and bread cubes in a large bowl. Add the thyme, salt, marjoram, pepper, poultry seasoning, and sage and toss well. Add the egg and pour in enough broth to moisten.
Pack the mixture lightly into the slow cooker. Cover it and cook it on a high setting for 45 minutes. Adjust the heat to a low setting. Cook the mixture for 4-8 hours.

Nutrition Information
Calories: 290 calories;;Total Carbohydrate: 25.2;Cholesterol: 78;Protein: 5.6;Total Fat: 19.1;Sodium: 901

128. Sweet Barbeque Beans

Serving: 10 | Prep: 30mins | Cook: 1hours20mins | Ready in:

Ingredients
- 6 slices bacon, chopped
- 1 pound ground beef
- 2 (16 ounce) cans baked beans with pork
- 1 (15.5 ounce) can navy beans, rinsed and drained
- 1 (15 ounce) can kidney beans, rinsed and drained
- 3/4 cup ketchup
- 3/4 cup packed brown sugar
- 3 tablespoons distilled white vinegar
- 2 tablespoons honey garlic sauce
- 2 tablespoons sweet and sour sauce
- 1 teaspoon onion powder
- 1 teaspoon garlic salt
- 1 teaspoon ground mustard
- 1 teaspoon Worcestershire sauce

Direction

In a big skillet, cook the bacon pieces until they turn crisp and brown. Move it out of the pan and put it to one side. Over the pan, crumble the ground beef up. Cook it until there isn't any hint of pink left in the meat, stirring throughout. Drain the grease. Move the bacon and ground beef into a slow cooker.
Followed by pouring in the navy beans, vinegar, brown sugar, ketchup, kidney beans and baked beans. Add Worcestershire sauce, mustard powder, garlic salt, onion powder, sweet and sour sauce and honey garlic sauce to season. Keep stirring until the mixture is thoroughly mixed together. Put the lid on. With the setting of the heat on high, cook for an hour then serve it.
Nutrition Information
Calories: 388 calories;Protein: 20.7;Total Fat: 9.7;Sodium: 1282;Total Carbohydrate: 56.9;Cholesterol: 41

129. Sweet And Sour Beans
Serving: 11 | Prep: | Cook: | Ready in:
Ingredients
1 pound bacon
3 onions, chopped
1 teaspoon garlic powder
1/2 teaspoon dry hot mustard
1/2 cup white wine vinegar
1 cup packed brown sugar
1 (15 ounce) can kidney beans, drained
1 (15 ounce) can lima beans, drained
1 (15 ounce) can butter beans
2 (15 ounce) cans baked beans
Direction
Cook bacon in big deep skillet till evenly brown over medium high heat. Drain; crumble. Put aside. Keep 2 tbsp. bacon fat.
Sauté onions in fat in pan till soft. Mix brown sugar, wine vinegar, dry mustard and garlic powder in then simmer it for 20 minutes.
Mix baked beans, butter beans, lima beans, kidney beans, bacon and onion mixture together in a big pot or slow cooker. Simmer for 70 minutes.
Nutrition Information
Calories: 440 calories;;Total Fat: 19.2;Sodium: 960;Total Carbohydrate: 55.4;Cholesterol: 28;Protein: 14.6

130. Swiss Corn Slow Cooker Casserole
Serving: 8 | Prep: 10mins | Cook: 4hours | Ready in:
Ingredients
cooking spray
1 (16 ounce) package frozen corn, thawed
1 pint heavy whipping cream
2 cups shredded Swiss cheese
2 eggs, lightly beaten
ground black pepper to taste
Direction
Spray cooking spray inside a slow cooker.
Mix eggs, Swiss cheese, cream and corn in a bowl; season using black pepper. Put corn mixture into the slow cooker.
Cook for 4-4 1/2 hours on Low till cheese melts and cooked through.
Nutrition Information
Calories: 376 calories;;Total Fat: 31.2;Sodium: 94;Total Carbohydrate: 14.9;Cholesterol: 153;Protein: 11.8

131. Tender Taters
Serving: 6 | Prep: 20mins | Cook: 4hours | Ready in:
Ingredients
3 pounds Yukon Gold potatoes, peeled and diced
1 pinch ground black pepper
1 (2.64 ounce) package country gravy mix
1/3 cup water
1 (12 fluid ounce) can evaporated skim milk
1/2 cup butter
Direction
In a slow cooker, put potatoes and sprinkle with black pepper. Stir water and the gravy mix together in a measuring cup until well combined. Next, pour this mixture over the potatoes, then pour in the evaporated milk. Stir to combine. Cover, and cook on low for 4 hours. When finished, allow to drain any excess liquid. Next, use a potato masher to mash the potatoes and stir in the butter.
Nutrition Information
Calories: 367 calories;;Sodium: 224;Total Carbohydrate: 48.4;Cholesterol: 43;Protein: 9.4;Total Fat: 15.9

132. Texas Style Baked Beans
Serving: 12 | Prep: 15mins | Cook: 2hours | Ready in:
Ingredients
1 pound ground beef
4 (16 ounce) cans baked beans with pork
1 (4 ounce) can canned chopped green chile peppers
1 small Vidalia onion, peeled and chopped
1 cup barbeque sauce
1/2 cup brown sugar
1 tablespoon garlic powder
1 tablespoon chili powder
3 tablespoons hot pepper sauce (e.g. Tabasco™), or to taste
Direction
Brown ground beef in a skillet over medium heat till not pink anymore; let the fat drain, and reserve.
Mix the barbeque sauce, onion, green chilies, baked beans and ground beef in a 3 1/2 quart or bigger slow cooker. Put hot pepper sauce, chili powder, garlic powder and brown sugar to season. Allow to cook for 2 hours on High, or for 4 to 5 hours on Low.
Nutrition Information
Calories: 360 calories;;Total Fat: 12.4;Sodium: 899;Total Carbohydrate: 50;Cholesterol: 43;Protein: 14.6

133. The Best Slow Cooker Baked Beans (Dad's Recipe)
Serving: 8 | Prep: 10mins | Cook: 9hours | Ready in:
Ingredients
1 (16 ounce) package dried navy beans
4 cups water, or more as needed
1/2 cup molasses
2 tablespoons brown sugar
1 teaspoon salt
3/4 teaspoon dry mustard
1/8 teaspoon ground black pepper
1/4 pound salt pork, thinly sliced
1 onion, sliced
Direction
Pour cool water over navy beans to cover by several inches in a large container; allow to soak for 8 hours to overnight. Drain off water and place beans into a pot; pour in enough water to cover beans.
Bring to a boil. Lower heat; simmer, covered for about 1 hour until beans become slightly tender.
In a mixing bowl, combine pepper, mustard, salt, brown sugar, molasses, and 4 cups water until no lumps remain.
Combine onion, salt pork, and beans in a slow cooker. Add molasses mixture and pour in water just enough to cover beans if necessary; mix well.
Cook for 8 to 10 hours on low setting.
Nutrition Information

Calories: 374 calories;;Sodium: 508;Total Carbohydrate: 54;Cholesterol: 12;Protein: 13.5;Total Fat: 12.4

134. The Best Slow Cooker Cream Corn

Serving: 20 | Prep: 5mins | Cook: 3hours | Ready in:
Ingredients
4 (16 ounce) packages frozen corn kernels
3 (8 ounce) packages cream cheese, cubed
1 cup butter, cut into pieces
1/2 cup white sugar
6 slices American cheese
1/2 cup whole milk
Direction
Combine milk, American cheese, sugar, butter, cream cheese, and corn in a 6-quart slow cooker. Cover the pot and choose low setting. Cook on Low for about 3 hours; stirring the mixture every half an hour. High setting with shorter time would not be recommended because milk and cheese burn easily.
Nutrition Information
Calories: 332 calories;;Sodium: 297;Total Carbohydrate: 25;Cholesterol: 70;Protein: 7.4;Total Fat: 24.5

135. Tomato And Bacon Creamed Corn Casserole

Serving: 16 | Prep: 20mins | Cook: 2hours | Ready in:
Ingredients
1 Reynolds® Slow Cooker Liner
4 (10 ounce) packages frozen whole-kernel corn, thawed*
1 1/2 cups half and half, light cream, or whole milk
1 cup chopped onion
1/2 cup finely shredded Parmesan cheese
1/4 cup butter, cut up
1/2 teaspoon salt
3/4 cup shredded Monterey Jack cheese
6 thick slices peppered bacon, crisp-cooked and chopped
1/2 cup chopped tomato
2 tablespoons snipped fresh basil
Direction
Line Reynolds® Slow Cooker Liner over the bottom of a 5- to 6-quart slow cooker.
In a blender, place 2 packages of corn and pour in milk or cream. Put the lid on and process until no lumps remain. Pour mixture into the prepared slow cooker.
Mix salt, butter, Parmesan cheese, onion, and remaining corn into the corn mixture in the cooker. Mix carefully using a rubber spatula until incorporated.
Cook, covered for 4 hours on low setting and 2 hours on high setting. Pour mixture into a serving dish to serve. Sprinkle with basil, tomato, bacon, and Monterey Jack cheese.
Nutrition Information
Calories: 178 calories;;Total Carbohydrate: 17.1;Cholesterol: 28;Protein: 7;Total Fat: 10.3;Sodium: 284

136. Western Style Baked Beans

Serving: 32 | Prep: 15mins | Cook: 3hours10mins | Ready in:
Ingredients
1 pound ground beef
2 (28 ounce) cans baked beans with pork
1 pound bacon, cooked and crumbled
1/2 pound cooked ham, chopped
2 tablespoons minced onion
1 tablespoon chili powder
1/4 cup ketchup
1/4 cup packed brown sugar
1 tablespoon molasses
1/4 cup water (optional)
Direction
In a big skillet, crumble the ground beef on medium-high heat and let it cook and stir for 5-10 minutes, until it has no visible pink color. Drain off the grease and place the beef into a 4-qt. or bigger slow cooker. Stir in the molasses, brown sugar, ketchup, chili powder, onion, ham, bacon and baked beans. Mix in water if it seems thick. Put on cover and let it cook for 6-8 hours on Low or 3 hours on High.
Nutrition Information
Calories: 186 calories;Protein: 11.6;Total Fat: 9.7;Sodium: 617;Total Carbohydrate: 13.5;Cholesterol: 32

137. Wild Rice Casserole I

Serving: 8 | Prep: 30mins | Cook: 4hours | Ready in:
Ingredients
2 onions, finely chopped
3 celery, thinly sliced
2 (6 ounce) packages dry instant long grain and wild rice mix
2 1/2 cups water
1 (10.75 ounce) can condensed cream of mushroom soup
1/2 cup butter
1/2 pound processed American cheese
1/2 cup sliced fresh mushrooms
Direction
Put the mushrooms, American cheese, butter, condensed cream of mushroom soup, water, rice mix, celery and onions in a slow cooker. Put cover and let it cook for 2-4 hours on high or 6-10 hours on low.
Nutrition Information
Calories: 408 calories;;Cholesterol: 57;Protein: 11.6;Total Fat: 23;Sodium: 1400;Total Carbohydrate: 39.5

Chapter 3: Main Dish Slow Cooker Recipes

138. Amazing Ribs

Serving: 12 | Prep: 30mins | Cook: 4hours40mins | Ready in:

Ingredients
6 pounds pork baby back ribs
1 pinch black pepper
1 pinch salt
1 pinch crushed red pepper
4 cups barbecue sauce
2 (12 ounce) bottles porter beer, room temperature

Direction
Into small portions, slice ribs with 2 or 3 bones each. Boil big pot of water. Add in to water a pinch each of crushed red pepper, black pepper and salt to season. Let ribs boil for 20 minutes in seasoned water. Drain, and let the ribs rest for about 30 minutes.
Meantime, preheat the outdoor grill for high heat. With barbecue sauce, coat the ribs lightly. Cook the ribs 5 to 10 minutes on each side on high heat to get a pleasant grilled look to them.
In a slow cooker, put grilled ribs. Add leftover barbecue sauce and a bottle of beer on the ribs; liquid must soak at least half of the ribs. Put cover, on high, cook for 3 hours. Each hour or so check ribs, if necessary, put extra beer to thin sauce. Mix to get the ribs over into the sauce. Once the meat is falling off the bone, the ribs are done. In the initial process ribs were cooked fully, while the remaining is about texture and flavor.

Nutrition Information
Calories: 524 calories;;Sodium: 1034;Total Carbohydrate: 33.7;Cholesterol: 117;Protein: 24.5;Total Fat: 29.6

139. Anna's Amazing Easy Pleasy Meatballs Over Buttered Noodles

Serving: 24 | Prep: 15mins | Cook: 3hours | Ready in:

Ingredients
2 (10.75 ounce) cans condensed cream of celery soup
2 (10.5 ounce) cans condensed French onion soup
1 (16 ounce) container sour cream
6 pounds frozen Italian-style meatballs
2 (16 ounce) packages uncooked egg noodles
1/2 cup butter

Direction
Combine sour cream, French onion soup, and cream of celery soup in a large slow cooker. Add meatballs and stir. Cook for 3-4 hours on high.
Boil a large pot with lightly salted water. Put in pasta and cook until al dente, or for 8-10 minutes; then drain the pasta. Toss the pasta together with the butter in a large bowl. Add sauce and meatballs on top of the cooked pasta and serve.

Nutrition Information
Calories: 492 calories;;Sodium: 591;Total Carbohydrate: 38.5;Cholesterol: 148;Protein: 25.9;Total Fat: 25.5

140. Apple Breakfast (Easy Slow Cooker Oatmeal)

Serving: 8 | Prep: 10mins | Cook: 5hours | Ready in:

Ingredients
4 cups rolled oats
1/2 cup white sugar
1 tablespoon ground cinnamon
1 teaspoon ground nutmeg
1 teaspoon ground ginger
1/2 teaspoon ground allspice
1/4 teaspoon ground cloves
2 1/2 cups water
1 1/2 cups sliced apple
1/2 cup vegetable oil
1 tablespoon molasses

Direction
In a slow cooker, combine cloves, allspice, ginger, nutmeg, cinnamon, sugar and oats. Stir in molasses, vegetable oil, apple slices and water until mixed thoroughly. Cook on Low for 5-7 hours.

Nutrition Information
Calories: 346 calories;;Total Fat: 16.5;Sodium: 6;Total Carbohydrate: 45.8;Cholesterol: 0;Protein: 5.5

141. Apple And Brown Sugar Corned Beef

Serving: 10 | Prep: 15mins | Cook: 4hours | Ready in:

Ingredients
4 cups apple juice
1/2 cup brown sugar
1 tablespoon prepared mustard
2 (3 pound) corned beef briskets with spice packets
20 small red potatoes, scrubbed
4 carrots, cut into chunks
2 onions, cut into 8 wedges
1 head cabbage, cored and cut into large chunks

Direction
Put apple juice in big slow cooker; mix mustard and brown sugar in. Mix till brown sugar dissolves; mix spice packet contents in. Lay briskets into apple juice mixture; put cabbage chunks, onions, carrots and red potatoes over. Push all ingredients into liquid. Cover; cook for 4-5 hours on high till corned beef is very tender/cook for 8-10 hours on low. Across grain, thinly slice meat; serve with veggies.

Nutrition Information
Calories: 672 calories;;Sodium: 1438;Total Carbohydrate: 87.2;Cholesterol: 117;Protein: 30.5;Total Fat: 23.5

142. Asian Bison Short Ribs

Serving: 6 | Prep: 20mins | Cook: 11hours | Ready in:

Ingredients
2 cups chopped onions
1 cup sliced carrots
1/3 cup all-purpose flour
1/2 teaspoon salt
1/4 teaspoon black pepper
4 pounds bison short ribs
1 tablespoon toasted sesame oil, or more to taste
1 cup beef broth
1/2 cup orange juice
1/4 cup soy sauce
3 tablespoons packed brown sugar
4 cloves garlic, minced
1/4 teaspoon cayenne pepper
2 tablespoons cornstarch
Salt and black pepper
Hot cooked rice
Chopped fresh cilantro

Direction
In a 5-quart or 6-quart slow cooker, insert the carrots and onions. In a big resealable plastic bag, mix 1/4 teaspoon of pepper, 1/2 teaspoon of salt and

flour together. From the bison short ribs, get rid of the fat by trimming. Slice them up into single rib portions if necessary. Use paper towels to pat them dry. Insert the bison short ribs into the plastic bag bit by bit. Shake them until well coated.

Pour the oil into an extremely big skillet then warm up at medium to high heat until heated. Insert the bison short ribs 1/2 by 1/2 at one time until evenly browned everywhere. If needed, pour in extra oil. Put them into a slow cooker atop the vegetables.

In a medium bowl, mix cayenne pepper, ginger, garlic, brown sugar, soy sauce, orange juice and broth together. Empty this out into the slow cover atop the vegetables and bison short ribs.

Leave the contents cooking with the cover on for 5-1/2-6 hours on high or for 11-2 hours on low. Move the vegetables and bison short ribs onto a serving platter with a slotted spoon. Keep the cooking liquid. Use foil to seal the vegetables and bison short ribs up in order to maintain the warmth. Get about three cups of the liquid after skimming the fat off of the cooking liquid. Get rid of the rest. Mix corn-starch with 3 cups of cooking liquid in a midsized saucepan, cooking and stirring at medium to high heat until it starts bubbling and thickening. Continue cooking and stirring for another 2 minutes. Add black pepper and extra salt to your liking. Before serving, put together with rice and scatter cilantro over the top.

143. Authentic Cochinita Pibil (Spicy Mexican Pulled Pork)

Serving: 6 | Prep: 25mins | Cook: 6hours20mins | Ready in:
Ingredients
1 red onion, sliced thin
3 habanero peppers, sliced
10 limes, juiced
salt to taste
3 ounces dried guajillo chile peppers, seeded and deveined
1 tablespoon vegetable oil
salt and pepper to taste
3 pounds boneless pork shoulder, cut into 1-inch cubes
3 cups fresh orange juice
1 cup white vinegar
1 bulb garlic, peeled
7 1/2 ounces achiote paste
Direction
In a bowl, mix together salt, lime juice, habanero peppers and onion; put a cover on and chill while cooking and preparing the pork. Wear rubber gloves while working with habanero peppers and do not touch your skin, nose or eyes while cutting the peppers.
In a bowl, put the guajillo peppers; cover the peppers with enough hot water. Soak the peppers for 10 minutes until they are tender.
In a big skillet heat oil over medium-high heat. Use pepper and salt to season the pork, cook in the hot oil for 15-20 minutes until entirely brown. Remove the pork to a slow cooker.
In a blender, mix together achiote paste, garlic, vinegar, orange juice and guajillo peppers; process until smooth. Pour the sauce onto the slow cooker with the pork cubes.

Cook on High for 6-8 hours until the pork is easy to fall apart. Transfer the pork to a serving dish and use 2 forks to shred. Pour over the shredded pork with the achiote sauce. For serving, put the onion-habanero salsa on top.
Nutrition Information
Calories: 468 calories;;Sodium: 368;Total Carbohydrate: 39.6;Cholesterol: 89;Protein: 27.1;Total Fat: 24.9

144. Awesome Pulled Pork BBQ

Serving: 10 | Prep: 15mins | Cook: 10hours15mins | Ready in:
Ingredients
1 (5 pound) boneless pork loin roast
1 pinch garlic powder, or to taste
1 pinch poultry seasoning, or to taste
salt to taste
ground black pepper to taste
1 large onion, quartered
1 apple, cored and quartered
3 stalks celery
1 (14.5 ounce) can chicken broth
Barbecue Sauce:
1/2 cup butter
2 cups chopped celery
1 1/2 cups chopped onion
4 cups ketchup
2 cups water
2/3 cup cider vinegar
1/2 cup brown sugar
1/4 cup Worcestershire sauce
2 tablespoons prepared mustard
1 tablespoon liquid smoke flavoring
1 tablespoon garlic powder
Direction
Put pork into a slow cooker; season with pepper, salt, poultry seasoning and garlic powder to taste. Add 3 celery stalks, apple and quartered onion; transfer chicken broth into the slow cooker.
Cook for approximately 8 hours till very tender on Low. Transfer pork onto a big platter; discard veggies and juice. Use a fork to shred pork; put back in the slow cooker.
As pork is cooking, prep barbecue sauce. Melt butter in a small Dutch oven or big saucepan on medium heat; mix and cook 1 1/2 cups onion and 2 cups celery for about 5 minutes till onion is translucent. Add 1 tbsp. garlic powder, liquid smoke, mustard, Worcestershire sauce, brown sugar, vinegar, water and ketchup; mix. Lower the heat to low; simmer for approximately 10 minutes till sauce is thick, occasionally mixing. Transfer barbecue sauce on top of shredded pork.
Keep cooking pork for about 2 hours till flavors merge on low heat.
Nutrition Information
Calories: 548 calories;;Total Carbohydrate: 44.2;Cholesterol: 131;Protein: 41.4;Total Fat: 23.5;Sodium: 1514

145. Bandito Slow Cooker Chili Dogs

Serving: 20 | Prep: 15mins | Cook: 4hours | Ready in:
Ingredients
2 (16 ounce) packages hot dogs
2 (15 ounce) cans chili without beans
1 (10.75 ounce) can condensed Cheddar cheese soup
3 tablespoons ketchup
1 (4 ounce) can chopped green chilies, drained

20 hot dog buns
1 cup shredded Cheddar cheese
1/4 cup chopped onion, or to taste
1 1/2 cups crushed corn chips (such as Fritos®)
Direction
Put hot dogs in a slow cooker. In a bowl, mix chopped green chilies, ketchup, Cheddar cheese soup, and chili; pour over the hot dogs. Next, cover the cooker, set to Low, and cook for 4-5 hours (if desired, you can cook longer).
Serve hot dogs on buns with about 2 tablespoons crushed corn chips, 1 tablespoon of shredded Cheddar cheese, 1 teaspoon of chopped onion, and a large spoonful of chili on top of them.
Nutrition Information
Calories: 385 calories;;Total Fat: 21.4;Sodium: 1172;Total Carbohydrate: 33.1;Cholesterol: 39;Protein: 14.7

146. Barbecued Pulled Pork With Sweet Sour Slaw

Serving: 6 | Prep: 25mins | Cook: 9hours | Ready in:
Ingredients
8 Ball Park® Hamburger Buns
1 (3 pound) boneless pork butt roast, trimmed and quartered
Pork Rub:
1/2 cup packed light brown sugar
1/2 cup sweet paprika
1 tablespoon garlic granules
1 tablespoon ground cumin
1 teaspoon ground cayenne
1/2 teaspoon ground ginger
1 teaspoon kosher salt
1/2 teaspoon ground black pepper
BBQ Sauce:
2 cups ketchup
1/2 cup brown sugar
3/4 cup apple cider vinegar
2 tablespoons plain mustard
1 tablespoon honey
1 tablespoon Worcestershire sauce
1 teaspoon liquid smoke flavoring
1/4 cup pork rub
Sweet Sour Slaw:
3/4 cup white balsamic vinegar
2 tablespoons olive oil
2 tablespoons brown sugar
2 teaspoons garlic granules
Kosher salt and ground black pepper, to taste
1 1/2 cups shredded red cabbage
1 1/2 cups shredded carrots
1 cup seeded, peeled, chopped cucumber
1/2 cup finely chopped Italian parsley
Direction
In a large bowl, blend all ingredients together to make rub. Use a fork to mix properly. Keep a quarter cup of the rub for making the barbecue sauce.
In a large Mason jar, blend all ingredients while stirring well to make sauce. Use a tight-fitting lid to cover then give it another good shake. Refrigerate overnight.
In a large casserole dish, add the pork rub.
Use a fork to pierce all over the pork several times. Cover all surfaces of the pork using the spice blend to rub into it.
Tightly wrap rubbed pork in plastic and let it refrigerate for 8 hours or overnight.

When it's cooking time, unwrap the pork then set in a slow-cooker.
Cover all surfaces of the pork by pouring on 1 cup of the Barbecue Sauce.
Cook while covering on Low for 9 to 11 hours or 5 to 7 hours on High, till softened.
Move the pork into a deep, large, wide casserole dish then let it cool for 15 - 20 minutes.
Use two large forks to shred the pork into bite-size pieces, eliminating the excess fat. Keep warm by covering.
In the pot, skim any fat left from the liquid. Move 2 - 3 tablespoons into a bowl then whisk in the leftover barbecue sauce.
Thoroughly mix and pour in more braising liquid for a thinner sauce if preferred.
In the oven, warm buns while turning over once at 400°, just till slightly toasty.
Pile pulled pork onto buns, add with some Barbecue Sauce and some Tangy Slaw (recipe below) on top then enjoy.
For the slaw: In a big bowl, whisk pepper, garlic, brown sugar, salt, oil and vinegar together.
Put in parsley, cucumber, carrots and cabbage, thoroughly mixing.
Let it sit for about 30 minutes while covering loosely with plastic.
Before serving, toss once and adjust seasonings, if wished.
Nutrition Information
Calories: 806 calories;;Sodium: 1781;Total Carbohydrate: 114.4;Cholesterol: 96;Protein: 35.5;Total Fat: 26.5

147. Barbeque Pork Two Ways

Serving: 8 | Prep: 15mins | Cook: 8hours | Ready in:
Ingredients
2 1/2 pounds pork shoulder
1/2 cup chopped onion
1 clove garlic, minced
1/4 cup brown sugar
1 teaspoon dry mustard
1/2 teaspoon salt
1/4 teaspoon ground black pepper
2 cups ketchup
1/4 cup Worcestershire sauce
Direction
Cut the boneless pork shoulder crosswise into 1/4 - inch slices. Partially freezing it will make cutting easier.
Mix Worcestershire sauce, ketchup, pepper, salt, dry mustard, brown sugar, garlic, onion, and sliced pork in the slow cooker; combine well and cover. Cook on low, stirring from time to time, for 6 to 8 hours until the meat is softened.
Or: Mix Worcestershire sauce, ketchup, pepper, salt, dry mustard, brown sugar, garlic, onion, and pork in a Dutch oven or large saucepan, blend well. Heat to a boil, lower the heat and cover. Simmer, stirring from time to time, for 2 1/2 to 3 hours until the pork is tender.
Nutrition Information
Calories: 279 calories;;Sodium: 965;Total Carbohydrate: 24.7;Cholesterol: 56;Protein: 15.8;Total Fat: 13.6

148. Barbeque Shredded Beef

Serving: 6 | Prep: 10mins | Cook: 8hours | Ready in:
Ingredients

1 cup chopped onion, or more to taste
1 (15 ounce) can tomato sauce
1/4 cup brown sugar
2 tablespoons vinegar
4 teaspoons chili powder
1 teaspoon soy sauce
1 teaspoon salt
1/2 teaspoon dry mustard
1 1/2 pounds boneless beef chuck roast
Direction
In a slow cooker, stir together mustard, salt, soy sauce, chili powder, vinegar, brown sugar, tomato sauce, and onion; add in roast. Coat the beef with onion mixture.
On high heat, cook for 7 hours. In the slow cooker, using a pair of forks to shred meat. Keep cooking for 1 more hour.
Nutrition Information
Calories: 235 calories;Protein: 15;Total Fat: 12.5;Sodium: 858;Total Carbohydrate: 16.3;Cholesterol: 51

149. Beef Roast In Red Wine (Carni Arrosto Al Vino Rosso)

Serving: 8 | Prep: 15mins | Cook: 8hours | Ready in:
Ingredients
1 small onion, very thinly sliced
3 1/2 pounds boneless beef chuck roast
1 teaspoon kosher salt
1 teaspoon freshly ground black pepper
4 large cloves garlic, very thinly sliced
2 cups dry red wine
2 (14.5 ounce) cans diced tomatoes, undrained
1 cup beef broth
1 tablespoon Worcestershire sauce
1 tablespoon dried rosemary
1 tablespoon dried oregano
1 tablespoon dried basil
2 teaspoons dried thyme
1 teaspoon kosher salt
1 teaspoon freshly ground black pepper
3 tablespoons tomato paste (optional)
Direction
Slice onions into half and put one of them at the bottom of a slow cooker. Use 1 teaspoon of black pepper and 1 teaspoon of kosher salt to season all sides, put the roast on top of the onions. Put garlic and the other half of the onion on top of the roast.
Mix 1 teaspoon black pepper, 1 teaspoon kosher salt, thyme, basil, oregano, rosemary, Worcestershire sauce, beef broth, diced tomatoes and red wine in a big bowl, dump the wine mixture on the roast. Put the lid on the slow cooker, set it to Low and cook for 8-10 hours until softened.
To thicken the sauce, whisk pan juices with tomato paste until thoroughly mixed. Set the cooker on high, cook for another 10 minutes.
Nutrition Information
Calories: 393 calories;;Total Fat: 22.6;Sodium: 866;Total Carbohydrate: 9.6;Cholesterol: 90;Protein: 25

150. Big V's Slow Cooker Pulled Pork

Serving: 6 | Prep: 15mins | Cook: 10hours | Ready in:
Ingredients
1 (12 fluid ounce) can or bottle beer
1/4 cup mustard, or to taste
1/4 cup honey
2 tablespoons Worcestershire sauce
2 tablespoons crushed garlic, or to taste
1 teaspoon cayenne pepper
1 teaspoon salt
3 pounds pork picnic roast
3/4 cup water (optional)
1 onion, chopped
Direction
In a bowl, stir together salt, cayenne pepper, garlic, Worcestershire sauce, honey, mustard and beer until the honey dissolves. Add a small amount of the beer marinade to a slow cooker; put in the pork. Pour over the pork with the leftover marinade. Put the cover on and chill overnight, flipping the pork sometimes.
In the slow cooker, cook the pork for 8 hours on Low, basting sometimes. If the pork appears dry, add water. Drop onion around pork and keep cooking for another 2 hours until the pork is very soft.
Use 2 forks to pull and shred the pork, disposing any fat pieces. Remove the pork to a serving dish. With a sieve, skim the leftover onion from the slow cooker and put to the pork.
Nutrition Information
Calories: 422 calories;;Total Fat: 23.1;Sodium: 786;Total Carbohydrate: 19.7;Cholesterol: 108;Protein: 28.5

151. Busy Mom Lasagna

Serving: 8 | Prep: 15mins | Cook: 4hours5mins | Ready in:
Ingredients
1 pound ground beef
1/2 cup diced onion
1 (16 ounce) jar spaghetti sauce, or more to taste
1/2 (8 ounce) package cream cheese, softened
1/2 (8 ounce) container sour cream
cooking spray
1 (12 ounce) package wide egg noodles
1 1/2 cups shredded mozzarella cheese
1 1/2 cups shredded Cheddar cheese
Direction
Heat a big skillet over medium heat. Cook while stirring the onion and beef in the hot skillet, for 5-7 minutes, until the onions becomes soft and the beef becomes brown. Strain and remove the grease.
In the skillet, put sour cream, cream cheese, and the spaghetti sauce. Stir well.
Spray the cooking spray onto a 5-quart slow cooker. In the slow cooker, layer the noodles, beef mixture and cheeses. Repeat the process, if needed, until the cooker is full.
Cook while covering for 2 hours on high. Turn to low and cook for approximately 2 more hours until the cheeses melt and the noodles become tender.
Nutrition Information
Calories: 533 calories;;Total Fat: 28.3;Sodium: 583;Total Carbohydrate: 40.4;Cholesterol: 128;Protein: 28.5

152. Cabbage Rolls II

Serving: 6 | Prep: 30mins | Cook: 9hours | Ready in:
Ingredients
12 leaves cabbage
1 cup cooked white rice
1 egg, beaten
1/4 cup milk
1/4 cup minced onion
1 pound extra-lean ground beef
1 1/4 teaspoons salt
1 1/4 teaspoons ground black pepper

1 (8 ounce) can tomato sauce
1 tablespoon brown sugar
1 tablespoon lemon juice
1 teaspoon Worcestershire sauce
Direction
Boil water in a big pot. Put in cabbage leaves and boil for 2 minutes. Drain water.
In a big bowl, mix egg, a cup of cooked rice, pepper, salt, ground beef, milk and onion. Put about 1/4 cup of meat mixture in the middle of each cabbage leaf. Roll up the leaf and tuck the ends. Put rolls in a slow cooker.
In a small bowl, mix together Worcestershire sauce, lemon juice, brown sugar and tomato sauce. Pour mixture on top of the cabbage rolls.
Cover and cook for 8-9 hours on Low.
Nutrition Information
Calories: 246 calories;;Total Fat: 10.8;Sodium: 748;Total Carbohydrate: 18.3;Cholesterol: 83;Protein: 19

153. Cajun Roast Beef

Serving: 8 | Prep: 15mins | Cook: 8hours | Ready in:
Ingredients
2 teaspoons garlic, minced
1/2 teaspoon prepared horseradish
1 teaspoon hot pepper sauce
1 teaspoon dried thyme
1/2 teaspoon salt
1/2 teaspoon ground black pepper
2 teaspoons Cajun seasoning
2 tablespoons olive oil
2 tablespoons malt vinegar
2 pounds beef eye of round roast
Direction
In a bowl, mix together malt vinegar, olive oil, Cajun seasoning, pepper, salt, thyme, hot pepper sauce, horseradish, and garlic until completely combined. Use a meat fork to pierce all over the beef roast. In a big resealable plastic bag, put the roast. Add the marinade and flip the roast to thoroughly coat. Chill overnight, flipping sometimes if you want.
Once ready to cook, in a slow cooker, put the roast together with the leftover marinade. Do not add water. Roast on Low until reaching the doneness you want, about 8-10 hours. A meat thermometer should display 135°F (57°C) for medium-rare. Take out of the slow cooker to a serving dish and let sit before cutting across the grain, about 15 minutes.
Nutrition Information
Calories: 148 calories;;Total Carbohydrate: 1.1;Cholesterol: 36;Protein: 13.4;Total Fat: 9.7;Sodium: 311

154. Carnitas With Pico De Gallo

Serving: 10 | Prep: 20mins | Cook: 18hours10mins | Ready in:
Ingredients
1 tablespoon olive oil
6 pounds boneless pork shoulder
1 cup ground cumin
4 dried New Mexico chiles, seeded and cut into 1/2 inch pieces
1 onion, quartered
6 cloves garlic, halved
1 jalapeno pepper, seeded and minced
6 cups water
6 tomatoes, chopped
1 onion, chopped
2 tomatillos, husked and chopped
2 jalapeno pepper, seeded and minced
1/3 cup lime juice
1 tablespoon salt
1/4 teaspoon ground black pepper
Direction
Heat olive oil in big skillet on medium high heat; sear pork in hot oil for 10 minutes till browned on all sides. Put in slow cooker with 1 minced jalapeno pepper, garlic, quartered onion, New Mexico chiles and cumin; put water in, cover; cook for 6-8 hours on high. Lower heat to low; cook for 12-16 hours till pork is easily shredded and tender. When cooked, transfer veggies and pork to big bowl; use 2 forks to finely shred. Mix enough cooking liquid in to moisten meat to your preference.
2-6 hours before carnitas are ready, prep pico de gallo. Mix 2 minced jalapeno peppers, tomatillos, onion and tomatoes in mixing bowl. Season with pepper, salt and lime juice; stir well. Refrigerate till needed.
Nutrition Information
Calories: 635 calories;;Sodium: 864;Total Carbohydrate: 14;Cholesterol: 174;Protein: 56.4;Total Fat: 38.9

155. Charley's Slow Cooker Mexican Style Pork

Serving: 12 | Prep: 10mins | Cook: 8hours10mins | Ready in:
Ingredients
1 (4 pound) boneless pork loin roast, trimmed of fat
1 teaspoon salt
1 teaspoon ground black pepper
2 tablespoons olive oil
1 large onion, chopped
1 1/4 cups diced green chile pepper
1 (5 ounce) bottle hot pepper sauce
1 teaspoon chili powder
1 teaspoon cayenne pepper
1 teaspoon garlic powder
2 cups water, or as needed
Direction
Season pork roast with ground black pepper and salt on all sides.
Heat olive oil over medium - high heat in a big skillet. Cook roast for 3 to 5 minutes per side in hot oil until browned; move to a slow cooker.
Top roast with garlic powder, cayenne pepper, chili powder, hot pepper sauce, chili pepper and chopped onion. Add enough water into the slow cooker to reach 1/3 of the way up the sides of the roast.
Cook for 6 hours on High, put in more water if the mixture becomes too dry. Decrease heat to Low then cook for another 2 to 4 hours, until meat is soft and falls apart. Move the roast to a bowl and shred the meat with 2 forks. Return the meat to the slow cooker with 2 cups of cooking liquid.
Nutrition Information
Calories: 162 calories;;Sodium: 303;Total Carbohydrate: 3.3;Cholesterol: 53;Protein: 18.2;Total Fat: 8.3

156. Cheesy Italian Tortellini

Serving: 6 | Prep: 15mins | Cook: 8hours15mins | Ready in:
Ingredients
1/2 pound ground beef
1/2 pound Italian sausage, casings removed

1 (16 ounce) jar marinara sauce
1 (4.5 ounce) can sliced mushrooms
1 (14.5 ounce) can Italian-style diced tomatoes, undrained
1 (9 ounce) package refrigerated or fresh cheese tortellini
1 cup shredded mozzarella cheese
1/2 cup shredded Cheddar cheese

Direction
In a large skillet, crumble the Italian sausage and the ground beef. Cook it on medium-high heat until the mixture has browned and drain. In a slow cooker, mix the mushrooms, ground meats, tomatoes and marinara sauce. Cover and for 7 to 8 hours cook on low heat.
Slowly stir in the tortellini, sprinkle cheddar cheese and mozzarella on the top. Cover, and for 15 more minutes cook on low, or until the tortellini turns tender.

Nutrition Information
Calories: 468 calories;;Total Fat: 24.1;Sodium: 1186;Total Carbohydrate: 35.2;Cholesterol: 82;Protein: 26.9

157. Chicken Delicious

Serving: 12 | Prep: 10mins | Cook: 4hours | Ready in:
Ingredients
10 skinless, boneless chicken breast halves
1 teaspoon fresh lemon juice
salt and pepper to taste
1/8 teaspoon celery salt
1 teaspoon paprika
1 (10.75 ounce) can condensed cream of mushroom soup
1 (10.75 ounce) can condensed cream of celery soup
1/3 cup dry sherry
1/4 cup grated Parmesan cheese

Direction
Wash chicken breasts and pat them dry. Use the paprika, celery salt, salt, pepper, and lemon juice to season to taste. Add into the slow cooker.
In the medium-sized bowl, combine celery and mushroom soups along with wine or sherry. Add the mixture on top of chicken breasts and dust with the grated Parmesan cheese.
Cook over LOW setting for 8 - 10 hours, OR over HIGH setting for 4 - 5 hours.

Nutrition Information
Calories: 154 calories;;Sodium: 479;Total Carbohydrate: 4.7;Cholesterol: 55;Protein: 20.5;Total Fat: 5.1

158. Chicken Livers Fandango

Serving: 4 | Prep: 45mins | Cook: 6hours | Ready in:
Ingredients
1/2 cup all-purpose flour for coating
1 teaspoon salt
1/4 teaspoon pepper
1 pound chicken livers, trimmed and cut into bite sized pieces
3 slices bacon
3 green onions, chopped
1 cup chicken stock
1 (10.75 ounce) can condensed golden mushroom soup
1 (4.5 ounce) can sliced mushrooms, drained
1/4 cup dry white wine

Direction
Combine together the pepper, salt and flour in a medium bowl. Into the seasoned flour, put the chicken livers, and coat by tossing.
In a big skillet over medium-high heat, put the bacon. Fry till crisp and browned. Take off to paper towels and allow to drain. From the livers, shake excess flour off, and fry using grease of bacon together with green onions till browned lightly on the outside. Into the skillet, put the chicken stock, and mix to scratch up some bits from the base.
To a slow cooker, put the mixture, and crumble in bacon. Mix in white wine, mushrooms and golden mushroom soup. Put cover, and let cook for 4 to 6 hours on Low. Put flour to thicken the gravy if wished prior serving.

Nutrition Information
Calories: 352 calories;;Sodium: 1729;Total Carbohydrate: 21.9;Cholesterol: 428;Protein: 24.1;Total Fat: 16.7

159. Christmas Morning Oatmeal

Serving: 4 | Prep: 15mins | Cook: 8hours | Ready in:
Ingredients
1/3 cup brown sugar
2 teaspoons ground cinnamon
1 teaspoon ground nutmeg
2 Granny Smith apples - peeled, cored, and sliced 1/4 inch thick
3/4 cup dried cranberries
1/4 cup butter, cut into pieces
2 cups regular rolled oats
2 cups water
1 cup apple juice
1 cup cranberry juice
1/4 teaspoon salt
3/4 cup candied walnuts (optional)

Direction
Get a bowl and stir in cinnamon, nutmeg, and brown sugar together. Mix in the cranberries and apple, make sure that the fruits are well coated by the sugar mixture. Place this in a slow cooker along with chopped butter. Combine together the water, cranberry juice, apple juice, salt and oatmeal in a bowl. Add this mixture into the slow cooker without stirring it together. Cook for 8 hours on low heat with cover.
Before serving this dish, make sure to stir the contents, and then serve on bowls. Garnish with candied walnuts if preferred.

Nutrition Information
Calories: 621 calories;Protein: 8.5;Total Fat: 26.5;Sodium: 246;Total Carbohydrate: 94.7;Cholesterol: 31

160. Classic Beef Stroganoff In A Slow Cooker

Serving: 4 | Prep: 15mins | Cook: 8hours | Ready in:
Ingredients
1 pound top round steak, trimmed
1 (8 ounce) package sliced fresh mushrooms
1 cup chopped onion
2 tablespoons Dijon mustard
2 tablespoons chopped fresh parsley
3 cloves garlic, minced
1/2 teaspoon salt
1/2 teaspoon dried dill
1/2 teaspoon freshly ground black pepper
1/3 cup all-purpose flour (spooned and leveled)
1 cup fat-free reduced-sodium beef broth

1 (8 ounce) container reduced-fat sour cream
2 cups hot cooked egg noodles
Direction
Slice steak diagonally across the grain into a quart-inch thick strip. Arrange mushrooms, steak, mustard, parsley, onion, garlic, dill, salt, and black pepper in a 3-quart slow cooker and stir well.
In a small bowl, add flour and gradually pour in broth, then whisk until blended. Pour into the slow cooker and stir well. Put on lid and cook for an hour over high heat. Adjust heat to low and continue cooking for 7 to 8 hours, until steak is tender.
Turn off slow cooker and take off the lid. Let the dish stand for 10 minutes. Add sour cream. Serve on top of noodles.
Nutrition Information
Calories: 441 calories;;Sodium: 560;Total Carbohydrate: 38.9;Cholesterol: 105;Protein: 32.6;Total Fat: 16.8

161. Classic Chulent

Serving: 8 | Prep: 15mins | Cook: 8hours | Ready in:
Ingredients
1/2 pound cubed beef brisket
6 potatoes, diced
1/4 cup dry kidney beans
1/2 cup barley
1 onion, chopped
2 cloves garlic, minced
2 tablespoons honey
1 tablespoon ketchup
1 tablespoon barbeque sauce
1 tablespoon soy sauce
1 tablespoon onion soup mix
1 tablespoon salt
1/4 teaspoon ground black pepper
1/2 teaspoon paprika
Direction
In a 6-quart slow cooker, blend the paprika, pepper, salt, onion soup mix, soy sauce, barbeque sauce, ketchup, honey, garlic, onion, kidney beans, potatoes, and beef brisket. Cook on High for 1 hour. After that, switch to Low and keep cooking for another 7 hours.
Nutrition Information
Calories: 267 calories;Protein: 9.5;Total Fat: 4.5;Sodium: 1086;Total Carbohydrate: 48.8;Cholesterol: 12

162. Corny Ham And Potato Scallop

Serving: 6 | Prep: 20mins | Cook: 8hours | Ready in:
Ingredients
5 potatoes, peeled and cubed
1 1/2 cups cubed cooked ham
1 (15 ounce) can whole kernel corn, drained
1/4 cup chopped green bell pepper
2 teaspoons instant minced onion
1 (10.75 ounce) can condensed Cheddar cheese soup
1/2 cup milk
3 tablespoons all-purpose flour
Direction
Mix together onion, green pepper, corn, ham and potatoes in a slow cooker. Stir flour, milk and soup together in a small bowl until smooth. Pour over vegetables and ham with the soup mixture, and then stir gently to coat well.
Place a cover and cook on low setting until potatoes are soft, for 8 hours.
Nutrition Information
Calories: 335 calories;;Sodium: 1030;Total Carbohydrate: 46.8;Cholesterol: 32;Protein: 13.6;Total Fat: 11.5

163. Country Cooking Slow Cooker Neck Bones

Serving: 8 | Prep: 15mins | Cook: 4hours | Ready in:
Ingredients
3 pounds pork neck bones
1 small onion, chopped
3 cloves garlic, minced, or more to taste
1 teaspoon salt (optional)
1 teaspoon dried thyme leaves
1 tablespoon distilled white vinegar
4 cups water
Direction
In a slow cooker, put neck bones. Sprinkle in thyme leaves, salt, garlic and onion. Pour in water and vinegar.
Cook, with cover, on High for 4 hours or until meat is tender.
Nutrition Information
Calories: 518 calories;;Cholesterol: 101;Protein: 19.1;Total Fat: 47.8;Sodium: 352;Total Carbohydrate: 1.3

164. Cream Of Mushroom And Soy Sauce Pork Chops

Serving: 6 | Prep: 5mins | Cook: 7hours | Ready in:
Ingredients
1/4 cup brown sugar
6 pork chops
1 (5 ounce) bottle soy sauce
1 (10.75 ounce) can condensed cream of mushroom soup
Direction
Use brown sugar to rub pork chops, then arrange them in a shallow dish and drizzle over with soy sauce. Cover and chill chops. Let them marinate for an hour.
Put into the crock of a slow cooker with the cream of mushroom soup. Take chops out of the soy sauce and put on top of soup.
Cover and cook on low setting for 6-8 hours, until extremely tender.
Nutrition Information
Calories: 193 calories;;Total Fat: 7.2;Sodium: 1995;Total Carbohydrate: 14.6;Cholesterol: 36;Protein: 17

165. Creamy Slow Cooker Chicken And Vegetables

Serving: 4 | Prep: 20mins | Cook: 5hours | Ready in:
Ingredients
1 (26 ounce) can condensed cream of chicken with herbs
1 cup chicken broth
2/3 cup sour cream
1 teaspoon minced garlic
1/2 teaspoon seasoned salt
1/2 teaspoon Italian seasoning
1/2 teaspoon onion powder
1/4 teaspoon dried chives
1 dash Worcestershire sauce
freshly ground black pepper to taste
1 pound skinless, boneless chicken tenders
1 parsnip, peeled and finely chopped, or more to taste
1 zucchini, thinly sliced

1 cup sliced fresh mushrooms
1/2 cup coarsely shredded carrots
2 green onions, finely chopped, or more to taste
Direction
In a slow cooker, blend pepper, Worcestershire sauce, chives, onion powder, Italian seasoning, seasoned salt, garlic, sour cream, chicken broth, and chicken soup. Add chicken, ensuring it is covered with liquid. Add green onions, carrots, mushrooms, zucchini, and parsnip. Put a cover on the slow cooker.
Cook on Low for about 5 hours until the chicken is not pink in the center anymore.
Nutrition Information
Calories: 419 calories;;Total Fat: 21.8;Sodium: 1696;Total Carbohydrate: 24.6;Cholesterol: 97;Protein: 31.2

166. Creole Pork Shanks With Sweet Potato Gravy

Serving: 4 | Prep: 25mins | Cook: 6hours | Ready in:
Ingredients
2 sweet potatoes
1 teaspoon vegetable oil
4 pork shanks, cut in half
1/2 teaspoon ground black pepper
1/4 teaspoon cayenne pepper
1/4 cup olive oil
1 medium onion, chopped
3 celery ribs, chopped
1 small green bell pepper, chopped
4 garlic cloves, minced
4 cups Swanson® Chicken Broth, plus more if needed
2 (14.5 ounce) cans diced tomatoes
3 bay leaves
1 teaspoon dried thyme
1/4 teaspoon cayenne pepper
1/2 teaspoon black pepper
Direction
Preheat an oven to 175°C/350°F; rub vegetable oil on sweet potatoes. In aluminum foil, wrap.
In preheated oven, put sweet potatoes; bake for 1 hour till soft. Peel then cut into 1-in. chunks when cool enough to handle.
Season all sides of pork shanks with cayenne pepper and black pepper.
Heat olive oil in big skillet on medium-high heat; cook all sides of shanks for 10 minutes in total till all sides are nicely browned. Put pork shanks into slow cooker.
Sauté garlic, bell pepper, celery and onion in skillet, scraping browned bits from the bottom; cook on medium heat for 5 minutes till soft.
Mix diced tomatoes and 4 cups of Swanson® Chicken Broth in; boil. Add thyme and bay leaves; simmer for 10 minutes till mixture slightly reduces. Put mixture into slow cooker with pork shanks; cook for 6 hours on high till tender. Put pork shanks onto a platter; to keep warm, tent with foil.
Take 1/2 veggies out of the cooking liquid; discard/keep for another use. Put all liquid and leftover veggies into a food processor/blender; put cooked sweet potato chunks in; process for 1 minute till smooth.
Add 2 tbsp. chicken broth at a time till you get your desired gravy consistency in case the gravy is too thick.
Put sweet potato gravy on top of pork shank servings.

Nutrition Information
Calories: 421 calories;;Total Fat: 19.5;Sodium: 2270;Total Carbohydrate: 27.9;Cholesterol: 81;Protein: 33.8

167. Crock Pot Cheesy Mushroom Chicken

Serving: 6 | Prep: 10mins | Cook: 8hours | Ready in:
Ingredients
6 skinless, boneless chicken breast halves
1 (10.75 ounce) can condensed cream of chicken soup
1 (10.75 ounce) can condensed cream of mushroom soup
1/2 cup cooking sherry
1 teaspoon minced garlic
1 teaspoon celery flakes
1/2 teaspoon paprika
1/2 cup grated Parmesan cheese
1 (8 ounce) can mushroom pieces, drained
Direction
In a slow cooker, put chicken breasts. Whisk paprika, celery flakes, garlic, sherry, cream of mushroom soup and cream of chicken soup in a mixing bowl. Mix in mushroom pieces and parmesan cheese; put on chicken.
Cook for 8 hours on low till sauce slightly reduces and chicken is tender.
Nutrition Information
Calories: 267 calories;;Total Carbohydrate: 12.6;Cholesterol: 71;Protein: 28.2;Total Fat: 10.4;Sodium: 1091

168. Crock Pot Portobello Chicken

Serving: 4 | Prep: 10mins | Cook: 6hours | Ready in:
Ingredients
4 frozen bone-in chicken breast halves
8 portobello mushroom caps
1 (8 ounce) bottle Italian-style salad dressing
1 (8 ounce) package angel hair pasta
Direction
In a slow cooker, place in the frozen chicken breasts and lay the mushroom caps on top of the chicken with half of the mushrooms facing up, then drizzle with the dressing over the chicken and mushrooms caps.
Cover the slow cooker, turning it on to a low setting, and cook for 6 hours until the chicken breasts are no longer pink at the bone and its juices run clear.
Minutes before you serve, heat a big pot of lightly salted water over high heat until it comes to a rolling boil, adding in the angel hair pasta and bring back to boiling. Boil the pasta uncovered, occasionally stirring, for 4-5 minutes until cooked through but still firm to the bite. Use a colander and drain well, setting it in the sink.
Portion out the hot, cooked pasta into 4 plates and top each with a chicken breast and two of the mushroom caps, drizzling with the sauce over the top.
Nutrition Information
Calories: 628 calories;;Sodium: 1155;Total Carbohydrate: 48.2;Cholesterol: 128;Protein: 58.6;Total Fat: 23

169. Cuban Style Pork And Sweet Potatoes

Serving: 6 | Prep: 15mins | Cook: 6hours | Ready in:
Ingredients
1 1/2 pounds sweet potatoes, cut into 1/2-inch cubes
1 pound pork, cut into 1-inch squares

1 (15 ounce) can diced tomatoes with green chile peppers
1/4 cup orange juice
1 1/2 tablespoons lime juice
2 cloves garlic, pressed
1/4 teaspoon ground cumin
1/4 teaspoon salt
1/4 teaspoon ground black pepper
1/4 cup chopped fresh cilantro, or to taste
Direction
In a slow cooker, combine together diced tomatoes along with green chile peppers, sweet potatoes, garlic, pork, orange juice, black pepper, lime juice, salt and cumin.
Let cook on Low heat for six hours. Stud with cilantro.
Nutrition Information
Calories: 266 calories;Protein: 17.4;Total Fat: 9.7;Sodium: 483;Total Carbohydrate: 27.3;Cholesterol: 48

170. Cyndee's Best Slow Cooker Italian Pot Roast

Serving: 6 | Prep: 20mins | Cook: 8hours | Ready in:
Ingredients
3 1/2 pounds top round steak
1 large onion, diced
2 celery ribs, finely chopped
1 red bell pepper, seeded and diced
1 green bell pepper, seeded and diced
1 (1 ounce) packet dry au jus mix
4 cups water, or amount to cover
Direction
In a slow cooker, position the pot roast. Put in the au jus mix, red and green bell peppers, celery, and onion, then cover the meat with enough water. Cook while covered on Low for 8 hours or until tender.
Nutrition Information
Calories: 504 calories;;Total Fat: 25;Sodium: 688;Total Carbohydrate: 8;Cholesterol: 161;Protein: 57.7

171. Dad's Home With The Kids Slow Cooker Roast

Serving: 8 | Prep: 10mins | Cook: 5hours40mins | Ready in:
Ingredients
1 (14 ounce) can beef broth
1/2 cup soy sauce
1/2 cup olive oil
1/3 cup lemon juice
5 tablespoons Worcestershire sauce
2 teaspoons minced garlic
2 tablespoons garlic powder, preferably roasted
2 tablespoons dried basil
2 tablespoons dried parsley
1 tablespoon ground black pepper
1 tablespoon vegetable oil
1 (5 pound) beef chuck roast, patted dry with paper towels
1 cup baby carrots
1 cup uncooked elbow macaroni
Direction
Add these liquids: Worcestershire sauce, lemon juice, olive oil, soy sauce and beef broth together with these dry ingredients: black pepper, parsley, basil, garlic powder and garlic into a blender. Close the lid and press the pulse button on your blender a few times, then start blending thoroughly for 20 seconds.

In a large skillet, add the vegetable oil and heat until hot over medium-high heat. When a faint wisp of smoke rises, add roast and brown it on all sides for 2-3 minutes each side. Transfer the roast into a slow cooker. Pour in the beef broth mixture in the blender, cover and cook in Medium setting.
Cook until desired tenderness for 5-6 hours, put the carrots in and cover the cooker and cook for 10 more minutes, then add the macaroni. Mix well. Keep simmering, covered for 20 minutes, until carrots and macaroni are tender. Cut the beef and serve with carrot, macaroni and sauce.
Nutrition Information
Calories: 648 calories;;Sodium: 1266;Total Carbohydrate: 18.1;Cholesterol: 129;Protein: 37.4;Total Fat: 46.8

172. Delicious Beef Tongue Tacos

Serving: 20 | Prep: 15mins | Cook: 8hours15mins | Ready in:
Ingredients
1 beef tongue
1/2 white onion, sliced
5 cloves garlic, crushed
1 bay leaf
salt to taste
3 tablespoons vegetable oil
5 Roma tomatoes
5 serrano peppers
salt to taste
1/2 onion, diced
2 (10 ounce) packages corn tortillas
Direction
In a slow cooker, put the beef tongue and pour water to cover. Add the bay leaf, garlic and slices of onion, then add salt to season. Put cover on and cook for 8 hours or overnight on low. Take out the tongue and shred the meat into strands.
In a skillet, heat the oil on medium heat. Cook the peppers and tomatoes in the hot oil until all sides become soft. Transfer the peppers and tomatoes in a blender and keep the oil on the heat, then add salt to season. Briefly blend until still a bit chunky. In the skillet, cook the diced onion until it becomes translucent; mix in the tomato mixture. Cook for an additional 5-6 minutes. Assemble the tacos by putting the shredded tongue meat into a tortilla and scooping the salsa on top of the meat.
Nutrition Information
Calories: 227 calories;;Total Fat: 14;Sodium: 46;Total Carbohydrate: 14;Cholesterol: 66;Protein: 11.4

173. Easy Corned Beef And Cabbage

Serving: 6 | Prep: 15mins | Cook: 8hours | Ready in:
Ingredients
1 onion, cut into wedges
4 potatoes, peeled and quartered
1 pound carrots, cut into large chunks
3 cups water
3 cloves garlic, minced
1 bay leaf
2 tablespoons sugar
2 tablespoons cider vinegar
1/2 teaspoon ground black pepper
1 (3 pound) corned beef brisket with spice packet, cut in half
1 small head cabbage, cut into wedges
Direction

Put carrots, potatoes and onion in 5-qt. slow cooker. Mix spice packet contents, vinegar, sugar, bay leaf, garlic and water; put on veggies. Put cabbage and brisket over.
Cover; cook till veggies and meat are tender for 8-9 hours on low. Before serving, remove bay leaf.
Nutrition Information
Calories: 647 calories;;Sodium: 2852;Total Carbohydrate: 45.8;Cholesterol: 123;Protein: 38.8;Total Fat: 34.3

174. Easy Ground Beef Stroganoff

Serving: 6 | Prep: 15mins | Cook: 1hours | Ready in:
Ingredients
2 pounds ground beef
2 onions, chopped
1 clove garlic, minced
1 (4.5 ounce) can mushrooms, drained
2 teaspoons salt
1/4 teaspoon ground black pepper
2 cups hot water
6 cubes beef bouillon
4 tablespoons tomato paste
1 1/2 cups water
4 tablespoons all-purpose flour
Direction
On medium-high heat, heat a big pan; sauté mushrooms, ground beef, garlic, and onions until the onion is golden brown. Sprinkle black pepper and salt.
Mix in tomato paste, bouillon cubes, and two cups of hot water in the meat mixture. Whisk flour and 1 1/2 cups of cold water together; mix into the pan. Turn to low heat and let it simmer for an hour.
Nutrition Information
Calories: 524 calories;;Total Fat: 40.5;Sodium: 1923;Total Carbohydrate: 11.3;Cholesterol: 129;Protein: 27.6

175. Easy Overnight Oatmeal

Serving: 8 | Prep: 10mins | Cook: 7hours | Ready in:
Ingredients
non-stick cooking spray
4 cups almond milk
2 cups steel-cut oats
2 cups chopped apples
1 cup raisins
1 cup chopped walnuts
1/2 cup brown sugar
2 tablespoons melted butter
1 teaspoon ground cinnamon
1/2 teaspoon salt
Direction
Use cooking spray to coat the inner part of a slow cooker.
In the prepared slow cooker, mix salt, cinnamon, butter, brown sugar, walnuts, raisins, apples, oats, and almond milk.
Cook for 7-8 hours on Low heat.
Nutrition Information
Calories: 434 calories;;Cholesterol: 8;Protein: 8.5;Total Fat: 16.4;Sodium: 252;Total Carbohydrate: 67.6

176. Easy Slow Cooker Carne Guisada

Serving: 8 | Prep: 30mins | Cook: 6hours | Ready in:
Ingredients
3 pounds chuck roast, cut into 1 1/2-inch cubes
3 medium potatoes, unpeeled and diced
1 medium onion, chopped
2 red bell peppers, cut into strips
3 cloves garlic, crushed
1/4 cup all-purpose flour
1/4 cup chili powder
1 teaspoon cumin
1 teaspoon salt
3 cups beef broth
Direction
In a large bowl, blend garlic, peppers, onion, potatoes and beef together. Combine salt, cumin, chili powder and flour in a small bowl. Toss beef mixture and flour mixture together to coat evenly. Bring mixture into a slow cooker, then add in enough beef broth until meat is barely covered in liquid. In case there isn't enough broth, fill the rest of the way with water as a substitute.
Cook beef for 6-8 hours on low until softened.
Nutrition Information
Calories: 366 calories;;Total Fat: 19.8;Sodium: 682;Total Carbohydrate: 22.7;Cholesterol: 77;Protein: 24

177. Easy Slow Cooker Chicken Curry With Potatoes And Coconut Milk

Serving: 4 | Prep: 15mins | Cook: 4hours | Ready in:
Ingredients
3 skinless, boneless chicken breasts, cubed
4 small (3 ounce) potatoes, peeled and cubed
1 red bell pepper, cored and sliced into 1/4-inch strips
1/2 onion, chopped
2 cups chicken broth
2 tablespoons mild curry powder
1 teaspoon red curry paste
1 teaspoon ground cumin
1 teaspoon salt, or more to taste
1/2 teaspoon cayenne pepper, or to taste
1 (14 ounce) can coconut milk
freshly ground black pepper
1/4 cup chopped fresh cilantro (optional)
Direction
In a slow cooker, mix together onion, bell pepper, potatoes and chicken.
In a bowl, mix together chicken broth, cayenne, 1 teaspoon salt , cumin, curry paste and curry powder and pour over ingredients in the slow cooker. Use a wooden spoon to mix well everything.
Close the slow cooker and cook for 4 to 5 hours on Low or 2 to 3 hours on High, until chicken gets tender. Pour in coconut milk 15 minutes before the cooking time runs out and keep cooking until heated through. Use salt and pepper to season and scatter on top with chopped cilantro to serve.
Nutrition Information
Calories: 387 calories;;Total Carbohydrate: 23.9;Cholesterol: 49;Protein: 22.5;Total Fat: 23.8;Sodium: 1248

178. Easy Slow Cooker Chicken Thighs With Honey

Serving: 4 | Prep: 15mins | Cook: 6hours10mins | Ready in:
Ingredients
1 teaspoon ground cumin
1/2 teaspoon dried thyme
1/2 teaspoon paprika
8 skinless, boneless chicken thighs

2 teaspoons vegetable oil
3 cloves garlic, finely chopped
1/4 cup good-quality honey
2 tablespoons Dijon mustard
1/2 cup chicken broth
salt and freshly ground black pepper to taste
Direction
In a small bowl, mix together the paprika, thyme and cumin and rub spice mix onto all sides of the chicken thighs.
In a frying pan, heat the oil on medium heat and cook the chicken for about 10 minutes, until all sides turn brown. In a slow cooker, put the chicken, then cover it with chopped garlic.
In a small bowl, mix together the mustard and honey and pour it on top of the chicken. Pour in the chicken broth, then close the slow cooker.
Let it cook for around 6 hours on low, until the chicken becomes cooked through. Sprinkle with pepper and salt to season.
Nutrition Information
Calories: 375 calories;;Sodium: 572;Total Carbohydrate: 20.4;Cholesterol: 192;Protein: 45.7;Total Fat: 11.5

179. Easy Slow Cooker Swiss Steak

Serving: 8 | Prep: 10mins | Cook: 9hours15mins | Ready in:
Ingredients
2 pounds beef stew meat, cut into 1-inch pieces
1/4 cup steak sauce (such as A1®)
1 onion, sliced
1 (14.5 ounce) can diced tomatoes
2 tablespoons flour
1/4 cup water
Direction
Put beef stew meat into the bottom of a slow cooker. Pour steak sauce on top of the beef along with tomatoes and onion.
Let it cook for 9-10 hours on Low.
In a small bowl, whisk flour into the water then stir into the liquid in slow cooker. Cook for 10-15 minutes until the liquid thickens.
Nutrition Information
Calories: 279 calories;;Cholesterol: 98;Protein: 34.6;Total Fat: 11.3;Sodium: 271;Total Carbohydrate: 7

180. Easy Sweet And Spicy Meatballs

Serving: 10 | Prep: 5mins | Cook: 4hours | Ready in:
Ingredients
3 (12 ounce) jars taco sauce
2 cups grape jelly
30 prepared meatballs
Direction
Pour grape jelly and taco sauce into a slow cooker; whisk properly to integrate the jelly into the sauce.
Carefully drop meatballs into the jelly sauce.
Cook on low for around 4 hours, till the meatballs are flavorful and tender and the sauce is warm.
Nutrition Information
Calories: 383 calories;;Total Carbohydrate: 56.2;Cholesterol: 70;Protein: 14.1;Total Fat: 10.8;Sodium: 708

181. Eaton's Easy Pulled Pork

Serving: 10 | Prep: 15mins | Cook: 8hours | Ready in:
Ingredients
1 onion, thinly sliced
4 1/2 pounds bone-in pork loin end roast
salt and ground black pepper to taste
3/4 cup cider vinegar
1/4 cup water
1/2 (18 ounce) bottle hickory brown sugar barbeque sauce
3 tablespoons brown sugar, or to taste
Direction
In the bottom of a slow cooker, arrange onion slices. Sprinkle pork with pepper and salt to season and pour over onion. Pour in water and vinegar.
Cook pork for 8 hours on Low. Bring pork to a platter and use 2 forks to shred. Take out and throw away about 1/2 the pork juices from slow cooker and mix in brown sugar, barbeque sauce, and shredded pork.
Nutrition Information
Calories: 270 calories;;Cholesterol: 71;Protein: 23.6;Total Fat: 12.1;Sodium: 341;Total Carbohydrate: 14.3

182. Egg, Spinach, And Mushroom Slow Cooker Casserole

Serving: 8 | Prep: 15mins | Cook: 6hours | Ready in:
Ingredients
1 (24 ounce) carton cottage cheese
6 eggs
1/3 cup all-purpose flour
3 tablespoons chopped onion
2 tablespoons melted butter
1/2 teaspoon salt
1/4 teaspoon ground black pepper
2 cups shredded Cheddar cheese
1 (8 ounce) package sliced fresh mushrooms
1 (7 ounce) bag fresh spinach
Direction
In a bowl, stir together pepper, salt, butter, onion, flour, eggs and cottage cheese. Stir in spinach, mushrooms and Cheddar cheese.
Into a slow cooker, put the mixture. Cook on Low with a cover, for 6 to 8 hours till eggs are firm.
Nutrition Information
Calories: 313 calories;;Total Carbohydrate: 9.1;Cholesterol: 190;Protein: 24.6;Total Fat: 20.1;Sodium: 760

183. Havana Slow Cooker Pork Tenderloin

Serving: 6 | Prep: 10mins | Cook: 6hours | Ready in:
Ingredients
1 onion, sliced
3 pounds pork tenderloin
3 tablespoons minced garlic
1/2 cup orange juice
3 tablespoons red wine vinegar
1 lemon, juiced
1 tablespoon ground cumin
1 tablespoon grill seasoning (such as Montreal Steak Seasoning®)
1 teaspoon salt
1 teaspoon ground red pepper
3 bay leaves
2 tablespoons grated lemon peel
Direction
Spread slices of onion on the bottom of a slow cooker and then place pork tenderloin on top. Drizzle garlic evenly atop pork and onion. Pour lemon juice, orange juice and vinegar atop pork. Drizzle cumin, lemon zest, grill seasoning, bay leaves, salt and red pepper atop pork.

Cover and let to cook on Low heat for about 6 to 7 hours until the pork is very tender. To serve, cut tenderloin into 1 1/2-inch pieces, spread on a platter and sprinkle juices all over the top.
Nutrition Information
Calories: 225 calories;;Cholesterol: 98;Protein: 36.1;Total Fat: 5.1;Sodium: 927;Total Carbohydrate: 7.3

184. Honey Ribs

Serving: 6 | Prep: 10mins | Cook: 5hours | Ready in:
Ingredients
1 (10.5 ounce) can beef broth
3 tablespoons honey mustard
1/4 cup honey
1/2 cup water
1/4 cup honey barbeque sauce
1/4 cup soy sauce
1/4 cup maple syrup
3 pounds baby back pork ribs
Direction
Combine the maple syrup, water, honey, beef broth, soy sauce, barbeque sauce, and honey mustard in the slow cooker's crook. Cut the ribs apart, making sure to leave an equal amount of meat on all of the sides of the bone. Arrange the ribs into the slow cooker so the ribs should be covered with the sauce. You may add a little water or beef broth to cover the ribs if the sauce isn't enough.
Cover the slow cooker; cook the ribs on high setting for 5 hours until they fall off easily from the bones.
Nutrition Information
Calories: 627 calories;Protein: 44.9;Total Fat: 37.7;Sodium: 1141;Total Carbohydrate: 29;Cholesterol: 170

185. Honey Baked Spiral Ham In The Slow Cooker

Serving: 12 | Prep: 10mins | Cook: 6hours8mins | Ready in:
Ingredients
cooking spray
1 (8 pound) spiral-cut ham, or more to taste
1/2 cup honey
1/2 cup brown sugar
2 tablespoons spicy brown mustard
1/2 teaspoon ground cinnamon
1/4 teaspoon ground nutmeg
1/3 cup water
2 tablespoons cornstarch
1 tablespoon water
Direction
Spritz cooking spray on the slow cooker insert and put the ham inside.
In a saucepan, mix together the nutmeg, cinnamon, mustard, brown sugar and honey on medium heat. Let it cook for 2-5 minutes, whisking thoroughly, until the ingredients are blended, and the sugar has melted. Take it out of the heat.
Pour the water in the bottom of the slow cooker, then pour the sauce on top of the ham; put cover.
Let it cook for 6-8 hours in the slow cooker on Low and baste it with juices coming from the bottom once every 1 hour.
Take out the ham from the slow cooker. Pour the juices coming from the bottom to the saucepan on medium heat. In a bowl, combine the water and cornstarch and pour on the saucepan. Let it cook for 6-8 minutes, until the mixture thickens and becomes a glaze. Use the glaze as a gravy or pour it on top of the ham.
Nutrition Information
Calories: 437 calories;;Sodium: 3005;Total Carbohydrate: 22.1;Cholesterol: 123;Protein: 56.3;Total Fat: 12.5

186. IPA Corned Beef

Serving: 10 | Prep: 10mins | Cook: 8hours | Ready in:
Ingredients
1 (4 pound) corned beef brisket with spice packet
1 tablespoon spicy brown mustard
2 cloves garlic, minced
22 fluid ounces IPA beer (such as Lagunitas® Wilco Tango Foxtrot)
Direction
Use spicy brown mustard to coat corned beef; put in slow cooker, fat-side down. Add seasoning packed and garlic to corned beef; put beer in, completely covering beef.
Cook for 8 hours on low. Take corned beef from slow cooker; rest before slicing across grain for 15 minutes.
Nutrition Information
Calories: 234 calories;;Total Carbohydrate: 3;Cholesterol: 80;Protein: 15.2;Total Fat: 15.5;Sodium: 943

187. Italian Beef In A Bucket

Serving: 12 | Prep: 5mins | Cook: 18hours | Ready in:
Ingredients
3 1/2 pounds rump roast
1 (12 ounce) jar pickled mixed vegetables
1 (16 ounce) jar pepperoncini
1 (.7 ounce) package dry Italian-style salad dressing mix
1 (10.5 ounce) can beef broth
Direction
Put the roast in a slow cooker (3 1/2 quarts in size) and add the beef broth, Italian dressing blend, pepperoncini and pickled mixed vegetables. Blend to mix, cover, and cook for 18 hours on low (18 hours - a light timer functions well if you do not want to stay up until midnight to switch it on).
To serve, take the roast out of the slow cooker. Cut it for sandwiches if necessary, but it usually breaks apart. In a bowl, put the pepperoncini and pickled vegetables to serve with the meat.
Nutrition Information
Calories: 301 calories;;Total Fat: 19.2;Sodium: 1240;Total Carbohydrate: 3.4;Cholesterol: 81;Protein: 26.9

188. Jennie's Heavenly Slow Cooker Chicken

Serving: 4 | Prep: 5mins | Cook: 4hours | Ready in:
Ingredients
2 tablespoons butter
1 (.7 ounce) package dry Italian-style salad dressing mix
1 (10.75 ounce) can condensed golden mushroom soup
1 (8 ounce) container chive and onion cream cheese
1/2 cup dry white wine
4 skinless, boneless chicken breast halves
Direction
In a saucepan, melt butter over medium heat, and mix in wine, cream cheese, mushroom soup, and salad dressing mix until the sauce mixture is

thoroughly blended, smooth, and hot. In the bottom of a slow cooker, put the chicken breasts; add pour the sauce mixture over the chicken. Put the lid on slow cooker and cook on Low setting for 4 hours until the chicken is soft.
Nutrition Information
Calories: 456 calories;;Total Carbohydrate: 13;Cholesterol: 133;Protein: 26;Total Fat: 28.3;Sodium: 1672

189. Jenny's Cuban Style Slow Cooker Chicken Fricassee

Serving: 8 | Prep: 15mins | Cook: 8hours | Ready in:
Ingredients
1 large onion, chopped
6 cloves garlic, chopped
1/2 green bell pepper, chopped
8 small whole peeled potatoes
1 (8 ounce) can tomato sauce
1/2 cup dry white wine
1/2 tablespoon cumin
1 leaf fresh sage
salt and pepper to taste
2 pounds chicken leg quarters
Direction
Mix potatoes, bell pepper, onion, and garlic in a medium bowl. Mix in wine and tomato sauce. Season with pepper, salt, cumin, and sage leaf. Transfer the chicken legs into the slow cooker and spread the mixture atop chicken. Cover and let cook on Low heat for about 6 to 8 hours until the juice runs clear.
Nutrition Information
Calories: 316 calories;;Total Fat: 14;Sodium: 245;Total Carbohydrate: 21;Cholesterol: 94;Protein: 23.3

190. Julia's Easy Slow Cooker Chicken

Serving: 5 | Prep: | Cook: | Ready in:
Ingredients
8 skinless, boneless chicken breast halves
4 potatoes, cubed
1 (10.75 ounce) can condensed cream of mushroom soup
1 1/3 cups milk
1 tablespoon cornstarch
1 (1 ounce) package dry onion soup mix
Direction
In a slow cooker, put potatoes and chicken pieces. Mix dry soup mix, cornstarch, milk and soup; put on potatoes and chicken. Cook on low for 8-10 hours. Serve.
Nutrition Information
Calories: 444 calories;Protein: 50.5;Total Fat: 7.5;Sodium: 1048;Total Carbohydrate: 41.9;Cholesterol: 115

191. Kalua Pig In A Slow Cooker

Serving: 12 | Prep: 10mins | Cook: 20hours | Ready in:
Ingredients
1 (6 pound) pork butt roast
1 1/2 tablespoons Hawaiian sea salt
1 tablespoon liquid smoke flavoring
Direction
Use a carving fork to pierce pork all over. Use salt to rub with and then the liquid smoke on meat. Transfer roast in a slow cooker.
Cook on low for 16-20 hours, covered, flipping once during cooking time. Take the meat from slow cooker and shred, putting drippings as necessary to dampen.
Nutrition Information
Calories: 243 calories;;Total Fat: 14.7;Sodium: 715;Total Carbohydrate: 0;Cholesterol: 82;Protein: 25.9

192. Kathy's Roast And Vegetables

Serving: 8 | Prep: 25mins | Cook: 8hours20mins | Ready in:
Ingredients
1 (3 pound) bottom round roast
ground black pepper to taste
garlic powder to taste
1 tablespoon vegetable oil
2 (10.75 ounce) cans condensed cream of mushroom soup
1 (1 ounce) package dry onion soup mix
5 carrots, peeled and sliced into 1 inch pieces
6 small new potatoes, halved
Direction
Use garlic powder and black pepper to season the roast. On medium heat, heat the oil in a big pot. Cook the roast until browned on all sides, about 20 minutes.
In a slow cooker, mix the onion soup mix and the mushroom soup together. Move the roast into slow cooker and surround the meat with potatoes and carrots. Cover it up and adjust the heat setting to low. Cook for 6 to 8 hours, stirring from time to time.
Nutrition Information
Calories: 310 calories;;Sodium: 952;Total Carbohydrate: 22.3;Cholesterol: 71;Protein: 26.6;Total Fat: 12.5

193. Kay Kay's Pulled Pork

Serving: 10 | Prep: 20mins | Cook: 6hours | Ready in:
Ingredients
3 tablespoons brown sugar
1 tablespoon salt
1 tablespoon paprika
1 tablespoon ground black pepper
1 tablespoon cayenne pepper
2 tablespoons white sugar
1 dash garlic powder
1 dash onion powder
1 (4 pound) pork shoulder roast (butt roast)
water to cover (optional)
1 (18 ounce) bottle barbeque sauce
Direction
In a bowl, stir together onion powder, garlic powder, white sugar, cayenne pepper, black pepper, paprika, salt and brown sugar until evenly blended. Rub over the pork with the spice mixture. Wrap plastic wrap around the pork to cover and chill for a minimum of 60 minutes, ideally overnight.
In a slow cooker, put the pork and pour in enough water to just cover the pork. Put the lid on and cook for 6-8 hours on Low or for 4 hours on High.
Remove the pork to a big bowl and use 2 forks to shred; dispose any excess fat, skin and bone. Strain and save the cooking liquid from the slow cooker. Put the shredded pork back into the slow cooker and mix in barbeque sauce.
Lower the heat to low and cook for another 2 hours. Moisten the pork to taste by pouring in an enough amount of the saved cooking liquid.
Nutrition Information
Calories: 339 calories;Protein: 18.8;Total Fat: 17.4;Sodium: 1319;Total Carbohydrate: 26;Cholesterol: 72

194. Low Fat Slow Cooker Glazed Meatloaf

Serving: 6 | Prep: 15mins | Cook: 7hours | Ready in:
Ingredients
cooking spray
1 1/2 pounds ground round beef
1 pound ground turkey breast
3/4 cup unseasoned dry bread crumbs
1 (1 ounce) package dry onion soup mix
1 tablespoon parsley flakes
1/2 teaspoon ground black pepper
1/4 teaspoon garlic powder
3 eggs, slightly beaten
1/4 cup ketchup
1 tablespoon Dijon mustard
3 tablespoons ketchup, or to taste
1 tablespoon brown sugar
Direction
Use cooking spray to grease a slow cooker.
In a bowl, mix together the turkey and ground round and mix until completely blended. Mix in the garlic powder, black pepper, parsley flakes, soup mix and breadcrumbs. Add mustard, 1/4 cup ketchup and eggs, then stir well. Shape the meat mixture into a loaf, then put it in a slow cooker. Let it cook for 6 hours on high, until no visible pink color in the middle. An inserted instant-read thermometer in the middle must read at least 70°C (160°F).
To make the glaze, in a small bowl, combine the brown sugar and 3 tbsp ketchup. Spread it on top of the meatloaf and keep on cooking for about 1 hour more, until the glaze becomes set.
Nutrition Information
Calories: 440 calories;;Total Fat: 19.2;Sodium: 887;Total Carbohydrate: 20.4;Cholesterol: 195;Protein: 44.3

195. Melt In Your Mouth Meat Loaf

Serving: 6 | Prep: 15mins | Cook: 5hours15mins | Ready in:
Ingredients
2 eggs
3/4 cup milk
2/3 cup seasoned bread crumbs
2 teaspoons dried minced onion
1 teaspoon salt
1/2 teaspoon rubbed sage
1/2 cup sliced fresh mushrooms
1 1/2 pounds ground beef
1/4 cup ketchup
2 tablespoons brown sugar
1 teaspoon ground mustard
1/2 teaspoon Worcestershire sauce
Direction
In a big bowl, mix mushrooms, sage, salt, onion, breadcrumbs, milk and eggs then crush ground beef on the mixture and stir it well until combined. Use the mixture to form a round loaf and put it on a 5-quart slow cooker. Cover it then adjust the setting to low and cook for 5-6 hours. It is ready when a meat thermometer registers at 71°F or 160°F.
In a small bowl, whisk Worcestershire sauce, mustard, brown sugar and ketchup together. Ladle this on the meat loaf and place it back in the slow cooker. Adjust the setting to low and cook until thoroughly heated, around 15 minutes. Leave it rest for 10 minutes before slicing.
Nutrition Information
Calories: 328 calories;;Sodium: 841;Total Carbohydrate: 18.4;Cholesterol: 136;Protein: 24.7;Total Fat: 16.9

196. Melt In Your Mouth Beef Cacciatore

Serving: 8 | Prep: 15mins | Cook: 6hours5mins | Ready in:
Ingredients
2 tablespoons olive oil
1 (2 1/2 pound) boneless beef chuck roast
3 tablespoons chopped garlic
salt and ground black pepper to taste
2 onions, cut into wedges and sliced
1 (28 ounce) can crushed tomatoes
1 (15 ounce) can diced tomatoes
1 1/2 cups water
1 green bell pepper, coarsely chopped
1 cup quartered fresh mushrooms
1 cup dry red wine (such as Cabernet or Merlot)
1 tablespoon white sugar
1 teaspoon fennel seed
1 teaspoon Italian seasoning
1 teaspoon dried thyme
Direction
In a big saucepan, heat olive oil over medium-high temperature. Include garlic and roast; season roast with pepper and salt. Cook roast about 5 minutes until all sides brown.
Move roast and garlic into a slow cooker; put in Italian seasoning, fennel seed, sugar, red wine, mushrooms, green bell pepper, water, diced tomatoes, crushed tomatoes, onions, and thyme. Cook over Low heat in 6 hours.
Nutrition Information
Calories: 349 calories;;Total Fat: 19.5;Sodium: 279;Total Carbohydrate: 18.9;Cholesterol: 65;Protein: 20

197. Monterey Spaghetti

Serving: 8 | Prep: | Cook: | Ready in:
Ingredients
4 ounces spaghetti, broken into pieces
1 egg
1 cup sour cream
1/4 cup grated Parmesan cheese
1/8 teaspoon crushed garlic
3 cups shredded Monterey Jack cheese
1 (10 ounce) package frozen chopped spinach, thawed and drained
1/2 (6 ounce) can French fried onions
Direction
Cook spaghetti in boiling salted water in a big pot until al dente. Strain.
Combine minced garlic, grated Parmesan cheese, and sour cream in a big bowl. Beat the egg in a small bowl, place to the large bowl and combine. Move to a slow cooker coated lightly with oil.
Into the slow cooker, combine 1/2 French fried onions, thawed spinach, 2 cups grated Monterey Jack cheese, and the cooked and drained spaghetti. Stir everything in the slow cooker just until combined. Put the lid on and cook for 3-4 hours on high, or 6-8 hours on low.
If cooking on low, adjust the heat to high during the final 30 minutes of cooking and top on the casserole with the rest of the French fried onions and grated Monterey Jack cheese. Once the cheese has melted, enjoy.
Nutrition Information

Calories: 369 calories;;Sodium: 406;Total Carbohydrate: 18.1;Cholesterol: 76;Protein: 16.1;Total Fat: 25.9

198. Mother's Pot Roast

Serving: 5 | Prep: 10mins | Cook: 7hours | Ready in:

Ingredients
2 1/2 pounds tip round roast
salt and pepper to taste
1 (15 ounce) can tomato sauce
1 onion, cut into thin strips
2 bay leaves
3 tablespoons all-purpose flour

Direction
Grease the slow cooker with a nonstick cooking spray. Season the roast with salt and pepper.
Transfer seasoned roast in the slow cooker pot with the fat side facing up. Add in tomato sauce and place onion rings all over. Stir in bay leaves then cover. Cook on high for 1 hour.
Reduce to low heat after an hour and cook for 6 to 8 hours more. Lift the meat carefully out of the pot and transfer to a warmed platter.
Strain drippings through a strainer into the medium-sized saucepan, then discard the solid material in strainer. Stir in flour to the liquid, then cook, stirring continuously on medium heat until the sauce thickens. Season according to taste with pepper and salt. Serve with the roast.

Nutrition Information
Calories: 552 calories;;Total Fat: 36.6;Sodium: 570;Total Carbohydrate: 10.2;Cholesterol: 150;Protein: 45.2

199. No Fuss Shredded Beef Tacos

Serving: 16 | Prep: 15mins | Cook: 6hours | Ready in:

Ingredients
1 large yellow onion, sliced into thin rings
1 (3 pound) boneless beef chuck roast, trimmed
2 (14.5 ounce) cans chili-seasoned diced tomatoes
1 (14 ounce) can beef broth
1 cup cold coffee
1 (4 ounce) can diced green chiles
2 jalapeno peppers, sliced (optional)
4 cloves garlic, chopped
1 teaspoon chili powder
1/2 teaspoon ground cumin
1/2 teaspoon salt
1/4 teaspoon ground black pepper

Direction
Layer 1/2 of the onion rings in the bottom of a slow cooker. Place the chuck roast over.
Pour in coffee, beef broth, and diced tomatoes. Stir in black pepper, salt, cumin, chili powder, garlic, jalapeno peppers, and diced green chiles. Spread the leftover onion rings atop the mixture.
Cook while covered on a low setting until the beef becomes really tender, 6-10 hours.
Move the chuck roast onto a bowl and shred the meat. Return into the sauce. Take out the onions and serve with the meat.

Nutrition Information
Calories: 148 calories;;Total Fat: 9.7;Sodium: 377;Total Carbohydrate: 3.3;Cholesterol: 39;Protein: 10.9

200. Not Barbecued Short Ribs

Serving: 12 | Prep: 10mins | Cook: 4hours | Ready in:

Ingredients
3 large onions, chopped
7 pounds beef short ribs, or more to taste
salt and ground black pepper to taste
3 cups water
2 (20 ounce) cans pineapple chunks in juice, undrained
1 1/2 cups brown sugar
7 tablespoons Worcestershire sauce
5 tablespoons ketchup
4 cloves garlic, minced, or more to taste
1 tablespoon dried sage
1 tablespoon dried thyme
1 1/2 teaspoons dry mustard

Direction
Into the base of slow cooker crock, scatter the onion. Put pepper and salt on short ribs to season; put on top of onion.
In a bowl, combine mustard, thyme, sage, garlic, ketchup, Worcestershire sauce, brown sugar, pineapple chunks with juice and water together; put on top of ribs.
Allow to cook for 4 hours on High, or for 6 to 8 hours on Low.

Nutrition Information
Calories: 740 calories;;Total Carbohydrate: 49.4;Cholesterol: 109;Protein: 26.1;Total Fat: 48.9;Sodium: 237

201. O'Kee's Healthy Gray Corned Beef Brisket From Scratch

Serving: 18 | Prep: 25mins | Cook: 2hours50mins | Ready in:

Ingredients
Brine:
8 cups water
1 1/4 cups kosher salt
2 tablespoons white sugar
Pickling Spice:
1 cinnamon stick, broken into pieces
12 whole juniper berries
8 whole cloves
8 whole allspice berries
1 teaspoon mustard seeds
1 teaspoon black peppercorns
1/2 teaspoon ground ginger
2 bay leaves, crumbled
1 (6 pound) beef brisket, or larger, as desired
Corned Beef Dinner:
water to cover
1 teaspoon sea salt
2 pounds celery root (celeriac), peeled and cut into cubes
2 pounds red potatoes, cut into cubes
1 pound rutabagas, peeled and cut into cubes
4 carrots - peeled, halved lengthwise, and cut into 1/2-inch strips
4 parsnips - peeled, halved lengthwise, and cut into 1/2-inch strips
2 onions, sliced
1 head cabbage, cut into eighths

Direction
In pot, boil 8 cups of water. Into the boiling water, mix sugar and salt till dissolved; turn off heat and put in crumbled bay leaves, ginger, peppercorns, mustard seeds, allspice berries, cloves, juniper berries and pieces of cinnamon stick.
Cool brine for a minimum of 1 hour to room temperature.

Put brisket in big glass or ceramic dish with sufficient depth to maintain brisket covered in brine. Add brine on top of brisket. Weigh brisket down by placing something over it and maintain it covered in liquid. Place plastic wrap on dish to tightly cover.
Place brisket in refrigerator to brine, monitoring brine amount daily for 7 to 10 days.
Take brisket out of brine and wash under cool running water. Throw away the brine.
In big crock of slow cooker, put the brisket; pour in sufficient cool water to submerge brisket by a few inches and add sea salt to taste.
Cook for 2 hours on High; put in onions, parsnips, carrots, rutabagas, red potatoes and celery root. Cooking for about half an hour on Low till brisket is hot and grey in middle and vegetables softens. An inserted instant-read thermometer into the middle should register 70 °C or 160 °F.
Transfer brisket onto a chopping board and tightly cover with aluminum foil.
Into slow cooker, place wedges of cabbage; keep cooking for 20 to 30 minutes till every vegetable is softened.
Cut corned beef into thin pieces and serve together with vegetables.
Nutrition Information
Calories: 318 calories;;Sodium: 6559;Total Carbohydrate: 28.9;Cholesterol: 61;Protein: 21.3;Total Fat: 13.5

202. Our Favorite Olive Beef
Serving: 8 | Prep: 15mins | Cook: 6hours | Ready in:
Ingredients
2 pounds boneless chuck roast
2 (14.5 ounce) cans stewed tomatoes, chopped
1 (8 ounce) jar pitted green olives, chopped, 1/3 of liquid reserved
8 kaiser rolls
Direction
In a crockpot, put in the stewed tomatoes, green olives with reserved liquid and chuck roast.
Let it cook for 6 hours on low setting until the roast falls off the bone with ease. Serve it on top of the Kaiser rolls.
Nutrition Information
Calories: 443 calories;;Total Fat: 25.8;Sodium: 1191;Total Carbohydrate: 27.7;Cholesterol: 81;Protein: 24.8

203. PHILLY Slow Cooker Beef Stroganoff
Serving: 4 | Prep: 15mins | Cook: 8hours | Ready in:
Ingredients
1 pound cubed stewing beef
1 cup chopped onions
1 cup chopped mushrooms
1/2 cup beef broth
1/2 cup PHILADELPHIA Herb Garlic Cream Cheese Spread
1 tablespoon flour
225 grams fettuccine, cooked, drained
Direction
In a slow cooker, combine the onions, mushrooms and meat together.
Mix in the broth. Put the lid onto the slow cooker. Let the mixture cook on low setting for 6-8 hours or on high setting for 3-4 hours.
Mix the flour and cream cheese spread together. Put the cream cheese mixture into the meat mixture right before serving time; mix the 2 mixtures until well-combined and the cream cheese has fully melted. Put it on top of the newly cooked pasta and mix until well-coated.
Nutrition Information
Calories: 532 calories;;Cholesterol: 90;Protein: 29;Total Fat: 25.1;Sodium: 287;Total Carbohydrate: 48.5

204. Parmesan Chicken I
Serving: 6 | Prep: 10mins | Cook: 5hours | Ready in:
Ingredients
6 tablespoons butter
1 (1 ounce) package dry onion soup mix
1 cup converted long-grain white rice
1/4 cup grated Parmesan cheese for topping
6 skinless, boneless chicken breasts
1 1/2 cups milk
2 (10.75 ounce) cans condensed cream of mushroom soup
salt to taste
ground black pepper to taste
Direction
In a medium-sized bowl, combine rice, cream of mushroom soup, milk, and onion soup mix.
In the bottom of a lightly oil-coated slow cooker, place chicken breasts. On each chicken breast, put 1 tablespoon margarine and add the soup mixture to all. Use pepper and salt to season to taste and sprinkle grated Parmesan cheese over.
Cook on high for 4-6 hours or on low for 8-10 hours.
Nutrition Information
Calories: 491 calories;Protein: 35.1;Total Fat: 21.5;Sodium: 1303;Total Carbohydrate: 37.5;Cholesterol: 107

205. Pot Roast With Balsamic Onions
Serving: 8 | Prep: 10mins | Cook: 6hours15mins | Ready in:
Ingredients
1 (2 1/2 pound) boneless beef chuck roast
1/8 teaspoon salt
1/8 teaspoon ground black pepper
1/2 teaspoon garlic powder
1 large onion, halved and sliced
1/2 cup balsamic vinegar
Direction
Sprinkle roast with garlic powder, pepper, and salt to season.
Over medium-high heat, heat a skillet. In hot skillet, cook roast for 3-5 minutes on each side until all sides turn brown.
In a slow cooker, place roast and sprinkle onion slices around roast. Spread vinegar over onions and roast.
Set the slow cooker to Low and cook roast for 6-8 hours until falling apart and tender. Shred meat and bring back to slow cooker with juices.
Nutrition Information
Calories: 232 calories;;Sodium: 81;Total Carbohydrate: 4.2;Cholesterol: 65;Protein: 16.8;Total Fat: 16

206. Pulled BBQ Pork Poutine
Serving: 8 | Prep: 30mins | Cook: 4hours | Ready in:
Ingredients
1 (2 pound) pork shoulder roast
1/2 teaspoon salt and pepper
7 tablespoons olive oil, divided
1 cup water

2 cups smoky barbeque sauce
4 russet potatoes, cut into wedges
1 cup Cheddar cheese curds
1 cup diced bread-and-butter pickles
Reynolds Wrap® Aluminum Foil
Reynolds® Slow Cooker Liner
Direction
Start preheating the grill to medium-high heat.
Flavor the pork on all sides with pepper and salt.
In a large frying pan, heat 1 tablespoon of olive oil and cook the pork shoulder for about 4 minutes each side until browned evenly on all sides.
In a slow cooker lined with a Reynolds(R) Slow Cooker Liner, place the pork and add BBQ sauce and water, then cook on low heat for 6 hours or high heat for 4 hours.
Break the pork apart using 2 forks until it is shredded, reserve warm.
Arrange a 1 1/2 - to a 2-feet-long sheet of Reynolds Wrap(R) Aluminum Foil on a table and put the potato wedges in the center of the foil.
Sprinkle on the leftover 6 tablespoons olive oil, flavor with pepper and salt, then fold up the outside of the foil to make a foil packet.
Put the packet directly on a medium-hot grill and cook until the potatoes are cooked through and browned for 25 to 30 minutes.
Serve the shredded pork over top of diced pickles, cheese curds, and potato wedges.
Nutrition Information
Calories: 547 calories;;Total Fat: 28.4;Sodium: 1123;Total Carbohydrate: 53.8;Cholesterol: 63;Protein: 18.9

207. Ropa Vieja In A Slow Cooker

Serving: 6 | Prep: 15mins | Cook: 7hours30mins | Ready in:
Ingredients
1 (2 pound) beef chuck pot roast
3 cloves garlic
2 red bell peppers, cut into large wedges
2 green bell peppers, cut into large wedges
1 yellow onion, cut into wedges
1 sweet onion, cut into wedges
1/2 (6 ounce) can tomato paste, or to taste
1/4 cup red wine vinegar
1/8 teaspoon garlic powder, or to taste
1/8 teaspoon seasoned salt, or to taste
salt and ground black pepper to taste
Direction
Pierce the beef roast to make it tender and let the flavors in; transfer to a slow cooker with sweet onions, yellow onions, green bell peppers, red bell peppers and garlic. Stir in red wine vinegar and tomato paste. Season with ground black pepper, salt, seasoned salt and garlic powder.
Cook on Low with a cover for 7-8 hours until beef becomes tender. Take the beef out; shred into long strands with 2 forks. Transfer the meat back to the slow cooker; mix with vegetables.
Cook for half an hour on Low until vegetables and meat become very tender.
Nutrition Information
Calories: 291 calories;;Total Fat: 17.3;Sodium: 179;Total Carbohydrate: 14.1;Cholesterol: 69;Protein: 19.7

208. Salsa Verde Pork

Serving: 6 | Prep: 5mins | Cook: 6hours10mins | Ready in:
Ingredients
1 tablespoon canola oil
1 (3 pound) boneless pork loin roast
11 ounces green salsa
Direction
In a big Dutch oven, heat oil on moderately high heat. In the hot oil, brown pork loin for 2-3 minutes each side, then remove roast to the crock of a slow cooker. Drizzle over pork with green salsa.
Cook pork on low setting for about 5 hours.
Use 2 forks to shred the pork into strands then stir with the sauce so the texture is slightly even. Keep on cooking on low setting for about 1-3 hours longer.
Nutrition Information
Calories: 313 calories;;Total Carbohydrate: 3.6;Cholesterol: 106;Protein: 38.5;Total Fat: 14.6;Sodium: 238

209. Sarge's EZ Pulled Pork BBQ

Serving: 10 | Prep: 10mins | Cook: 8hours | Ready in:
Ingredients
1 (5 pound) pork butt roast
salt and pepper to taste
1 (14 ounce) can beef broth
1/4 cup brewed coffee
Direction
Halve the roast. Rub pepper and salt onto each half and put in the slow cooker. Pour over the meat with coffee and broth.
Set the slow cooker to Low and put the cover on. Cook until the roast is fork-tender, or about 6-8 hours.
Carefully transfer the roast to a cutting board. Use a fork to remove the meat from the bone. If you want to finely cut your roast, you can then use a cleaver to chop it.
Nutrition Information
Calories: 270 calories;;Sodium: 196;Total Carbohydrate: 0;Cholesterol: 85;Protein: 23.4;Total Fat: 18.8

210. Shredded Tri Tip For Tacos In The Slow Cooker

Serving: 12 | Prep: 15mins | Cook: 8hours | Ready in:
Ingredients
cooking spray
1 (3 pound) beef tri-tip roast, fat layer left untrimmed
2 teaspoons garlic pepper seasoning (such as SuzyQ's Santa Maria Valley Style Seasoning®), or to taste
2 tablespoons olive oil
2 tablespoons minced garlic
2 onions, chopped
2 teaspoons ground ancho chile pepper
2 teaspoons cayenne pepper
2 teaspoons ground black pepper
1 1/2 cups white wine
1 (28 ounce) can crushed tomatoes
1 tablespoon chopped fresh cilantro, or to taste
Direction
Use cooking spray to spray the inside of the slow cooker. Season tri-tip roast with garlic pepper seasoning on both sides.
Heat up a big heavy pan with olive oil atop a medium heat and sear the roast on all sides until fully browned, 5 minutes each side. Place the roast in the slow cooker with the fatty-side up.

Cook and stir onions and garlic in the hot pan until they turn golden brown for roughly 10 minutes, then season with black pepper, cayenne pepper, and ancho chile pepper. Place the seasoned onions and garlic over the roast and pour in crushed tomatoes and white wine. Cover and set the cooker on a low setting; cook until soft, around 8 hours.
Take the roast out of the cooker and use a sharp knife to trim the fatty layer (it should cut easily if meat is tender). Place the roast back into the cooker and use 2 forks to shred the meat. You can remove some of the liquid if you want. Stir in cilantro to serve.
Nutrition Information
Calories: 300 calories;;Total Fat: 11.9;Sodium: 207;Total Carbohydrate: 10.3;Cholesterol: 105;Protein: 32.1

211. Simple Slow Cooker Pulled Pork

Serving: 6 | Prep: 10mins | Cook: 6hours | Ready in:
Ingredients
1 tablespoon salt
1 tablespoon ground black pepper
1 tablespoon paprika
1 tablespoon garlic powder
1 (2 1/2 pound) boneless pork loin roast
1 1/2 cups diet cola-flavored carbonated beverage
1 1/2 cups ketchup
2 tablespoons liquid smoke flavoring
6 Portuguese rolls, split
Direction
In a small bowl, whisk garlic powder, paprika, black pepper, and salt until mixed well, then rub onto the pork loin to completely coat. Place the loin into a slow cooker.
Whisk ketchup and cola in a bowl and stir in the liquid smoke, then pour mixture over the pork.
Cook on low setting for 6-7 hours or on high setting for 3-4 hours. Use 2 forks to shred the pork and serve on Portuguese rolls.
Nutrition Information
Calories: 692 calories;;Total Carbohydrate: 77.1;Cholesterol: 90;Protein: 42.2;Total Fat: 23.6;Sodium: 2588

212. Slow Cooker 5 Ingredient Ham

Serving: 10 | Prep: 5mins | Cook: 6hours | Ready in:
Ingredients
1 (5 pound) bone-in ham
1 (8 ounce) can pineapple chunks in juice
1/2 cup spicy brown mustard
2 1/2 tablespoons honey, or more to taste
2 tablespoons minced garlic
Direction
In a slow cooker, put in ham.
In a bowl, combine garlic, honey, mustard and pineapple chunks. Pour over ham and spread out.
Cook for 6 to 8 hours on Low until the ham can be shredded easily with 2 forks.
Nutrition Information
Calories: 594 calories;;Sodium: 262;Total Carbohydrate: 9;Cholesterol: 164;Protein: 40.1;Total Fat: 43.2

213. Slow Cooker Adobo Chicken

Serving: 6 | Prep: 30mins | Cook: 8hours | Ready in:
Ingredients
1 small sweet onion, sliced
8 cloves garlic, crushed
3/4 cup low sodium soy sauce
1/2 cup vinegar
1 (3 pound) whole chicken, cut into pieces
Direction
In a slow cooker, put the chicken. Combine vinegar, soy sauce, garlic, and onion in a small bowl, and add to the chicken. Cook for 6-8 hours on low.
Nutrition Information
Calories: 254 calories;;Sodium: 1121;Total Carbohydrate: 5.3;Cholesterol: 61;Protein: 23;Total Fat: 14.7

214. Slow Cooker Barbecue Goose Sandwich

Serving: 3 | Prep: 5mins | Cook: 6hours | Ready in:
Ingredients
2 tablespoons butter
1 clove garlic, minced
1 small yellow onion, sliced
1 goose breast
1 1/2 tablespoons Worcestershire sauce
2 cups chicken broth
Direction
In a big saucepan, melt butter over medium heat. Add onion and garlic and sauté for 5 minutes. Put in goose breast and brown on both sides until turning brown, or about 5 minutes.
In a slow cooker, put the goose breast and pour in Worcestershire sauce. Cover with chicken broth (about 2 cups) and cook on High setting until the meats separate from the bone, or about 6-8 hours. Use a fork to shred and toss with your desired barbecue sauce.
Nutrition Information
Calories: 190 calories;Protein: 9;Total Fat: 15.2;Sodium: 162;Total Carbohydrate: 4.4;Cholesterol: 51

215. Slow Cooker Barbecued Ribs

Serving: 12 | Prep: 15mins | Cook: 3hours | Ready in:
Ingredients
1 (28 ounce) can chunky tomato sauce
1/3 cup brown sugar
2 tablespoons red wine vinegar
1 tablespoon chili powder
1 tablespoon soy sauce
2 teaspoons ground cumin
1 teaspoon paprika
1 teaspoon garlic powder
1/2 teaspoon salt
1 pinch cayenne pepper
6 pounds pork spareribs, cut into serving-size pieces
Direction
In a bowl, mix cayenne pepper, salt, garlic powder, paprika, cumin, soy sauce, chili powder, red wine vinegar, brown sugar and tomato sauce together.
Into the slow cooker, put the sparerib portions and add the sauce on top of ribs. Let cook for 3 to 4 hours on High or for 6 to 8 hours on Low.
Nutrition Information
Calories: 431 calories;Protein: 30;Total Fat: 30.4;Sodium: 615;Total Carbohydrate: 8.5;Cholesterol: 120

216. Slow Cooker Beef Enchiladas

Serving: 16 | Prep: 10mins | Cook: 7hours | Ready in:
Ingredients
4 pounds beef chuck roast
1 large onion, sliced thin
5 cloves garlic, minced

2 (10 ounce) cans red enchilada sauce
1 cup MUSSELMAN'S® Apple Butter
1/2 cup cayenne pepper sauce
1 teaspoon salt
16 flour tortillas
3 cups shredded Monterey Jack cheese or "Mexican blend" cheese

Direction

In a large slow cooker, arrange the beef roast and cover with a teaspoon of salt, cayenne sauce, apple butter, enchilada sauce, garlic and sliced onions. Place the lid on top and set the slow cooker to low to cook for 10-12 hours, or 5-7 hours on high until the roast is fork-tender.
Remove the beef roast from the sauce, then transfer onto a cutting board. Use 2 forks to shred and combine the shredded meat back into the sauce. Keep it warm until ready to carry on.
Set an oven to 400°F and start preheating. Spoon the meat into the tortillas, then roll.
In a large 10x15-inch baking dish, arrange each enchilada. Spread the rest of the sauce on top of the beef enchilada recipe when the meat and tortillas are used up, then add the shredded cheese to cover.
Bake until the cheese bubbles and melts, 10-15 minutes. Serve it warm with fresh toppings you choose.

Nutrition Information

Calories: 447 calories;;Cholesterol: 70;Protein: 23.8;Total Fat: 21.4;Sodium: 801;Total Carbohydrate: 39.1

217. Slow Cooker Beef Tinga

Serving: 8 | Prep: 15mins | Cook: 5hours15mins | Ready in:

Ingredients

2 tablespoons vegetable oil
2 1/2 pounds beef chuck, cut into 2-inch cubes
1 large onion, diced
5 cloves garlic, pressed
1/2 pound chorizo sausage
1 (14 ounce) can dark red kidney beans, rinsed
1 (14 ounce) can diced tomatoes
14 fluid ounces water
1 (6 ounce) can tomato paste
6 chipotle chiles in adobo sauce, finely chopped
3 cups tomato juice, or as needed
1 pinch salt and ground black pepper to taste

Direction

In a big skillet, heat oil over medium-high heat. Cook and mix beef chuck for 5 minutes till browned on every side. Put the garlic and onion; cook and mix for 3 to 5 minutes till aromatic and softened. To a slow cooker, place the mixture.
Using the same skillet, cook and mix chorizo for 5 minutes till crumbly and browned. Put to slow cooker. To the slow cooker, put diced tomatoes and kidney beans; with water, fill an empty can and put in on top of beans. Mix in chipotle chili peppers and tomato paste. To fill the slow cooker, add in sufficient tomato juice.
Allow to cook on Low for 5 to 7 hours till sauce is thick and beef is very soft.

Nutrition Information

Calories: 470 calories;;Total Fat: 30.4;Sodium: 1093;Total Carbohydrate: 20.6;Cholesterol: 89;Protein: 28.4

218. Slow Cooker Blackberry Pork Tenderloin

Serving: 6 | Prep: 10mins | Cook: 4hours | Ready in:

Ingredients

1 (2 pound) pork tenderloin
1 teaspoon salt
1 teaspoon ground black pepper
1 tablespoon dried rubbed sage
1 tablespoon crushed dried rosemary, or to taste
1 (16 ounce) jar seedless blackberry jam
1/4 cup honey
2 tablespoons dry red wine (such as Cabernet Sauvignon, Merlot, or a blend)
1/2 cup dry red wine (such as Cabernet Sauvignon, Merlot, or a blend)
2 tablespoons honey
1 cup fresh blackberries

Direction

Use rosemary, sage, pepper and salt to season all sides of the pork tenderloin. Put the tenderloin into a slow cooker, and pour 2 tablespoons of red wine, 1/4 cup honey and the blackberry jam over the pork. Set the cooker to Low, and cook for 4 to 5 hours until the pork becomes very tender.
Add the fresh blackberries, 2 tablespoons of honey and 1/2 cup red wine to a saucepan about 15 minutes before serving time. Bring to a boil over medium-low heat, and simmer for about 15 minutes until the sauce slightly thickens and some of the berries burst.
To serve, slice the tenderloin and drizzle blackberry-wine sauce over slices.

Nutrition Information

Calories: 417 calories;;Total Fat: 3.4;Sodium: 441;Total Carbohydrate: 70.4;Cholesterol: 65;Protein: 24

219. Slow Cooker Breakfast Casserole

Serving: 10 | Prep: 15mins | Cook: 6hours5mins | Ready in:

Ingredients

cooking spray
1 pound bulk Italian sausage
1 (26 ounce) package frozen hash-brown potatoes
1 (16 ounce) package shredded mozzarella cheese
12 eggs
1 cup milk
1 tablespoon ground mustard
1 teaspoon salt
1/2 teaspoon ground black pepper

Direction

Grease the whole bottom of the inside of a slow cooker crock using cooking spray.
Place a large skillet on medium-high heat. Cook while stirring sausage in the hot skillet for 5-7 minutes till browned and crumbly; strain and discard grease.
Cover the bottom of the slow cooker crock with hash-brown potatoes. Arrange cooked sausage on top. Sprinkle the sausage with mozzarella cheese; stir.
In a large bowl, beat eggs till smooth; include in milk; beat to integrate. Mix pepper, salt and mustard into the egg mixture then, stream over the potato mixture. Cook on low for 6-8 hours.

Nutrition Information

Calories: 386 calories;;Sodium: 1009;Total Carbohydrate: 17.5;Cholesterol: 272;Protein: 27.1;Total Fat: 27.1

220. Slow Cooker Chicken Curry

Serving: 4 | Prep: 20mins | Cook: 8hours | Ready in:
Ingredients
1 pound cubed skinless, boneless chicken breast meat
2 large potatoes, cubed
1 (10.5 ounce) can condensed chicken broth
2 1/2 cups water
2 tablespoons curry powder
1/2 (10 ounce) package frozen mixed stir-fry vegetables
1 tablespoon cornstarch
Direction
Combine curry powder, water, broth, potatoes, and chicken in a slow cooker.
Cook for 4 hours on high setting or 8 hours on low setting.
Add vegetables during the last hour of cooking time (last 30 minutes if cooking on high setting). Dissolve cornstarch into some of the cooking broth and stir into the mixture in the cooker just after adding vegetables. Keep cooking, covered until done.
Nutrition Information
Calories: 260 calories;;Total Fat: 2.9;Sodium: 570;Total Carbohydrate: 25.1;Cholesterol: 67;Protein: 33

221. Slow Cooker Chicken Curry With Coconut Milk

Serving: 3 | Prep: 10mins | Cook: 4hours10mins | Ready in:
Ingredients
2 boneless chicken breasts, cubed
1 (14.5 ounce) can diced tomatoes
1/2 (14 ounce) can coconut milk
2 medium carrots, sliced
1 onion, finely chopped
1 clove garlic, minced
2 tablespoons mild curry paste
1 tablespoon finely ground almonds
1 small bunch chopped fresh cilantro
1 tablespoon cornstarch
1 tablespoon water, or as needed
1/4 cup sliced almonds
1 1/2 cups uncooked white rice
Direction
Mix together 4/5 of the cilantro, ground almonds, curry paste, garlic, onion, carrots, coconut milk, tomatoes and chicken in a slow cooker and close the lid.
Cook on high for about 4 hours, until chicken is cooked through. If sauce is too thin, in a small bowl, stir cornstarch with water and blend into the sauce. Cook for 10 minutes more.
In the meantime, bring 3 cups water and rice to a boil in a saucepan. Lower the heat to medium-low, cover up, and let it simmer for 20 to 25 minutes until the rice gets tender and water has been absorbed.
Serve the curry over rice, use the rest of cilantro and sliced almonds to sprinkle.
Nutrition Information
Calories: 707 calories;;Total Fat: 21.9;Sodium: 584;Total Carbohydrate: 97.6;Cholesterol: 43;Protein: 28.4

222. Slow Cooker Chicken Marsala

Serving: 6 | Prep: 15mins | Cook: 4hours | Ready in:
Ingredients
1 tablespoon olive oil
2 cloves garlic cloves, minced
1/4 cup all-purpose flour
salt and ground black pepper to taste
3 pounds skinless, boneless chicken breast, cut into 2-inch cubes
12 ounces sliced white mushrooms
1 cup Marsala wine
2 tablespoons water (optional)
1 tablespoon cornstarch (optional)
1 tablespoon chopped fresh parsley for garnish
Direction
In the bowl of a slow cooker, combine garlic and olive oil.
In a bowl, combine pepper, salt, and flour. Add the flour mixture to a big resealable plastic bag; put the chicken into a bag, close and shake so the flour mixture can coat the chicken. In the slow cooker, put sliced mushrooms and the coated chicken.
In a small skillet, heat Marsala wine over medium-high heat for 2-3 minutes until decreased; add to the slow cooker and put the lid on.
Cook in the slow cooker for 4-5 hours on low setting until the chicken has fully cooked and the sauce has thickened. If the sauce is overly thin, in a small bowl, stir together cornstarch and water and gradually add to the chicken mixture. Cook in the slow cooker for 15 minutes on high setting until thickened. Adjust the seasonings to taste, use parsley to garnish and enjoy.
Nutrition Information
Calories: 374 calories;;Sodium: 155;Total Carbohydrate: 13;Cholesterol: 132;Protein: 54.9;Total Fat: 5.3

223. Slow Cooker Chicken And Dumplings

Serving: 8 | Prep: 10mins | Cook: 6hours | Ready in:
Ingredients
4 skinless, boneless chicken breast halves
2 tablespoons butter
2 (10.75 ounce) cans condensed cream of chicken soup
1 onion, finely diced
2 (10 ounce) packages refrigerated biscuit dough, torn into pieces
Direction
In a slow cooker, put onion, soup, butter, and chicken; cover with sufficient water.
Cover and cook on High for 5-6 hours. Transfer torn biscuit dough into the slow cooker when there is 30 minutes before serving. Cook until the dough is not raw inside anymore.
Nutrition Information
Calories: 385 calories;;Sodium: 1245;Total Carbohydrate: 37;Cholesterol: 45;Protein: 18.1;Total Fat: 18

224. Slow Cooker Corned Beef Style Brisket

Serving: 8 | Prep: 20mins | Cook: 8hours | Ready in:
Ingredients
1 small onion, minced
3 cloves garlic, minced
1/2 cup Dijon mustard
2 tablespoons apple cider vinegar
3 bay leaves, crumbled
8 whole black peppercorns, crushed
1 tablespoon pickling salt
1 teaspoon chopped fresh parsley
1 teaspoon celery seed

1 (4 pound) beef brisket
1 cup water
4 carrots, peeled and cut into 1-inch chunks
1/2 small head cabbage, sliced into strips
Direction
Mix celery seed, parsley, salt, peppercorns, bay leaves, vinegar, mustard, garlic and onion in bowl then cover; refrigerate it for 24 hours.
Rub mixture on brisket; tightly wrap then refrigerate overnight.
Cook brisket: Put in slow cooker with water then cover; cook for 5 hours on low. Add cabbage and carrots; cook for 3 hours till brisket is tender.
Nutrition Information
Calories: 339 calories;;Sodium: 1348;Total Carbohydrate: 11.2;Cholesterol: 92;Protein: 27.8;Total Fat: 19.6

225. Slow Cooker Country Style Spareribs

Serving: 8 | Prep: 30mins | Cook: 10hours | Ready in:
Ingredients
4 pounds pork spareribs
salt and pepper to taste
1 onion, chopped
1 green bell pepper, chopped
2 stalks celery, chopped
2 (8 ounce) cans tomato sauce
3 tablespoons brown sugar
2 tablespoons white wine vinegar
1/4 cup lemon juice
2 tablespoons Worcestershire sauce
Direction
Season the ribs to taste with pepper and salt. Brown ribs on every side in a big skillet over moderately-high heat.
In the base of a slow cooker, put 1/2 of celery, green pepper and onion. Top vegetables with half of ribs, then redo the layer with the rest of vegetables and ribs. Mix together the Worcestershire sauce, lemon juice, vinegar, brown sugar and tomato sauce in a medium bowl. Over the top of ribs, put the mixture. Place a cover, and allow to cook for an hour on High. Turn to Low, and let cook for 8 to 9 hours longer.
Nutrition Information
Calories: 442 calories;;Cholesterol: 120;Protein: 29.9;Total Fat: 30.2;Sodium: 584;Total Carbohydrate: 11.8

226. Slow Cooker Cranberry Chicken

Serving: 4 | Prep: 5mins | Cook: 4hours | Ready in:
Ingredients
4 skinless, boneless chicken breast halves
1 (16 ounce) bottle Catalina salad dressing
1 (14.5 ounce) can whole berry cranberry sauce
1 envelope onion soup mix
Direction
In the bottom of a slow cooker, put chicken breasts. Drizzle the chicken with onion soup mix, cranberry sauce, and salad dressing.
Cook for 4-6 hours on Low.
Nutrition Information
Calories: 740 calories;;Sodium: 1810;Total Carbohydrate: 70.5;Cholesterol: 61;Protein: 23.4;Total Fat: 41

227. Slow Cooker Cranberry And Muscadine Pork Roast

Serving: 8 | Prep: 10mins | Cook: 6hours | Ready in:
Ingredients
1 (5 pound) boneless pork loin roast, trimmed of fat
1 (750 milliliter) bottle muscadine red wine
1 (12 ounce) package fresh cranberries
1 tablespoon minced garlic
1/2 teaspoon salt
1/4 teaspoon ground black pepper
Direction
In the crock of a slow cooker, put the pork roast. Pour over the roast with wine, add garlic and cranberries. Use pepper and salt to season all the ingredients.
Cook for 6-8 hours on Low.
Nutrition Information
Calories: 502 calories;;Cholesterol: 134;Protein: 46;Total Fat: 22.9;Sodium: 231;Total Carbohydrate: 8

228. Slow Cooker Dump And Go Cheesy Chicken

Serving: 5 | Prep: 5mins | Cook: 6hours | Ready in:
Ingredients
6 skinless, boneless chicken breast halves
2 (11 ounce) cans condensed cream of Cheddar cheese soup
1/2 cup milk
salt and pepper to taste
1 teaspoon garlic powder
Direction
Spray cooking spray over a slow cooker. Add chicken breasts. Combine milk and soup in a medium-sized bowl, and add to the chicken. Season to taste with pepper and salt, add garlic powder.
Cook for approximately 6 hours on High. Note: Do not remove the lid during cooking.
Nutrition Information
Calories: 321 calories;;Total Carbohydrate: 11.8;Cholesterol: 113;Protein: 38.9;Total Fat: 12.4;Sodium: 1034

229. Slow Cooker Ham

Serving: 24 | Prep: 15mins | Cook: 8hours | Ready in:
Ingredients
2 cups packed brown sugar
1 (8 pound) cured, bone-in picnic ham
Direction
On the bottom of a slow cooker crock, spread about 1 1/2 cups brown sugar and then put ham with the flat side down inside the slow cooker. Trim a bit if necessary, to make it fit. Rub remaining brown sugar over ham with your hands. Cover the cooker and let it cook on Low for 8 hours.
Nutrition Information
Calories: 360 calories;Protein: 25.8;Total Fat: 20.1;Sodium: 1425;Total Carbohydrate: 18;Cholesterol: 74

230. Slow Cooker Honey Garlic Chicken

Serving: 10 | Prep: 20mins | Cook: 4hours | Ready in:
Ingredients
1 tablespoon vegetable oil
10 boneless, skinless chicken thighs
3/4 cup honey
3/4 cup lite soy sauce
3 tablespoons ketchup
2 cloves garlic, crushed
1 tablespoon minced fresh ginger root
1 (20 ounce) can pineapple tidbits, drained with juice reserved
2 tablespoons cornstarch
1/4 cup water
Direction

In a skillet, heat oil on medium heat, then cook chicken thighs in hot oil until just browned evenly on every sides. Transfer thighs into a slow cooker. Combine reserved pineapple juice, ginger, garlic, ketchup, soy sauce and honey in a bowl. Add into slow cooker.
Cook, covered, over high heat, about 4 hours. Mix in pineapple tidbits, then serve.
In a small bowl, combine water and cornstarch. Take thighs out of the slow cooker. Combine the rest of the sauce in the slow cooker with cornstarch mixture until thickened. Pour sauce on top of the chicken to serve.

Nutrition Information
Calories: 235 calories;;Total Fat: 6;Sodium: 724;Total Carbohydrate: 34.4;Cholesterol: 42;Protein: 13

231. Slow Cooker Kielbasa And Beer

Serving: 8 | Prep: 10mins | Cook: 6hours | Ready in:
Ingredients
2 pounds kielbasa sausage, cut into 1 inch pieces
1 (12 fluid ounce) can or bottle beer
1 (20 ounce) can sauerkraut, drained
Direction
Mix the beer, sauerkraut and sausage together in a slow cooker. Allow the mixture to cook for 5-6 hours on low setting until the sausage has softened and bulged.

Nutrition Information
Calories: 383 calories;;Cholesterol: 75;Protein: 14.7;Total Fat: 31.1;Sodium: 1491;Total Carbohydrate: 7.8

232. Slow Cooker Lancaster County Pork And Sauerkraut

Serving: 6 | Prep: 20mins | Cook: 6hours | Ready in:
Ingredients
1 (4 pound) pork loin roast
1 teaspoon caraway seeds
salt and pepper to taste
2 cups sauerkraut with liquid
Direction
If needed, cut pork loin to fit in slow cooker. Use caraway seeds to season and pepper and salt to taste. Put sauerkraut on roast.
Cook for 1 hour on high then for 5-6 hours on low. The roast's internal temperature should be at least 63°C/145°F.

Nutrition Information
Calories: 245 calories;;Cholesterol: 105;Protein: 36.8;Total Fat: 8.5;Sodium: 582;Total Carbohydrate: 3.5

233. Slow Cooker Lasagna II

Serving: 10 | Prep: 30mins | Cook: 2hours | Ready in:
Ingredients
1 (16 ounce) package lasagna noodles
1 pound lean ground beef
1 1/2 (26 ounce) jars spaghetti sauce
2 cups shredded mozzarella cheese
1/2 cup grated Parmesan cheese
1 (8 ounce) container ricotta cheese
2 eggs
2 cups shredded mozzarella cheese
Direction
Fill lightly salted water into in a big pot and bring water to a rolling boil on high heat. When water is boiling, stir in lasagna noodles and bring back to a boil. Cook pasta without a cover for 7 minutes while stirring sometimes, until pasta is softened a bit yet still not cooked through. Drain pasta well in a colander set in the sink.
In a big skillet, cook and stir ground beef on medium-high heat until beef is browned, then drain and stir in sauce. Put aside. Mix together in a separate bowl with eggs, ricotta cheese, Parmesan cheese and 2 cups of mozzarella cheese.
Add in the bottom of a slow cooker with 1/2 cup of the sauce mixture and use a layer of noodles to cover. Sprinkle over noodles with 1/4 of the cheese mixture, then scoop over cheese with about a quarter of the leftover sauce. Repeat layering as above and finish with a layer of sauce, then put the 2 leftover cups of mozzarella cheese on top. Cook on high setting for about 2-3 hours or low setting for about 8-9 hours.

Nutrition Information
Calories: 521 calories;Protein: 33.1;Total Fat: 20.6;Sodium: 861;Total Carbohydrate: 50.3;Cholesterol: 110

234. Slow Cooker Lengua (Beef Tongue)

Serving: 6 | Prep: 10mins | Cook: 8hours5mins | Ready in:
Ingredients
1 beef tongue
1/2 onion
2 cloves garlic, or more to taste
1 bay leaf
salt and ground black pepper to taste
water to cover
1 tablespoon butter
Direction
In the crock of a slow cooker, put bay leaf, garlic, onion and beef tongue; season with salt generously. Pour in enough water to cover the beef mixture. Cook for 8 hours on low.
Transfer the beef tongue onto a work surface; allow to cool slightly. Peel the outer layer of the skin from the beef tongue; remove the rough end. Chop the meat into bite-sized pieces.
Place a skillet on medium heat; heat butter; cook while stirring for 5-10 minutes, or till the beef tongue meat becomes tender. Season with pepper and salt.

Nutrition Information
Calories: 492 calories;;Sodium: 123;Total Carbohydrate: 1.2;Cholesterol: 224;Protein: 32.1;Total Fat: 38.8

235. Slow Cooker London Broil

Serving: 8 | Prep: 10mins | Cook: 10hours | Ready in:
Ingredients
2 pounds flank steak
1 (10.75 ounce) can condensed cream of mushroom soup
1 (10.75 ounce) can condensed tomato soup
1 (1 ounce) package dry onion soup mix
Direction
In the bottom of a slow cooker, add meat. You may need to slice meat to make it fit the slow cooker. Combine tomato soup and mushroom together in a medium bowl, then drizzle over beef. Sprinkle over top with the dry onion soup mix.
Place a cover and cook on low setting, about 8-10 hours.

Nutrition Information
Calories: 198 calories;;Total Fat: 11.1;Sodium: 801;Total Carbohydrate: 9.8;Cholesterol: 36;Protein: 14.9

236. Slow Cooker Mexican Chicken And Rice

Serving: 6 | Prep: 10mins | Cook: 3hours20mins | Ready in:
Ingredients
3 cups chicken broth
1 1/2 cups converted long-grain white rice
1/2 large white onion, sliced
1 (24 ounce) jar salsa
1 (4 ounce) can chopped green chilies
1 (1 ounce) packet dry taco seasoning mix, divided
2 skinless, boneless chicken breast halves
1 (15 ounce) can black beans, drained
Direction
Into a slow cooker, add the chicken stock, then mix in half the taco seasoning, green chilies, salsa, onion, and rice. Rub the chicken breasts with the rest of taco seasoning, position into the cooker. Put the lid on the cooker, then adjust to high setting.
Cook for around 3 hours till the rice is thickened and nearly all the liquid has been absorbed. Change the cooker to warm setting for about 20 minutes before serving time. Take the chicken breasts out, then slice. Stir the black beans and chicken into the slow cooker. Move the lid back to the cooker, let the beans heat, and serve.
Nutrition Information
Calories: 340 calories;;Total Carbohydrate: 61.8;Cholesterol: 23;Protein: 18.2;Total Fat: 1.9;Sodium: 2006

237. Slow Cooker Orange Chicken

Serving: 4 | Prep: 15mins | Cook: 6hours | Ready in:
Ingredients
1 pound skinless, boneless chicken breast halves
12 fluid ounces orange-flavored carbonated beverage
1/2 cup soy sauce
1 cup uncooked long grain white rice
2 cups water
Direction
In a slow cooker, put the chicken and add soy sauce and orange-flavored carbonated beverage.
Put the lid on the slow cooker and cook the chicken for 5-6 hours on Low.
Boil water and rice in a saucepan. Lower the heat to low, put a cover on and simmer for 20 minutes. Enjoy the cooked chicken with the rice.
Nutrition Information
Calories: 357 calories;;Sodium: 1868;Total Carbohydrate: 53;Cholesterol: 59;Protein: 27.8;Total Fat: 2.7

238. Slow Cooker Overnight Breakfast Casserole

Serving: 12 | Prep: 30mins | Cook: 8hours | Ready in:
Ingredients
2 (12 ounce) packages Johnsonville® Original Breakfast Sausage
1 cup chopped green onions
1 sweet red bell pepper, chopped
1 (4 ounce) can diced mild green chilies
1/4 cup chopped fresh cilantro
1 (30 ounce) package frozen shredded hash brown potatoes
1 1/2 cups shredded Cheddar cheese
12 eggs
1 cup milk
1/2 teaspoon salt
1/8 teaspoon pepper
Direction
Cook sausage following the package instructions; slice into slices, about 1/4-in. each slice; put aside.
Mix cilantro, chilies, red pepper, and green onions together in a bowl; put aside.
Spray vegetable cooking spray over the inside of a 5-6-qt. slow cooker. Layer into the crock with 1/3 hash browns, the sausage, and the green onion mixture then cheese. Repeat these layers twice. Combine pepper, salt, milk, and eggs in a bowl; add over the layered ingredients.
Put the lid on and cook on low until a thermometer displays 160°F when you insert it into the middle, about 7-8 hours. Enjoy.
Nutrition Information
Calories: 389 calories;;Total Fat: 28.9;Sodium: 1026;Total Carbohydrate: 17.9;Cholesterol: 239;Protein: 23.6

239. Slow Cooker Pepper Steak II

Serving: 6 | Prep: 10mins | Cook: 8hours | Ready in:
Ingredients
2 tablespoons olive oil
3 pounds beef sirloin, sliced into strips
1 tablespoon minced garlic
1 onion, chopped
1/2 cup soy sauce
1 teaspoon salt
1/2 teaspoon ground black pepper
2 teaspoons white sugar
3 green bell peppers, cut into strips
1 tablespoon cornstarch
1/4 cup cold water
Direction
Heat the oil over medium heat in a big skillet. Put in the steak strips, then brown quickly on both sides; put in the garlic when cooking the steak. Move the steak and its juices to a slow cooker. Put in the sugar, pepper, salt, soy sauce and onion. Cook for 6 to 8 hours on Low, covered, until the meat is fork tender. Put in the green peppers an hour before the end of the cooking time. Mix the cold water and cornstarch together. Put into the slow cooker in the last few minutes, then cook until the sauce is thickened.
Nutrition Information
Calories: 430 calories;Protein: 39.5;Total Fat: 25.4;Sodium: 1678;Total Carbohydrate: 9.2;Cholesterol: 121

240. Slow Cooker Philly Steak Sandwich Meat

Serving: 4 | Prep: 15mins | Cook: 8mins | Ready in:
Ingredients
1/2 large onion, sliced
3 cloves garlic, chopped
1 pound beef sirloin, cut into 2-inch strips, or more to taste
1/2 teaspoon ground cumin
1/2 teaspoon ground black pepper
1/2 teaspoon chili powder
1/2 teaspoon onion powder
1/2 teaspoon garlic powder
1/4 teaspoon paprika
1/4 teaspoon dried thyme
1/4 teaspoon dried marjoram
1/4 teaspoon dried basil
2 tablespoons bourbon whiskey (such as Jim Beam®)
1 teaspoon soy sauce

1 teaspoon prepared mustard
1 teaspoon Worcestershire sauce
1/2 teaspoon hot sauce (such as Frank's Red Hot ®)
1 (12 fluid ounce) can or bottle beer (such as Budweiser®)
2 cubes beef bouillon
Direction
Into the bottom of a slow cooker, spread garlic and onion. Spread beef on top of garlic and onion. Drizzle garlic powder, cumin, chili powder, basil, black pepper, onion powder, marjoram, paprika, and thyme on top of beef. Add Worcestershire sauce, bourbon, mustard, hot sauce and soy sauce on top. Add beer on top of beef mixture and top with beef bouillon cubes.
Cook for 8 hours on low while stirring after every hour or so (or cook on high for 4 hours).
Nutrition Information
Calories: 251 calories;;Total Fat: 10.6;Sodium: 602;Total Carbohydrate: 7.6;Cholesterol: 60;Protein: 20.1

241. Slow Cooker Pork Loin Roast With Apple Cranberry Rice

Serving: 10 | Prep: 15mins | Cook: 6hours | Ready in:
Ingredients
1 (5 pound) boneless pork loin roast
2 teaspoons olive oil
1 tablespoon herbes de Provence (optional)
salt and ground black pepper to taste
4 cups cooked rice
1 large yellow onion, chopped
2 Granny Smith apples, chopped
1 1/2 cups dried cranberries
1 teaspoon salt
1/4 teaspoon ground black pepper, or to taste
Direction
In a big slow cooker, put the pork roast; drizzle olive oil over. Sprinkle herbes de Provence over, use black pepper and salt to season to taste.
In a bowl, combine 1/4 teaspoon black pepper, 1 teaspoon salt, cranberries, apples, onion and rice. Spoon the rice mixture around and over the pork. Put the cover on and cook for 8-10 hours on Low or for 6 hours on High.
Nutrition Information
Calories: 488 calories;;Cholesterol: 108;Protein: 38.7;Total Fat: 19.9;Sodium: 317;Total Carbohydrate: 37.5

242. Slow Cooker Pork And Sauerkraut With Apples

Serving: 6 | Prep: 10mins | Cook: 4hours5mins | Ready in:
Ingredients
6 thick-cut pork chops
4 tart apples, peeled and sliced
1 large onion, sliced
water to cover
1 quart sauerkraut
1/2 teaspoon fennel seed, or to taste
Direction
Over medium-high heat, heat a large skillet and then brown the pork chops in hot skillet for about 2 to 3 minutes on each side. Drain the chops.
Into the bottom of a slow cooker, spread onion and apples and then add the browned pork chops on top.
Add in plenty of water to cover the bottom of slow cooker crock.
Cook on Low for 6 hours or on High for 3 hours. Add fennel seed and sauerkraut into the pork chop mixture. Let to cook for one more hour.
Nutrition Information
Calories: 400 calories;;Sodium: 1103;Total Carbohydrate: 21.8;Cholesterol: 95;Protein: 37.2;Total Fat: 18.4

243. Slow Cooker Pork With Mushrooms And Barley

Serving: 6 | Prep: 20mins | Cook: 8hours | Ready in:
Ingredients
3 cloves garlic, finely chopped
1 teaspoon salt
6 pork chops
1/2 cup barley
8 ounces white mushrooms, sliced
1/2 onion, chopped
2 (14 ounce) cans chicken broth
1/2 cup water
2 teaspoons Worcestershire sauce
1 bay leaf
1 pinch salt and ground black pepper to taste
Direction
Rub 1 tsp. salt and chopped garlic into porkchops. Put barley in slow cooker; top using porkchops. Cover using chopped onion and white mushrooms. Add few grinds of fresh black pepper, salt, bay leaf, Worcestershire sauce, water and chicken broth. Put slow cooker on low; cover. Cook for 8 hours.
Nutrition Information
Calories: 236 calories;;Cholesterol: 68;Protein: 28.8;Total Fat: 6.3;Sodium: 1077;Total Carbohydrate: 14.9

244. Slow Cooker Pulled Pork

Serving: 8 | Prep: 10mins | Cook: 7hours | Ready in:
Ingredients
1 (2 pound) pork tenderloin
1 (12 fluid ounce) can or bottle root beer
1 (18 ounce) bottle your favorite barbecue sauce
8 hamburger buns, split and lightly toasted
Direction
In a slow cooker, put the pork tenderloin; drizzle root beer over the meat. Cook while covered on low for 6 - 7 hours until thoroughly cooked and the pork can be easily shredded. Note: the actual length of time depends on individual slow cooker. Let drain well. Mix in barbecue sauce. Serve with hamburger buns.
Nutrition Information
Calories: 335 calories;;Sodium: 990;Total Carbohydrate: 49.4;Cholesterol: 49;Protein: 21.2;Total Fat: 5

245. Slow Cooker Pulled Pork Roast

Serving: 8 | Prep: 10mins | Cook: 10hours | Ready in:
Ingredients
1 (3 1/2) pound pork butt roast
1 tablespoon chili powder
1 tablespoon vegetable oil
2 teaspoons pepper
2 teaspoons ground cumin
2 teaspoons coriander
2 teaspoons paprika
1 teaspoon allspice
1/2 teaspoon salt
2 cloves garlic, minced

1 1/2 cups Heinz Tomato Ketchup
1 cup Heinz® Apple Cider Vinegar
1/2 cup fancy molasses
1/3 cup Heinz® Mustard
2 teaspoons cornstarch
Soft rolls

Direction

Discard all string from the roast and trim away excess fat. In a bowl, put chili powder; mix in garlic, salt, allspice, paprika, coriander, cumin, pepper, chili and oil to form a paste. Rub all over the whole pork; thoroughly work the spice mixture into the meat. Let the meat marinate for a minimum of 30 minutes or overnight. Remove the roast to a slow cooker.

Stir together mustard, molasses, vinegar and ketchup. Add the mixture onto the roast and cook on low until very soft, or about 8-10 hours.

Remove the roast to a big bowl; remove any fat you can see. Separate the meat into long strands with 2 forks. Pour off 1 1/2 cups of the cooking juices and drain into a saucepan. Mix in cornstarch and boil. Cook until bubbly and thick while whisking. Put the shredded meat back into the slow cooker, mix to blend with the leftover cooking juices. Put the meat on soft rolls to enjoy, drizzle the thickened sauce mixture over to taste.

Nutrition Information

Calories: 503 calories;;Total Carbohydrate: 49.3;Cholesterol: 78;Protein: 24.8;Total Fat: 22.8;Sodium: 934

246. Slow Cooker Red Curry Beef Pot Roast

Serving: 6 | Prep: 15mins | Cook: | Ready in:

Ingredients

1 (2 1/2 pound) boneless beef chuck roast
salt and ground black pepper to taste
2 teaspoons vegetable oil
1 onion, chopped
1 teaspoon red curry paste, or to taste
2 teaspoons ground cumin
1 teaspoon ground coriander
2 cups chicken broth
1 (14 ounce) can coconut milk
1 (10 ounce) can diced tomatoes and green chiles
3 tablespoons Asian fish sauce, or to taste
1/4 cup brown sugar
4 cloves garlic, minced
1 tablespoon tomato paste
1 (3 inch) piece fresh ginger root, peeled and sliced
1 lime, juiced
2 bay leaves
1 1/2 pounds small potatoes, halved
4 small heads baby bok choy, sliced in 2-inch sections, green leaves intact
1 1/2 teaspoons cornstarch
1 tablespoon water
For garnish:
1/4 cup chopped roasted peanuts, or to taste
1/4 cup chopped fresh cilantro, or to taste

Direction

Season the beef chuck roast generously with pepper and salt.

On high heat, heat a big skillet and put in vegetable oil. Brown the roast on every side in the hot oil, around 2 minutes on each side. Take the pan off the heat.

Put chopped onions in the slow cooker and put the browned roast over the onions.

Place red chili paste in the hot skillet. Put coriander and cumin. Rub and blend the mixture into the hot oil with the back of a spoon. Put the skillet on medium heat.

Put in the chicken stock and bring the heat to high. Mix in the coconut milk. Place in diced tomatoes along with the fish sauce, green chiles, minced garlic, sliced ginger, brown sugar and tomato paste. Mix in the lime juice. Bring it to a boil.

Place the mixture on the pot roast and put bay leaves in. Mix the ingredients to distribute it in the slow cooker. Put a cover on the slow cooker and set it on low. Cook for 7-8 hours until fork-tender.

Take the meat out of the broth. If you want, skim some fat on the broth's surface.

Put the bok choy and potatoes in the broth; mix. Cover and put the heat on high. Cook for about 12 minutes until the potatoes are tender.

Mix water and cornstarch together in a small dish until it dissolves. Mix into the broth mixture.

Slice the meat into big chunks and put it in the slow cooker and mix. Cover the slow cooker and cook on high for about 12 minutes until the meat's completely heated and the broth gets a bit thick.

Place into serving bowls and put cilantro and chopped peanuts on top.

Nutrition Information

Calories: 625 calories;;Sodium: 960;Total Carbohydrate: 42.2;Cholesterol: 86;Protein: 30.1;Total Fat: 39

247. Slow Cooker Roast Beef

Serving: 6 | Prep: 5mins | Cook: 22hours | Ready in:

Ingredients

1/3 cup soy sauce
1 (1 ounce) package dry onion soup mix
3 pounds beef chuck roast
2 teaspoons freshly ground black pepper

Direction

Pour the dry onion soup mix and soy sauce into the slow cooker, then stir well. Put the chuck toast into the slow cooker, then pour water until the top 1/2-inch of the roast is not covered. Sprinkle with ground pepper.

Put on cover and let it cook for 22 hours on low.

Nutrition Information

Calories: 555 calories;;Total Carbohydrate: 4.4;Cholesterol: 161;Protein: 40.4;Total Fat: 40.8;Sodium: 1369

248. Slow Cooker Sauerkraut And Sausage

Serving: 5 | Prep: 15mins | Cook: 4hours | Ready in:

Ingredients

1 (20 ounce) can sauerkraut
1/4 cup brown sugar
1 1/2 pounds ground pork sausage
1 onion, sliced

Direction

Mix the brown sugar and sauerkraut in a medium bowl and then transfer to a slow cooker. Spread the onion and sausage on top of the sauerkraut.

Cook for 2 hours on high, checking for dryness, and adding more water if need be. Switch to low setting and then cook for 2 more hours on low.

Nutrition Information

Calories: 640 calories;;Total Fat: 55.1;Sodium: 1653;Total Carbohydrate: 19;Cholesterol: 93;Protein: 17.2

249. Slow Cooker Shoyu Pork

Serving: 8 | Prep: 10mins | Cook: 8hours | Ready in:
Ingredients
1 (4 pound) pork butt roast
1 (8 ounce) can tomato sauce
1 cup white sugar
1 cup soy sauce
1 cup sake
3 cloves garlic, crushed
Direction
In the bottom of a slow cooker, put pork roast. In a bowl, put garlic, sake, soy sauce, sugar, and tomato sauce, mix together until the sugar melts. Put the mixture on the pork roast. Put the cover on the slow cooker and cook for 8-10 hours on Low.
Nutrition Information
Calories: 427 calories;;Total Fat: 17.6;Sodium: 2008;Total Carbohydrate: 30.8;Cholesterol: 97;Protein: 27.5

250. Slow Cooker Shredded Venison For Tacos

Serving: 7 | Prep: 15mins | Cook: 45mins | Ready in:
Ingredients
1 (1.25 ounce) package taco seasoning mix
1/4 cup all-purpose flour
3 pounds venison roast
2 teaspoons cayenne pepper, or to taste
2 tablespoons vegetable oil
1 1/2 cups water
Direction
Mix cayenne pepper to taste, flour and 1/2 taco seasoning; coat meat in this mixture. In a big skillet, heat oil on medium-high heat. Put roast into oil; brown all sides well.
Put meat into slow cooker with water. Cook for 8 hours on low setting or for 5 hours on high setting. Shred with a fork when meat is done. Season to your taste.
Nutrition Information
Calories: 403 calories;;Total Fat: 10.8;Sodium: 449;Total Carbohydrate: 7.1;Cholesterol: 235;Protein: 64.1

251. Slow Cooker Sloppy Swiss Steak

Serving: 6 | Prep: 20mins | Cook: 8hours20mins | Ready in:
Ingredients
2 pounds boneless beef round steak, cut into 6-ounce pieces
1/2 teaspoon seasoned salt (such as LAWRY'S®), or to taste
1/2 teaspoon paprika, or to taste
2/3 cup all-purpose flour
2 tablespoons vegetable oil, or as needed
1 large green bell pepper, cut into strips
1 large onion, cut into strips
1 large carrot, chopped
1 (10 ounce) can diced tomatoes with green chile peppers (such as RO*TEL®), undrained
1/2 (15 ounce) can sloppy joe sauce (such as Manwich®)
1 tablespoon Worcestershire sauce
2 cloves garlic, minced
1/2 cup red wine
Direction
Scatter paprika and seasoned salt onto each side of the steak pieces. Put the flour into a low-sided dish and use it to coat the meat thoroughly on both sides. Use the tenderizing side of a meat mallet to pound the flour into both sides of meat.
In a big skillet, heat vegetable oil on medium heat. Cook both sides of steaks well until browned, 5 minutes on each side. In a slow cooker, place the steaks in and layer with green bell pepper, carrot and onion strips. Combine Worcestershire sauce, wine, garlic, sloppy Joe sauce, and diced tomatoes with green chiles; then pour this mixture over the steak and vegetables.
Place the lid on the slow cooker. Adjust the setting to low and cook for 8 to 10 hours. It is done when the sauce is thoroughly blended and thick and the steaks are tender.
Nutrition Information
Calories: 466 calories;;Cholesterol: 136;Protein: 57.6;Total Fat: 12.4;Sodium: 695;Total Carbohydrate: 24.4

252. Slow Cooker Spanish Rice

Serving: 6 | Prep: 20mins | Cook: 6hours5mins | Ready in:
Ingredients
2 pounds ground beef or chuck
1 (28 ounce) can whole peeled tomatoes
2 green bell peppers, chopped
1 cup water
1 (8 ounce) can tomato sauce
2 onions, chopped
1 cup uncooked converted rice
2 1/2 teaspoons salt
2 1/2 teaspoons chili powder
2 teaspoons Worcestershire sauce
Direction
Put ground beef into a large skillet. Cook and regularly stir the beef on medium-high heat until it gets brown color and crumbles, 5-7 minutes. Drain and remove any grease. Put the beef into a slow cooker.
Add Worcestershire sauce, chili powder, salt, rice, onions, tomato sauce, water, green pepper and tomatoes into the slow cooker. Whisk really well. Put the lid on and let the mixture cook on Low until the rice gets tender, 6 – 8 hours.
Nutrition Information
Calories: 399 calories;;Total Fat: 17.7;Sodium: 1429;Total Carbohydrate: 38.1;Cholesterol: 69;Protein: 22.1

253. Slow Cooker Tender And Yummy Round Steak

Serving: 6 | Prep: 20mins | Cook: 10hours | Ready in:
Ingredients
3 potatoes, peeled and quartered
1 onion, chopped
6 carrots, peeled and sliced into 1 inch pieces
2 pounds boneless round steak
1 (1 ounce) package dry onion soup mix
1 (10.75 ounce) can condensed cream of mushroom soup
3/4 cup water
Direction
Put in a slow cooker the carrots, onion, and potatoes. Slice the steak into 6 pieces and top the vegetables

with meat. Mix the water, soup and soup mix in a mixing bowl; add over the beef.
Cover, then cook for 7 to 10 hours on Low.
Nutrition Information
Calories: 393 calories;;Cholesterol: 81;Protein: 33.8;Total Fat: 13.6;Sodium: 829;Total Carbohydrate: 33.1

254. Slow Cooker Texas Pulled Pork

Serving: 8 | Prep: 15mins | Cook: 5hours | Ready in:
Ingredients
1 teaspoon vegetable oil
1 (4 pound) pork shoulder roast
1 cup barbeque sauce
1/2 cup apple cider vinegar
1/2 cup chicken broth
1/4 cup light brown sugar
1 tablespoon prepared yellow mustard
1 tablespoon Worcestershire sauce
1 tablespoon chili powder
1 extra large onion, chopped
2 large cloves garlic, crushed
1 1/2 teaspoons dried thyme
8 hamburger buns, split
2 tablespoons butter, or as needed
Direction
In the bottom of a slow cooker, add the vegetable oil. Put the pork roast into the slow cooker; add chicken broth, apple cider vinegar and the barbecue sauce. Mix in thyme, garlic, onion, chili powder, Worcestershire sauce, yellow mustard and the brown sugar. Cover up and cook on high for 5 to 6 hours, until the roast shreds easily with a fork.
Take the roast out of the slow cooker, and use two forks to shred the meat. Put back the shredded pork to the slow cooker, and mix the meat into the juices. Spread the butter on the inside of both halves of hamburger buns. Toast the buns in a skillet over medium heat with butter side down, until golden brown. Spoon the pork into the toasted buns.
Nutrition Information
Calories: 527 calories;;Total Fat: 23.1;Sodium: 730;Total Carbohydrate: 45.5;Cholesterol: 98;Protein: 31.9

255. Slow Cooker Texas Smoked Beef Brisket

Serving: 4 | Prep: 10mins | Cook: 6hours | Ready in:
Ingredients
Brisket Rub:
3 tablespoons smoked paprika
2 tablespoons ground black pepper
2 tablespoons kosher salt
1 tablespoon brown sugar
1 tablespoon chili powder
1 teaspoon ground cumin
1 1/2 pounds beef brisket
Barbeque Sauce:
3/4 cup barbeque sauce
1/4 cup water (optional)
1 tablespoon Worcestershire sauce
1/4 teaspoon liquid smoke flavoring
1/2 onion, sliced into rings
Direction
Mix cumin, chili powder, brown sugar, salt, pepper and paprika in bowl; evenly rub on brisket's surface.
Put brisket in big resealable plastic bag then refrigerate for 30 minutes-overnight.
Mix liquid smoke, Worcestershire sauce, water and barbeque sauce in bottom of slow cooker; lay the brisket into sauce mixture. Put onions over brisket.
Cook for 6-7 hours on low till brisket is very tender; before shredding/slicing, rest brisket for 10 minutes. Serve with sauce from slow cooker.
Nutrition Information
Calories: 342 calories;Protein: 21.5;Total Fat: 16.1;Sodium: 3520;Total Carbohydrate: 28.7;Cholesterol: 69

256. Slow Cooker Tropical Chicken

Serving: 6 | Prep: 20mins | Cook: 6hours | Ready in:
Ingredients
4 skinless, boneless chicken breast halves, cut into bite size pieces
4 sweet potatoes, peeled and cut into chunks
1 onion, chopped
1 (20 ounce) can pineapple chunks with juice
1/2 cup raisins
2 tablespoons Jamaican jerk seasoning
1 tablespoon grated lime zest
2 teaspoons Worcestershire sauce
1 teaspoon ground ginger
1 teaspoon ground cumin
1 teaspoon dried thyme
Direction
In a slow cooker, place the onion, sweet potatoes and chicken.
In a bowl, mix together the raisins, jerk seasoning, pineapple chunks with juice, lime zest, ginger, Worcestershire sauce, and cumin till well combined. Pour onto the chicken mixture. Sprinkle with thyme. Cover and set to Low.
Cook for up to 6 hours or once the chicken and vegetables turn tender.
Nutrition Information
Calories: 361 calories;;Sodium: 601;Total Carbohydrate: 68.3;Cholesterol: 41;Protein: 19.6;Total Fat: 2.1

257. Slow Cooker Venison Burritos

Serving: 8 | Prep: 15mins | Cook: 6hours | Ready in:
Ingredients
1 1/2 pounds boneless venison round steak
1 (16 ounce) jar salsa
1 (15 ounce) can black beans
1 (15.25 ounce) can Mexicorn, drained
1 (3 ounce) package cream cheese, cubed
8 (12 inch) flour tortillas, warmed
1 (8 ounce) package shredded Mexican cheese blend
Direction
In bottom of slow cooker, cover venison steaks with salsa. Throw away 1/2 liquid from black beans. Pour beans into slow cooker with Mexicorn.
Put slow cooker on low. Cook till venison easily pulls apart using a fork, about 6-8 hours.
Break meat up to bite-sized pieces. Mix cream cheese cubes in till melted. Put tortilla onto work surface. Spoon some filling halfway between middle and bottom edge of tortilla. Use back of a spoon to flatten filling to a rectangle shape. Sprinkle some Mexican cheese blend on filling. Fold bottom of tortilla snugly over the filling. Fold in right and left edges. Roll burrito up to the top edge, making a tight cylinder. Repeat with the leftover ingredients.
Nutrition Information

Calories: 658 calories;;Sodium: 1540;Total Carbohydrate: 74.6;Cholesterol: 103;Protein: 36.4;Total Fat: 24.1

258. Slow Cooker Venison Sloppy Joes

Serving: 4 | Prep: 5mins | Cook: 8hours | Ready in:
Ingredients
1/4 pound bacon
2 pounds venison stew meat
1 large yellow onion, chopped
1/2 cup brown sugar
1/4 cup wine vinegar
1 tablespoon ground cumin
1 teaspoon chili powder
2 tablespoons minced garlic
1 tablespoon prepared Dijon-style mustard
1 cup ketchup
salt and pepper to taste
Direction
Cook bacon in big deep skillet on medium high heat till browned evenly. Take out of skillet; crumble. Put aside. In bacon grease, brown stew meat for flavor. Mix pepper, salt, ketchup, garlic, mustard, chili powder, cumin, vinegar, sugar and onion in slow cooker well. Add venison and bacon; mix together. Cook on low setting for at least 8 hours. Separate meat with a fork to sloppy joe-style and thick barbecue.
Nutrition Information
Calories: 538 calories;Protein: 51.8;Total Fat: 18.4;Sodium: 1071;Total Carbohydrate: 41.1;Cholesterol: 191

259. Slow Cooker Wieners In Wiener BBQ Sauce

Serving: 7 | Prep: 10mins | Cook: 1hours | Ready in:
Ingredients
2 pounds hot dogs
1 (18 ounce) jar grape jelly
1 (8 ounce) jar prepared mustard
1 tablespoon brown sugar
1 tablespoon apple cider vinegar
Direction
In a slow cooker, add the wieners. Mix together cider vinegar, brown sugar, mustard and grape jelly in a medium bowl. Blend well and drizzle over the wieners.
On low setting, cook wieners for a minimum of an hour prior to serving.
Nutrition Information
Calories: 633 calories;;Cholesterol: 67;Protein: 16.8;Total Fat: 39.6;Sodium: 1813;Total Carbohydrate: 53.9

260. Slow Cooked Turkey Legs

Serving: 4 | Prep: 15mins | Cook: 7hours30mins | Ready in:
Ingredients
3 tablespoons poultry seasoning
1 1/2 teaspoons salt
1/2 teaspoon ground black pepper
4 turkey legs
1 cube vegetable bouillon
1 cup water
Direction
In a bowl, combine pepper, salt, and poultry seasoning. Rub over the turkey legs. Chill in the fridge for 8 hours to overnight.
In a bowl, put bouillon cube in water to dissolve. Pour into the slow cooker.
Shape aluminum foil into a coil form with a height at least 1-inch. Line the bottom of the slow cooker with it. On the aluminum foil, put the turkey legs, above the liquid.
Cook on Low for 7 1/2 hours until the meat begins to fall apart.
Nutrition Information
Calories: 421 calories;;Total Fat: 12.7;Sodium: 1118;Total Carbohydrate: 2;Cholesterol: 304;Protein: 70.6

261. Slow Cooker Posole

Serving: 8 | Prep: 20mins | Cook: 6hours35mins | Ready in:
Ingredients
1 tablespoon canola oil
1 (2 pound) boneless pork loin roast, cut into 1-inch cubes
2 (14.5 ounce) cans enchilada sauce
2 (15.5 ounce) cans white hominy, drained
1 onion, sliced
1/2 cup green chilies, diced
4 cloves garlic, minced
1/2 teaspoon cayenne pepper, or to taste
2 teaspoons dried oregano
1/4 cup cilantro, chopped
1/2 teaspoon salt
Direction
Heat the canola oil over high heat in a skillet. Put in the pork; cook and mix for 5 minutes or just until all sides of the meat are browned.
Put the meat in a 4-quart slow cooker. Pour enchilada sauce over. Top with oregano, cayenne pepper, garlic, chilies, onion and hominy. Put enough water to fill the slow cooker.
Cover and cook for 6 to 7 hours on High. Mix in the salt and cilantro. Cook for another 30 minutes on Low.
Nutrition Information
Calories: 241 calories;;Sodium: 671;Total Carbohydrate: 25.7;Cholesterol: 40;Protein: 16.8;Total Fat: 7.7

262. Sour Cream Pork Chops

Serving: 6 | Prep: 15mins | Cook: 8hours30mins | Ready in:
Ingredients
6 pork chops
salt and pepper to taste
garlic powder to taste
1/2 cup all-purpose flour
1 large onion, sliced 1/4 inch thick
2 cubes chicken bouillon
2 cups boiling water
2 tablespoons all-purpose flour
1 (8 ounce) container sour cream
Direction
Sprinkle garlic powder, pepper and salt on the pork chops to season, then dredge it in half a cup of flour. Brown the chops lightly in a fry pan with a small amount of oil on medium heat.
In a slow cooker, put the pork chops and put the slices of onion on top. In boiling water, dissolve the bouillon cubes and pour on top of the pork chops. Put cover and let it cook for 7-8 hours on Low.
Set an oven to preheat to 95°C (200°F).
Once the pork chops have been cooked, move the chops to the oven to keep it warm. Be cautious as the

chops are so tender that it might fall apart. Blend the sour cream with 2 tbsp flour in a small bowl, then stir into the meat juices. Increase the slow cooker to high heat for 15-30 minutes or until the sauce becomes a bit thick. Serve the sauce on top of the pork chops.
Nutrition Information
Calories: 257 calories;;Total Fat: 14.4;Sodium: 487;Total Carbohydrate: 14.3;Cholesterol: 54;Protein: 16.8

263. Southern Barbeque Pulled Beef Sandwiches
Serving: 8 | Prep: 20mins | Cook: 7hours30mins | Ready in:
Ingredients
cooking spray
1/2 cup beef broth
1 teaspoon liquid smoke flavoring
1 tablespoon olive oil
1 (4 pound) boneless beef chuck roast
3 tablespoons barbeque seasoning (such as Grill Mates® Smokehouse Maple)
2 tablespoons Worcestershire sauce
2 cups barbeque sauce
8 Kaiser rolls, split
Direction
Use cooking spray to cover the inside of a 6-quart oval slow cooker crock.
In a small bowl, add liquid smoke and beef broth then mix together. Transfer the mixture to the prepared crock.
Add drizzles of olive oil on top of the beef chuck roast. Season the roast by rubbing in barbeque seasoning and gently put the meat into the liquid mixture in the slow cooker. Add drizzles of Worcestershire sauce over the roast.
Cook on Low until the meat is tender and can be separated easily, 7 to 8 hours. Transfer roast to a cutting board and use a pair of forks to tear the roast into strands.
Drain liquid from the slow cooker crock, keeping 1/2 cup of the liquid and throwing away the remaining.
In a bowl, mix barbeque sauce with the 1/2 cup of liquid that we keep.
Put shredded beef back to the slow cooker. Stir the meat with drizzles of the barbeque sauce mixture. Cook on High until bubbles form, about 30 minutes.
Put spoons of beef onto split Kaiser rolls.
Nutrition Information
Calories: 580 calories;;Total Fat: 29.3;Sodium: 2105;Total Carbohydrate: 45.7;Cholesterol: 103;Protein: 30.9

264. Spanish Chicken
Serving: 8 | Prep: 15mins | Cook: 6hours | Ready in:
Ingredients
2 pounds boneless chicken thighs
1 quart boiling water
1/2 teaspoon salt
5 onions, cut into 2 inch pieces
5 large green bell peppers, cut into 2 inch pieces
1 (8 ounce) jar chili sauce
1 (15 ounce) can tomato sauce
1 cup ketchup
Direction
Add chicken into a big slow cooker. Add in enough boiling water to totally cover the chicken, and put in half tsp. of salt. Keep it covered, and set slow cooker to HIGH. Cook till the chicken meat becomes white.

Put in onions and peppers. Let it simmer for roughly 10 minutes or till peppers and onions become slightly soft. Mix in ketchup, chili sauce, and tomato sauce. Keep it covered, set slow cooker to LOW, and cook for roughly 6 hours.
Nutrition Information
Calories: 342 calories;Protein: 23.3;Total Fat: 17.7;Sodium: 850;Total Carbohydrate: 24;Cholesterol: 95

265. Sunday Sticky Chicken
Serving: 5 | Prep: 20mins | Cook: 1hours | Ready in:
Ingredients
1 cup all-purpose flour
1 teaspoon seasoned salt
ground black pepper to taste
1 (4 pound) whole chicken, cut into pieces
1/4 cup vegetable oil
2 cups milk
1 (14.5 ounce) can chicken broth
1 tablespoon cornstarch
1/4 cup water
Direction
Start preheating the oven to 175°C (350°F).
Mix the ground black pepper, seasoned salt and the flour in a big resealable plastic bag. Put the chicken parts into the bag and shake until coated.
Add the oil to a big skillet over medium-high heat. Add the chicken parts into the hot oil and quickly cook until all sides are a bit browned. Move the chicken parts to a Dutch oven. Put in broth and milk and cover.
Bake for an hour at 175°C (350°F).
Take away from the oven and move the chicken to a serving dish. Mix the water and cornstarch in a different small bowl. Stir well until cornstarch is dissolved. Pour a little of the cornstarch mixture at a time to the liquid in the Dutch oven until it reaches the consistency you want. Pour the prepared gravy over the chicken or serve alongside.
Nutrition Information
Calories: 696 calories;;Sodium: 709;Total Carbohydrate: 25.6;Cholesterol: 169;Protein: 56.6;Total Fat: 39

266. Sweet Ham Recipe
Serving: 24 | Prep: 10mins | Cook: 8hours | Ready in:
Ingredients
1 (7 pound) canned ham
2 cups orange juice
1/2 cup water
1 (20 ounce) can crushed pineapple
3 tablespoons brown sugar
Direction
Add the ham into slow cooker. Add the pineapple, water, and orange juice on top of ham. Scatter the brown sugar along top and sides. Keep covered, and cook over Low heat for 8 hours.
Nutrition Information
Calories: 220 calories;;Total Fat: 9.9;Sodium: 1691;Total Carbohydrate: 7.5;Cholesterol: 50;Protein: 24

267. Sweet And Savory Brisket
Serving: 6 | Prep: 10mins | Cook: 8hours | Ready in:
Ingredients
1 (3 pound) beef brisket, visible fat trimmed
1 cup ketchup
1/4 cup grape jelly
1 envelope dry onion soup mix
1/2 teaspoon ground black pepper

Direction
Across grain, cut brisket in half; put 1/2 in slow cooker. Spread 1/2 ketchup and grape jelly; sprinkle 1/2 dry onion soup mix. Put leftover brisket piece over 1st piece; repeat spreading with leftover onion soup mix, grape jelly and ketchup. Into cooker, sprinkle black pepper.
Cover cooker; cook for 8-10 hours on low till meat is very tender.
Nutrition Information
Calories: 372 calories;;Sodium: 922;Total Carbohydrate: 22.3;Cholesterol: 91;Protein: 27.3;Total Fat: 19.3

268. Sweet And Savory Slow Cooker Pulled Pork

Serving: 10 | Prep: 20mins | Cook: 6hours15mins | Ready in:
Ingredients
1 (4.5 pound) bone-in pork shoulder roast
1 cup root beer
2 1/2 tablespoons light brown sugar
2 teaspoons kosher salt
1/2 teaspoon ground black pepper
1 1/2 teaspoons ground paprika
1/2 teaspoon dry mustard
1/2 teaspoon onion powder
1/4 teaspoon garlic salt
1/4 teaspoon celery salt
1/4 teaspoon ground cinnamon
1/4 teaspoon ground ginger
1/4 teaspoon ground nutmeg
1/3 cup balsamic vinegar
1 1/2 cups root beer
1 1/2 fluid ounces whiskey
1/4 cup brown sugar
1 tablespoon olive oil
3/4 cup prepared barbecue sauce
10 hamburger buns, split
Direction
In a large plastic bag, put the pork shoulder roast, then drizzle the meat with 1 cup of root beer; squeeze all the air out of the bag. Seal the bag, then refrigerate for 6 hours till overnight.
On the following day, in a bowl, stir the nutmeg, ginger, cinnamon, celery salt, garlic salt, dry mustard, onion powder, paprika, black pepper, kosher salt, and light brown sugar together.
Take the meat out of the marinade, shake off the excess. Rub spice mixture all over the meat, use plastic wrap to wrap, then refrigerate for half an hour to 2 hours.
In a bowl, mix the brown sugar, whiskey, 1 1/2 cups of root beer, and balsamic vinegar together; stir until the sugar dissolves.
In a frying pan, heat the olive oil over medium-high heat, then sear all sides of the meat for around 3 minutes each side until the meat forms a brown crust. Add the seared meat to a slow cooker. Drizzle the meat with the balsamic vinegar-root beer mixture, adjust the slow cooker to High, then cook for 6 - 8 hours.
Take the roast out of the slow cooker, use 2 forks to shred the meat. Debone and discard all except for 1 cup of liquid in the slow cooker. Move the shredded meat back to the cooker, stir in the barbecue sauce, then allow to sit on Low until ready to serve. Serve piled on buns.
Nutrition Information
Calories: 485 calories;;Total Fat: 19.1;Sodium: 985;Total Carbohydrate: 45.5;Cholesterol: 81;Protein: 28.5

269. Sweet And Sour Beef

Serving: 4 | Prep: 5mins | Cook: 6hours10mins | Ready in:
Ingredients
1 pound cubed beef stew meat
3 cups cold water
3/4 cup vinegar
9 tablespoons soy sauce
9 tablespoons brown sugar
5 tablespoons cornstarch
Direction
Heat the deep skillet on medium heat; mix and cook beef in the hot skillet for 7-10 minutes till fully brown. Put beef into a slow cooker.
Whisk cornstarch, brown sugar, soy sauce, vinegar and water till smooth; put on beef.
Cook on low for 6-8 hours till sauce is thick and beef is tender.
Nutrition Information
Calories: 321 calories;;Total Carbohydrate: 41.8;Cholesterol: 60;Protein: 23.1;Total Fat: 6.5;Sodium: 2090

270. Tangy Slow Cooker Pork Roast

Serving: 8 | Prep: 10mins | Cook: 6hours | Ready in:
Ingredients
1 large onion, sliced
2 1/2 pounds boneless pork loin roast
1 cup hot water
1/4 cup white sugar
3 tablespoons red wine vinegar
2 tablespoons soy sauce
1 tablespoon ketchup
1/2 teaspoon black pepper
1/2 teaspoon salt
1/4 teaspoon garlic powder
1 dash hot pepper sauce, or to taste
Direction
On the bottom of a slow cooker, evenly arrange onion slices, and then top the onion with the roast.
Combine hot sauce, garlic powder, salt, black pepper, ketchup, soy sauce, vinegar, sugar and water in a bowl; add onto the roast.
Put the cover on and cook for 3-4 hours on High or for 6-8 hours on Low.
Nutrition Information
Calories: 210 calories;Protein: 24.6;Total Fat: 7.7;Sodium: 483;Total Carbohydrate: 9.4;Cholesterol: 66

271. Two Corn Chicken Posole

Serving: 6 | Prep: 10mins | Cook: 4hours | Ready in:
Ingredients
2 cups diced onion
1 tablespoon minced garlic
1 1/2 teaspoons ground cumin
1 teaspoon dried oregano
1 teaspoon chili powder
1 (28 ounce) can green enchilada sauce
1 (29 ounce) can hominy, rinsed and drained
1 (15.25 ounce) can Del Monte® Whole Kernel Corn, drained
1 (14.5 ounce) can Del Monte® Diced Tomatoes, not drained
2 cups College Inn® Chicken Broth
3 pounds boneless, skinless chicken thighs
Topping Options:

Shredded cabbage
Sliced jalapeno chile
Diced avocado
radishes, sliced
Shredded Monterey Jack cheese
Chopped cilantro
Lime juice
Direction
In a 6- to 7-quart slow cooker, mix together all ingredients except chicken. Add chicken and press down to cover with mixture. Cook, covered, for 8 to 10 hours on LOW or 4 to 5 hours on HIGH.
Remove chicken and use a fork to shred. Remove chicken back to stew.
Place stew in bowls and serve with toppings as desired.
Nutrition Information
Calories: 557 calories;;Sodium: 882;Total Carbohydrate: 37.4;Cholesterol: 162;Protein: 44.3;Total Fat: 25.5

272. Vegetarian Slow Cooker Meal
Serving: 6 | Prep: 5mins | Cook: 5hours | Ready in:
Ingredients
1 (32 fluid ounce) container vegetable broth
1 (16 ounce) package frozen cheese-filled tortellini
1 (8 ounce) package cream cheese, cut into pieces
1 (8 ounce) package fresh spinach
1 cup sliced crimini ('baby bella') mushrooms
Direction
In a slow cooker stir mushrooms, spinach, cream cheese, tortellini and vegetable broth together. For 5 to 6 hours, cook on low heat.
Nutrition Information
Calories: 398 calories;;Total Fat: 20;Sodium: 733;Total Carbohydrate: 40.8;Cholesterol: 74;Protein: 15.5

273. Verenike Casserole For The Slow Cooker
Serving: 8 | Prep: 10mins | Cook: 5hours | Ready in:
Ingredients
1 (24 ounce) carton cottage cheese
3 eggs, beaten
1 cup sour cream
2 cups evaporated milk
2 cups cubed cooked ham
1 teaspoon salt
1/2 teaspoon ground black pepper
7 uncooked lasagna noodles, or as needed
Direction
In a bowl, combine together the sour cream, cottage cheese, ham, eggs, evaporated milk, pepper and salt until mixed well. Spread about 1/2 of the mixture into the bottom of a slow cooker. Spread a layer of noodles atop cottage cheese mixture and break as needed to fit. Add the remaining cottage cheese mixture on top.
Cook 5 to 6 hours on Low until noodles are cooked through.
Nutrition Information
Calories: 419 calories;;Total Fat: 23.2;Sodium: 1179;Total Carbohydrate: 25.4;Cholesterol: 132;Protein: 27.3

274. Waikiki Style Meatballs
Serving: 6 | Prep: 15mins | Cook: 3hours30mins | Ready in:
Ingredients
1 1/2 pounds ground beef
2/3 cup plain breadcrumbs
1/3 cup minced onion
1/4 cup milk
1 egg
1 1/2 teaspoons salt
2 tablespoons cornstarch
1/2 cup brown sugar
1 (15 ounce) can pineapple chunks, juice reserved
1/3 cup vinegar
1/3 cup chopped green bell pepper
Direction
Turn the oven to 350°F (175°C) to preheat.
In a bowl, well combine together salt, egg, milk, onion, bread crumbs, and ground beef. Form the mixture into balls and place onto a cookie sheet.
In the preheated oven, bake for 25 minutes, or until the bottoms of the meatballs turn brown. Remove to a slow cooker.
In the bottom of a saucepan, mix together brown sugar and cornstarch and heat on low heat. Add vinegar and the reserved pineapple juice; whisk until smooth. Boil the mixture for exactly 1 minute, and then take away from heat. In the slow cooker, pour the mixture over the meatballs.
Add green bell pepper and pineapple chunks to the slow cooker.
In the slow cooker, cook the mixture on Low for 3-4 hours, or until the flavors are fully blended.
Nutrition Information
Calories: 393 calories;;Total Fat: 15.1;Sodium: 757;Total Carbohydrate: 41.8;Cholesterol: 101;Protein: 22.5

275. Zesty Pulled Pork Sandwiches
Serving: 4 | Prep: 10mins | Cook: 4hours30mins | Ready in:
Ingredients
1 1/2 cups barbeque sauce, or more as desired
1/2 cup chopped white onion
1/4 cup ketchup
1/4 cup brown sugar
1 teaspoon salt
1 teaspoon ground black pepper
1/2 teaspoon chili powder
1 pound boneless pork loin, quartered
4 onion rolls, halved
Direction
In a slow cooker, stir chili powder, black pepper, salt, brown sugar, ketchup, onion, and barbeque sauce; put in the pork loin and coat with the sauce. Cook on High, covered, for about 4 1/2 hours, until pork is very soft. Use 2 forks to shred the pork. Keep warm on Low until it's ready to serve.
Then serve on onion rolls.
Nutrition Information
Calories: 504 calories;;Total Fat: 9;Sodium: 2089;Total Carbohydrate: 78.6;Cholesterol: 53;Protein: 25.7

Chapter 4: Dessert Slow Cooker Recipes

276. Alexander's Chocolate Covered Peanuts

Serving: 28 | Prep: 15mins | Cook: 2mins | Ready in:
Ingredients
18 ounces white almond bark, broken into pieces
2 cups chocolate chips, or more to taste
24 ounces lightly salted peanuts, or more to taste
Direction
In a slow cooker, add almond bark. On High, stir from time to time until mostly melted, for about 2 minutes. Reduce the heat to Low. Mix in chocolate chips until thoroughly dark, for about 30 seconds. Add the peanuts.
Drop the peanut clusters onto a parchment paper-lined countertop by a spoonful to test if they are chunky and thick. Mix in more chocolate chips and peanuts if it is too runny and loose.
Use parchment paper to line 4 to 5 baking sheets. Use a melon baller to put spoonfuls of the peanut clusters on top. Let harden for about 1 hour.
Nutrition Information
Calories: 286 calories;;Sodium: 199;Total Carbohydrate: 21.2;Cholesterol: 0;Protein: 7.7;Total Fat: 22.8

277. Amazing Slow Cooker Chocolate Cake

Serving: 12 | Prep: 20mins | Cook: 3hours | Ready in:
Ingredients
2 cups white sugar
1 3/4 cups all-purpose flour
3/4 cup unsweetened cocoa powder
1 1/2 teaspoons baking soda
1 1/2 teaspoons baking powder
1 teaspoon salt
2 eggs
1 cup milk
1/2 cup vegetable oil
2 teaspoons vanilla extract
1 cup boiling water
Direction
Grease crock of a large slow cooker with cooking spray.
Stir together the salt, baking powder, baking soda, cocoa, flour and sugar in a medium bowl. In a different small bowl, stir together vanilla, oil, milk and eggs until well blended. Mix in the boiling water. Put in the dry with wet ingredients and stir well.
In a prepared slow cooker, pour the cake batter. Set slow cooker on Low setting. Cook for 3 hours, until the cake's top has no wet spots and has pulled away from of the crock's sides. Switch off the slow cooker and let the cake rest about 30 minutes prior to serving.
Nutrition Information
Calories: 313 calories;;Total Fat: 11.3;Sodium: 434;Total Carbohydrate: 51.4;Cholesterol: 33;Protein: 4.7

278. Ashley And Whitney's Apple Cherry Cobbler

Serving: 6 | Prep: | Cook: | Ready in:
Ingredients
1 Reynolds® Slow Cooker Liner
1/2 cup granulated sugar
4 teaspoons quick-cooking tapioca
1 teaspoon apple pie spice
1 1/2 pounds cooking apples, peeled, cored and cut into 1/2-inch slices
1 (16 ounce) can pitted tart cherries
1/2 cup dried cherries
Spiced Triangles:
1 tablespoon sugar
1/2 teaspoon apple pie spice
1 (8 ounce) package refrigerated crescent rolls
1 tablespoon melted butter
Ice cream, such as butter pecan or cinnamon; or half-and-half; or light cream (optional)
Direction
Line a crockery cooker of 3 1/2 or 4-quarts using Reynolds(R) Slow Cooker Liner. Put in apple pie spice, tapioca, and sugar; mix.
Mix in the dried cherries, undrained canned cherries and apple slices until blended.
Cover; cook for 6 to 7 hours on low-heat setting or for 3 to 3 1/2 hours on high setting.
Spiced Triangles: Mix 1/2 teaspoon apple pie spice and 1 tablespoon sugar together in a bowl.
Unroll 1 package (8) of refrigerated crescent rolls. Split triangles. Brush with 1 tablespoon of melted butter on top and dust with sugar-cinnamon mixture. Slice every triangle into 3 triangles. Put on an ungreased baking sheet.
Bake for 8 to 10 minutes in a 375°F oven, until the bottoms are lightly browned. Transfer to cool on a wire rack.
Split cherry-apple mixture among 6 to 8 shallow dessert plates to serve.
If desired, add with ice cream and Spiced Triangles or half-and-half on top of it.
Nutrition Information
Calories: 414 calories;;Total Fat: 12.6;Sodium: 333;Total Carbohydrate: 71.6;Cholesterol: 15;Protein: 5

279. Bread Pudding In The Slow Cooker

Serving: 6 | Prep: 10mins | Cook: 3hours | Ready in:
Ingredients
8 cups cubed bread
1 cup raisins (optional)
2 cups milk
4 eggs
1/4 cup butter, melted
1/4 cup white sugar
1/2 teaspoon vanilla extract
1/4 teaspoon ground nutmeg
Direction
Put raisins and bread in a slow cooker.
Whisk nutmeg, vanilla extract, sugar, butter, eggs and milk in a bowl; put on raisins and bread. Toss to coat evenly.
Cook on low for 3 hours till inserted knife near the middle exits clean.
Nutrition Information
Calories: 396 calories;;Sodium: 455;Total Carbohydrate: 57.9;Cholesterol: 151;Protein: 11.4;Total Fat: 14.3

280. Chocolate Cherry Slow Cooker Cake

Serving: 8 | Prep: 10mins | Cook: 4hours | Ready in:
Ingredients
1 (18.25 ounce) box red velvet cake mix
2 eggs
1/2 cup water

1/2 cup sour cream
1 (3.9 ounce) package instant chocolate fudge pudding mix
1 (21 ounce) can cherry pie filling
1 cup semisweet chocolate chips
Direction
Coat the crock of slow cooker with cooking spray. Mix chocolate pudding blend with sour cream, water, eggs and cake mix in a bowl using an electric hand mixer until smooth. Mix in the chocolate chips and cherry pie filling; drizzle into the greased crock.
Cook for about 4 hours on Low until set in the center.
Nutrition Information
Calories: 558 calories;;Cholesterol: 53;Protein: 6.5;Total Fat: 16.9;Sodium: 628;Total Carbohydrate: 99.5

281. Chocolate Pudding Cake IV

Serving: 16 | Prep: 10mins | Cook: 50mins | Ready in:
Ingredients
1 (18.25 ounce) package chocolate cake mix
1 (3.9 ounce) package instant chocolate pudding mix
2 cups sour cream
4 eggs
1 cup water
3/4 cup vegetable oil
1 cup semisweet chocolate chips
Direction
Set oven to 175 °C (350 ° F) to preheat. Prepare a 10-inch Bundt(R) pan, grease and flour it.
Combine pudding mix and cake mix in a large bowl. In the center, make a well and pour oil, water, eggs, and sour cream. On low speed, beat until combined. Scrape bowl and beat on medium speed about 4 minutes. Mix in chocolate chips. Transfer batter to prepared pan.
Bake in the prepared oven until a toothpick comes out clean from the center, about 45 to 50 minutes. Allow to cool in pan for 10 minutes, then take out and place on a serving plate. Serve warm.
Alternate cooking directions: Coat a 5-quart slow cooker with nonstick cooking spray and pour in batter. Cook with a cover on low for 6 hours. Divide into individual dishes.
Nutrition Information
Calories: 384 calories;;Total Fat: 25.8;Sodium: 398;Total Carbohydrate: 37.5;Cholesterol: 59;Protein: 5

282. Gluten Free Slow Cooker Chocolate Lava Cake

Serving: 10 | Prep: 15mins | Cook: 2hours30mins | Ready in:
Ingredients
Cake:
1 (16 ounce) package gluten-free chocolate cake mix
2/3 cup milk
2 eggs, lightly beaten
1/3 cup vegetable oil
2/3 cup boiling water
Pudding:
2 avocados, halved and pitted
1 cup almond milk, or as needed
1/2 cup honey
1/2 cup unsweetened cocoa powder
1/2 teaspoon vanilla extract
2 cups semisweet chocolate chips
Direction
In a large bowl, pour the cake mix. Create a well in the middle, then add vegetable oil, eggs, and milk; mix until thoroughly combined. Add the boiling water to the batter, then stir to combine.
Spread the batter into a slow cooker.
In a food processor, combine vanilla extract, cocoa powder, honey, almond milk, and avocados; process until the consistency of pudding. Spread the batter in a slow cooker. Top with chocolate chips.
Cook on High for around 2 and a half hours until edges pull away from the cooker's sides.
Nutrition Information
Calories: 564 calories;;Total Fat: 26;Sodium: 412;Total Carbohydrate: 81.1;Cholesterol: 34;Protein: 7.5

283. Heaven In A Slow Cooker

Serving: 8 | Prep: 5mins | Cook: 3hours | Ready in:
Ingredients
1 (19.8 ounce) package fudge brownie mix
1 (17.5 ounce) pouch chocolate chip cookie mix
4 eggs, beaten
1/2 cup butter, melted
Direction
In a slow cooker, combine butter, eggs, chocolate chip cookie mix, and fudge brownie mix.
Cook for 3 hours on Low.
Nutrition Information
Calories: 746 calories;;Total Fat: 40.1;Sodium: 508;Total Carbohydrate: 93;Cholesterol: 149;Protein: 9.5

284. Meadowwood Tapioca Pudding

Serving: 8 | Prep: 15mins | Cook: 2hours30mins | Ready in:
Ingredients
4 cups whole milk
2/3 cup white sugar
2 teaspoons vanilla extract
1/2 teaspoon salt
1/2 cup small tapioca pearls
3 egg yolks
Direction
In a slow cooker, stir tapioca pearls, salt, vanilla extract, sugar and milk until the sugar is dissolved. Switch the cooker to high setting, cover with a lid, then cook for 2 hours (Switch to low setting, then cook for 4 hours, if preferred. Mix pudding occasionally while cooking).
In a bowl, put egg yolks and stir until smooth. Blend egg yolks with about 1 tablespoon of hot pudding until thoroughly mixed; keep gradually mixing hot tapioca pudding into egg yolks, slowly increase the amount of pudding blended in until the pudding and yolks total about 2 cups. Slowly pour the yolk mixture into the slow cooker with pudding until mixed, stirring continuously for 5 minutes until the egg yolks have thickened the pudding.
Put the lid back on the cooker, then keep cooking on high setting for another 30 minutes (or another hour on a low setting) until the pudding reaches desired degree of thickness.
Nutrition Information
Calories: 190 calories;;Total Fat: 5.6;Sodium: 198;Total Carbohydrate: 29.8;Cholesterol: 89;Protein: 5

285. Pumpkin Pie Pudding

Serving: 8 | Prep: 15mins | Cook: 4hours | Ready in:

Ingredients
1 cup brown sugar
3/4 cup biscuit baking mix
2 tablespoons ground cinnamon
2 tablespoons ground nutmeg
2 teaspoons ground cloves
2 teaspoons ground ginger
3 tablespoons butter, cubed
1 (12 fluid ounce) can evaporated milk
2 eggs
1 (15 ounce) can solid pack pumpkin puree
1/4 cup applesauce
1 tablespoon vanilla extract
Direction
Gently grease a small (1-quart) slow cooker.
In a food processor, combine ginger, cloves, nutmeg, cinnamon, baking mix, and brown sugar. Pulse 3 to 4 times until mixed. Put in eggs, evaporated milk, and butter, and pulse 5 to 6 times until blended. Add vanilla extract, applesauce, and pumpkin puree and process for 30 seconds until smooth.
In the prepared slow cooker, pour the pumpkin mixture. Heat on Low for 4 hours until very thick.
Nutrition Information
Calories: 315 calories;Protein: 6.5;Total Fat: 12;Sodium: 378;Total Carbohydrate: 47.3;Cholesterol: 72

286. Reindeer Poop

Serving: 60 | Prep: 10mins | Cook: 1hours30mins | Ready in:
Ingredients
1 (16 ounce) package white candy coating, coarsely chopped
1 (4 ounce) bar German sweet chocolate, chopped
1 (16 ounce) package semi-sweet chocolate chips
2 (16 ounce) jars dry roasted peanuts
Direction
In a slow cooker, add peanuts, chocolate chips, German sweet chocolate, and white candy coating. Turn the cooker to Low, gently heat the candy with a cover for one and a half hours without stirring. Stir the mixture after 1 1/2 hours and spoon out by teaspoons onto waxed paper. Let cool and set for 45 minutes.
Nutrition Information
Calories: 174 calories;;Sodium: 129;Total Carbohydrate: 13.6;Cholesterol: 2;Protein: 4.4;Total Fat: 12.8

287. Rice Pudding In A Slow Cooker

Serving: 8 | Prep: 10mins | Cook: 2hours | Ready in:
Ingredients
1 cup uncooked glutinous white rice
1 cup white sugar
2 (12 fluid ounce) cans evaporated milk
1 teaspoon vanilla extract
1 ounce cinnamon stick
1 teaspoon ground nutmeg
Direction
Put in a slow cooker the nutmeg, cinnamon stick, vanilla, evaporated milk, sugar and rice. Cover and cook on Low, mixing occasionally, for 1 1/2 hours. Discard cinnamon stick, then serve warm.
Nutrition Information
Calories: 321 calories;;Total Fat: 7.5;Sodium: 102;Total Carbohydrate: 56.4;Cholesterol: 27;Protein: 8.2

288. Slow Cooked Apple Brown Betty

Serving: 6 | Prep: 20mins | Cook: 3hours | Ready in:
Ingredients
3 cups apples - peeled, cored and diced
10 slices bread, cubed
1/2 teaspoon ground cinnamon
1/4 teaspoon ground nutmeg
1/8 teaspoon salt
3/4 cup brown sugar
1/2 cup butter, melted
Direction
Put apples into the crock of a slow cooker. Toss brown sugar, salt, nutmeg, cinnamon and bread cubes in a medium bowl. Add the mixture on the top of apples and give a drizzle of melted butter. Cover up and cook on Low until apples are tender, or for 3 hours.
Nutrition Information
Calories: 349 calories;;Cholesterol: 41;Protein: 3.5;Total Fat: 16.9;Sodium: 447;Total Carbohydrate: 47.7

289. Slow Cooker Apple Cinnamon Bread Pudding

Serving: 8 | Prep: 15mins | Cook: 3hours | Ready in:
Ingredients
4 Granny Smith apples - peeled, cored, and chopped
3 cups 1-inch bread cubes
4 large eggs
2 (12 fluid ounce) cans evaporated skim milk
3/4 cup packed brown sugar
2 teaspoons ground cinnamon
1 teaspoon nutmeg
Direction
Mix bread and apples in slow cooker crock.
Beat eggs in bowl; mix nutmeg, cinnamon, brown sugar and milk in. Put on bread and apples.
Cook for 3-4 hours on high till custard forms.
Nutrition Information
Calories: 261 calories;;Total Fat: 3.4;Sodium: 257;Total Carbohydrate: 48.1;Cholesterol: 96;Protein: 11.3

290. Slow Cooker Apple Crisp

Serving: 6 | Prep: 30mins | Cook: 2hours | Ready in:
Ingredients
1 cup all-purpose flour
1/2 cup light brown sugar
1/2 cup white sugar
1/2 teaspoon ground cinnamon
1/4 teaspoon ground nutmeg
1 pinch salt
1/2 cup butter, cut into pieces
1 cup chopped walnuts
1/3 cup white sugar, or to taste
1 tablespoon cornstarch
1/2 teaspoon ground ginger
1/2 teaspoon ground cinnamon
6 cups apples - peeled, cored and chopped
2 tablespoons lemon juice
Direction
Put salt, nutmeg, half a teaspoon of cinnamon, half a cup of white sugar, brown sugar and flour in a bowl then mix together. Use a fork or fingers to mix the flour mixture with butter till coarse crumbs form. Put in walnuts and stir then set aside.
Whisk half a teaspoon of cinnamon, ginger, cornstarch, a third of a cup of sugar together. Put the

apples in a slow cooker, stir in the cornstarch mixture then toss with lemon juice. Use the walnut crumb topping to sprinkle on top. Put a lid on cooker and cook on Low for 4 hours or on High for 2 hours till apples become soft. Uncover the slow cooker partially for about an hour to let the topping harden.
Nutrition Information
Calories: 593 calories;;Total Fat: 28.9;Sodium: 116;Total Carbohydrate: 83.8;Cholesterol: 41;Protein: 5.8

291. Slow Cooker Apples With Cinnamon And Brown Sugar

Serving: 4 | Prep: 20mins | Cook: 3hours | Ready in:
Ingredients
1 Reynolds® Slow Cooker Liner
4 medium tart baking apples (such as Granny Smith, Braeburn, or Jonathan), cored
1/4 cup regular rolled oats
1/4 cup raisins
2 tablespoons packed brown sugar
1 tablespoon butter, chopped
1/2 teaspoon ground cinnamon
2/3 cup apple juice
Direction
Use a Reynolds® Slow Cooker Liner to line a 5- to 6-quart slow cooker.
Lay apples in the prepared slow cooker. Mix cinnamon, butter, brown sugar, raisins and oats in a small bowl. Use a spoon to transfer mixture into the centers of apples, using a narrow metal spatula or the back of the spoon to pat in mixture. Pile any remaining oat mixture on top of apples. Add apple juice around apples in the cooker.
Put the lid on and cook for 3 hours on low.
Move apples to serving bowls and use cooking liquid to drizzle over.
Nutrition Information
Calories: 191 calories;;Sodium: 27;Total Carbohydrate: 43;Cholesterol: 8;Protein: 1.5;Total Fat: 3.3

292. Slow Cooker Bananas Foster

Serving: 4 | Prep: 10mins | Cook: 2hours | Ready in:
Ingredients
4 bananas, peeled and sliced
4 tablespoons butter, melted
1 cup packed brown sugar
1/4 cup rum
1 teaspoon vanilla extract
1/2 teaspoon ground cinnamon
1/4 cup chopped walnuts
1/4 cup shredded coconut
Direction
Layer cut bananas in the bottom of slow cooker.
In a small bowl, mix cinnamon, vanilla, rum, brown sugar and butter; drizzle over bananas.
Cover and cook for 2 hours on Low. Top bananas with coconut and walnuts in the last 30 minutes of cooking.
Nutrition Information
Calories: 539 calories;;Sodium: 101;Total Carbohydrate: 83.7;Cholesterol: 31;Protein: 3;Total Fat: 20.6

293. Slow Cooker Cherry Cobbler

Serving: 6 | Prep: 15mins | Cook: 2hours | Ready in:
Ingredients
1 (21 ounce) can cherry pie filling
1 cup all-purpose flour
1/4 cup white sugar
1 1/2 teaspoons baking powder
1/4 teaspoon salt
1/4 cup butter, melted
1/2 cup milk
1/2 teaspoon vanilla extract
Direction
Use cooking spray to coat the inside of the slow cooker. Add the cherry pie filling. Stir the salt, baking powder, sugar, and flour together in a medium bowl. Create a well in the middle, then pour in vanilla, milk, and melted butter. Stir until thoroughly blended. Pour evenly over the cherry pie filling. Cook while covered on High for 1 and a half hours to 2 hours or till a toothpick pinned into the topping comes out clean.
Nutrition Information
Calories: 302 calories;;Total Fat: 8.3;Sodium: 300;Total Carbohydrate: 53.3;Cholesterol: 22;Protein: 3.3

294. Slow Cooker Cherry Delight

Serving: 8 | Prep: 10mins | Cook: 3hours | Ready in:
Ingredients
2 (21 ounce) cans cherry pie filling
1 (18.25 ounce) box yellow cake mix
1/2 cup unsalted butter, melted
Direction
Pour the cherry pie filling into a 2-quart slow cooker. In a bowl, mix butter together with yellow cake mixture. Distribute over pie filling in the slow cooker. Cook on Low for 3 to 4 hours until soft and bubbly.
Nutrition Information
Calories: 552 calories;;Total Fat: 19.1;Sodium: 453;Total Carbohydrate: 92.1;Cholesterol: 32;Protein: 3.5

295. Slow Cooker Chocolate Candy

Serving: 48 | Prep: 5mins | Cook: 3hours | Ready in:
Ingredients
2 pounds dry roasted peanuts
4 (1 ounce) squares German sweet chocolate
1 (12 ounce) bag semi-sweet chocolate chips
2 1/2 pounds white almond bark
Direction
In slow cooker, respectively, layer white almond bark, chocolate chips, German chocolate squares and peanuts.
Switch slow cooker to low then cook for 3 hours. Do not mix.
Mix the mixture until smooth using the wooden spoon. Drop by tablespoonfuls into miniature muffin cups. Cool for 30 minutes, until hardened.
Nutrition Information
Calories: 269 calories;;Total Fat: 21.7;Sodium: 156;Total Carbohydrate: 21;Cholesterol: 0;Protein: 6.7

296. Slow Cooker Fruit Cobbler

Serving: 8 | Prep: 10mins | Cook: 3hours | Ready in:
Ingredients
cooking spray
2 cups frozen peach slices
2 cups mixed frozen berries
2 tablespoons cornstarch
1 teaspoon vanilla extract
1/2 cup brown sugar
1/2 teaspoon ground cinnamon

1/2 teaspoon nutmeg
1 (18.25 ounce) package white cake mix
1/2 cup melted butter
Direction
Grease lightly a slow cooker with cooking spray. In the slow cooker, blend together berries and peaches; dust with cornstarch and toss to coat.
Mix vanilla into the berry combination; put in nutmeg, cinnamon and brown sugar. Pour cake mix atop berry blend then pour with melted butter.
Cook for 3 to 3 1/2 hours in the slow cooker on high, until bubbling.
Nutrition Information
Calories: 511 calories;;Sodium: 514;Total Carbohydrate: 84.7;Cholesterol: 31;Protein: 3.7;Total Fat: 18.8

297. Slow Cooker Peach Cobbler

Serving: 6 | Prep: 15mins | Cook: 4hours | Ready in:
Ingredients
3/4 cup old-fashioned oats
3/4 cup white sugar
2/3 cup brown sugar
1/2 cup all-purpose baking mix (such as Bisquick®)
3/4 teaspoon ground cinnamon
5 fresh peaches - peeled, pitted, and sliced
Direction
Grease the inside of a 3- to 4-quart slow cooker crock. In a bowl, combine cinnamon, baking mix, brown sugar, white sugar, and oats; mix in peaches and add mixture to greased slow cooker.
Cook for 4 hours on Low.
Nutrition Information
Calories: 258 calories;;Sodium: 134;Total Carbohydrate: 59;Cholesterol: 0;Protein: 2.1;Total Fat: 2.2

298. Slow Cooker Peach Upside Down Cake

Serving: 8 | Prep: 30mins | Cook: 2hours | Ready in:
Ingredients
3 (15 ounce) cans sliced peaches in heavy syrup, drained well
5 tablespoons butter, melted
2/3 cup packed light brown sugar
1 teaspoon cinnamon
1/2 teaspoon nutmeg
1 1/2 sticks butter, softened
1 cup white sugar
2 large eggs
1/2 teaspoon pure almond extract
2 cups flour
2 teaspoons baking powder
1/2 teaspoon salt
1 cup whole milk
Direction
Distribute the peach slices between several layers of paper towels, then allow to dry for 20 minutes, gently pushing occasionally and replacing any soaked towels.
In the meantime, pour the melted butter over the bottom of an oval slow cooker (6 quarts in size). In a bowl, mix nutmeg with cinnamon and brown sugar; dust atop butter.
Place peaches on brown sugar in a tight layer. (To fit them all in, you may need a partial second layer).
In a big bowl, beat white sugar with softened butter using an electric mixer for 3 minutes until light and fluffy. Beat in eggs, one by one; beat well after each addition. Beat in the almond extract.
In a separate bowl, stir salt, baking powder, and flour together. Process in batches, alternately mix milk and flour mixture into the egg blend, starting and ending with the flour blend. Stir the batter until well mixed. Spoon over peaches and evenly spread.
Drape paper towels on top of slow cooker (to soak up any condensation while baking), cover using a lid. Cook on High for 2 to 2 1/2 hours until a wooden skewer placed into the middle comes out clean. Uncover and discard paper towels. Remove ceramic liner from the slow cooker with oven mitts; then let cool for 10 minutes. Run a knife around the cake's edges and flip on a serving platter carefully.
Nutrition Information
Calories: 654 calories;;Sodium: 486;Total Carbohydrate: 100.8;Cholesterol: 114;Protein: 6.8;Total Fat: 27.2

299. Slow Cooker Peanut Butter Fudge Cake

Serving: 8 | Prep: 15mins | Cook: 1hours45mins | Ready in:
Ingredients
1 1/2 cups all-purpose flour
1/2 cup packed brown sugar
1 teaspoon baking powder
1 teaspoon baking soda
1/4 teaspoon salt
1 cup chunky peanut butter
3/4 cup sour cream (not reduced-fat)
3 tablespoons butter, melted
2 tablespoons boiling water
1 cup semisweet chocolate chips
3/4 cup white sugar
6 tablespoons unsweetened cocoa powder
3/4 cup whole milk, warmed
1 teaspoon vanilla extract
Direction
In a bowl, stir together salt, baking soda, baking powder, brown sugar and flour. In a large bowl, stir boiling water, butter, sour cream and peanut butter together (mixture is going to be very thick). Toss the flour blend into peanut butter blend until fully mixed; mix in chocolate chips.
Grease a 6-quart oval slow cooker generously. In the slow cooker, distribute the batter evenly.
In a small bowl, stir vanilla with milk, cocoa powder and white sugar until smooth. Drizzle over the batter. Cover and cook for 1 1/2 to 2 hours on High until the sides of the cake start pulling away from the ceramic liner and appear solid (the middle will still be soft).
Nutrition Information
Calories: 608 calories;Protein: 13.4;Total Fat: 32.5;Sodium: 507;Total Carbohydrate: 74.7;Cholesterol: 23

300. Slow Cooker Tapioca Pudding

Serving: 8 | Prep: 5mins | Cook: 3hours | Ready in:
Ingredients
4 cups milk
2/3 cup white sugar
1/2 cup small pearl tapioca
2 eggs, lightly beaten
Direction
In a slow cooker, stir eggs, tapioca, sugar, and milk together. Cook with a cover on Low for 6 hours or on Medium for 3 hours, mixing occasionally. Serve warm.

Nutrition Information
Calories: 191 calories;;Total Fat: 5.2;Sodium: 66;Total Carbohydrate: 30.3;Cholesterol: 59;Protein: 6.5

301. Slow Cooker Vanilla Tapioca Pudding

Serving: 14 | Prep: 5mins | Cook: 6hours | Ready in:
Ingredients
1/2 gallon whole milk
1 1/3 cups white sugar
1 cup small pearl tapioca
4 eggs, lightly beaten
1 teaspoon vanilla extract
Direction
In a slow cooker crock, mix the eggs together with tapioca, sugar and milk.
Cook on Low for 6 hours, mixing once per hour. Mix vanilla into pudding.
Nutrition Information
Calories: 218 calories;;Total Carbohydrate: 35.1;Cholesterol: 67;Protein: 6.3;Total Fat: 6;Sodium: 76

302. Slow Cooker Peanut Butter Fudge Cake

Serving: 8 | Prep: 20mins | Cook: 1hours30mins | Ready in:
Ingredients
1 1/2 cups all-purpose flour
1/2 cup packed brown sugar
1 teaspoon baking powder
1 teaspoon baking soda
1/4 teaspoon salt
1 cup chunky peanut butter
3/4 cup sour cream
3 tablespoons butter, melted
2 tablespoons boiling water
1 cup semisweet chocolate chips
1 serving cooking spray
3/4 cup whole milk, warmed
3/4 cup white sugar
6 tablespoons unsweetened cocoa powder
1 teaspoon vanilla extract
Direction
In a small bowl, whisk salt, baking soda, baking powder, brown sugar, and flour together.
In a big bowl, stir boiling water, butter, sour cream, and peanut butter till thick. Blend peanut butter mixture and flour mixture together until batter is thoroughly mixed; fold in chocolate chips.
Use cooking spray to generously coat the liner of a 6-quart oval slow cooker. Pour batter evenly in the slow cooker.
In a small bowl, whisk vanilla extract, cocoa powder, white sugar, and milk till smooth. Spread over batter.
Cook on High for 1 and a half hours to 2 hours until edges of the cake are about to pull away from liner and look solid (but the core will remain soft).
Nutrition Information
Calories: 610 calories;;Cholesterol: 23;Protein: 13.3;Total Fat: 32.8;Sodium: 507;Total Carbohydrate: 74.7

303. Stef's Slow Cooker Creme Brulee

Serving: 4 | Prep: 20mins | Cook: 2hours | Ready in:
Ingredients
4 egg yolks
1/4 cup white sugar
1/4 teaspoon salt
1 2/3 cups heavy whipping cream
2 teaspoons vanilla extract
4 teaspoons white sugar
Direction
In a bowl, whisk together salt, 1/4 cup of sugar and yolks until smooth, then whisk in vanilla extract and cream gently. Strain into a liquid measuring cup with the custard mixture.
Use a folded kitchen towel to line the bottom of a 6-qt. oval slow cooker to make a flat surface so ramekins do not slide around. Place on the towel with four 4-oz. ramekins, then fill enough water into the slow cooker to reach halfway up sides of ramekins.
Put evenly into ramekins with custard. Drape over top of the slow cooker with paper towels to absorb any condensation during baking process, then place a lid to cover securely.
Cook on low setting for 2 hours, until custard is set yet still jiggles a bit.
Remove ramekins to a rack to cool thoroughly for 45 minutes, then chill the custards without a cover for a minimum of 3 hours, until cold.
Sprinkle over each ramekin with 1 tsp. of sugar and gently shake to distribute sugar evenly. Use a culinary torch to heat the sugar for a minute, until browned and melted.
Nutrition Information
Calories: 465 calories;;Total Fat: 41.1;Sodium: 191;Total Carbohydrate: 20.3;Cholesterol: 341;Protein: 4.7

304. Triple Coconut Cake

Serving: 8 | Prep: 30mins | Cook: 1hours25mins | Ready in:
Ingredients
Cake:
1 cup white sugar
1/2 cup refined coconut oil
1 stick unsalted butter
3 large eggs
2 cups flour
1 teaspoon baking powder
1/4 teaspoon salt
1/2 cup full-fat coconut milk
Frosting:
4 ounces cream cheese
1/2 stick unsalted butter
1 1/2 cups confectioners' sugar
1/4 teaspoon salt
1/2 teaspoon vanilla extract
1/2 cup toasted sweetened coconut flakes
Direction
In a large bowl, beat butter, coconut oil, and sugar together using an electric mixer until thoroughly combined. Put in eggs, one by one, beating well after each addition.
In a bowl, whisk salt, baking powder, and flour together. Working in batches, blend the flour mixture into the butter mixture, alternately with the coconut milk until just combined.
Use a cooking spray to generously coat a 6-quart oval slow cooker, then use parchment paper to line the base. In the slow cooker, pour the batter evenly.
Drape paper towels atop the slow cooker (to soak up any condensation during baking), then use lid to cover. Cook on High for 1 hour to 1 and a half hours till a wooden skewer pinned into the middle of cake comes out clean.

Take the lid and paper towels away. Use oven mitts to take ceramic liner out of the slow cooker, then allow to cool for 10 minutes. On a serving platter, carefully turn the cake out, then allow to cool completely for around 1 hour.
For the frosting: In a bowl, beat butter and cream cheese together using an electric mixer on high speed for around 3 minutes until fluffy and light. Beat in a little powdered sugar at a time until thoroughly combined. Beat in vanilla and salt.
Frost the top of the cake, then put coconut flakes on top to serve.
Nutrition Information
Calories: 761 calories;;Sodium: 285;Total Carbohydrate: 79.7;Cholesterol: 131;Protein: 7.9;Total Fat: 47.7

305. Unbelievably Easy Slow Cooker Black Forest Cake

Serving: 10 | Prep: 5mins | Cook: 3hours | Ready in:
Ingredients
1/2 cup butter
1 (8 ounce) can crushed pineapple, drained and juice reserved
1 (21 ounce) can cherry pie filling
1 (18.25 ounce) package chocolate cake mix
Direction
Melt the butter in a small saucepan then blend in reserved juice from the pineapple can. Put the mixture aside.
On the bottom of a slow cooker, distribute the crushed pineapple in a layer. Spoon cherry pie filling on top of the pineapple in an even layer, then empty the dry cake mix into the slow cooker on top of cherry filling. Mix the pineapple juice blend and butter then pour over the dry cake mix.
Set slow cooker to Low then cook for 3 hours. In bowls, spoon the dessert into bowls and allow to cool for 5 minutes for the hot pie filling to cool prior to serving.
Nutrition Information
Calories: 385 calories;Protein: 3.5;Total Fat: 17.3;Sodium: 503;Total Carbohydrate: 57.9;Cholesterol: 24

306. Warm Berry Compote

Serving: 6 | Prep: 10mins | Cook: 1hours35mins | Ready in:
Ingredients
6 cups frozen mixed berries
1/2 cup white sugar
1 1/2 teaspoons finely grated orange zest
1/4 cup orange juice
2 tablespoons cornstarch
2 tablespoons water
Direction
In a slow cooker, mix juice with zest, sugar and berries. Cook on high for about 1 1/2 hours until bubbling.
In a cup, mix the water and cornstarch together until completely dissolved. Mix into berry blend. Cook with a cover for another 5 to 10 minutes until thickened. Serve warm or at room temperature.
Nutrition Information
Calories: 140 calories;;Sodium: 1;Total Carbohydrate: 37.3;Cholesterol: 0;Protein: 1.1;Total Fat: 0.5

307. Warm Chocolate Peanut Butter Pudding Cake

Serving: 12 | Prep: 15mins | Cook: 1hours30mins | Ready in:
Ingredients
cooking spray
1 1/2 cups all-purpose flour
1/2 cup brown sugar
1 teaspoon baking powder
1 teaspoon baking soda
1 cup creamy peanut butter
3/4 cup sour cream
3 tablespoons butter, melted
1 teaspoon almond extract
2 tablespoons boiling water
3/4 cup white sugar
6 tablespoons unsweetened cocoa powder
2 cups boiling water
2 tablespoons chocolate syrup
Direction
Grease the inside of a slow cooker with cooking spray. In a bowl, mix together baking soda, baking powder and flour. In a different bowl, stir in 2 tablespoons boiling water with almond extract, melted butter, sour cream and peanut butter until smooth. To create a very thick batter, mix the peanut butter mixture with flour mixture. Scoop batter into a prepared slow cooker.
In a bowl, mix 2 cups of boiling water, cocoa powder and white sugar until mixed completely. Pour the chocolate mixture over the batter in a slow cooker. Cook on High for 1 1/2 hours, until cake starts pulling away from the cooker's sides and feels firm on top. Let cool prior to serving for 15 minutes. Pour with chocolate syrup.
Nutrition Information
Calories: 327 calories;;Total Fat: 17.3;Sodium: 278;Total Carbohydrate: 38.8;Cholesterol: 14;Protein: 8.1

Chapter 5: Soup And Stew Slow Cooker Recipes

308. African Sweet Potato Stew

Serving: 10 | Prep: 30mins | Cook: 6hours15mins | Ready in:

Ingredients
1 onion, chopped
2 small jalapeno peppers, seeded and chopped
3 cloves garlic, minced
2 teaspoons minced fresh ginger
2 teaspoons ground cumin
1/2 teaspoon salt
1/4 teaspoon ground coriander
1/4 teaspoon ground cinnamon
1/8 teaspoon red pepper flakes
4 cups water
2 1/2 pounds sweet potatoes, peeled and chopped into 2-inch pieces
2 (15 ounce) cans diced tomatoes, drained
2 (15 ounce) cans chickpeas, drained and rinsed
1/4 cup peanut butter
1 (15 ounce) can sliced green beans, drained

Direction
Into the big slow cooker, add red pepper flakes, cinnamon, coriander, salt, cumin, ginger, garlic, jalapeno peppers and onion. Add in water and mix to combine. Whisk in peanut butter, chickpeas, tomatoes, and sweet potatoes.
Set cooker to the Medium High, cover it, and cook for roughly 6 hours or till the sweet potatoes become soft and stew becomes thick. Mix in the green beans and keep on cooking, covered, for 15-20 minutes or till beans are thoroughly heated.

Nutrition Information
Calories: 231 calories;;Sodium: 569;Total Carbohydrate: 43.1;Cholesterol: 0;Protein: 7.4;Total Fat: 4.2

309. Alison's Slow Cooker Vegetable Beef Soup

Serving: 10 | Prep: 10mins | Cook: 8hours | Ready in:

Ingredients
1 1/2 pounds cubed beef stew meat
2 cups water
1 small onion, chopped
1 (28 ounce) can crushed tomatoes
1 (16 ounce) package frozen mixed vegetables
2 potatoes, peeled and cubed
10 cubes beef bouillon, crumbled
2 teaspoons ground black pepper
1 tablespoon salt
1 tablespoon dried basil

Direction
In a slow cooker, put beef. Add water. Mix in potatoes, mixed vegetables, tomatoes, and onion. Use basil, salt, pepper, and bouillon to season. Cook for 8 hours on low.

Nutrition Information
Calories: 228 calories;;Sodium: 1717;Total Carbohydrate: 21.2;Cholesterol: 38;Protein: 15.4;Total Fat: 9.3

310. Amelia's Slow Cooker Brunswick Stew

Serving: 8 | Prep: 30mins | Cook: 8hours | Ready in:

Ingredients
1 tablespoon vegetable oil
1 pound country style pork ribs
1 onion, chopped
1 roasted chicken, deboned and shredded
1 (28 ounce) can diced tomatoes
3/4 cup ketchup
1/2 (10 fluid ounce) bottle steak sauce
1/2 cup cider vinegar
2 tablespoons Worcestershire sauce
1 tablespoon hot sauce
1 lemon, juiced
2 cubes chicken bouillon
1/2 tablespoon ground black pepper
1 (15 ounce) can whole kernel corn, undrained
1 cup frozen lima beans, thawed

Direction
In a skillet, heat vegetable oil on medium heat. Brown all sides of ribs. Put in a slow cooker. Put onion in skillet. Cook until they're tender. Put into slow cooker.
In the slow cooker, put in pepper, chicken bouillon, lemon, hot sauce, Worcestershire sauce, cider vinegar, steak sauce, ketchup and tomatoes.
Cook on high, covered, for 6 hours. Take out ribs. Throw bones then shred. Put meat back in slow cooker. Mix in lima beans and corn. Cook on high for 2 hours, covered.

Nutrition Information
Calories: 405 calories;;Total Fat: 17.1;Sodium: 1281;Total Carbohydrate: 31.4;Cholesterol: 91;Protein: 32.1

311. Award Winning White Chicken Chili

Serving: 10 | Prep: 10mins | Cook: 8hours3mins | Ready in:

Ingredients
1 1/4 pounds skinless, boneless chicken breast
2 (15 ounce) cans great Northern beans
1 (15 ounce) can white corn
1 (14 ounce) can chicken broth
1 (10.5 ounce) can cream of chicken soup
1 (4 ounce) can chopped green chile peppers
1 (1.25 ounce) package taco seasoning
1/2 cup sour cream
1/2 cup shredded pepper Jack cheese, or to taste

Direction
Into a slow cooker, layer chicken, great Northern beans and corn.
In a bowl, put together taco seasoning, green chile peppers, chicken soup and chicken broth; put atop chicken mixture.
Cover and cook for 8 to 10 hours on Low till chicken is not pink anymore in the middle. Mix in pepper Jack cheese and sour cream; cover and cook for 3 to 5 minutes till cheese melts.

Nutrition Information
Calories: 179 calories;;Total Fat: 7.7;Sodium: 933;Total Carbohydrate: 12.5;Cholesterol: 45;Protein: 14.6

312. Babushka's Slow Cooker Root Vegetable And Chicken Stew

Serving: 10 | Prep: 40mins | Cook: 7hours10mins | Ready in:

Ingredients
2 ½ pounds skin-on, bone-in chicken thighs
1 yellow onion, coarsely chopped
1 red onion, coarsely chopped
4 stalks celery with some leaves, coarsely chopped

4 mediums red potatoes - peeled, halved, and cubed
1 rutabaga - peeled, halved, and cubed
2 mediums turnips - peeled, halved, and cubed
2 mediums carrots, peeled and sliced
1 ½ cups cremini mushrooms, coarsely chopped
4 cloves garlic, peeled and crushed
2 teaspoons salt
1 teaspoon herbes de Provence
1 teaspoon onion powder
1 teaspoon garlic powder
freshly ground black pepper
1 (32 fluid ounce) container vegetable broth
Direction
On medium low heat, heat a sauté pan. In batches, cook chicken thighs, 2-3 minutes per side, until skin begins to brown. Do not overcook. Meat should be raw and pink inside. Put chicken in a bowl, keeping juices in the pan.
In the pan, sauté celery and onion for 5 minutes until edges brown and is translucent. Put in a big bowl. Add in garlic, mushrooms, carrots, turnips, rutabaga and potatoes to celery-onion mixture. Sprinkle on pepper, garlic powder, onion powder, herbes de Provence and salt. Mix and stir veggies until coated.
In a slow cooker, put 1/2 of veggie mixture. Add 1/2 of chicken. Layer leftover chicken and veggies on top.
Put vegetable broth on mixture in the slow cooker. Cook for 7 hours on low, stirring gently every several hours if you want.
Take chicken from stew with tongs. Cool. Separate bones and skin from meat. Shred meat. Put meat back in slow cooker.
Nutrition Information
Calories: 296 calories;Protein: 21.4;Sodium: 756;Total Carbohydrate: 26.2;Cholesterol: 64;Total Fat: 11.8

313. Bachelor's Stew

Serving: 6 | Prep: | Cook: | Ready in:
Ingredients
2 pounds lean beef chuck, trimmed and cut into 1 inch cubes
1/3 cup dried bread crumbs
1 teaspoon salt
1/8 teaspoon ground black pepper
1 yellow onion
3 carrots, cut into thick strips
4 stalks celery, chopped
1 teaspoon dried basil
1/3 cup quick-cooking tapioca
1 (4.5 ounce) can sliced mushrooms
1 teaspoon soy sauce
2 (10.75 ounce) cans condensed tomato soup
1 cup beef broth
Direction
Combine breadcrumbs with pepper and salt, then toss with beef. In a slow cooker, place coated beef cubes and add celery, basil, onion, carrots, soy sauce, tapioca, tomato soup, mushrooms, and broth. Stir well, cook on high setting while covered for 3 to 5 hours or on low for 10 to 12 hours.
Nutrition Information
Calories: 510 calories;;Total Fat: 29.3;Sodium: 1415;Total Carbohydrate: 31.4;Cholesterol: 107;Protein: 30.3

314. Beef And Barley Soup I

Serving: 16 | Prep: 20mins | Cook: 8hours | Ready in:
Ingredients
2 beef soup bones
2 tablespoons kosher salt
5 stalks celery
1 onion, quartered
1/2 teaspoon ground black pepper
2 'bouqet garni' spice balls
1/2 pound baby carrots
1/4 cup fresh parsley
11 cloves garlic, peeled
1 cup barley
Direction
In a big slow cooker, put beef bones. Add garlic, parsley, carrots, pepper, bouquets garnis, onion, celery stalks, and salt. Pour in hot water, leaving 2 inches headspace. Put a cover on and cook over high heat, about 6 hours, mixing sometimes.
Add barley and cook until you can easily remove the meat from bones, about another 2 hours, mixing sometimes.
Take out and dispose parsley, celery, bouquets garnis, and onion.
Move to bones to a plate and strip the meat off bones, make sure to leave the gristle and cartilage intact.
Return the meat to the soup, whisk and enjoy.
Nutrition Information
Calories: 58 calories;;Total Fat: 0.4;Sodium: 744;Total Carbohydrate: 12.3;Cholesterol: 0;Protein: 1.9

315. Beer Beef Stew II

Serving: 12 | Prep: 30mins | Cook: 8hours | Ready in:
Ingredients
2 tablespoons vegetable oil
3 1/2 pounds beef stew meat, cut into 1 1/2 inch pieces
1 cup all-purpose flour
2 large potatoes, chopped
1 cup chopped carrots
3/4 cup chopped celery
3/4 cup chopped onion
3 cloves garlic, chopped
1 tablespoon dried basil
1 tablespoon dried thyme
1 cup chili sauce
1 cup beer
1/4 cup brown sugar
Direction
In the skillet, heat oil on medium heat. Into the big resealable plastic bag, add flour and beef stew meat and shake to coat. Move the coated meat into skillet and cook till browned or for roughly 60 seconds.
In the slow cooker, combine garlic, onion, celery, carrots and potatoes. Add the browned beef on top of vegetables and use thyme and basil to season.
Whisk brown sugar, beer and chili sauce in the bowl and add on top of the meat in slow cooker.
Keep the slow cooker covered and cook for 8 hours on Low setting or for 2 hours on High setting.
Nutrition Information
Calories: 421 calories;;Total Fat: 20.5;Sodium: 376;Total Carbohydrate: 32.4;Cholesterol: 73;Protein: 24.9

316. Beer Baked Irish Beef

Serving: 6 | Prep: | Cook: | Ready in:
Ingredients
6 slices bacon, diced
1/3 cup all-purpose flour
1 teaspoon salt

1/2 teaspoon ground black pepper
1 teaspoon ground allspice
2 1/2 pounds cubed beef stew meat
4 carrots, peeled and cut diagonally into 1-inch pieces
4 large onions, cut into eighths
2 cloves garlic, chopped
1/4 cup minced fresh parsley
1 teaspoon dried rosemary, crushed
1 teaspoon dried marjoram
1 bay leaf
1 (12 fluid ounce) can or bottle Irish stout beer

Direction

In a large nonstick skillet, place the bacon and cook until crisp and brown over medium heat. Remove the bacon pieces; set aside, leaving the drippings in the skillet.

In a large plastic zipper bag, place the black pepper, flour, allspice, and salt, then shake a few times to combine. Place the beef stew meat into the pocket and shake to cover the meat. In the skillet, place the meat pieces with the bacon drippings and cook until all sides are brown.

Remove to a slow cooker the browned meat and add the bay leaf, parsley, carrots, onions, marjoram, rosemary, and garlic to the cooker.

Pour the beer into the skillet and boil over medium-low heat, scraping all the browned bits from the bottom of the skillet. Pour the beer over the meat and vegetables in the slow cooker. Cook on medium setting while covered for 4 to 5 hours until the meat is very tender.

Remove the bay leaf before serving and sprinkle the stew with the reserved pieces of bacon.

Nutrition Information
Calories: 576 calories;;Sodium: 729;Total Carbohydrate: 19.7;Cholesterol: 123;Protein: 36.4;Total Fat: 38.5

317. Beezie's Black Bean Soup

Serving: 10 | Prep: 1hours | Cook: 5hours | Ready in:

Ingredients
1 pound dry black beans
1 1/2 quarts water
1 carrot, chopped
1 stalk celery, chopped
1 large red onion, chopped
6 cloves garlic, crushed
2 green bell peppers, chopped
2 jalapeno pepper, seeded and minced
1/4 cup dry lentils
1 (28 ounce) can peeled and diced tomatoes
2 tablespoons chili powder
2 teaspoons ground cumin
1/2 teaspoon dried oregano
1/2 teaspoon ground black pepper
3 tablespoons red wine vinegar
1 tablespoon salt
1/2 cup uncooked white rice

Direction

Put beans in a big pot and fill it with water 3 times the volume of the beans. Boil for 10 minutes on medium-high heat. Cover then take off heat. Let it sit for an hour. Drain then rinse.

Mix 1 1/2 qt. fresh water and soaked beans in a slow cooker. Cook on high for 3 hours, covered.

Mix in tomatoes, lentils, jalapeno pepper, bell peppers, garlic, onion, celery, and carrot. Season with salt, red wine vinegar, black pepper, oregano, cumin and chili powder. Cook for 2-3 hours on low. Mix rice into slow cooker at the final 20 minutes of cooking. Puree half of soup in a food processor or blender. Pour back into pot then serve.

Nutrition Information
Calories: 231 calories;;Total Fat: 1.2;Sodium: 851;Total Carbohydrate: 43.4;Cholesterol: 0;Protein: 12.6

318. Best Italian Sausage Soup

Serving: 8 | Prep: 30mins | Cook: 6hours | Ready in:

Ingredients
1 1/2 pounds sweet Italian sausage
2 cloves garlic, minced
2 small onions, chopped
2 (16 ounce) cans whole peeled tomatoes
1 1/4 cups dry red wine
5 cups beef broth
1/2 teaspoon dried basil
1/2 teaspoon dried oregano
2 zucchini, sliced
1 green bell pepper, chopped
3 tablespoons chopped fresh parsley
1 (16 ounce) package spinach fettuccine pasta
salt and pepper to taste

Direction

Cook sausage on medium heat till brown in big pot; use slotted spoon to remove. On paper towels, drain. Drain fat from pan; keep 3 tbsp.

Cook onion and garlic for 2-3 minutes in reserved fat; mix oregano, basil, broth, wine and tomatoes in. Put in slow cooker; mix parsley, bell pepper, zucchini and sausage in.

Cover; cook for 4-6 hours on low.

Boil pot of lightly salted water; in boiling water, cook pasta for 7 minutes till al dente. Drain water; put pasta in slow cooker. Simmer for several minutes; before serving, season with pepper and salt.

Nutrition Information
Calories: 436 calories;;Total Carbohydrate: 43.5;Cholesterol: 33;Protein: 21;Total Fat: 17.8;Sodium: 1609

319. Best No Bean Chili

Serving: 8 | Prep: 15mins | Cook: 2hours10mins | Ready in:

Ingredients
1 cup strong brewed coffee
1 (14.5 ounce) can diced tomatoes
1 (12 fluid ounce) can or bottle porter-style beer
2 (6 ounce) cans tomato paste
1 cup beef broth
1/2 cup brown sugar
1/4 cup ketchup-style chili sauce (such as Heinz®)
1/4 cup chopped jalapeno peppers
1 tablespoon ground cumin
1 tablespoon cocoa powder
2 teaspoons ground ancho chile powder
1 teaspoon oregano
1 teaspoon cayenne pepper
1 teaspoon ground coriander
1 teaspoon salt
2 teaspoons vegetable oil
2 pounds extra lean ground beef
2 onions, chopped
3 cloves garlic, minced
1/2 cup cornmeal

Direction

Add coffee into a slow cooker and set to high setting; put in salt, coriander, cayenne pepper, oregano, chile powder, cocoa powder, cumin, jalapeno peppers, chili sauce, brown sugar, beef broth, tomato paste, beer and diced tomatoes.
In a big skillet, heat oil on moderate heat. Cook and stir garlic, onions and ground beef in the skillet for 7-10 minutes until the beef is browned thoroughly, then put the mixture into the slow cooker.
Add cornmeal into the slow cooker gradually while stirring to ensure no lumps.
Lower heat to low and cook for about 2 hours.
Nutrition Information
Calories: 449 calories;;Total Carbohydrate: 40.8;Cholesterol: 79;Protein: 29;Total Fat: 18;Sodium: 1004

320. Black Lentil Veggie Soup

Serving: 6 | Prep: 25mins | Cook: 4hours10mins | Ready in:
Ingredients
1 1/2 cups black lentils
2 quarts vegetable broth
3 cups diced tomatoes
10 carrots, peeled and diced
1 onion, cut into 1/2-inch dice
2 small turnips, peeled and diced
1 green bell pepper, diced
3 tablespoons unsalted butter
2 tablespoons minced ginger
2 cloves garlic, minced
1/2 teaspoon ground coriander
1/2 teaspoon ground cumin
salt to taste
Direction
Transfer black lentils covered with 4 cups water into a microwave-safe bowl; microwave for 5 minutes till soft. Mix; if needed, add more water. Microwave for another 5 minutes. Drain; rinse.
Mix together salt, cumin, coriander, garlic, ginger, butter, green bell pepper, turnips, onion, carrots, tomatoes and vegetable broth in a big slow cooker; mix in lentils.
Cook for 4-6 hours on high till carrots are tender.
Nutrition Information
Calories: 164 calories;Protein: 3.8;Total Fat: 6.7;Sodium: 879;Total Carbohydrate: 21.8;Cholesterol: 15

321. Black Eyed Pea Bratwurst Stew

Serving: 8 | Prep: 15mins | Cook: 3hours | Ready in:
Ingredients
2 pounds bratwurst sausages, cut into thirds
2 (15 ounce) cans black-eyed peas, rinsed and drained
2 (9 ounce) packages frozen cut green beans, thawed
2 cups cubed potatoes
1 cup chopped onion
2 cloves garlic, minced
1 (32 fluid ounce) container chicken stock
2 tablespoons hot Buffalo wing sauce (such as Frank's® REDHOT Buffalo Wing Sauce), or to taste
2 tablespoons ketchup
1 tablespoon Worcestershire sauce
1/2 teaspoon ground thyme
salt and ground black pepper to taste
1/4 cup all-purpose flour (optional)
1 cup water (optional)
Direction
In the slow cooker, put black pepper, salt, thyme, Worcestershire sauce, ketchup, Buffalo wing sauce, chicken stock, garlic, onion, potatoes, green beans, black-eyed peas and bratwurst sausages.
Cook on high heat for 3-4 hours, until the soup is thickened and the vegetables become tender.
If you prefer a thick stew, blend water and flour together until smooth in a blow. Transfer the mixture into the stew; keep simmering for about 5 minutes, until thickened.
Nutrition Information
Calories: 530 calories;;Total Carbohydrate: 37.9;Cholesterol: 69;Protein: 21.5;Total Fat: 32.1;Sodium: 1909

322. Bull Riders All Beef Chili

Serving: 8 | Prep: 30mins | Cook: 8hours | Ready in:
Ingredients
1 tablespoon olive oil
1 1/2 pounds cubed beef stew meat
1 large eggplant, diced
5 tablespoons mild chili powder
1/4 cup dried oregano
1 teaspoon paprika
1 teaspoon ground black pepper
2 cups water
3 cubes beef bouillon
1 (6 ounce) can tomato paste
3 tablespoons all-purpose flour
1 teaspoon sea salt
Direction
Heat a big cast-iron skillet on moderate high heat until it starts to smoke a little. Add olive oil and tilt the pan to coat. Put in beef cubes, then cook and stir to brown all sides. Once the meat is pretty much browned, season with pepper, paprika, oregano and chili powder. Stir beef to coat well with all spices and keep on browning until spices become aromatic. Transfer all of the beef from the pan to a 3 1/2-qt. slow cooker.
Add water into the skillet and watch out as it will sizzle. Stir in beef bouillon and scrape all the spice and bits of beef off of the bottom of the pan. Once the bouillon is dissolved and the pan's bottom is clear, add the liquid. Combine tomato paste and eggplant with the chili. Put more water if needed until the amount of liquid in the cooker is within 1/2 in. of the top.
Cover and cook on high setting for about 3-4 hours or on low setting for about 6-8 hours. If you have time, cooking on low heat is recommended. Sift in the flour and mix in along with salt twenty minutes before serving. Let it cook until thickened. Serve together with preferred chili toppings.
Nutrition Information
Calories: 246 calories;;Total Carbohydrate: 14.2;Cholesterol: 47;Protein: 16.8;Total Fat: 14.6;Sodium: 799

323. Busy Day Slow Cooker Chili

Serving: 8 | Prep: 10mins | Cook: 6hours5mins | Ready in:
Ingredients
1 pound ground beef
1 (15 ounce) can kidney beans, rinsed and drained
1 (14.5 ounce) can diced tomatoes
2 (14.5 ounce) cans Mexican-style stewed tomatoes
1 green bell pepper, chopped
1 (4 ounce) can diced green chile peppers

2 tablespoons chili powder
2 cloves garlic, minced
1 teaspoon sea salt
ground black pepper to taste
1 (8 ounce) can whole kernel corn (no salt added), drained
Direction
Heat a big skillet on moderate high heat. In the hot skillet, cook and stir beef for 5-7 minutes until crumbly and browned, then drain and get rid of grease. Put the beef to slow cooker.
Stir in black pepper, sea salt, garlic, chili powder, green chile peppers, green bell pepper, stewed tomatoes, diced tomatoes and kidney beans.
Cook on low setting for 5 1/2 to 7 1/2 hours. Stir corn into the chili and keep on cooking for a half hour longer.
Nutrition Information
Calories: 220 calories;;Sodium: 953;Total Carbohydrate: 24.6;Cholesterol: 34;Protein: 15;Total Fat: 7.7

324. Cabbage Beef Soup

Serving: 10 | Prep: 20mins | Cook: 8hours | Ready in:
Ingredients
2 tablespoons vegetable oil
1 pound ground beef
1/2 large onion, chopped
5 cups chopped cabbage
2 (16 ounce) cans red kidney beans, drained
2 cups water
24 ounces tomato sauce
4 beef bouillon cubes
1 1/2 teaspoons ground cumin
1 teaspoon salt
1 teaspoon pepper
Direction
Heat the oil on medium-high heat in the big stock pot. Put in the onion and ground beef, and cook till the beef becomes crumbly and browned-well. Drain off the fat, and move the beef into the slow cooker. Put in the pepper, salt, cumin, bouillon, tomato sauce, water, kidney beans and cabbage. Mix to the dissolve the bouillon, and keep covered.
Cook over low setting for 6-8 hours, or over high setting for 4 hours. Mix once in a while.
Nutrition Information
Calories: 211 calories;;Total Carbohydrate: 20.3;Cholesterol: 28;Protein: 14.1;Total Fat: 8.7;Sodium: 1154

325. Cabbage Patch Stew

Serving: 4 | Prep: 20mins | Cook: 7hours | Ready in:
Ingredients
1 pound lean ground beef
1 onion, chopped
1 (15 ounce) can ranch-style beans
1/4 teaspoon ground cumin
3 cloves garlic, minced
2 1/2 cups chopped cabbage
1 green bell pepper, chopped
1 (14.5 ounce) can stewed tomatoes, with liquid
2 stalks celery, chopped
1/4 cup picante sauce
1 cup water
salt to taste
freshly ground pepper, to taste
Direction
Brown ground beef with onion on medium heat in the skillet. Drain off fat.
In the crock pot, mix green pepper, cabbage, garlic, cumin, and ranch-style beans. Mix in beef mixture, water, picante sauce, celery, and stewed tomatoes. Season to taste with pepper and salt.
Keep it covered and cook for 6 - 8 hours.
Nutrition Information
Calories: 374 calories;Protein: 29.9;Total Fat: 14.3;Sodium: 914;Total Carbohydrate: 31.2;Cholesterol: 74

326. Cabbage Soup

Serving: 6 | Prep: 20mins | Cook: 5hours | Ready in:
Ingredients
1/2 head cabbage, chopped
4 leaves Swiss chard, torn into several pieces
3 leaves kale, torn into several pieces
4 green onions, chopped
1/2 cup chopped red bell pepper
1/2 cup thin carrot slices
1/2 cup chopped celery
3 cubes chicken bouillon
3/4 cup chopped bacon
1 teaspoon dried marjoram
1 tablespoon dried parsley
1 teaspoon dried sage
water, to cover
Direction
In a food processor, finely chop the celery, cabbage, carrot, chard, bell pepper, green onions, and kale; move to a slow cooker. Put in sage, chicken bouillon, parsley, marjoram, and bacon. Pour in just enough water over the ingredients to fill the cooker up to the crock's brim.
Cook for 5hrs on High.
Nutrition Information
Calories: 158 calories;;Cholesterol: 16;Protein: 5.7;Total Fat: 10.6;Sodium: 877;Total Carbohydrate: 11.6

327. Campbell's® Slow Cooker Chicken And Dumplings

Serving: 8 | Prep: 20mins | Cook: 8hours | Ready in:
Ingredients
1 1/2 pounds skinless, boneless chicken breasts, cut into 1-inch pieces
2 medium Yukon Gold potatoes, cut into 1-inch pieces
2 cups whole baby carrots
2 stalks celery, sliced
2 (10.75 ounce) cans Campbell's® Condensed Cream of Chicken Soup (Regular or 98% Fat Free)
1 cup water
1 teaspoon dried thyme leaves, crushed
1/4 teaspoon ground black pepper
2 cups all-purpose baking mix
2/3 cup milk
Direction
Put celery, carrots, potatoes and chicken into a 6-qt. slow cooker.
In a small bowl, mix together black pepper, thyme, water and soup. Pour the soup mixture over the vegetables and chicken.
Cook with a cover on low till the chicken is cooked through, about 7-8 hours.
In a medium bowl, blend milk and the baking mix. Use a spoon to spread the batter over the chicken mixture. Turn the heat up to high. Tilt the cover to

vent; cook for half an hour, or till the dumplings are cooked in the center.
Nutrition Information
Calories: 330 calories;;Sodium: 994;Total Carbohydrate: 34.3;Cholesterol: 52;Protein: 22.1;Total Fat: 11.7

328. Cauliflower Potato Soup
Serving: 4 | Prep: 15mins | Cook: 3hours10mins | Ready in:
Ingredients
1 head cauliflower, stemmed and chopped
2 large red potatoes, cut into 1-inch pieces
5 baby carrots, cut into 1/2-inch slices, or more to taste
2 teaspoons dried onion flakes, or to taste
water, or as needed
1 cube chicken bouillon
1 (10.75 ounce) can condensed cream of chicken soup
1/2 cup milk
1/2 (8 ounce) package cream cheese
1 tablespoon bacon bits, or more to taste
1/4 cup chopped fresh parsley, or more to taste
1/2 cup shredded Cheddar cheese
Direction
In a pot, mix onion flakes, carrots, potatoes, and cauliflower; cover with enough water and stir in chicken bouillon cube. Simmer and cook for about 10 minutes till cauliflower turns soft.
Move vegetable mixture and 1 cup of cooking liquid to a slow cooker. Blend bacon bits, cream cheese, milk, and cream of chicken soup into vegetable mixture.
Cook on Low, stirring once in a while, for 2.5 hours. Mix parsley into soup and go on cooking for half an hour to 1.5 hours until flavors blend and vegetable are softened. Dust with shredded Cheddar cheese.
Nutrition Information
Calories: 417 calories;;Sodium: 1090;Total Carbohydrate: 46.1;Cholesterol: 56;Protein: 15.9;Total Fat: 20.3

329. Caveman Chili
Serving: 8 | Prep: 20mins | Cook: 6hours15mins | Ready in:
Ingredients
2 pounds ground pork
8 thick slices bacon, chopped
1 (14.5 ounce) can diced tomatoes, drained
1 onion, chopped
3 small green bell peppers, chopped
1 (6 ounce) can tomato paste
1 (1.25 ounce) package chili seasoning (such as McCormick®)
1 pinch garlic powder, or more to taste
1 pinch onion powder, or more to taste
salt and ground black pepper to taste
1 pinch ground cayenne pepper, or more to taste
Direction
In a frying pan, put the pork over medium heat, then sprinkle with pepper and salt. Let it cook and stir for about 5-7 minutes, until it becomes crumbly and brown. Drain and get rid of the grease. Move the pork to a slow cooker.
In the hot frying pan, put the bacon and let it cook for about 10 minutes on medium-high heat until browned evenly. Drain and get rid of the grease. Move the bacon to the slow cooker.

In the slow cooker, mix the tomato paste, green bell pepper, onion and drained tomatoes, then add the cayenne pepper, pepper, salt, onion powder, garlic powder and seasoning packet. Mix to incorporate. Let it cook for about 6 hours on low, until the flavors have blended.
Nutrition Information
Calories: 357 calories;;Total Fat: 22;Sodium: 1031;Total Carbohydrate: 12.2;Cholesterol: 87;Protein: 27.4

330. Chad's Slow Cooker Taco Soup
Serving: 20 | Prep: 20mins | Cook: 8hours20mins | Ready in:
Ingredients
1 pound ground beef
1 pound bulk hot pork sausage
1 (28 ounce) can crushed tomatoes
1 (15.25 ounce) can whole kernel corn with red and green bell peppers (such as Mexicorn®), drained and rinsed
1 (14.5 ounce) can black beans, rinsed and drained
1 (14 ounce) can kidney beans, rinsed and drained
1 (1 ounce) package ranch dressing mix
1 (1 ounce) package taco seasoning mix
1 onion, chopped
1 green bell pepper, chopped
1 red bell pepper, chopped
1 (14.5 ounce) can diced tomatoes with green chile peppers (such as RO*TEL®), undrained
1/2 cup chili sauce
2 fresh jalapeno peppers, diced
1 (12 fluid ounce) can or bottle dark beer
ground black pepper to taste
Direction
In a large skillet, brown the ground beef completely over medium heat; let drain. Place into a slow cooker.
In a big skillet, brown the sausage completely over medium heat; let drain. Place the beef to a slow cooker.
Put black pepper, beer, jalapeno peppers, chili sauce, green chile peppers, diced tomatoes, red bell pepper, green bell pepper, onion, taco seasoning mix, ranch dressing mix, kidney beans, black beans, corn, and crushed tomatoes in the slow cooker. Turn the heat of slow cooker to low and cook for 8 to 10 hours, or if you want, set the heat to high and cook for 4 to 6 hours.
Nutrition Information
Calories: 195 calories;;Total Fat: 8.1;Sodium: 839;Total Carbohydrate: 19.4;Cholesterol: 27;Protein: 10.9

331. Chane's Beer And Rye Beef Stew
Serving: 10 | Prep: 30mins | Cook: 7hours | Ready in:
Ingredients
1/3 cup rye flour
1/3 cup whole wheat flour
2 1/2 teaspoons ground black pepper, divided
2 1/2 teaspoons dried thyme, divided
2 teaspoons caraway seeds, divided
1 teaspoon garlic powder
1 teaspoon dried basil
3 pounds cubed beef stew meat
1 (14 ounce) can Italian-style crushed tomatoes
1 large onion, cut into chunks
2 tablespoons coarse kosher salt
3 cloves garlic, pressed
1 (12 ounce) bottle beer

1 (14 ounce) package frozen carrots, celery, and onions
1 (10 ounce) package frozen chopped green bell pepper
1 (6 ounce) can tomato paste
1 (5 ounce) can sliced mushrooms, drained
1 cup beef broth
1 (.75 ounce) packet dry brown gravy mix
1 1/2 tablespoons chipotle-flavored hot sauce (such as Tabasco®)
1 tablespoon white sugar

Direction
In a large resealable plastic bag, mix 1 teaspoon ground pepper, rye flour, 1 teaspoon thyme, basil, 1 teaspoon caraway seeds, whole wheat flour, and garlic powder. Add beef, a handful at a time, to the bag and toss to coat.
Transfer beef into a large slow cooker. Add salt, garlic, remaining 1 and 1/2 teaspoon thyme, 1 teaspoon caraway seeds, onion, and crushed tomatoes. Pour in beer.
Cover and cook for 3 to 4 hours on Low setting. Stir stew. Mix in frozen carrot mixture, tomato paste, mushrooms, green bell pepper, gravy mix, beef broth, sugar, and hot sauce.
Cover and cook on Low setting until beef is tender and flavors combine for another 4 hours. Add the remaining 1 1/2 teaspoon pepper to season.

Nutrition Information
Calories: 526 calories;;Total Fat: 27.9;Sodium: 1779;Total Carbohydrate: 25.5;Cholesterol: 118;Protein: 40.9

332. Cheddar Bratwurst Stew

Serving: 6 | Prep: 10mins | Cook: 3hours | Ready in:
Ingredients
6 bratwurst sausages, cut into 2-inch pieces
1 (15 ounce) can green beans, drained
1 (10.75 ounce) can condensed cream of mushroom soup
1 red bell pepper, cut into strips
1 onion, chopped
8 small red potatoes, cut into bite-size chunks
1 (8 ounce) package shredded Cheddar cheese
1 cup water
salt and ground black pepper to taste

Direction
In a slow cooker, combine the green beans, bell pepper, red potatoes, onion, bratwurst sausages, Cheddar cheese, water, and cream of mushroom soup. Season the mixture with salt and black pepper. Set the cooker on High and let it cook for 3 hours until the potatoes are tender.

Nutrition Information
Calories: 646 calories;;Total Fat: 39;Sodium: 1502;Total Carbohydrate: 48.6;Cholesterol: 91;Protein: 25.6

333. Cheesy Brat Stew For The Slow Cooker

Serving: 6 | Prep: 15mins | Cook: 3hours | Ready in:
Ingredients
6 bratwurst links, browned and cut into 1/2 inch slices
4 medium potatoes, peeled and cubed
1 tablespoon dried minced onion
1 (15 ounce) can green beans, drained
1 small red bell pepper, seeded and chopped
2 cups shredded Cheddar cheese
1 (10.75 ounce) can cream of mushroom soup
2/3 cup water

Direction
In a slow cooker, place the potatoes, bratwurst, green beans, minced onion, Cheddar cheese, red pepper, water and mushroom soup. Cover while cooking on medium for 3 hours, or until potatoes are fork-tender.

Nutrition Information
Calories: 604 calories;Protein: 24.8;Total Fat: 40.4;Sodium: 1487;Total Carbohydrate: 35.1;Cholesterol: 102

334. Chicken Broth In A Slow Cooker

Serving: 5 | Prep: 15mins | Cook: 10hours | Ready in:
Ingredients
2 1/2 pounds bone-in chicken pieces
6 cups water
2 stalks celery, chopped
2 carrots, chopped
1 onion, quartered
1 tablespoon dried basil

Direction
In the slow cooker, put basil, onion, carrots, celery, water and chicken pieces.
Set the cooker on low; cook for 8-10 hours. Before using, drain and discard the vegetables. You may debone the chicken and use the meat in the soup.

Nutrition Information
Calories: 247 calories;;Total Fat: 14.8;Sodium: 99;Total Carbohydrate: 5.8;Cholesterol: 61;Protein: 21.7

335. Chicken Gumbo Over Rice

Serving: 6 | Prep: 35mins | Cook: 7hours25mins | Ready in:
Ingredients
1/4 cup olive oil, divided
1/2 pound Italian sausage, cut into 1/4-inch slices
1/4 cup all-purpose flour
1 pound skinless, boneless chicken breasts, cut into 1/2-inch strips
1 cup chopped onion
1 cup diced green bell pepper
1 cup chopped celery
2 tablespoons minced jalapeno peppers
1 teaspoon ground paprika
1 1/2 cups 1/4-inch fresh okra slices
1 cup chicken broth
1/2 cup white wine
2 cups cooked white rice

Direction
Heat 2 tbsp. oil in big skillet on medium heat and add sausage. Mix and cook for about 10 minutes till browned. Put on paper towel-lined plate with a slotted spoon.
In skillet, heat leftover 2 tbsp. oil. Add flour; cook, constantly whisking, for 8-10 minutes till dark brown. Add paprika, jalapeno peppers, celery, green bell pepper, onion and chicken; mix and cook for 7-8 minutes till onion is soft.
In a slow cooker, pour chicken mixture, then mix white wine, chicken broth, okra, and cooked sausage,. Cover. Cook for 7-8 hours on low till flavors merge. Serve on rice.

Nutrition Information
Calories: 373 calories;;Cholesterol: 55;Protein: 22.5;Total Fat: 18.1;Sodium: 526;Total Carbohydrate: 25.2

336. Chicken Soup With Drop In Noodles

Serving: 4 | Prep: 45mins | Cook: 8hours | Ready in:
Ingredients
2 skinless, boneless chicken breasts
2 1/2 tablespoons mixed vegetable flakes
1 bay leaf
1 teaspoon dried parsley
1/4 teaspoon dried tarragon
3/4 teaspoon celery salt
1 onion, chopped
1/2 cup frozen diced carrots
2 (14.5 ounce) cans chicken broth
2 teaspoons chicken bouillon powder
salt to taste
2 cups all-purpose flour
1 tablespoon shredded Cheddar cheese
2 eggs
1 tablespoon milk
Direction
Put chicken breasts in a big slow cooker. Cover, 3/4 of the way full, with cold water. Add onion, celery salt, tarragon, parsley, bay leaf and vegetable flakes; cook for 8 hours on low or 6 hours minimum on high. Add chicken broth, chicken bouillon and carrots 1 hour before serving; begin creating drop-in noodles.
Boil 4-6-qt. of salted water in a big stockpot. Mix cheese and flour in a mixing bowl. Create a well in the middle of flour mixture; drop in milk and eggs. Mix till it looks like peas and dough crumbles with a fork; add milk if too dry, add flour if too moist. Drop pea-size dough pieces into boiling water; cook for 20 minutes then drain. Rinse noodles in cold water.
Ladle soup into serving bowls when veggies in soup become tender and noodles are finished; drop in noodles. Serve.
Nutrition Information
Calories: 401 calories;;Total Fat: 6.1;Sodium: 1418;Total Carbohydrate: 55.1;Cholesterol: 130;Protein: 29.1

337. Chicken Stew With Pepper And Pineapple

Serving: 4 | Prep: | Cook: | Ready in:
Ingredients
1 pound skinless, boneless chicken breast halves - cut into cubes
4 cups carrots, cut into 1 inch pieces
1/2 cup chicken broth
1 tablespoon minced fresh ginger root
1 tablespoon packed brown sugar
2 tablespoons soy sauce
1/2 teaspoon ground allspice
1/2 teaspoon hot pepper sauce
1 tablespoon cornstarch
1 (8 ounce) can pineapple chunks, juice reserved
1 red bell pepper, diced
Direction
In a 1 1/2- to-4-qt. crock pot slow cooker, combine pepper sauce, allspice, soy sauce, brown sugar, ginger root, broth, carrots and chicken. Cover, cook for 7-8 hours on low heat setting or until chicken is no longer pink in the middle and vegetables are tender.
Blend reserved pineapple juice with cornstarch; stir into chicken mixture gradually. Mix in bell pepper and pineapple. Cover, cook for about 15 minutes longer on high heat, or until lightly bubbly and thickened.

Nutrition Information
Calories: 249 calories;;Total Fat: 2;Sodium: 723;Total Carbohydrate: 28.6;Cholesterol: 66;Protein: 29.1

338. Chicken Tortilla Soup In The Slow Cooker

Serving: 12 | Prep: 15mins | Cook: 4hours10mins | Ready in:
Ingredients
1 tablespoon olive oil
4 skinless, boneless chicken breast halves, cut into cubes
1 large onion, chopped
2 (16 ounce) cans refried beans
2 (15 ounce) cans corn, drained
1 (14.5 ounce) can chicken broth, or more as needed
1 (1 ounce) package taco seasoning
1 cup picante sauce
1/8 teaspoon garlic powder
shredded Cheddar cheese, or as needed
Direction
Heat the olive oil on medium high heat in the skillet. Cook and stir the onion and chicken in the hot oil for 7-10 minutes or till juices come out clear and chicken middle part is not pink anymore.
Whisk together garlic powder, picante sauce, taco seasoning, chicken broth, corn and refried beans together in the slow cooker; put in onion and chicken mixture.
Cook over Low heat for 3-5 hours or till chicken can be flaked easily using 2 forks. Shred the chicken in soup using 2 forks. Keep cooking for 60 minutes longer. Pour into the bowls and add Cheddar cheese on top.
Nutrition Information
Calories: 242 calories;;Total Carbohydrate: 28.8;Cholesterol: 38;Protein: 16.7;Total Fat: 7.4;Sodium: 958

339. Chicken And Pumpkin Goulash

Serving: 6 | Prep: 30mins | Cook: 4hours25mins | Ready in:
Ingredients
2 (14.5 ounce) cans diced tomatoes
1 tablespoon brown sugar
2 tablespoons olive oil
1 onion, chopped
1 teaspoon ground ginger
1 teaspoon ground cinnamon
1 teaspoon ground cumin
1 tablespoon ground coriander
1 1/2 pounds skinless, boneless chicken breast halves, cut into bite size pieces
1 (15 ounce) can garbanzo beans, drained and rinsed
3 pounds fresh pumpkin, peeled and cut into 3/4-inch cubes
salt, or to taste
1 teaspoon cornstarch (optional)
1/4 cup water (optional)
Direction
Set the slow cooker to high and place brown sugar and diced tomatoes into the cooker; stir to combine. In a nonstick skillet over medium-high, heat olive oil; cook and stir onion for about 10 minutes until lightly browned. Mix in the cumin, ginger, coriander, and cinnamon; cook and stir for about 2 minutes until the spices release their fragrance. Add the chicken, cook and stir until chicken is not pink anymore. Into the chicken mixture, add the garbanzo beans; bring to a

simmer. Transfer to the slow cooker and mix with tomatoes.
In the same skillet, place pumpkin; decrease heat to medium. Cook for about 10 minutes while stirring frequently until the pumpkin is hot and some pieces are slightly browned. Place the pumpkin in the cooker, then cover.
Cook the stew for 1 hour on the High setting; decrease to Low setting and cook for 3 to 4 more hours until pumpkin is tender. Spice with salt and black pepper. If stew appears to be too watery, mix the cornstarch with water until smooth in a small cup and stir into the stew. Cook until thickened for approximately 30 minutes.

Nutrition Information
Calories: 330 calories;;Total Fat: 7.9;Sodium: 696;Total Carbohydrate: 37.2;Cholesterol: 59;Protein: 28.4

340. Chorizo Chili

Serving: 8 | Prep: 15mins | Cook: 3hours15mins | Ready in:
Ingredients
2 teaspoons olive oil, or as needed
1/4 cup chopped onion
2 cloves garlic, minced
1 pound ground beef
12 ounces chorizo sausage
1 (14 ounce) can diced tomatoes
1 (14 ounce) can prepared chili
1 (14 ounce) can butter beans
3/4 cup tomato sauce
1 tablespoon chili powder
1 tablespoon salt-free seasoning blend (such as Mrs. Dash® Chipotle seasoning)
salt and ground black pepper to taste
Direction
In a skillet, heat olive oil on moderate heat, then cook and stir garlic and onion for 5 minutes in the hot oil until softened. Stir into onion mixture the chorizo sausage and ground beef, then cook for 10-15 minutes until not pink anymore while stirring and breaking the meat apart.
Combine in a slow cooker the black pepper, salt, chipotle seasoning blend, chili powder, tomato sauce, butter beans, chili, diced tomatoes and ground beef-chorizo mixture.
Cook on high heat for about 3 to 4 hours until flavors combine.

Nutrition Information
Calories: 434 calories;;Sodium: 1193;Total Carbohydrate: 17.4;Cholesterol: 81;Protein: 25.7;Total Fat: 29.3

341. Christina's Slow Cooker Chili

Serving: 16 | Prep: 20mins | Cook: 6hours5mins | Ready in:
Ingredients
3 pounds ground beef
2 (14.5 ounce) cans diced tomatoes, or more to taste
2 (6 ounce) cans tomato paste
1/4 cup chili powder
2 tablespoons dried oregano
2 tablespoons ground cumin
1 tablespoon chipotle pepper powder
1 tablespoon cayenne pepper
3 (14.5 ounce) cans kidney beans, rinsed and drained
4 cups chopped onions
4 cups chopped bell peppers
3 jalapeno peppers, chopped
2 cloves garlic, minced, or more to taste
Direction
At a moderately high level of heat, heat a big skillet and add the beef. For 5 to 7 minutes, cook the beef, stirring, until it starts to crumble and brown then drain the grease and get rid of it.
In a slow cooker, combine tomato paste and diced tomatoes, followed by cayenne pepper, chipotle pepper powder, cumin, oregano and chilli powder. Over the tomato mixture, layer garlic, jalapeno peppers, bell peppers, onions, kidney beans and ground beef. For 3 hours, leave it cooking at a high setting then adjust the setting to low heat. Continue cooking for at least 3 hours until the flavors blend together. If desired, insert additional diced tomatoes.

Nutrition Information
Calories: 306 calories;;Total Carbohydrate: 24.4;Cholesterol: 52;Protein: 20.7;Total Fat: 14.4;Sodium: 487

342. Classic Slow Cooker Corn Chowder

Serving: 8 | Prep: 15mins | Cook: 4hours | Ready in:
Ingredients
3 cups milk
2 (14.75 ounce) cans cream-style corn
2 (10.75 ounce) cans condensed cream of mushroom soup
2 (4 ounce) cans chopped green chiles
2 cups frozen corn
2 cups frozen shredded hash brown potatoes
2 cups cubed cooked ham
1 large onion, chopped
2 tablespoons butter
2 tablespoons hot sauce
2 teaspoons dried parsley
1 teaspoon chili powder
salt and ground black pepper to taste
Direction
In a slow cooker, combine the cream-style corn, chopped green chiles, cream of mushroom soup, frozen corn, onion, hash brown potatoes, ham, butter, parsley, hot sauce, and chili powder. Add salt and black pepper to season. Cover then cook for 4 hours on High or for 6 hours on Low.

Nutrition Information
Calories: 376 calories;;Sodium: 1716;Total Carbohydrate: 47.1;Cholesterol: 34;Protein: 14.9;Total Fat: 18.7

343. Coconut Chicken Curry Stew

Serving: 6 | Prep: 30mins | Cook: 6hours5mins | Ready in:
Ingredients
cooking spray
2 pounds skinless, boneless chicken thighs, cut into 1-inch pieces
6 cups chopped carrots
4 cups chopped onion
12 cloves garlic, minced
2 tablespoons freshly grated ginger
2 (14.25 ounce) cans low-sodium chicken broth
2 cups light coconut milk
2 tablespoons curry powder
1 teaspoon salt
1/2 cup chopped fresh cilantro
2 tablespoons lime juice
Direction

Place a nonstick skillet coated with cooking spray over medium high heat. Add chicken pieces, cook for about 3 minutes until light brown in color, remember to stir while cooking. Drain off all excess fat.
In the bottom of a slow cooker, spread ginger, garlic, onion, carrots and chicken.
Whisk together salt, curry powder, coconut milk and chicken broth in a bowl; add to the slow cooker.
Cook for 6 to 8 hour on Low or 3 to 4 hours on High.
Stir in lime juice and cilantro.
Nutrition Information
Calories: 455 calories;;Total Fat: 23.9;Sodium: 645;Total Carbohydrate: 28.8;Cholesterol: 96;Protein: 31.1

344. Collard Kielbasa Soup

Serving: 24 | Prep: 20mins | Cook: 1hours | Ready in:
Ingredients
1 quart water
2 (16 ounce) packages kielbasa sausage, sliced into 1/2 inch pieces
4 medium potatoes, peeled and diced
2 pounds frozen, chopped collard greens, thawed
3 (14.5 ounce) cans great Northern beans
1/4 cup diced bacon
1 clove garlic, minced
1 small onion, diced
1 green bell pepper, diced
salt and pepper to taste
Direction
Add the kielbasa and water to the soup pot, keep covered, and boil on high heat. Lower the heat to low, and let simmer for half an hour. Mix in the diced potatoes, and let simmer for 15 - 20 minutes longer. Put in the beans and greens, let simmer for 20 minutes more.
When beans and greens are being cooked, position the saucepan on medium heat. Mix in bacon, and cook till melting out some fat. Mix in the bell pepper, onions and garlic; cook till bacon becomes nearly crisp. Drain off as much grease as possible, and pour mixture into the simmering soup, and cook for 15 – 20 more minutes. Use the pepper and salt to season.
Nutrition Information
Calories: 227 calories;;Cholesterol: 26;Protein: 10.5;Total Fat: 11.6;Sodium: 406;Total Carbohydrate: 21.2

345. Colleen's Slow Cooker Jambalaya

Serving: 12 | Prep: 20mins | Cook: 8hours | Ready in:
Ingredients
1 pound skinless, boneless chicken breast halves - cut into 1 inch cubes
1 pound andouille sausage, sliced
1 (28 ounce) can diced tomatoes with juice
1 large onion, chopped
1 large green bell pepper, chopped
1 cup chopped celery
1 cup chicken broth
2 teaspoons dried oregano
2 teaspoons dried parsley
2 teaspoons Cajun seasoning
1 teaspoon cayenne pepper
1/2 teaspoon dried thyme
1 pound frozen cooked shrimp without tails
Direction
Blend tomatoes with juice, sausage, chicken, broth, celery, green bell pepper, onion in a slow cooker. Put in thyme, cayenne pepper, Cajun seasoning, parsley, and oregano to season.
Cover and cook on Low for 7-8 hours or cook on High for 3-4 hours. Mix in shrimp during the last 1/2 hour of cook time.
Nutrition Information
Calories: 235 calories;;Total Fat: 13.6;Sodium: 688;Total Carbohydrate: 6.1;Cholesterol: 99;Protein: 20.2

346. Colorado Buffalo Chili

Serving: 6 | Prep: 30mins | Cook: 8hours10mins | Ready in:
Ingredients
1 pound ground buffalo
1/2 teaspoon ground cumin
1 pinch cayenne pepper, or to taste
1 (10 ounce) can diced tomatoes with green chiles
1 (10.75 ounce) can tomato soup
1 (14.5 ounce) can kidney beans, drained
1 (15 ounce) can chili beans, drained
1/2 medium onion, chopped
1/2 teaspoon minced garlic
1 Anaheim chile pepper, chopped
1 poblano chile pepper, chopped
2 tablespoons chili powder
1 teaspoon red pepper flakes
1 1/2 teaspoons ground cumin
1/2 teaspoon cayenne pepper
salt and ground black pepper to taste
Direction
Cook the buffalo in a frying pan on medium heat until it becomes brown. Drizzle on half a tsp of cumin and a pinch of cayenne pepper to taste. Drain the grease.
Mix together the buffalo, tomato soup, tomatoes with green chiles, kidney beans, onion, chili beans, garlic, poblano chile pepper, Anaheim chile pepper, red pepper flakes, chili powder, 1 1/2 tsp of cumin, salt, half a tsp of cayenne pepper and black pepper in slow cooker. Let it cook on low for 8 hours or overnight.
Nutrition Information
Calories: 219 calories;;Cholesterol: 39;Protein: 22.3;Total Fat: 2.8;Sodium: 725;Total Carbohydrate: 29.8

347. Cozy Cottage Beef Stew Soup

Serving: 8 | Prep: 20mins | Cook: 6hours | Ready in:
Ingredients
3/4 pound beef stew meat, cut into 1 inch cubes
2 onions, diced
3 cloves garlic, minced
1 large stalk celery, minced
2 carrots, finely chopped
1/4 pound green beans, cut into 1 inch pieces
8 ounces fresh mushrooms, coarsely chopped
3 potatoes, peeled and diced
1 (14.5 ounce) can crushed tomatoes
1 (8 ounce) can tomato sauce
1 bay leaf
1/2 teaspoon ground black pepper
1/2 teaspoon dried thyme
1/4 teaspoon dried marjoram
2 (14.5 ounce) cans fat-free chicken broth
1/2 cup all-purpose flour
2 (10.5 ounce) cans beef consomme
Direction
In a slow cooker, combine beef, onions, garlic, celery, carrots, green beans, mushrooms, and potatoes. Add

tomato sauce and tomatoes. Season with marjoram, thyme, pepper, and bay leaf. Blend together flour and chicken broth. Transfer beef consomme and chicken broth mixture back to the slow cooker, then stir. Cook on Low while covered for 6 - 10 hours. Throw away bay leaf before use.
Nutrition Information
Calories: 293 calories;;Sodium: 814;Total Carbohydrate: 33.4;Cholesterol: 37;Protein: 22.4;Total Fat: 8.4

348. Crabmeat And Asparagus Soup

Serving: 6 | Prep: 10mins | Cook: 45mins | Ready in:
Ingredients
1 (10 ounce) can asparagus tips, drained
2 (6 ounce) cans crabmeat, drained and flaked
2 tablespoons fish sauce
1 tablespoon oyster sauce
1 cup chopped fresh spinach
1 cup diced firm tofu
2 teaspoons dried oregano
1 clove garlic, crushed
Direction
Combine the fish sauce, garlic, asparagus, tofu, crabmeat, spinach and oregano in a slow cooker. Add water enough to cover the mixture, about 2 inches. Cook on High setting with cover for 45 minutes, or until the spinach has cooked down dramatically and aromatic.
Nutrition Information
Calories: 100 calories;;Cholesterol: 50;Protein: 16.2;Total Fat: 3;Sodium: 695;Total Carbohydrate: 2.7

349. Creamy Slow Cooker Beef Stroganoff

Serving: 16 | Prep: 25mins | Cook: 5hours10mins | Ready in:
Ingredients
1 cup Shamrock Farms® Premium Sour Cream
3 tablespoons vegetable oil, divided
1 pound white mushrooms, trimmed and cut into thick slices
1 pinch salt
1 large white onion, minced
1/4 cup tomato paste
6 cloves garlic, minced
2 teaspoons dried thyme
1/3 cup all-purpose flour
1 1/2 cups low-sodium beef broth
1/2 cup dry white wine
1/3 cup soy sauce
2 bay leaves
4 pounds boneless beef chuck roast, trimmed of excess fat and cut into 1 1/2-inch chunks
salt and ground black pepper to taste
1 tablespoon Dijon mustard
1/2 teaspoon dried dill
Direction
Put a 12-inch skillet on medium heat. Pour in 1 tablespoon oil. Then add mushrooms and sprinkle a pinch of salt on top. Cook mushrooms for 5 – 10 minutes or until mushrooms soften. Transfer mushrooms into a 5-quart slow cooker.
Heat 2 tablespoon oil in the empty 12-inch skillet. Then put thyme, garlic, tomato paste, onion into the skillet. Cook everything until onion have softened, keep stirring while cooking, about 5 – 10 minutes. Fold in flour and cook for 1 more minute.

Add in broth, wine and whisk, remove any browned pieces. Make sure to keep whisking until there are no flour lumps left. Transfer the mixture into the slow cooker. Add soy sauce, bay leaves and stir.
Use salt and pepper to season beef chunks. Put the seasoned beef chunks into the slow cooker, cover the whole chunk in the sauce.
Put the lid on and cook till the beef is tender, 5 – 7 hours on High or 9 – 11 hours on Low. Skim from the top any formed fat. Remove bay leaves.
Transfer 1 cup of cooking liquid from slow cooker to a bowl. Whisk in mustard and Shamrock Farms Premium Sour Cream. Put the mixture back to the slow cooker and stir well to mix. Season with dill, pepper and more salt to taste.
Nutrition Information
Calories: 246 calories;Protein: 15.8;Total Fat: 16.8;Sodium: 426;Total Carbohydrate: 6.5;Cholesterol: 57

350. Creamy Slow Cooker Potato Cheese Soup

Serving: 18 | Prep: 30mins | Cook: 5hours | Ready in:
Ingredients
1/4 cup butter
1/2 white onion, chopped
1/4 cup all-purpose flour
2 cups water
2 large carrots, diced
4 stalks celery, diced
1 tablespoon dried, minced garlic
salt and pepper to taste
1 cup milk
2 tablespoons chicken soup base
1 cup warm water
5 pounds russet potatoes, peeled and cubed
1 bay leaf
1 cup shredded Cheddar cheese
6 slices crisp cooked bacon, crumbled
Direction
Put butter in a big saucepan and melt over medium heat. Add onion in butter and cook until translucent. Put in flour and stir till smooth; stir in pepper, salt, garlic, celery, carrots and 2 cups of water slowly. Cook through; add milk and stir. Put chicken base into 1 cup of warm water and dissolve, then pour into vegetable mixture.
Put potatoes into the slow cooker and add heated vegetable mixture into the potatoes. Put bay leaf into the pot.
Cook, covered, for 8 hours on Low or 5 hours on High. Take out bay leaf. Put 4 cups of soup in a food processor or blender and puree; stir pureed soup into contents in slow cooker. Add bacon and cheese, and stir till cheese is melted.
Nutrition Information
Calories: 180 calories;;Total Carbohydrate: 26.7;Cholesterol: 17;Protein: 5.4;Total Fat: 6;Sodium: 366

351. Creamy Vegetable Soup

Serving: 12 | Prep: | Cook: | Ready in:
Ingredients
1 onion, chopped
1/4 cup butter, melted
3 sweet potatoes, peeled and diced
3 zucchini, chopped
1 1/2 cups fresh broccoli, chopped
3 (14 ounce) cans chicken broth

2 potatoes, peeled and shredded
1/2 teaspoon celery seed
2 teaspoons salt
1 teaspoon ground cumin
2 cups milk
Direction
Combine broccoli, zucchini, sweet potatoes, margarine or butter, and onion in a slow cooker. Add chicken broth and whisk. Add ground cumin, salt, celery seed, and potatoes and whisk.
Put a cover on and cook for 8-10 hours on low. Pour in milk and cook for 30-60 minutes. Enjoy.
Nutrition Information
Calories: 133 calories;;Total Carbohydrate: 18.5;Cholesterol: 16;Protein: 4.1;Total Fat: 5.1;Sodium: 930

352. Crock Pot® Chicken Chili
Serving: 5 | Prep: 10mins | Cook: 6hours | Ready in:
Ingredients
1 (16 ounce) jar green salsa (salsa verde)
1 (16 ounce) can diced tomatoes with green chile peppers
2 (15 ounce) cans white beans, drained
1 (14.5 ounce) can chicken broth
1 (14 ounce) can corn, drained
1 onion, chopped
1/2 teaspoon dried oregano
1/4 teaspoon ground cumin
salt and ground black pepper to taste
3 skinless, boneless chicken breasts
Direction
In a slow cooker, combine the black pepper, salt, cumin, oregano, onion, corn, chicken broth, white beans, green chile peppers, diced tomatoes and green salsa together. Set chicken breasts over the mixture. Cook for 6 to 8 hours on Low till the chicken effortlessly shreds with 2 forks.
To a cutting board, put chicken and shred completely; in slow cooker with chili, put the chicken back then mix.
Nutrition Information
Calories: 386 calories;;Sodium: 1338;Total Carbohydrate: 62.9;Cholesterol: 37;Protein: 28.8;Total Fat: 2.9

353. Crocked Tater Tot® Soup
Serving: 10 | Prep: 10mins | Cook: 4hours | Ready in:
Ingredients
1 (32 ounce) package frozen bite-size potato nuggets (such as Tater Tots®)
2 cups milk
1 (10 ounce) can cream of mushroom soup
1 cup shredded Cheddar cheese
1 cup sour cream
1 cup chopped cooked ham
1/2 cup finely chopped onion
salt and ground black pepper to taste
Direction
In the slow cooker, mix pepper, salt, onion, ham, sour cream, Cheddar cheese, cream of mushroom soup, milk and potato nuggets.
Cook over High heat, mixing once in a while, for 4 hours or you can cook on Low heat for 5-7 hours.
Nutrition Information
Calories: 334 calories;;Sodium: 838;Total Carbohydrate: 28.5;Cholesterol: 33;Protein: 10.3;Total Fat: 22.2

354. Dan's Slow Cooker Ham And White Bean Soup
Serving: 12 | Prep: 45mins | Cook: 7hours | Ready in:
Ingredients
1 pound ham, diced
2 (15 ounce) cans black beans, rinsed and drained
2 (14.5 ounce) cans great Northern beans, rinsed and drained
1 (14 ounce) can quartered artichoke hearts, drained
1 (14.25 ounce) can baby corn, drained and cut into pieces
2 (4.5 ounce) cans sliced mushrooms, drained
1 (4 ounce) can chopped green chilies (optional)
1 bunch celery, chopped
2 large potatoes, peeled and chopped
1 large carrot, diced
1 large leek, chopped
4 large cloves garlic, chopped
2 tablespoons chopped fresh rosemary
1 tablespoon chopped fresh parsley
1 tablespoon chopped fresh thyme
1/2 cup brown sugar
1 teaspoon Creole seasoning
1 tablespoon white pepper
1 tablespoon ground black pepper
1 tablespoon salt
1 pinch cayenne pepper, or more to taste
2 tablespoons dry red wine
water to cover
Direction
Heat a big skillet on medium high heat; mix and cook diced ham in the hot skillet for 5 minutes till brown. Put ham in a slow cooker.
Put red wine, cayenne pepper, salt, black pepper, white pepper, Creole seasoning, brown sugar, thyme, parsley, rosemary, garlic, leek, carrot, potatoes, celery, green chilies, mushrooms, baby corn, artichoke hearts, great Northern beans and black beans into slow cooker.
Put sufficient water in the slow cooker to cover all ingredients.
Heat the slow cooker till boiling on high. Lower heat to low; cook for 7 hours.
Nutrition Information
Calories: 355 calories;;Total Fat: 7.8;Sodium: 1766;Total Carbohydrate: 52.8;Cholesterol: 21;Protein: 19.5

355. Diego's Special Beef Stew
Serving: 6 | Prep: 20mins | Cook: 8hours15mins | Ready in:
Ingredients
1 pound cubed beef stew meat
1 tablespoon all-purpose flour
2 tablespoons olive oil
2 teaspoons butter
1 medium yellow onion, thinly sliced
1/4 cup red wine
1 beef bouillon cube
1 cup hot water
1 large potato, cubed
1/2 cup baby carrots
1/2 teaspoon rosemary
1/2 teaspoon dried thyme
1/2 tablespoon garlic powder
1/2 teaspoon ground black pepper
1/4 cup water
2 dashes Worcestershire sauce

Direction
Add the cubed beef and flour into the resealable plastic bag. Seal up and shake to equally coat the beef with flour. In the skillet, heat oil on medium heat and brown the beef on all sides. Move into the slow cooker.
In skillet, melt butter on medium heat and cook the onion till softened. Move into a slow cooker along with beef. Add wine to skillet to deglaze, then add wine to the slow cooker.
Dissolve cube of beef bouillon in 1 cup of hot water and add to the slow cooker. Add carrots and potato into the slow cooker and use pepper, garlic powder, thyme and rosemary to season. Whisk in Worcestershire sauce and the rest of water. Pour in extra water if necessary to cover all of the ingredients.
Keep the slow cooker covered and cook stew for 7 - 8 hours on Low heat.
Nutrition Information
Calories: 272 calories;;Total Fat: 16.2;Sodium: 200;Total Carbohydrate: 15.5;Cholesterol: 45;Protein: 14.2

356. Different Ham And Potato Soup

Serving: 6 | Prep: 15mins | Cook: 5hours | Ready in:
Ingredients
1 meaty ham bone
3 potatoes, cubed
1 (8 ounce) package baby carrots
1 (6 ounce) can tomato paste
1 tablespoon chicken bouillon granules
2 teaspoons Creole seasoning
2 teaspoons Italian seasoning
6 cups water, or as needed to cover
Direction
Arrange the carrots, potatoes, and ham bone into a slow cooker. Put Italian seasonings, Creole seasonings, chicken bouillon granules, and tomato paste on top.
As necessary, cover with water; cook on High for 5-6 hours until the carrots and potatoes become soft. Occasionally stir.
Nutrition Information
Calories: 124 calories;;Sodium: 609;Total Carbohydrate: 27.9;Cholesterol: 1;Protein: 3.9;Total Fat: 0.5

357. Easy Slow Cooker Butternut Squash Soup

Serving: 8 | Prep: 20mins | Cook: 8hours10mins | Ready in:
Ingredients
1 tablespoon olive oil
2 onions, chopped
2 teaspoons dried rosemary
1/2 teaspoon ground black pepper
5 cups vegetable stock
1 butternut squash - peeled, seeded, and cut into cubes
2 Granny Smith apples - peeled, cored, and chopped
salt to taste
1 cup shredded Swiss cheese
1/2 cup finely chopped walnuts
Direction
In a big frying pan, heat oil over medium heat. Stir and cook onions in the hot oil for 5-10 minutes until tender. Mix in black pepper and rosemary, move the mixture to a slow cooker. Add apples, butternut squash, and vegetable stock to the slow cooker.
Cook for 8 hours on Low (or 4 hours on high).
Put the oven rack approximately 6-inch from the heat source and start preheating the oven's broiler.
With an immersion blender, puree the soup until smooth. Or you can add the soup to a food processor and puree in batches until smooth. Use salt to season.
Pour the soup into oven-safe bowls and sprinkle over the top with walnuts and Swiss cheese.
Cook the soup under the preheated broiler for 1-2 minutes until the cheese is bubbly and hot.
Nutrition Information
Calories: 206 calories;Protein: 6.7;Total Fat: 10.8;Sodium: 223;Total Carbohydrate: 24.5;Cholesterol: 12

358. Easy Slow Cooker Cauliflower Soup With Cheese

Serving: 4 | Prep: 10mins | Cook: 4hours | Ready in:
Ingredients
1 large head cauliflower, cut into florets
1 3/4 cups shredded Cheddar cheese
1 onion, diced
1 teaspoon English mustard
3 bay leaves
salt and freshly ground black pepper to taste
6 1/3 cups hot chicken broth
Direction
In a slow cooker, mix pepper, salt, bay leaves, mustard, onion, Cheddar cheese, and cauliflower. Add the hot chicken broth.
Cook on High setting for 4 hours until the flavors are mixed thoroughly. Discard the bay leaves. Put the mixture in a blender. Close the lid and use a potholder to keep it down; pulse until smooth.
Nutrition Information
Calories: 307 calories;;Sodium: 2254;Total Carbohydrate: 19.3;Cholesterol: 62;Protein: 19.2;Total Fat: 17.8

359. Easy Slow Cooker Chicken Soup

Serving: 6 | Prep: 10mins | Cook: 6hours | Ready in:
Ingredients
2 cups water
1 (10.75 ounce) can condensed cream of mushroom soup
4 skinless, boneless chicken breast halves
1 onion, chopped
1 cup chopped celery
1 cup chopped carrots
3 small baby bell peppers, chopped
1 (1 ounce) package dry onion soup mix (such as Lipton®)
Direction
In a slow cooker, combine together onion soup, baby bell peppers, carrots, celery, onion, chicken, cream of mushroom soup, and water.
Choose Low setting and cook for 6-8 hours. Use 2 forks to shred chicken and mix soup well.
Nutrition Information
Calories: 165 calories;;Sodium: 809;Total Carbohydrate: 13;Cholesterol: 41;Protein: 17.2;Total Fat: 4.8

360. Easy Slow Cooker Chicken And Dumplings

Serving: 8 | Prep: 20mins | Cook: 5hours | Ready in:
Ingredients

1/4 cup water, or as needed
1 teaspoon poultry seasoning
salt and ground black pepper to taste
4 skinless, boneless chicken breast halves
1 (10.75 ounce) can low-sodium chicken broth, divided
1 large onion, finely diced
3 carrots, chopped
4 stalks celery, chopped
2 tablespoons butter
1 (10.75 ounce) can reduced-fat condensed cream of celery soup (such as Campbell's®)
1 (10.75 ounce) can reduced-fat condensed cream of chicken soup (such as Campbell's® Healthy Request)
1/2 teaspoon dried rosemary
1 (10 ounce) package refrigerated biscuit dough, torn into pieces

Direction
In a bowl, blend together black pepper, salt, poultry seasoning, and water. Put in chicken, toss to coat.
Transfer half of the chicken broth to a slow cooker; put in poultry seasoning mixture and chicken.
Arrange in a layer the onion over chicken, then put carrots over, and place celery atop. Dot butter on the surface of vegetables; then pour chicken soup and celery soup over vegetables; place rosemary over top.
Cook for 3h 30 min – 4h 30 min on High. Take chicken out of the slow cooker, use 2 forks to shred.
Bring shredded chicken back to the slow cooker. In the chicken mixture, put biscuit dough pieces. Cook for 1h 30 min on High.

Nutrition Information
Calories: 270 calories;;Sodium: 755;Total Carbohydrate: 27.3;Cholesterol: 44;Protein: 16.1;Total Fat: 10.6

361. Easy Slow Cooker White Chicken Chili

Serving: 24 | Prep: 15mins | Cook: 8hours | Ready in:

Ingredients
3 (15.5 ounce) cans great Northern beans, undrained
2 (15.5 ounce) cans pinto beans, undrained
2 (15.25 ounce) cans corn, undrained
3 onions, diced
2 (14 ounce) cans chicken broth
1 rotisserie chicken, boned and cubed
2 (4 ounce) cans diced green chile peppers, undrained
1 tablespoon hot pepper sauce
2 teaspoons dried oregano
2 teaspoons ground cumin
1 teaspoon garlic powder
salt and ground black pepper to taste

Direction
In a slow cooker, mix pepper, salt, garlic powder, cumin, oregano, hot pepper sauce, green chile peppers, rotisserie chicken, chicken broth, onions, corn, pinto beans and great Northern beans.
Cook for 8 hours on Low till flavors blend.

Nutrition Information
Calories: 201 calories;;Cholesterol: 23;Protein: 14.3;Total Fat: 4.5;Sodium: 512;Total Carbohydrate: 27.4

362. Easy Sweet Chili

Serving: 6 | Prep: 5mins | Cook: 8hours10mins | Ready in:

Ingredients
1 pound ground beef
6 cloves garlic, finely chopped - or more to taste
2 tablespoons dried oregano
2 teaspoons chili powder
1 tablespoon dried basil
2 (15 ounce) cans light red kidney beans, drained and rinsed
2 (15 ounce) cans dark red kidney beans, drained and rinsed
3 (14.5 ounce) cans diced tomatoes
2 (15 ounce) cans corn
3 tablespoons white sugar
salt and ground black pepper to taste

Direction
At moderate heat, crumble ground beef down into the skillet. Add basil, chilli powder, oregano and garlic into the beef. Cook for 7 to 10 minutes, stirring until the beef turns entirely brown.
In the crock of a slow cooker, mix corn, diced tomatoes, dark red and light red kidney beans together, followed by stirring in the cooked ground beef into the bean mixture.
At medium-low setting, cook the mixture for 2 hours.
Mix sugar into the chilli. Proceed to cook for as long as possible, for a minimum of 6 hours. Before serving, add black pepper and salt to season.

Nutrition Information
Calories: 567 calories;;Cholesterol: 47;Protein: 33.8;Total Fat: 11.8;Sodium: 1392;Total Carbohydrate: 85.3

363. Easy Venison Stew

Serving: 6 | Prep: 10mins | Cook: 8hours | Ready in:

Ingredients
2 pounds venison stew meat
1 (10.75 ounce) can condensed cream of mushroom soup
1 (10.75 ounce) can condensed golden mushroom soup
1/2 onion, chopped
4 carrots, cut into 1 inch pieces

Direction
Mix carrots, onion, golden mushroom soup, cream of mushroom soup and venison in a slow cooker. Cover.
Cook for 6-8 hours on low setting.

Nutrition Information
Calories: 278 calories;;Sodium: 794;Total Carbohydrate: 12.2;Cholesterol: 131;Protein: 36.8;Total Fat: 8.2

364. Eggplant Stew

Serving: 6 | Prep: 20mins | Cook: 8hours | Ready in:

Ingredients
2 (15 ounce) cans diced tomatoes
1 eggplant, peeled, quartered, and cut into rounds
2 yellow squash, halved and sliced
2 zucchini, cut into rounds
1 cup water
1 large onion, sliced and quartered
1 (4 ounce) can sliced mushrooms with juice
1 tablespoon extra-virgin olive oil
1 tablespoon chopped garlic
1 tablespoon dried oregano
salt to taste

Direction
Mix salt, oregano, garlic, olive oil, sliced mushrooms, onion, water, zucchini, yellow squash, eggplant and diced tomatoes in 6-qt. slow cooker.
Cook for 8 hours on low till eggplant is tender.

Nutrition Information

Calories: 109 calories;;Total Fat: 2.8;Sodium: 338;Total Carbohydrate: 18.1;Cholesterol: 0;Protein: 4

365. Emily's Broccoli Cheese Soup

Serving: 6 | Prep: 15mins | Cook: 3hours5mins | Ready in:
Ingredients
2 cups low-sodium chicken stock
1 (10.75 ounce) can reduced-fat, reduced-sodium cream of chicken soup (such as Campbell's® Healthy Request)
2 tablespoons cornstarch
1 tablespoon Montreal steak seasoning
1 teaspoon freshly ground black pepper
1 teaspoon Italian seasoning
1 teaspoon garlic powder
2 tablespoons canola oil
1 large head broccoli, cut into bite-size pieces
1 cup grated carrots
1 small onion, finely diced
1/2 cup shredded reduced-fat Cheddar cheese
6 tablespoons reduced-fat sour cream
Direction
Into the slow cooker set, mix together the garlic powder, Italian seasoning, black pepper, steak seasoning, cornstarch, chicken soup and chicken stock.
Heat the canola oil on medium high heat in the skillet. Cook and stir the onion, carrots and broccoli in the hot oil for roughly 5 minutes or till the onion turns translucent. Move the broccoli mixture into the slow cooker.
Cook over Low heat for 3 - 4 hours; put in the Cheddar cheese and mix till melts. Pour the soup into the bowls and add a dollop of the sour cream on top of each portion.
Nutrition Information
Calories: 167 calories;;Total Fat: 8.7;Sodium: 791;Total Carbohydrate: 16.3;Cholesterol: 12;Protein: 7.1

366. Emma's Slow Cooker Clam Chowder

Serving: 4 | Prep: 20mins | Cook: 8hours10mins | Ready in:
Ingredients
1/4 pound bacon, diced
1 (28 ounce) can diced tomatoes with juice
2 (6.5 ounce) cans chopped clams with juice
3 large potatoes, diced
1 large onion, chopped
2 carrots, thinly sliced
3 stalks celery with leaves, thinly sliced
1 tablespoon chopped fresh parsley
1 1/2 teaspoons salt
1 1/2 teaspoons ground black pepper
1 teaspoon dried thyme leaves
1 bay leaf
Direction
Set heat to medium-high. Cook the bacon in a big, deep skillet, while stirring for 10 minutes to an even brown color. Drain the fat and add the cooked bacon into a slow cooker.
Add the clams, tomatoes, potatoes, onions, celery, carrots, parsley, thyme, bay leaf, salt and pepper into the slow cooker. Put the lid on and set it on low. Let the vegetables cook for 8-10 hours until tender and the flavors fully combine.
Nutrition Information

Calories: 476 calories;;Sodium: 1561;Total Carbohydrate: 67.8;Cholesterol: 72;Protein: 35.3;Total Fat: 6.1

367. Ez's Slow Cooker Hot Chili

Serving: 8 | Prep: 10mins | Cook: 2hours | Ready in:
Ingredients
1 onion, chopped
1 green bell pepper, chopped
1 clove garlic, minced
2 tablespoons olive oil
2 pounds ground beef
4 (11.5 ounce) cans tomato-vegetable juice cocktail
1 (10.75 ounce) can condensed tomato soup
1 (16 ounce) can chili beans, drained
1/8 teaspoon cayenne pepper
3 tablespoons chili powder
1 tablespoon soy sauce
1 cup water
Direction
Sauté together garlic, green bell pepper and onion in oil in a big skillet on moderate heat until softened, about 5 minutes. Stir in beef and cook until it turns brown. Put the mixture to a slow cooker.
Put water, soy sauce, chili powder, cayenne pepper, chili beans, soup and tomato-vegetable juice into the slow cooker.
Cover and cook on low heat for about 2 hours.
Nutrition Information
Calories: 508 calories;;Total Fat: 35.1;Sodium: 1096;Total Carbohydrate: 25.5;Cholesterol: 97;Protein: 24.6

368. Fall French Onion Soup

Serving: 6 | Prep: 20mins | Cook: 10hours | Ready in:
Ingredients
4 large onions, thinly sliced
2 Granny Smith apples - peeled, cored and chopped
1/2 cup butter, divided
2 tablespoons olive oil
4 cups chicken broth
1 1/2 cups apple cider
2 tablespoons brandy (optional)
1 tablespoon ground cinnamon
1 tablespoon white sugar
1/2 cup shredded Gouda cheese
6 (1 inch thick) slices French bread
Direction
In a slow cooker set on Low, melt 1/2 butter. Add apples and onions, put a cover on and cook for 6 to 8 hours on Low.
Once the cooking has ended and onions and apples are tender, add apple cider, chicken broth, and brandy. Turn the slow cooker to High and cook until simmering, about 1-2 hours.
Start preheating the oven's broiler. Combine the leftover butter, sugar, and cinnamon. Spread on each bread slice with this mixture. On a cookie sheet, put the bread with the cinnamon side turning up, and broil for 3 minutes until toasted. Take out of the oven; turn the slices over so the cinnamon side turns down. Sprinkle over the top with Gouda cheese and put back to the broiler until the cheese melts.
Pour the soup into serving bowls and put the toasted slices on top with the cheese side turning up. Enjoy.
Nutrition Information
Calories: 417 calories;;Total Fat: 23.3;Sodium: 397;Total Carbohydrate: 43.5;Cholesterol: 52;Protein: 7.5

369. Fisherman's Catch Chowder

Serving: 4 | Prep: 15mins | Cook: 8hours | Ready in:
Ingredients
1 1/2 pounds cod fillets, cubed
1 (16 ounce) can whole peeled tomatoes, mashed
1 (8 ounce) jar clam juice
1/2 cup chopped onion
1/2 cup chopped celery
1/2 cup chopped carrots
1/2 cup dry white wine
1/4 cup chopped fresh parsley
1/4 teaspoon dried rosemary
1 teaspoon salt
3 tablespoons all-purpose flour
3 tablespoons butter, melted
1/3 cup light cream
Direction
Blend together the clam juice, wine, cod, tomatoes, celery, onion, carrots, parsley, salt, and rosemary, in a slow cooker. Cover the saucepan. For up to 7 or 8 hours, cook on Low heat. Or heat through on High for up to 3 or 4 hours.
An hour before you serve, combine the butter, light cream and flour in a small bowl. Then add it into the slow cooker and let the consistency thicken.
Nutrition Information
Calories: 343 calories;;Sodium: 1064;Total Carbohydrate: 14.7;Cholesterol: 117;Protein: 34.6;Total Fat: 14.4

370. Five Star Venison Stew

Serving: 12 | Prep: 30mins | Cook: 10hours10mins | Ready in:
Ingredients
2 pounds cubed venison
1/2 (16 ounce) bottle French salad dressing (such as Wishbone®)
seasoned salt to taste
1 pinch salt and black pepper to taste (optional)
2 tablespoons all-purpose flour
1/4 cup vegetable oil
1 (6 ounce) can tomato paste
2 (14 ounce) cans beef broth
2/3 cup water
3 tablespoons brown sugar
1 tablespoon Worcestershire sauce
1/4 teaspoon mustard powder
1/4 teaspoon paprika
1 clove garlic, minced
1 (1 ounce) package dry onion soup mix
4 potatoes, peeled and cut into 1-inch pieces
4 carrots, peeled and cut in chunks
3 stalks celery, sliced
1 large onion, chopped
1 (10 ounce) package frozen peas, thawed
1 (10 ounce) package frozen Brussels sprouts, thawed (optional)
Direction
In a non-metallic bowl, mix French salad dressing and venison till venison is coated evenly. Use plastic wrap to cover bowl. Marinate overnight in the fridge. Take venison out of the marinade; squeeze excess off. Put venison cubes into clean bowl. Throw away leftover marinade. Season venison with pepper, salt and seasoned salt. Sprinkle flour; toss till coated.
In a big skillet, heat vegetable oil on medium-high heat. Add venison cubes; cook for 10 minutes till all sides are golden brown. As venison cubes brown, whisk beef broth and tomato paste in a slow cooker till tomato paste dissolves. Mix browned venison cubes, Brussels sprouts, peas, chopped onion, celery, carrots, potatoes, onion soup mix, garlic, paprika, mustard powder, Worcestershire sauce, brown sugar and water in.
Cover. Cook for 10-12 hours on low till carrots, potatoes and venison are tender.
Nutrition Information
Calories: 357 calories;;Sodium: 820;Total Carbohydrate: 32.8;Cholesterol: 64;Protein: 23.2;Total Fat: 15.5

371. German Texas Chili

Serving: 12 | Prep: 25mins | Cook: 6hours20mins | Ready in:
Ingredients
1/4 cup olive oil
4 red onions, chopped
6 chipotle peppers in adobo sauce, chopped, or to taste
1 pound hot pork sausage (such as Jimmy Dean®)
2 1/2 pounds ground turkey
2 (28 ounce) cans crushed tomatoes with juice (such as Hunt's®)
1 (28 ounce) can Italian-style diced tomatoes (such as Hunt's® Diced Tomatoes with Basil, Garlic and Oregano)
1 (12 fluid ounce) can or bottle beer
1 tablespoon garlic powder
1 1/2 teaspoons kosher salt
1 tablespoon ground black pepper
3 tablespoons ground cumin
1 tablespoon chili powder
1/4 cup paprika
1/4 cup brown sugar
4 cinnamon sticks
12 whole cloves
Direction
In a very large skillet, heat the olive oil over medium heat, cook the chipotle peppers and onions for about 10 minutes until the onions become translucent. Put turkey and the hot sausage into the skillet, cook until brown, using a spoon to chop up the meat into crumbles while cooking, 10 to 15 more minutes. Using a spoon, transfer the meat mixture to a large slow cooker, getting rid of excess grease. Stir the brown sugar, paprika, chili powder, cumin, black pepper, kosher salt, garlic powder, beer, Italian-style diced tomatoes and crushed tomatoes into the meat mixture until combined thoroughly.
Using a piece of cheesecloth, wrap the cloves and cinnamon sticks tightly, then place the bundle into the slow cooker. On low setting, cook for 6 to 8 hours. Get rid of the cheesecloth bundle before serving.
Nutrition Information
Calories: 402 calories;;Cholesterol: 92;Protein: 28.1;Total Fat: 21.1;Sodium: 956;Total Carbohydrate: 26

372. Gram's Irish Stew

Serving: 10 | Prep: 20mins | Cook: 3hours30mins | Ready in:
Ingredients
1 teaspoon vegetable oil
4 pounds cubed beef stew meat
2 teaspoons sage
10 potatoes, peeled and cubed
4 carrots, diced

1 (4 ounce) can sliced mushrooms, drained
1 small onion, chopped
1 teaspoon celery seed
1 teaspoon Worcestershire sauce
1 teaspoon ground black pepper
1 cube beef bouillon
salt to taste
water to cover
1 tablespoon cornstarch, or as needed
1/4 cup warm water
Direction
In the skillet, heat oil on medium high heat. Put beef into oil and use sage to season; cook beef till browned on all sides; drain.
Into the slow cooker, add beef bouillon, pepper, Worcestershire sauce, celery seed, onion, mushrooms, carrots, potatoes and beef; use salt to season. Add enough water to cover the mixture. Switch the slow cooker to HIGH and cover. Cook for 4 - 5 hours, mixing once in a while.
In a small-sized bowl, mix warm water and cornstarch together till smooth; mix through stew. Let stew cook for 15-20 minutes or till thick.
Nutrition Information
Calories: 746 calories;;Total Fat: 40.1;Sodium: 281;Total Carbohydrate: 43.1;Cholesterol: 160;Protein: 51.2

373. Grandma B's Bean Soup

Serving: 8 | Prep: 15mins | Cook: 10hours | Ready in:
Ingredients
1 pound dry navy beans
3 carrots, peeled and shredded
2 medium potatoes, peeled and diced
3 stalks celery, sliced
1 medium onion, diced
2 cups cubed cooked ham
Direction
In a slow cooker, put beans; cover with sufficient water. Soak 6-8 hours or all night.
Drain beans, bring back to slow cooker. Pour in water to cover, stir in ham, onion, celery, potatoes, and carrots.
Cover the slow cooker, cook soup for 3 hours and 30 minutes on High. Switch to Low, keep cooking at least 6 hours and 30 minutes. The soup is more flavorful if being cooked longer and longer.
Nutrition Information
Calories: 324 calories;;Total Carbohydrate: 47.2;Cholesterol: 19;Protein: 18.5;Total Fat: 7.2;Sodium: 465

374. Great Aunt Nina's Noodles And Chicken

Serving: 12 | Prep: 30mins | Cook: 8hours | Ready in:
Ingredients
2 carrots, sliced
2 onions, sliced
2 stalks celery, cut into 1 inch pieces
1 (4 pound) whole chicken
1 teaspoon salt
1/2 teaspoon ground black pepper
1/2 cup white wine
1/4 teaspoon dried basil
2 eggs, beaten
1/4 cup water
1 pinch salt
2 tablespoons shortening
1 cup all-purpose flour, or as needed
2 quarts low salt chicken broth
Direction
Place celery, onions, and carrots in a slow cooker's bottom. Place the whole chicken over the veggies and add pepper and salt to season. Add white wine and sprinkle with basil. Cook, covered for 8 to 10 hours on Low.
Combine flour, shortening, salt, water, and eggs in a medium bowl until a stiff dough is formed. Mix in as much flour as possible with a fork, then knead the dough with your hands right in the bowl to combine with as much flour as it can. Allow the dough to rest for a few minutes.
Roll out the dough onto an oiled 1/8-inch-thick board. Cut into 1/2-inch wide and 3-inch-long strips using a pie crust cutter or pizza cutter. Lightly sprinkle with flour, and let strips dry for a few hours while chicken cooks.
Once chicken is cooked, transfer vegetables and meat to a platter. Pour juices into a large pot and mix in 2 quarts of chicken broth. Bring to a boil and stir in noodles. Cook until noodles are tender, about 10 minutes. In the meantime, separate meat from chicken and shred. Discard chicken bones and skin. Once noodles are cooked perfectly, add vegetables back to the pot, and put in shredded chicken meat. Enjoy.
Nutrition Information
Calories: 423 calories;;Total Fat: 26.1;Sodium: 377;Total Carbohydrate: 10.9;Cholesterol: 147;Protein: 32.3

375. Greek Style Beef Stew

Serving: 6 | Prep: 35mins | Cook: 15mins | Ready in:
Ingredients
1 tablespoon olive oil
1 pound cubed beef stew meat
1 onion, peeled and chopped
1 large clove garlic, minced
1/4 cup red wine
2 tablespoons red wine vinegar
1/2 cup fat-free reduced-sodium beef broth
1 tablespoon tomato paste
1/2 teaspoon dried rosemary
1/2 teaspoon dried oregano
6 whole black peppercorns
2 bay leaves
1 teaspoon ground cumin
1/8 teaspoon ground cinnamon
1 pinch ground cloves
1/4 teaspoon ground black pepper
1 1/2 teaspoons light brown sugar
1 (28 ounce) can whole plum tomatoes, undrained and quartered
1/2 cup water
2 potatoes, peeled and cut into 2-inch pieces
2 carrots, peeled and sliced
salt to taste (optional)
Direction
In a 5-qt pressure cooker, heat olive on medium-high heat. Cook and stir half of the beef until all sides are well browned. Use a slotted spoon to remove the beef; set aside. Cook the remaining beef, set aside.
Sauté chopped onion in the pressure cooker for a minute. Stir in garlic and cook for another minute. Add tomato paste, beef broth, red wine vinegar, and red wine; stir well.

Use a spice grinder or mortar and pestle to crush peppercorns, oregano, and rosemary. Put the crushed spice with brown sugar, bay leaves, black pepper, cumin, cloves, and cinnamon in the cooker. Add the tomatoes and their juice; swish half cup water on the can and add water in the cooker. Place carrots, potatoes, and return the browned meat to the pressure cooker. The 5-quart pot should be half full and a bit soupy. The potato will dissolve a bit and will thicken it after cooking. Cover the pot and secure the lid.

On high heat, bring the pot and set the pressure to high. Turn heat to low to maintain the full pressure, cook for 15 minutes. Turn off heat and naturally release the pressure. Season stew with salt to taste.

Nutrition Information
Calories: 289 calories;;Total Fat: 13;Sodium: 367;Total Carbohydrate: 26.8;Cholesterol: 42;Protein: 15.9

376. Gringo Posole

Serving: 10 | Prep: 20mins | Cook: 3hours45mins | Ready in:

Ingredients
1 cup water, or more as needed to cover
1 tablespoon vegetable oil, or as needed
1/2 pound pork stew meat, cut into 1-inch pieces
1 green bell pepper, coarsely chopped
1 red bell pepper, coarsely chopped
1 onion, finely chopped
2 cloves garlic, minced
2 cubes beef bouillon
2 (10 ounce) cans diced tomatoes with green chile peppers (such as RO*TEL®), undrained
1 (15.5 ounce) can white hominy, undrained
1 (15.5 ounce) can yellow hominy, undrained
1 tablespoon ground cumin
1 teaspoon ground red pepper
1 teaspoon ground black pepper

Direction
Add the water to the slow cooker, and set the cooker on High heat to pre heat. Heat the vegetable oil on medium heat in the big skillet, and brown the pork on all of the sides, mixing once in a while, for roughly 10 minutes. Add browned pork into hot water in the slow cooker, leaving the oil in the skillet. Cook and stir garlic, onion, red and green bell peppers on medium low heat in the hot skillet for roughly 5 minutes or till onion turns translucent. Move the vegetables into the slow cooker. Drop in the bouillon cubes. Pour in water as needed to barely cover the ingredients, set the cooker to Medium heat, and cook for 1.5-2 hours or till veggies soften.
Add in diced tomatoes along with the chiles, and combine by stirring. Cook for 60 minutes more; mix in black pepper, red pepper, cumin, and hominy with liquid, and cook for 60 minutes longer.

Nutrition Information
Calories: 149 calories;;Cholesterol: 14;Protein: 6.7;Total Fat: 5.8;Sodium: 595;Total Carbohydrate: 17.7

377. Ham Bone Chowder

Serving: 6 | Prep: 15mins | Cook: 6hours45mins | Ready in:

Ingredients
1 meaty ham bone, fat trimmed
1 (32 fluid ounce) container chicken stock
1 onion, chopped
2 tablespoons chopped garlic
6 red potatoes, cubed
4 large carrots, chopped
1 tablespoon chopped fresh parsley
2 teaspoons ground cumin
1 cup frozen corn
1 cup milk
salt and ground black pepper to taste

Direction
In a slow cooker, put the ham bone in and top it with onion, chicken stock, and garlic.
Cook for 6 to 8 hours on Low.
Take the ham bone out of the slow cooker, separate the meat from the bone then shred the meat. Put the meat back to the slow cooker and throw the bone away. Toss in the potatoes, parsley, carrots, and cumin to the soup.
Cook the soup on High for about 45 minutes, until the potatoes are tender. Stir in the frozen corn.
Take 1 cup of soup and put it into a blender then add in the milk. Cover the blender and hold the lid down then start to blend by pulsing a few times before leaving it on to blend. Put the blended soup back to the slow cooker and stir. Add salt and pepper to season.

Nutrition Information
Calories: 112 calories;;Sodium: 510;Total Carbohydrate: 21.9;Cholesterol: 4;Protein: 4.3;Total Fat: 1.8

378. Ham Bone Soup

Serving: 4 | Prep: 30mins | Cook: 6hours | Ready in:

Ingredients
1 ham bone with some meat
1 onion, diced
1 (14.5 ounce) can peeled and diced tomatoes with juice
1 (15.25 ounce) can kidney beans
3 potatoes, cubed
1 green bell pepper, seeded and cubed
4 cups water
6 cubes chicken bouillon

Direction
In a 3 quart or larger slow cooker, combine the tomatoes, onion, green pepper, ham bone, kidney beans, and potatoes. Place bouillon cubes in water and dissolve. Pour the dissolved cubes into the slow cooker.
Cover the slow cooker and let it cook on High setting until warm. Adjust the heat to Low. Cook for 5-6 hours longer.

Nutrition Information
Calories: 266 calories;;Total Fat: 1;Sodium: 2136;Total Carbohydrate: 53.3;Cholesterol: 1;Protein: 11.4

379. Ham Bone And Vegetable Soup

Serving: 12 | Prep: 20mins | Cook: 4hours | Ready in:

Ingredients
2 tablespoons bacon grease
1 large onion, diced
2 carrots, peeled and diced
3 stalks celery, diced
2 cloves garlic, crushed
3 potatoes, diced
8 cups hot water
8 cubes chicken bouillon
1 ham bone
1 (14 ounce) can diced tomatoes

1/2 (16 ounce) package frozen corn
1 (8 ounce) can tomato sauce
1 teaspoon black pepper
1/2 teaspoon salt
Direction
Melt the bacon grease on medium high heat in the big skillet. Cook and stir the garlic, celery, carrots and onion in the hot bacon grease for roughly 5 minutes or till the veggies soften a bit and fragrant. Mix the potatoes to the onion mixture; cook and stir for roughly 10 minutes or till turning golden.
Mix together the chicken bouillon and hot water in the slow cooker till the bouillon dissolves; put in the salt, black pepper, tomato sauce, corn, diced tomatoes, ham bone, and onion mixture.
Cook the soup in slow cooker set on Low heat for 4 - 6 hours. Take the ham bone out of the soup and allow it to stand till becoming cool enough to handle. Remove the meat from ham bone and mix the meat into the soup.
Nutrition Information
Calories: 108 calories;;Total Fat: 2.8;Sodium: 1042;Total Carbohydrate: 18.8;Cholesterol: 3;Protein: 3

380. Hamburger Corn Soup
Serving: 6 | Prep: 10mins | Cook: 6hours5mins | Ready in:
Ingredients
1 pound ground beef
1 large onion
2 (15.25 ounce) cans sweet corn, undrained
2 (15 ounce) cans sweet cream-style corn
3 potatoes, peeled and cubed
2 teaspoons dried parsley
water, as needed
2 teaspoons salt, or to taste
1 teaspoon ground black pepper
Direction
Over medium-high heat, heat a large skillet, add onion and beef. Cook while stirring for about 5 minutes until the beef turns brown. Place the beef and onion into a slow cooker. Then add parsley, sweet corn, potatoes and cream-style corn. Add plenty of water into the slow cooker to fill it completely.
Cover the cooker and cook the corn mixture for about 6 hours on Low until the potatoes become very tender. Add pepper and salt.
Nutrition Information
Calories: 458 calories;;Sodium: 1711;Total Carbohydrate: 77.1;Cholesterol: 46;Protein: 21.7;Total Fat: 11

381. Hamburger Soup II
Serving: 6 | Prep: 15mins | Cook: 10mins | Ready in:
Ingredients
1 1/2 pounds lean ground beef
2 large potatoes, sliced
2 stalks celery, sliced
salt and pepper to taste
2 onions, thinly sliced
1 (15 ounce) can peas
3 small carrots, sliced
1 (10.75 ounce) can condensed tomato soup
1 1/4 cups water
Direction
In a big, deep frying pan, put ground beef. Cook on medium-high heat until turning brown evenly. Strain, break apart and put aside.
Cover the bottom of a slow cooker with a layer of potatoes. Sprinkle over the potatoes with celery, and place ground beef in 1 layer. Use pepper and salt to season each layer. Add peas, onions, and carrots. Stir together water and tomato soup, and put on top. Put a cover on and cook for 6-8 hours on low.
Nutrition Information
Calories: 492 calories;;Sodium: 530;Total Carbohydrate: 41;Cholesterol: 85;Protein: 26.4;Total Fat: 24.7

382. Harvest Pork Stew
Serving: 6 | Prep: 40mins | Cook: 1hours | Ready in:
Ingredients
2 tablespoons butter or oil
1 1/2 pounds boneless pork, cut into 1/2-inch cubes
2 cloves garlic, minced
1 medium onion, chopped
3 cups chicken broth
1/2 teaspoon salt
1/4 teaspoon dried rosemary, crushed
1/4 teaspoon rubbed sage
1 bay leaf
3 cups frozen, cubed butternut squash
2 MacIntosh apples, cored and cubed
2 large potatoes, peeled and cubed (optional)
2 cups carrots, peeled and diced (optional)
Direction
Melt the butter over medium-high heat in a big skillet. Add the pork and cook until all sides are lightly browned. Stir in the onion and garlic; continue to cook until the pork is firm and no longer pink and the onion has softened for 5 minutes.
Place the onions and pork in a big saucepan. Pour in the chicken broth and season with salt, sage, bay leaf, and rosemary. Bring to a boil, lower heat to medium-low; cover and simmer for 20 minutes.
Stir in the potatoes, carrots, butternut squash, and apples. Return to a simmer, then cook without a cover until the squash and apples are tender for about 20 minutes. Discard the bay leaf and serve.
Nutrition Information
Calories: 465 calories;;Cholesterol: 80;Protein: 27.4;Total Fat: 21.3;Sodium: 365;Total Carbohydrate: 42.6

383. Hearty Beef Stew
Serving: 4 | Prep: 20mins | Cook: 6hours | Ready in:
Ingredients
1 pound cubed beef stew meat
1/4 cup all-purpose flour
1 tablespoon paprika
salt and pepper to taste
2 cups beef broth
1 1/2 tablespoons teriyaki sauce
1 onion, chopped
3 carrots, sliced
1 stalk celery, sliced
2 potatoes, cubed
1/2 pound mushrooms, quartered
2 cloves garlic, minced
1 bay leaf
Direction
Put beef stew meat into a slow cooker. Combine pepper, salt, paprika and flour in a small bowl; pour the mixture over beef stew meat, stirring to cover.

Mix in bay leaf, garlic, potatoes, mushrooms, celery, carrots, onion, teriyaki sauce and beef broth.
Cook on low with a cover for 6 hours, stirring sometimes.
Nutrition Information
Calories: 319 calories;;Sodium: 735;Total Carbohydrate: 19.9;Cholesterol: 62;Protein: 23.5;Total Fat: 16.3

384. Hearty Ham Bone Black Bean Soup

Serving: 4 | Prep: 10mins | Cook: 5hours51mins | Ready in:
Ingredients
1 ham bone with some meat
1 drizzle olive oil
3 stalks celery with leaves, chopped, or more to taste
1/2 onion, chopped
4 cloves garlic, crushed
1/2 (12 ounce) package baby carrots
1 cup fingerling potatoes, or to taste
1 small red bell pepper, seeded and chopped (optional)
4 cups water
1 (19 ounce) can black beans, drained and rinsed
1 (12 fluid ounce) can vegetable juice (such as V8®)
1 (11 ounce) can canned corn (such as Green Giant Niblets®), drained (optional)
2 tomatoes, chopped
2 tablespoons chopped green chilies
2 teaspoons ground cumin
salt and ground black pepper to taste
Direction
In a big slow cooker, put in ham bone.
Heat olive oil in a big saucepan on medium high heat; sauté garlic, onion and celery for 5 minutes till onion is translucent. Transfer ham mixture over the ham bone in slow cooker.
Sauté red bell pepper, potatoes and carrots in same saucepan for 1 minute till coated in oil. Put veggies into the slow cooker; add black pepper, salt, cumin, green chiles, tomatoes, corn, vegetable juice, black beans and water. Cover; cook for 45-60 minutes till soup is warm on high. Lower the heat to low; keep cooking for 5-6 hours.
Take ham bone out of the soup. Separate meat from bone; put it back into soup. Discard bone. Cover the soup; refrigerate for 8 hours – overnight. On top of soup, discard the thick fat; reheat.
Nutrition Information
Calories: 310 calories;;Total Carbohydrate: 60.8;Cholesterol: 0;Protein: 13.5;Total Fat: 2.3;Sodium: 1140

385. Hearty Lentil And Sausage Soup

Serving: 10 | Prep: 15mins | Cook: 4hours15mins | Ready in:
Ingredients
1/2 pound bulk pork sausage
8 cups water
2 (14.5 ounce) cans chicken broth
1 (28 ounce) can diced tomatoes
1 (16 ounce) package dry lentils, rinsed
1 large onion, chopped
1 stalk celery, finely chopped
1 cup shredded carrot
1 tablespoon chopped garlic
1 tablespoon garlic powder
1 tablespoon chopped fresh parsley
1/2 teaspoon dried oregano
1/2 teaspoon black pepper
1/4 teaspoon dried basil
1 pinch dried rosemary
salt to taste
1 1/2 cups diced cabbage
Direction
In a big pot, heat oil medium-high heat. Crumble sausage into pieces and add to the pot, stir and cook for 5-7 minutes until very browned.
Move the cooked sausage to a slow cooker. Add garlic, carrot, celery, onion, lentils, tomatoes, chicken broth, and water. Use salt, rosemary, basil, pepper, oregano, parsley, and garlic powder to season the mixture.
Cook for 4 hours on Low, until the lentils are soft.
Mix into the soup with cabbage; keep cooking for 15-20 minutes until cabbage is tender.
Nutrition Information
Calories: 258 calories;;Total Fat: 5.6;Sodium: 697;Total Carbohydrate: 34.7;Cholesterol: 15;Protein: 16.4

386. Hearty Slow Cooked Beef Stew

Serving: 6 | Prep: 20mins | Cook: 4hours | Ready in:
Ingredients
2 pounds beef stew meat, trimmed and cut into 1-inch cubes
1 (15 ounce) can new potatoes, drained and quartered
1 onion, chopped
1 cup chopped carrot
1 (8 ounce) can tomato sauce
1 cup water
1 cup dry red wine
2 beef bouillon cubes
1 (1 ounce) package dry onion soup mix (such as Lipton®)
1 teaspoon dried rosemary
1 teaspoon garlic powder
1 teaspoon salt
1 pinch ground black pepper
2 tablespoons cornstarch
3 tablespoons cold water
Direction
Add carrot, onion, potatoes and beef stew meat to the crock of a slow cooker. Put pepper, salt, garlic powder, rosemary, onion soup mix, beef bouillon cubes, red wine, water and tomato sauce into the beef mixture; stir gently.
Combine cornstarch with water until dissolved; toss softly into the beef mixture.
Cook on High for 4 hours.
Nutrition Information
Calories: 324 calories;;Total Fat: 9.1;Sodium: 1518;Total Carbohydrate: 22.5;Cholesterol: 80;Protein: 30.3

387. Hearty Vegan Slow Cooker Chili

Serving: 15 | Prep: 45mins | Cook: 5hours10mins | Ready in:
Ingredients
1 tablespoon olive oil
1 green bell pepper, chopped
1 red bell pepper, chopped
1 yellow bell pepper, chopped
2 onions, chopped
4 cloves garlic, minced
1 (10 ounce) package frozen chopped spinach, thawed and drained
1 cup frozen corn kernels, thawed

1 zucchini, chopped
1 yellow squash, chopped
6 tablespoons chili powder
1 tablespoon ground cumin
1 tablespoon dried oregano
1 tablespoon dried parsley
1/2 teaspoon salt
1/2 teaspoon ground black pepper
2 (14.5 ounce) cans diced tomatoes with juice
1 (15 ounce) can black beans, rinsed and drained
1 (15 ounce) can garbanzo beans, drained
1 (15 ounce) can kidney beans, rinsed and drained
2 (6 ounce) cans tomato paste
1 (8 ounce) can tomato sauce, or more if needed
1 cup vegetable broth, or more if needed
Direction
In a big skillet, put olive oil and cook in medium fire; mix in onions and garlics for 8 to 10 minutes until brown. Add red, yellow and green bell peppers. In a slow cooker, transfer the mixture. Combine corn, yellow squash, cumin, parsley, black pepper, black beans, kidney beans, spinach, zucchini, chili powder, oregano, salt, tomatoes, tomato paste, tomatoes and garbanzo beans until thoroughly mixed. Put vegetable broth and tomato sauce over the mixture. Let vegetables cook in the cooker in low heat for 4 to 5 hours until vegetables are tender. Adjust the seasoning; add more tomato sauce and vegetable broth if chili is too thick to achieve preferred thickness. Continue to cook for another 1 to 2 hours until flavors are completely blended.
Nutrition Information
Calories: 134 calories;;Total Fat: 2.4;Sodium: 617;Total Carbohydrate: 24.8;Cholesterol: 0;Protein: 6.3

388. Hobo Ground Beef And Vegetable Soup

Serving: 6 | Prep: 15mins | Cook: 8hours | Ready in:
Ingredients
1 (32 fluid ounce) container beef broth, or more if needed
1 pound ground sirloin beef
1 (15.25 ounce) can whole kernel corn, drained
1 (15 ounce) can green beans, drained
1 (15 ounce) can peas, drained
1 (14 ounce) can tomato sauce
3 carrots, cut into bite-size pieces
2 potatoes, peeled and cut into bite-size pieces
1 onion, chopped
1 large stalk celery, cut into bite-size pieces
1 clove garlic, minced
1 1/2 tablespoons chopped fresh parsley
1/2 teaspoon celery seed
2 bay leaves
salt and ground black pepper to taste
Direction
In a slow cooker, stir together bay leaves, celery seed, parsley, garlic, celery, onion, potatoes, carrots, tomato sauce, peas, green beans, corn, ground sirloin, and beef broth.
Heat on Low for 4 hours. Pour in the broth if more moisture is needed. Keep on cooking for 4 more hours. Use black pepper and salt to season.
Nutrition Information
Calories: 354 calories;;Total Carbohydrate: 45.9;Cholesterol: 46;Protein: 22.4;Total Fat: 10.4;Sodium: 1465

389. Homemade Chili

Serving: 12 | Prep: 10mins | Cook: 4hours13mins | Ready in:
Ingredients
2 tablespoons olive oil
1 large onion, chopped
2 cloves garlic, minced, or more to taste
2 pounds lean ground beef
2 (16 ounce) cans kidney beans, rinsed and drained
1 (28 ounce) can diced tomatoes
1 (15 ounce) can tomato puree
1 cup water
1 (4 ounce) can chopped green chile peppers
2 tablespoons mild chili powder
2 teaspoons salt
2 teaspoons ground cumin
1 teaspoon ground black pepper
Direction
In a big skillet, heat oil on moderate low heat. Put in garlic and onion, then cook and stir for 5 minutes, until onion is translucent. Put in ground beef, then cook and stir for 8 to 10 minutes until browned. Move beef mixture to a 6-qt. slow cooker. Stir in black pepper, cumin, salt, chili powder, green chili peppers, water, tomato puree, diced tomatoes and kidney beans.
Cook on low setting for 4-6 hours until flavors blend.
Nutrition Information
Calories: 274 calories;;Total Fat: 13.3;Sodium: 959;Total Carbohydrate: 19.6;Cholesterol: 46;Protein: 18.8

390. Homemade Potato Soup

Serving: 8 | Prep: 25mins | Cook: 12hours | Ready in:
Ingredients
6 medium white potatoes, peeled and chopped
2 onions, chopped
1 carrot, peeled and diced
3 stalks celery, diced
1 tablespoon oil-packed minced garlic
4 cubes chicken bouillon
1 quart water
1 tablespoon parsley flakes
1 tablespoon salt-free herb seasoning blend
1 tablespoon Italian seasoning
1 1/2 cups soy milk
2 cups chopped broccoli
Direction
Put bouillon cubes, oil-packed garlic, celery, carrot, onions, and potatoes in a slow cooker. Add water, and use Italian seasoning, herb seasoning blend, and parsley to season.
Put the lid on the slow cooker, and cook the soup on low for 10-12 hours or on high for 3-4 hours. Once the soup has 30 minutes left to cook, mix in soy milk. In a steamer basket fitted in a pot of boiling water, put broccoli, and steam until soft but not mushy, about 5 minutes. Add to the soup and enjoy.
Nutrition Information
Calories: 171 calories;;Total Fat: 1.5;Sodium: 640;Total Carbohydrate: 35;Cholesterol: 1;Protein: 5.9

391. Hungarian Goulash II

Serving: 6 | Prep: 15mins | Cook: 10hours15mins | Ready in:
Ingredients
2 pounds beef chuck roast, cubed

1 large onion, diced
1/2 cup ketchup
2 tablespoons Worcestershire sauce
1 tablespoon brown sugar
2 teaspoons salt
2 teaspoons Hungarian sweet paprika
1/2 teaspoon dry mustard
1 1/4 cups water, divided
1/4 cup all-purpose flour
Direction
Cook the beef in a slow cooker, covering it with onion. Mix together the Worcestershire sauce, ketchup, salt, brown sugar, paprika, mustard, and 1 cup water in a separate medium bowl. Pour this mixture on top of the beef and onions then cover it.
Cook this on low heat with cover until the meat is tender, for about 9 to 10 hours.
Combine flour and 1/4 cup of water to make a paste and stir it into the goulash. Cook it for 10 to 15 minutes on high or until the sauce is already thick.
Nutrition Information
Calories: 281 calories;;Sodium: 1100;Total Carbohydrate: 15.3;Cholesterol: 69;Protein: 19.2;Total Fat: 15.8

392. It's Chili By George!!

Serving: 10 | Prep: 10mins | Cook: 1hours45mins | Ready in:
Ingredients
2 pounds lean ground beef
1 (46 fluid ounce) can tomato juice
1 (29 ounce) can tomato sauce
1 (15 ounce) can kidney beans, drained and rinsed
1 (15 ounce) can pinto beans, drained and rinsed
1 1/2 cups chopped onion
1/4 cup chopped green bell pepper
1/8 teaspoon ground cayenne pepper
1/2 teaspoon white sugar
1/2 teaspoon dried oregano
1/2 teaspoon ground black pepper
1 teaspoon salt
1 1/2 teaspoons ground cumin
1/4 cup chili powder
Direction
In a large deep skillet add ground beef. Cook over medium-high heat until evenly brown. Drain and break up the beef.
Add to a large pot over high heat, combine the ground beef, onions, bell pepper, tomato juice, tomato sauce, kidney beans, pinto beans, cayenne pepper, sugar, cumin, chili powder, oregano, ground black pepper and salt, bring to a boil then turn heat to low. Simmer for 1 1/2 hours. (Note: If using a slow cooker, add all the ingredients and cook on low for 8 to 10 hours.)
Nutrition Information
Calories: 305 calories;;Total Fat: 13.7;Sodium: 1267;Total Carbohydrate: 25.5;Cholesterol: 55;Protein: 22.3

393. Jamie's Pulled Pork Chili

Serving: 8 | Prep: 15mins | Cook: 7hours | Ready in:
Ingredients
2 (10.75 ounce) cans fat-free, low-sodium chicken broth
2 cups diced tomatoes
1 cup drained and rinsed kidney beans
1 large onion, chopped
2 tablespoons chili powder
2 teaspoons ground cumin
1 (2 pound) pork shoulder roast
1 (8 ounce) package shredded Cheddar cheese (such as Kraft®)
1 1/4 cups sour cream
Direction
In a slow cooker, mix tomatoes, cumin, chicken broth, chili powder, kidney beans and onion. Mix pork shoulder in then place cover on.
Let it cook for 10-12 hours on low or 7 hours on high. Take out pork shoulder and cut meat into shreds; then put back in the slow cooker and stir. Garnish with sour cream and Cheddar cheese.
Nutrition Information
Calories: 396 calories;;Sodium: 448;Total Carbohydrate: 12.1;Cholesterol: 91;Protein: 23.4;Total Fat: 28.1

394. Jay's Spicy Slow Cooker Turkey Chili

Serving: 8 | Prep: 20mins | Cook: 8hours | Ready in:
Ingredients
2 pounds ground turkey
1 (1.25 ounce) package taco seasoning mix
1 yellow onion, chopped
1 (14.5 ounce) can crushed tomatoes, drained
1 (15 ounce) can kidney beans, drained and rinsed
1 (10.75 ounce) can condensed tomato soup
1/2 (15 ounce) can black beans, drained and rinsed
1/4 cup chili powder
3 canned green chile peppers, sliced
1 tablespoon diced peppers from adobo sauce with chipotle peppers, or more to taste
2 teaspoons chile-garlic sauce (such as Sriracha®)
1 teaspoon ground black pepper
1 teaspoon salt
1 teaspoon dried basil
1 teaspoon paprika
1 teaspoon cayenne pepper
Direction
Over medium-high heat, heat a big skillet. In hot skillet, cook and mix ground turkey for 5 to 7 minutes till crumbly and browned; let drain and throw the grease. Into the ground turkey, mix taco seasoning till equally coated.
In a slow cooker, combine cayenne pepper, paprika, basil, salt, black pepper, chili-garlic sauce, chipotle peppers from adobo sauce, green chili peppers, chili powder, black beans, tomato soup, kidney beans, crushed tomatoes, onion and seasoned ground turkey.
Allow to cook on Low for 8 to 9 hours or approximately 4 hours on High.
Nutrition Information
Calories: 309 calories;;Total Fat: 9.9;Sodium: 1595;Total Carbohydrate: 28.1;Cholesterol: 84;Protein: 28.9

395. Jerre's Black Bean And Pork Tenderloin Slow Cooker Chili

Serving: 8 | Prep: 10mins | Cook: 10hours | Ready in:
Ingredients
1 1/2 pounds pork tenderloin, cut into 2 inch strips
1 small onion, coarsely chopped
1 small red bell pepper, coarsely chopped
3 (15 ounce) cans black beans
1 (16 ounce) jar salsa
1/2 cup chicken broth
1 teaspoon dried oregano
1 teaspoon ground cumin

2 teaspoons chili powder
Direction
Mix together chili powder, cumin, oregano, chicken broth, salsa, black beans, red pepper, onion and pork tenderloin in a slow cooker. Set cooker to low setting and cook for about 8-10 hours.
Before serving, break up pieces of cooked pork to thicken the chili.
Nutrition Information
Calories: 245 calories;;Total Fat: 2.8;Sodium: 1045;Total Carbohydrate: 31.9;Cholesterol: 37;Protein: 24

396. Kale Soup With Portuguese Sausage

Serving: 20 | Prep: 15mins | Cook: 10hours | Ready in:
Ingredients
1 quart beef stock
1 quart chicken stock
2 (14.5 ounce) cans white beans, rinsed and drained
1/2 onion, unchopped
3 cloves whole garlic cloves
2 teaspoons kosher salt
1 teaspoon ground black pepper
2 sprigs fresh thyme
1/2 pound Portuguese andouille sausage, sliced
2 bunches kale, torn into small pieces
1 stalk celery, diced
2 carrots, chopped, or more to taste
1/4 teaspoon garlic salt, or to taste
Direction
In a slow cooker, mix together thyme, black pepper, salt, garlic cloves, onion half, beans, chicken stock, and beef stock; cook for 8 hours to overnight on Low. Take out the garlic and onion and dispose. Choose the 'Keep Warm' setting on the slow cooker. Add the andouille sausage to the stock mixture; keep cooking for 1 hour until the sausage is aromatic. Mix garlic salt, carrots, celery, and kale into the soup, cook for another 1 hour until the carrots are soft.
Nutrition Information
Calories: 122 calories;;Cholesterol: 7;Protein: 6.9;Total Fat: 4.1;Sodium: 499;Total Carbohydrate: 15.8

397. Kas' Chili

Serving: 10 | Prep: 15mins | Cook: 7hours7mins | Ready in:
Ingredients
2 pounds ground beef
2 green bell peppers, chopped
2 onions, chopped
2 (15.25 ounce) cans kidney beans, rinsed and drained
1 (15 ounce) can black beans
1 (8 ounce) can tomato sauce
2 (14.5 ounce) cans diced tomatoes
1 tablespoon minced garlic
2 1/2 tablespoons chili powder
1 1/2 teaspoons paprika
1 tablespoon dried oregano
1 teaspoon dried rosemary
1 teaspoon ground coriander
1 teaspoon garlic powder
1 1/2 teaspoons salt
2 tablespoons ground cumin
1/4 cup chopped fresh cilantro
2 bay leaves
Direction

Put a big skillet on moderate high heat. Cook in the hot skillet the ground beef for 7-10 minutes until browned thoroughly, then drain.
In a slow cooker, mix together diced tomatoes, tomato sauce, black beans, kidney beans, onions, bell peppers and drained beef. Cook on high setting for a half hour. Stir into the beef mixture the bay leaves, cilantro, cumin, salt, garlic powder, coriander, rosemary, oregano, paprika, chili powder and garlic. Lower heat to low and cook for 6 1/2 hours more.
Nutrition Information
Calories: 289 calories;;Total Fat: 12.1;Sodium: 855;Total Carbohydrate: 23;Cholesterol: 57;Protein: 22

398. Kathy's Perfect Turkey Bisque

Serving: 4 | Prep: 10mins | Cook: 8hours35mins | Ready in:
Ingredients
2 teaspoons vegetable oil
1 turkey thigh with skin
1 cup Merlot wine
2 cups water
1 teaspoon dried thyme leaves
1/2 teaspoon dried rosemary
1/4 teaspoon poultry seasoning
1/4 teaspoon salt
1/8 teaspoon ground black pepper
1 (8 ounce) can tomato sauce (such as Del Monte®)
1/2 cup half-and-half cream
1 tablespoon cream sherry, or as desired (optional)
Direction
Heat vegetable oil in a skillet on medium heat. Cook both sides of turkey thigh, 8 minutes per side, till brown. Remove then discard skin; put thigh in skillet. Cook, 8 more minutes, till skinless side becomes golden brown. Remove turkey thigh; put Merlot wine into skillet. Scrape and dissolve drippings and browned flavor bits from bottom of skillet into wine; boil. Reduce wine for 10 minutes to 1/2 cup.
Put turkey thigh in slow cooker; put pepper, salt, poultry seasoning, rosemary, thyme, water and reduced wine. Cover cooker; put on low. Cook for 4 hours. Mix tomato sauce in; cook for 4 more hours. Remove turkey thigh; separate meat from bone. Put meat into slow cooker; simmer. Put half-and-half in. Mix cream sherry into soup; serve.
Nutrition Information
Calories: 266 calories;;Total Fat: 9.2;Sodium: 528;Total Carbohydrate: 6.3;Cholesterol: 115;Protein: 27.2

399. Kelly's Slow Cooker Beef, Mushroom, And Barley Soup

Serving: 6 | Prep: 20mins | Cook: 6hours | Ready in:
Ingredients
1 (32 ounce) carton beef stock
1 (8 ounce) can tomato sauce
1 cup water
1/2 onion, diced
3/4 cup diced carrots
1 cup barley
1 (6 ounce) package sliced fresh mushrooms
4 cloves garlic, minced
2 pounds beef sirloin, cut into chunks
1 pinch garlic salt, or to taste
salt and ground black pepper to taste
2 bay leaves
Direction

In a slow cooker, stir the beef stock, garlic, mushrooms, barley, carrot, onion, tomato sauce, and water together.

Dust black pepper, salt, and garlic salt to season the beef chunks; add to the beef stock mixture. Put bay leaves into the slow cooker.

Cook on Low heat for about 6 hours, until the soup is thickened and the beef is tender.

Take out and omit the bay leaves to serve.

Nutrition Information
Calories: 359 calories;;Total Fat: 10.3;Sodium: 381;Total Carbohydrate: 31.7;Cholesterol: 65;Protein: 34.6

400. Kyera's Hearty Beef Borscht

Serving: 16 | Prep: 45mins | Cook: 6hours | Ready in:
Ingredients
2 pounds beef oxtail
2 onions, diced
2 cups diced carrots
1 head cabbage, diced
1 cup diced celery (optional)
1/2 cup pearled barley
1 (1 ounce) package dry onion soup mix
1 teaspoon dried dill weed
1 teaspoon ground cinnamon
1 bay leaf
4 cups water, or enough to cover
1 bunch beets with greens - scrubbed, beets diced, and greens chopped
salt and ground black pepper to taste
1 cup sour cream

Direction
In a large slow cooker, put water, bay leaf, cinnamon, dill, onion soup mix, barley, celery, cabbage, carrots, onions and oxtail. Cook for around 5 hours on low, until the meat is tender.

Take the meat and bones out of the slow cooker; allow to cool for 10 minutes on a plate, till easily handled. Cut into small pieces; take the meat back to the soup; discard bones. Skim fat from the soup and discard the bay leaf.

Mix into soup the beet greens and beets; cook for 1 hour on low until the beets turn tender. Taste with pepper and salt; put 1 tablespoon of sour cream on top of each bowl. Serve.

Nutrition Information
Calories: 238 calories;;Total Fat: 11;Sodium: 333;Total Carbohydrate: 16;Cholesterol: 69;Protein: 20.3

401. Leek And Potato Chowder

Serving: 6 | Prep: 10mins | Cook: 3hours15mins | Ready in:
Ingredients
3 leeks
6 tablespoons butter, divided
1/4 cup all-purpose flour
2 (15 ounce) cans chicken broth
5 small red potatoes, peeled and diced
2 slices crispy cooked bacon, chopped
salt and ground black pepper to taste
1/2 cup water as needed
1 cup half-and-half

Direction
Make leeks clean by cutting off the tips and roots of the leaves. Cut vertically from the root end to the tops, being cautious to avoid cutting through entirely. The leeks will now open like the pages of a book and you can clean all the mud between the leaves under the faucet. Cut cleaned leeks into quarter-inch strips.

Put 1/2 butter in a skillet and melt over medium-high heat. Sauté the leeks in hot butter for 3-5 minutes till they are wilted.

Put the leftover butter in the same skillet and melt over low heat. Whisk flour into the melted butter slowly till mixture forms a dough clump. Pour chicken broth gradually into the skillet, whisking continuously till broth is incorporated completely; stream atop the mixture in the slow cooker. Put potatoes and bacon in the slow cooker. Add pepper and salt to season; stir well.

Cook on Low until the potatoes are soft, stirring water into the mixture if it becomes too thick, a minimum of 2 hours. Stir half-and-half into the mixture and keep on cooking for 1 hour longer.

Nutrition Information
Calories: 326 calories;Protein: 7;Total Fat: 18.1;Sodium: 865;Total Carbohydrate: 35.3;Cholesterol: 52

402. Leftover Ham And Shrimp Slow Cooker Gumbo

Serving: 12 | Prep: 15mins | Cook: 4hours40mins | Ready in:
Ingredients
1 clove garlic, minced
1 teaspoon ground turmeric
1 teaspoon chili powder
1 teaspoon dried basil
1/2 teaspoon cayenne pepper
1/4 cup butter
1 onion, minced
2 cups frozen cooked peeled and deveined jumbo shrimp
3 cups chopped leftover honey-baked, spiral-cut ham
1 ham bone
2 (15 ounce) cans black beans
1 (14.5 ounce) can diced tomatoes
1 cup coconut milk

Direction
Place a small saucepan on medium heat, stir in cayenne pepper, basil, chili powder, turmeric and garlic for about 1 minute, until aromatic. Liquefy butter into the mixture; include in onion; cook for about 5 minutes, until the onion is translucent and softened. Transfer the onion mixture to the slow cooker; keep as much butter in the saucepan as possible.

Raise the heat under the saucepan to medium-high. Sauté in frozen shrimp for about 2 minutes in hot butter until just firm; transfer to the slow cooker. Put tomatoes, black beans, ham bone and ham to the slow cooker.

Cook on Low for 6-8 hours or on High for 4-6 hours, until the ham is falling off from the bones. Discard the ham bones; stir in coconut milk to the mixture; keep cooking on Low for about 30 minutes, until the coconut milk is warmed.

Nutrition Information
Calories: 241 calories;;Total Carbohydrate: 18.4;Cholesterol: 81;Protein: 19.4;Total Fat: 9.8;Sodium: 869

403. Leftover Turkey Soup (Slow Cooker)

Serving: 8 | Prep: 20mins | Cook: 10hours | Ready in:
Ingredients
2 quarts chicken broth

1 turkey carcass, skin and meat removed
1 onion, quartered
2 carrots, halved lengthwise
3 celery stalks, halved lengthwise
2 bay leaves
1 cup chopped carrots
1/3 cup chopped celery
1/4 cup chopped onion
2 cups penne pasta
3 cups chopped cooked turkey
1 (10.75 ounce) can condensed cream of mushroom soup (optional)
Direction
In the slow cooker, whisk the bay leaves, celery halves, carrot halves, onion quarters, turkey carcass, and chicken broth.
Cook over High heat for 4 hours. Gently strain off the broth, remove the solids, and move the broth into the bowl. Wash the slow cooker.
Add the broth back to the slow cooker; put in the chopped onion, chopped celery, and chopped carrots. Cook over Low heat for 3 hours. Put the penne pasta into the slow cooker; cook for 2.5 hours longer. Whisk the cream of the mushroom soup and turkey meat into the soup and cook for half an hour longer.
Nutrition Information
Calories: 1877 calories;;Cholesterol: 426;Protein: 92.5;Total Fat: 140.8;Sodium: 1541;Total Carbohydrate: 54.5

404. Lemon Salmon Soup

Serving: 8 | Prep: 15mins | Cook: 5hours | Ready in:
Ingredients
2 pounds potatoes, peeled and cubed
1 pound salmon fillets
water to cover
2 tablespoons butter
1 tablespoon lemon zest
1 1/2 teaspoons salt
ground black pepper to taste
1 pinch dried oregano
1 pinch dried thyme
1 pinch dried basil
2 cups milk
Direction
Layer the potatoes and salmon into the bottom of the slow cooker. Add enough water to the slow cooker to cover. Put in the basil, thyme, oregano, pepper, salt, lemon zest, and butter. Keep loosely covered and cook over Low heat for 4 - 5 hours. Mix in milk and cover securely; cook for 1 – 2 more hours.
Nutrition Information
Calories: 227 calories;;Sodium: 515;Total Carbohydrate: 23.1;Cholesterol: 38;Protein: 16.5;Total Fat: 7.5

405. Lentil Soup With Garlicky Vinaigrette

Serving: 6 | Prep: 15mins | Cook: 6hours10mins | Ready in:
Ingredients
2 tablespoons olive oil
1 cup chopped onion
3/4 cup diced celery
3/4 cup diced carrots
2 cloves garlic, finely chopped
2 teaspoons kosher salt
3/4 cup tomato sauce
2 cups green or brown lentils
2 cups water

4 cups low-sodium chicken or vegetable broth
1 bay leaf
1 sprig fresh thyme
1 teaspoon balsamic or sherry vinegar
Vinaigrette:
1/4 cup olive oil
2 tablespoons balsamic or sherry vinegar
1 clove garlic, minced
1/2 teaspoon salt
Direction
In a big frying pan, heat oil over medium heat. Cook garlic, carrots, celery, and onion with salt for 10 minutes, mixing sometimes until the vegetables are brown and limp. Move the vegetables to a slow cooker with vinegar, thyme, bay leaf, broth, water, lentils, and tomato sauce. Cook for 6 hours on Low. To prepare the vinaigrette, stir together salt, garlic, vinegar, and olive oil.
Season the soup with salt, and then drizzle over each bowl with vinaigrette to serve.
Nutrition Information
Calories: 392 calories;;Total Fat: 14.6;Sodium: 1102;Total Carbohydrate: 46.6;Cholesterol: 3;Protein: 19.7

406. Low Carb Cream Of Broccoli Soup

Serving: 16 | Prep: 15mins | Cook: 4hours16mins | Ready in:
Ingredients
2 (14 ounce) cans chicken broth
1 (8 ounce) package cream cheese
1 cup shredded Cheddar cheese
1/4 cup butter
1 tablespoon minced onion flakes
1 pint heavy whipping cream
1 (10 ounce) can chicken chunks, or more to taste
3 heads broccoli, broken into florets
Direction
In a big pot, mix together onion flakes, butter, Cheddar cheese, cream cheese, and chicken broth over medium heat; stir and cook for 3-5 minutes until smooth. Add chicken and heavy cream, lightly simmer.
Insert a steamer into a saucepan and fill using water until just beneath the steamer's bottom. Boil the water. Put in broccoli, put a cover on and steam for 4-5 minutes until soft. Move to a colander to strain the excess liquid.
In a slow cooker, add the chicken broth mixture, then put in broccoli.
Cook on low for 4 hours until the flavors blend.
Nutrition Information
Calories: 258 calories;;Total Fat: 22.8;Sodium: 458;Total Carbohydrate: 5.5;Cholesterol: 83;Protein: 9.1

407. Luscious Lima Bean Soup II

Serving: 8 | Prep: 15mins | Cook: 7hours | Ready in:
Ingredients
3 slices bacon
4 cups frozen lima beans
1 (15 ounce) can butter beans, undrained
2 potatoes, diced
2 stalks celery, chopped
2 small onions, chopped
3 carrots, sliced
1/4 cup butter
1/2 tablespoon dried marjoram
1 teaspoon salt

1/2 teaspoon pepper
3 (14 ounce) cans chicken broth
Direction
Cook bacon in skillet over medium heat till crisp and evenly brown. Drain; crumble.
Mix together butter, carrots, onions, celery, potatoes, butter beans and liquid, lima beans and cooked bacon in slow cooker. Season with pepper, salt and marjoram. Put chicken broth in.
Cover the slow cooker. Cook on low for 7 hours.
Nutrition Information
Calories: 326 calories;;Total Fat: 11.4;Sodium: 1381;Total Carbohydrate: 43.7;Cholesterol: 26;Protein: 13

408. Main Line Chicken Chili
Serving: 8 | Prep: 25mins | Cook: 4hours | Ready in:
Ingredients
1 1/2 pounds skinless, boneless chicken meat, cut into bite-size pieces
1 (15 ounce) can kidney beans, drained (retain half the liquid)
1 (15 ounce) can black beans, drained (retain half the liquid)
1 large onion, chopped
1 green bell pepper, chopped
1 (6 ounce) can tomato paste
1 (14.5 ounce) can stewed tomatoes
1/2 cup mango salsa
2 tablespoons rice vinegar
1 bay leaf
1 teaspoon smoked paprika, or to taste
1/2 teaspoon salt
1 tablespoon chili powder
ground black pepper to taste
Direction
Into a slow cooker add chicken meat, black beans with half their liquid, kidney beans with half their liquid, green pepper, onion, stewed tomatoes, tomato paste, mango salsa, rice vinegar, bay leaf, chili powder, smoked paprika, salt and black pepper and stir well to combine. Cook and cover for 1 hour on high setting; stir the chili. Reduce to low heat and cook another 3 to 4 hours.
Nutrition Information
Calories: 212 calories;;Sodium: 747;Total Carbohydrate: 26;Cholesterol: 36;Protein: 16.7;Total Fat: 5.4

409. Maine Venison Stew
Serving: 8 | Prep: 20mins | Cook: 9hours | Ready in:
Ingredients
2 pounds venison stew meat
8 medium potatoes, peeled and cubed
3 medium onions, diced
3 stalks celery, diced
8 large carrots, peeled and diced
3 cubes beef bouillon
2 (14.5 ounce) cans beef broth
2 tablespoons browning and seasoning sauce
2 cups frozen green peas (optional)
2 cups fresh mushrooms, sliced (optional)
salt and pepper to taste
1/2 cup cornstarch
1 cup water
Direction
Place venison, onions, celery, carrots, bouillon, broth, seasoning sauce and potatoes in a slow cooker. Add enough water to cover the ingredients. Set cooker on high and cook until stew boils. Reduce heat and continue cooking on low for 8 to 10 hours until venison is tender.
Spoon off all fat from the surface of stew and stir in mushrooms (if using) and peas; season to taste with salt and pepper. In a bowl whisk together water and cornstarch. Stir the cornstarch mixture into the stew. Continue cooking and set on high heat until the stew thickens and the peas have warmed through.
Nutrition Information
Calories: 407 calories;;Cholesterol: 86;Protein: 32.6;Total Fat: 3.4;Sodium: 876;Total Carbohydrate: 61.9

410. Make Ahead Slow Cooker Beef Stew
Serving: 6 | Prep: 30mins | Cook: 4hours | Ready in:
Ingredients
1/3 cup all-purpose flour
1 teaspoon Spanish smoked paprika
1/2 teaspoon seasoned salt
1/2 teaspoon ground black pepper
2 pounds beef chuck, cut into 1-inch cubes
1 tablespoon olive oil
1 onion, chopped
1 (8 ounce) package mushrooms, chopped
3 potatoes, diced
5 carrots, sliced
2 stalks celery, chopped
2 cloves garlic, minced
1/4 cup Marsala wine
1 tablespoon Worcestershire sauce
3 (10.5 ounce) cans organic beef broth
1 (14.5 ounce) can crushed tomatoes
1 (1 ounce) package dry onion soup mix
1 teaspoon Spanish smoked paprika, or to taste
salt and ground black pepper to taste
2 tablespoons cornstarch (optional)
2 tablespoons water (optional)
Direction
In a big resealable plastic bag, mix together 1/2 teaspoon of black pepper, seasoned salt, 1 teaspoon of smoked paprika, and flour. Add beef, and close the bag. Shake the bag well so that the seasoned flour can coat the beef.
In a big frying pan, heat olive oil over medium-high heat. Remove any the excess seasoning from the beef by shaking it off, and then mix the beef into the hot frying pan with mushrooms and onion. Cook while stirring until the beef is not pink anymore and turns brown evenly. Strain and remove and extra fat.
In a slow cooker, put the beef mixture. Add Worcestershire sauce, Marsala wine, garlic, celery, carrots, and potatoes to the beef mixture in the cooker. Add tomatoes and beef broth to the cooker, and mix in 1 additional teaspoon of smoked paprika and onion soup mix. Cook on low for 10-12 hours and on high for 4-6 hours. Use black pepper and salt to season to taste.
If you want a thicker stew, in a small bowl, mix together water and cornstarch. Slowly mix the mixture into the stew until thickened.
Nutrition Information
Calories: 467 calories;;Total Fat: 20.6;Sodium: 1110;Total Carbohydrate: 43.8;Cholesterol: 69;Protein: 25.3

411. Maverick Moose Chili
Serving: 12 | Prep: 15mins | Cook: 8hours10mins | Ready in:

Ingredients
1 pound ground moose
1 (28 ounce) can diced tomatoes with green chile peppers
2 (15 ounce) cans chili beans, undrained
2 (14 ounce) cans kidney beans, rinsed and drained
2 (14.5 ounce) cans pinto beans, rinsed and drained
2 (2.25 ounce) cans sliced black olives
1 white onion, chopped
1 green bell pepper, chopped
1 (1.25 ounce) package chili seasoning mix
Direction
In a big skillet, brown the ground moose on moderate high heat.
Mix in a slow cooker the bell pepper, onion, olives, pinto beans, kidney beans, chili beans, diced tomatoes and moose, then stir in the chili seasoning. Set the slow cooker to low setting and cook for 8-12 hours.
Nutrition Information
Calories: 241 calories;;Sodium: 1309;Total Carbohydrate: 39;Cholesterol: 19;Protein: 18.8;Total Fat: 3

412. Meat Lovers' Vegetarian Chili

Serving: 12 | Prep: 40mins | Cook: 6hours15mins | Ready in:
Ingredients
6 tablespoons olive oil, divided
2 large red bell peppers, seeded and chopped
2 poblano peppers, seeded and chopped
1 large onion, chopped
5 cloves garlic, minced
1 jalapeno pepper, seeded and minced, or more to taste
2 cups hot vegetable broth
2 cups texturized vegetable protein (TVP)
3 tablespoons nutritional yeast
1 (32 ounce) can canned diced tomatoes, undrained
2 (15 ounce) cans kidney beans, drained and rinsed
1 (15 ounce) can black beans, drained and rinsed
1/2 cup beer
1 (6 ounce) can tomato paste
1/2 cup cider vinegar
3 tablespoons soy sauce
3 tablespoons lemon juice
2 tablespoons chili powder
2 tablespoons unsweetened cocoa powder
4 teaspoons seasoned salt
1 tablespoon Worcestershire sauce
1 tablespoon paprika
1 tablespoon ground cumin
2 teaspoons dried oregano
1 teaspoon liquid smoke flavoring
1 teaspoon ground black pepper
1 teaspoon white sugar
Direction
Use a skillet to heat 3 tablespoons of olive oil on medium low heat. Add in the bell peppers, onion, poblano peppers, jalapeno and garlic. Cook for 15 minutes while stirring until tender. Transfer the mixture into a slow cooker.
Mix together the TVP and hot vegetable broth in a mixing bowl. Mix for 5 minutes until the liquid is well absorbed. Add it to the slow cooker.
Mix in the slow cooker the diced tomatoes, black beans, kidney beans, beer, tomato paste, soy sauce, vinegar, chili powder, lemon juice, seasoned salt, cocoa powder, paprika, oregano, cumin, Worcestershire sauce, black pepper, liquid smoke and sugar. Mix well.
Let the chili cook in the slow cooker for 6-10 hours on low or 4-5 hours on high.
Nutrition Information
Calories: 300 calories;;Sodium: 1347;Total Carbohydrate: 32.7;Cholesterol: 0;Protein: 25;Total Fat: 9.1

413. Mexican Chocolate Chili

Serving: 6 | Prep: 15mins | Cook: 2hours30mins | Ready in:
Ingredients
1 pound ground round
1 cup chopped onion
1 cup hot water
2 (14.5 ounce) cans diced tomatoes with garlic, undrained
1 (15 ounce) can kidney beans, rinsed and drained
1 (15 ounce) can black beans, rinsed and drained
1 (14.5 ounce) can whole kernel corn, drained
1/3 cup semisweet chocolate chips
2 teaspoons chili powder
1 tablespoon ground cumin
1/2 teaspoon dried oregano
1 teaspoon salt
Direction
In a big saucepan, mix together onion and ground round on moderate high heat. Cook while stirring for 5 minutes until beef is browned.
Put the onions and cooked beef to a slow cooker. Stir in salt, oregano, cumin, chili powder, chocolate chips, corn, black beans, kidney beans, tomatoes and water. Cook on high setting for 20 minutes until chili starts to bubble. Lower heat to low and cook for 2 hours until thickened.
Nutrition Information
Calories: 276 calories;;Sodium: 978;Total Carbohydrate: 37.3;Cholesterol: 25;Protein: 16.4;Total Fat: 7.9

414. Mile High Green Chili

Serving: 8 | Prep: 30mins | Cook: 4hours30mins | Ready in:
Ingredients
4 fresh tomatillos - husked, peeled, and halved
3 Anaheim chile peppers - seeded and halved
3 jalapeno peppers - seeded and halved lengthwise
1 medium onion, halved
1 green bell pepper, seeded and halved lengthwise
1 tablespoon olive oil, or as needed
salt to taste
1 tablespoon olive oil
1 1/2 cups pork shoulder, cut into 1-inch chunks
salt and ground black pepper to taste
2 tomatoes, chopped
4 cloves garlic, chopped
1 beef bouillon cube
1/2 (12 fluid ounce) can or bottle lager-style beer
2 tablespoons chopped fresh oregano
1 tablespoon chopped fresh parsley
1 tablespoon ground cumin
1 teaspoon chili powder
4 ounces cream cheese at room temperature
Direction
Preheat oven to 220 degrees C/425 degrees F.

Put green bell pepper, onion, jalapenos, Anaheim chiles and halved tomatillos on a baking sheet. Drizzle 1 tbsp. olive oil on veggies.
Roast veggies in the preheated oven for 30 minutes until they get brown spots. Cool. Chop veggies to bite-sized pieces.
In a big skillet, heat 1 more tbsp. olive oil on high heat. Pan-fry pork for 12 minutes until brown, sprinkling meat with black pepper and salt while you cook. Put pork cubes in a slow cooker. Mix in roasted veggies. Mix in chili powder, cumin, parsley, oregano, beer, beef bouillon cube, garlic and tomatoes. Set cook on low, cook, covered, for 1-8 hours until pork is really tender.
Half hour prior to serving, put cream cheese in a bowl. Mix 1 tbsp. chili liquid until combined. Mix in chili broth, 1 tbsp. at a time, until cream cheese is nearly liquid. Mix cream cheese mixture back into chili.
Nutrition Information
Calories: 174 calories;;Sodium: 210;Total Carbohydrate: 8.6;Cholesterol: 32;Protein: 7.6;Total Fat: 12

415. Miner's Chili

Serving: 12 | Prep: 30mins | Cook: 8hours | Ready in:
Ingredients
1 pound lean ground beef
1 onion, chopped
3 stalks celery, diced
1 green bell pepper, chopped
3 (14.5 ounce) cans peeled and diced tomatoes
2 (15 ounce) cans dark red kidney beans
1 (15 ounce) can light red kidney beans
1 (16 ounce) jar hot salsa
4 teaspoons white sugar
1/2 teaspoon cayenne pepper
2 tablespoons chili powder
1 1/2 teaspoons dried basil
1 1/2 teaspoons dried oregano
Direction
Heat beef in a big skillet over medium heat until brown. Cook bell pepper, onion and celery until veggies become tender.
In a slow cooker, mix kidney beans, tomatoes, salsa and beef mixture. Spice it with oregano, cayenne, sugar, chili powder and basil. Let it cook in low for 8 hours. Place in the refrigerator for 8 hours or overnight, reheat then serve.
Nutrition Information
Calories: 239 calories;;Total Carbohydrate: 26.1;Cholesterol: 28;Protein: 14.3;Total Fat: 8.6;Sodium: 657

416. Mixed Beans And More

Serving: 10 | Prep: 15mins | Cook: 4hours30mins | Ready in:
Ingredients
1 1/2 cups dried black beans, rinsed
1 1/2 cups dried pinto beans, rinsed
1 1/2 cups dried kidney beans, rinsed
1 pound andouille sausage, chopped
1 pound lean ground beef
1 large onion, chopped
1 bell pepper, chopped
2 cloves cloves garlic, minced
1 cup corn (optional)
3/4 cup salsa
3/4 cup tomato-based chili sauce
2 tablespoons white vinegar
1 cup water
salt and ground black pepper to taste
Direction
In a large container with several inches of cool water, combine pinto beans, kidney beans, and black beans, and soak it for at least 12 hours. Transfer the beans into a large pot. Bring them to boil, and then cook for 30 minutes until the beans are soft and heated through. Remove pot from heat and allow the beans to cool and drain.
Combine and stir bell pepper, beef, garlic, onion, and sausage in a large skillet. Let it cook over medium high heat for 5-10 minutes until the meat was all brown. Drain and remove excess fat.
In a slow cooker, mix water, beans, chili sauce, sausage mixture, corn, vinegar, and salsa.
Set it on High setting and allow it to cook for at least 4 hours, stirring it for some time. Flavor it with ground black pepper and salt.
Nutrition Information
Calories: 574 calories;;Sodium: 843;Total Carbohydrate: 65.6;Cholesterol: 56;Protein: 34.4;Total Fat: 19.9

417. Mo's Spicy Beef Stew

Serving: 6 | Prep: 20mins | Cook: 4hours10mins | Ready in:
Ingredients
all-purpose flour
1 pinch garlic salt, or to taste
ground black pepper to taste
2 1/2 pounds beef stew meat, cut into cubes
1 tablespoon olive oil, or more if needed
3 cups water
1 (1.5 ounce) package dry beef stew seasoning mix
2 large potatoes, cut into cubes
1 small onion, chopped
1 (10 ounce) can diced tomatoes with green chile peppers (such as RO*TEL®)
1 teaspoon hot pepper sauce (such as Frank's RedHot®)
1 cup frozen corn
Direction
In a shallow dish, combine black pepper, garlic salt, and flour.
To coat properly, press carefully the beef cubes into the flour blend.
In a skillet, heat the olive oil over medium heat; working in batches, stir and cook the beef in the heated oil for around 5 minutes for each batch until completely browned. Use a slotted spoon to transfer the browned beef to a bowl when all beef gets browned.
In a slow cooker, stir together the beef stew seasoning mix and water until the seasoning has been dissolved in the liquid. Add the hot pepper sauce, green chile peppers with diced tomatoes, onion, potatoes, and the browned beef.
Cook on high for 3 1/2 - 4 1/2 hours. Put in the frozen corn and keep on cooking for 30 more minutes until the corn becomes hot.
Nutrition Information
Calories: 436 calories;;Total Carbohydrate: 38.3;Cholesterol: 100;Protein: 39;Total Fat: 13.4;Sodium: 934

418. Mom's Chicken And Dumplings (Slow Cooker Version)

Serving: 6 | Prep: 20mins | Cook: 6hours | Ready in:
Ingredients
4 (14.5 ounce) cans chicken broth
3 (12.5 fl oz) cans chunk chicken (such as Kirkland®), drained and broken into chunks
4 baking potatoes, peeled and cubed
4 carrots, sliced
2 cups chopped broccoli
1 cup water
2 tablespoons quick-mixing flour (such as Wondra®)
salt and cracked black pepper to taste
2 1/4 cups all-purpose baking mix (such as Bisquick®)
2/3 cup milk
Direction
In a slow cooker, mix broccoli, carrots, potatoes, chicken and chicken broth together.
In a bowl, blend quick –mixing flour and water till a paste-like consistency is reached; mix into the slow cooker mixture. Season with pepper and salt.
Cook on low for 5 hours. In a bowl, blend milk and baking mix together. Drop teaspoonful of the milk mixture into the slow cooker on top of chicken mixture. Keep cooking; turn the dumplings once, till they are cooked through, about 1 more hour.
Nutrition Information
Calories: 649 calories;;Total Carbohydrate: 62.9;Cholesterol: 117;Protein: 47.8;Total Fat: 22.2;Sodium: 2692

419. Mom's Italian Beef Barley Soup

Serving: 6 | Prep: 10mins | Cook: 5hours | Ready in:
Ingredients
2 pounds cubed beef chuck roast
5 cups water
4 cubes beef bouillon, crumbled
1/2 onion, chopped
1 (8 ounce) can tomato sauce
3/4 cup uncooked pearl barley
salt and pepper to taste
Direction
Combine beef, pepper, salt, barley, tomato sauce, onion, bouillon, and water in a slow cooker.
Cover up and cook on Low heat for about 5 hours.
Nutrition Information
Calories: 512 calories;;Sodium: 884;Total Carbohydrate: 35.4;Cholesterol: 107;Protein: 29.7;Total Fat: 27.8

420. Nikki's Creamy Crock Pot Potato Soup

Serving: 6 | Prep: 30mins | Cook: 3hours10mins | Ready in:
Ingredients
3 slices bacon, cooked and crumbled
4 red potatoes, peeled and cut into 1/2 inch chunks
1/4 cup butter
1/2 onion, chopped
3 cloves garlic, coarsely chopped
1/2 cup milk
1/4 cup all-purpose flour
3 cups milk
1 cup sour cream
1/4 cup shredded Cheddar cheese
1/4 cup grated Parmesan cheese
2 tablespoons seasoned salt
1 tablespoon chopped fresh parsley
1 tablespoon crushed red pepper flakes
1/2 teaspoon celery salt
1/2 teaspoon dried basil
chives for garnish (optional)
Direction
Preheat a big slow cooker by turning to High setting and using the lid to cover it.
Add cut-up potatoes to the microwave-safe bowl, and microwave on High till potatoes are cooked and steaming hot, roughly 8 minutes.
While potatoes are being cooked, add butter to preheated slow cooker, and cook and stir garlic and onions till onions become golden in color, roughly 5 minutes. Mix in half cup milk, and mix in flour till becoming smooth. Slowly mix in the rest 3 cups milk, and allow mixture to come to simmer in slow cooker. Let simmer till soup starts to thicken, roughly 10 minutes.
Mix in dried basil, celery salt, red pepper flakes, parsley, seasoned salt, Parmesan cheese, Cheddar cheese, sour cream, crumbled bacon and hot cooked potatoes. Whisk to mix soup well, lower slow cooker setting to Low, keep it covered, and cook for 3 hours, mixing once in a while. Drizzle with chives and serve.
Nutrition Information
Calories: 429 calories;Protein: 13.7;Total Fat: 23.5;Sodium: 1366;Total Carbohydrate: 42.5;Cholesterol: 61

421. No Peek Beef Stew

Serving: 6 | Prep: 28mins | Cook: 8hours | Ready in:
Ingredients
2 pounds beef stew meat, cut into 1 inch cubes
1 (10.5 ounce) can condensed French onion soup
1 (10.75 ounce) can condensed cream of mushroom soup
1 (4.5 ounce) can mushrooms, drained
1/2 cup dry red wine
Direction
In the slow cooker, mix together dry red wine, mushrooms, condensed cream of mushroom soup, condensed French onion soup and beef stew meat.
Cook with a cover for 8 hours on Low.
Nutrition Information
Calories: 382 calories;;Total Fat: 24.3;Sodium: 904;Total Carbohydrate: 9.3;Cholesterol: 85;Protein: 27

422. Old Fashioned Beef Stew

Serving: 8 | Prep: 20mins | Cook: 6hours | Ready in:
Ingredients
2 pounds cubed beef stew meat
4 cups boiling water
1 tablespoon lemon juice
1 teaspoon Worcestershire sauce
1 clove garlic, crushed
1 onion, diced
1 bay leaf
1 tablespoon salt
1 teaspoon sugar
1/2 teaspoon ground black pepper
1/2 teaspoon paprika
1/8 teaspoon ground allspice
6 potatoes, cubed
2 carrots, sliced
1/2 cup whole kernel corn
Direction
Mix garlic, Worcestershire sauce, lemon juice, boiling water and the stew meat together in a slow cooker.
Blend in the allspice, paprika, ground pepper, sugar,

salt, bay leaf and onion. Put in the corn, carrots and potatoes.
Cook on HIGH, 2 hours.
Turn the slow cooker down to LOW and cook for 3 and 1/2 hours. Discard bay leaves. Serve.
Nutrition Information
Calories: 444 calories;;Sodium: 969;Total Carbohydrate: 28.6;Cholesterol: 99;Protein: 33.6;Total Fat: 21.3

423. Old Fashioned Onion Soup
Serving: 8 | Prep: 15mins | Cook: 4hours | Ready in:
Ingredients
3 pounds onions, sliced
1/2 cup butter, melted
7 slices French or Italian-style bread
4 1/2 cups chicken broth
Direction
In a slow cooker, place butter and sliced onions and mix until the onions are coated thoroughly. Stir in the chicken broth and bread.
Cover and cook on HIGH 4 to 5 hours or on LOW for 10-18 hours, occasionally stirring. During the last hour, stir well.
Nutrition Information
Calories: 255 calories;;Cholesterol: 31;Protein: 7.3;Total Fat: 12.8;Sodium: 660;Total Carbohydrate: 28.8

424. Old School Bean Soup With Wheat Berries
Serving: 12 | Prep: 20mins | Cook: 5hours | Ready in:
Ingredients
1 ham bone
water to cover
8 ounces dried navy beans
8 ounces cranberry beans
8 ounces wheat berries
1 tablespoon celery salt
1 tablespoon dried thyme
1 tablespoon dried oregano
2 dashes Worcestershire sauce, or to taste
fresh cracked black pepper to taste
8 ounces dried lentils
salt and ground black pepper to taste
2 ripe tomatoes, diced
1 ripe avocado, diced
2 green onions, sliced, or more to taste
Direction
In a slow cooker, arrange the ham bone. Cover with enough water. Cook on low for 12-15 hours until stock releases fragrance.
In a large container, combine wheat berries, cranberry beans, and navy beans, and pour several inches of cool water to cover; soak for 8 hours to overnight. Let drain.
Take the ham bone out from the stock. Add in wheat berries and beans. Stir in black pepper, Worcestershire sauce, oregano, thyme, and celery salt. Cook on High for around 4 hours until the beans become tender but al dente.
Add the lentils into the slow cooker and stir. Cook on High for around an hour until tender. Use black pepper and salt to season. Place green onions, avocado and diced tomatoes on top to serve.
Nutrition Information
Calories: 721 calories;;Total Carbohydrate: 144.7;Cholesterol: 0;Protein: 33.1;Total Fat: 5.7;Sodium: 398

425. Paleo Chili You Won't Miss The Beans
Serving: 10 | Prep: 30mins | Cook: 6hours10mins | Ready in:
Ingredients
1 tablespoon extra-virgin olive oil
1 large yellow onion, chopped
2 cloves garlic, chopped
2 pounds ground beef
1 pound bulk Italian sausage
2 (15 ounce) cans diced tomatoes
1 (6 ounce) can tomato paste
2 zucchini, diced
4 carrots, peeled and diced
2 red bell peppers, seeded and chopped
3 stalks celery, chopped
1 green chile pepper, seeded and chopped
2 tablespoons chili powder
4 teaspoons beef bone broth powder
1 tablespoon Worcestershire sauce
1 tablespoon dried oregano
2 teaspoons hot sauce
1 teaspoon paprika
1 teaspoon ground cumin
1 teaspoon dried basil
1 teaspoon salt
1 teaspoon ground black pepper
1 teaspoon cayenne pepper
Direction
Place a skillet over medium heat and heat the olive oil. Stir in garlic and onion. Stir while cooking for 5 minutes, or until the onion is translucent and soft. Stir in sausage and ground beef; cook for 5 to 7 minutes, or until meat is browned and crumbly. Transfer the mixture to a slow cooker.
In the slow cooker, stir the mixture above with cayenne pepper, black pepper, salt, basil, cumin, paprika, hot sauce, oregano, Worcestershire sauce, broth powder, chili powder, green chile pepper, celery, carrots, red bell peppers, zucchini, tomato paste, and diced tomatoes. Cook for 6 to 8 hours on Low, or until vegetables are tender.
Nutrition Information
Calories: 390 calories;;Total Carbohydrate: 17.1;Cholesterol: 74;Protein: 24.3;Total Fat: 24.9;Sodium: 1198

426. Pareve Cholent
Serving: 6 | Prep: 20mins | Cook: 11hours | Ready in:
Ingredients
1 cup dry kidney beans
1/2 cup dry white beans
1/2 cup barley
2 large potatoes, peeled and cubed
1 large sweet potato, peeled and cubed
1 large onion, cut into chunks
2 cloves garlic, minced
2/3 cup ketchup
1/4 cup barbeque sauce
1/4 cup soy sauce
1/4 cup brown sugar
2 teaspoons garlic powder
2 teaspoons onion powder
2 teaspoons paprika
2 teaspoons ground black pepper
1 tablespoon salt
4 cups water, or more as needed to cover
Direction

In the slow cooker, mix together water, salt, pepper, paprika, onion powder, garlic powder, brown sugar, soy sauce, barbeque sauce, ketchup, garlic, onion, sweet potato, potatoes, barley, white beans and kidney beans; mix properly. Cook for 3 hours on High, then lower the heat to Low and keep cooking overnight, until the beans become tender.

Nutrition Information
Calories: 465 calories;;Total Fat: 1.3;Sodium: 2244;Total Carbohydrate: 98.9;Cholesterol: 0;Protein: 18.3

427. Potato And Corn Chowder (Freezer Dump Meal)

Serving: 6 | Prep: 10mins | Cook: 8hours | Ready in:
Ingredients
1 1/2 pounds red potatoes, diced
1 (16 ounce) package frozen corn
3 tablespoons almond flour
1 teaspoon dried thyme
1 teaspoon dried oregano
1/2 teaspoon garlic powder
1/2 teaspoon onion powder
salt and ground black pepper to taste
6 cups chicken stock
1/4 cup coconut milk
2 tablespoons ghee (clarified butter)
Direction
Put corn, almond flour, red potatoes, oregano, thyme, garlic and onion powders, pepper, and salt in a freezer bag. Freeze it until you're ready to use it.
To prepare, pour the bagged ingredients in a slow cooker or pot with chicken stock, ghee, and coconut milk. Cook slowly on low heat for 8 hours or until potatoes are very soft.
Nutrition Information
Calories: 237 calories;;Sodium: 722;Total Carbohydrate: 36.4;Cholesterol: 12;Protein: 6.1;Total Fat: 9.6

428. Pozole In A Slow Cooker

Serving: 12 | Prep: 30mins | Cook: 8hours25mins | Ready in:
Ingredients
2 pasilla chile peppers - stems, seeds, and veins removed
2 ancho chile peppers - stems, seeds, and veins removed
2 guajillo chile peppers - stems, seeds, and veins removed
water, to cover
1 teaspoon cumin seeds
2 cloves garlic
1/2 white onion, chopped
5 Roma tomatoes, chopped
1 (3 1/2) pound pork shoulder, cut into several large pieces
salt to taste
2 bay leaves
4 cups chicken stock
2 (15.5 ounce) cans white hominy, rinsed and drained
Direction
In a small pot, toast cumin over medium-high heat for 1-2 minutes until aromatic, make sure not to burn. Add guajillo chile peppers, ancho chile peppers, and pasilla chile peppers to the pot. Fully cover the peppers with enough water. Put tomatoes, onion, and garlic cloves on top of the chiles. Put a cover on the pot, lower the heat to low, and bring the mixture to a simmer, about 10 minutes. Take away from heat and let the mixture cool. In a blender, add the mixture to puree until smooth.
In the bottom of a slow cooker, place the pork. Use salt to season liberally. Put bay leaves in the slow cooker and add the pureed chile pepper mixture to the pork.
Cook for 8-9 hours or overnight on Low. Remove as much fat from the top as you can. Transfer to pork to a bowl or cutting board, using 2 forks to shred. Put the shredded pork back into the slow cooker and stir with the sauce.
In a big pot, mix the shredded pork with hominy, chicken stock, and sauce over medium heat. Cook for 10-15 minutes until the stock is hot. Enjoy hot.
Nutrition Information
Calories: 240 calories;;Total Fat: 13.6;Sodium: 427;Total Carbohydrate: 13.6;Cholesterol: 52;Protein: 15.4

429. Pretty Easy Chili

Serving: 4 | Prep: 15mins | Cook: 6hours5mins | Ready in:
Ingredients
1 pound ground beef
1 onion, chopped
3 cloves garlic, chopped
2 (15 ounce) cans pinto beans, drained
1 (28 ounce) can whole peeled tomatoes, broken apart by hand
1 (15 ounce) can tomato sauce
1 (10.75 ounce) can tomato soup (optional)
2 tablespoons chili powder
2 tablespoons white sugar
2 tablespoons Italian seasoning
2 teaspoons garlic salt
1 pinch cracked black pepper to taste
4 fluid ounces beer
Direction
Heat a big skillet on moderate high heat. Cook and stir garlic, onion and beef for 5 to 7 minutes in the hot skillet until crumbly and browned; drain and get rid of grease. Put the beef mixture to a slow cooker. Stir into the beef mixture the tomato soup, tomato sauce, tomatoes and pinto beans.
Combine together in a bowl with pepper, garlic salt, Italian seasoning, sugar and chili powder, then stir into the beef mixture. Put in beer.
Cook on low setting for about 6 to 8 hours.
Nutrition Information
Calories: 551 calories;;Total Fat: 21.4;Sodium: 2706;Total Carbohydrate: 61;Cholesterol: 70;Protein: 31.5

430. Pulled Pork Chili

Serving: 8 | Prep: 20mins | Cook: 9hours | Ready in:
Ingredients
1 (1 1/2-pound) whole pork loin
1/4 cup red chile paste
1 tablespoon hot sauce
1 teaspoon ground cumin
1 teaspoon ground chili powder
1 (16 ounce) can tomato sauce
1 (16 ounce) can low-sodium chicken broth
1 (16 ounce) can low-sodium great northern beans
6 slices bacon, cut into 1-inch pieces
1/2 cup wild rice
1/4 cup diced onion

1/4 cup diced jalapeno pepper
1 cup shredded Monterey Jack cheese
Direction
In a slow cooker, add the pork loin. Combine together in a small bowl the chili powder, cumin, hot sauce and red chile paste. Rub pork with the chile paste mixture.
In a big bowl, stir together jalapeno pepper, onion, wild rice, bacon, beans, chicken broth and tomato sauce, then put into the slow cooker and coat the pork.
Cook on low setting for 9-10 hours until flavors are blended. Take the cooked pork out of the sauce and use 2 forks to shred the meat. Move it back to the slow cooker and combine well.
Put the shredded Monterey Jack cheese on top of individual servings.
Nutrition Information
Calories: 347 calories;;Total Fat: 13.4;Sodium: 703;Total Carbohydrate: 30.2;Cholesterol: 61;Protein: 29

431. Pumpkin Pulled Pork Chili
Serving: 10 | Prep: 30mins | Cook: 8hours51mins | Ready in:
Ingredients
2 pounds boneless pork loin
1 onion, finely chopped
1 (12 fluid ounce) can dark ale
1 (8 ounce) can tomato sauce
2 tablespoons chili powder
1 tablespoon ground cumin
6 cups water
2 pounds pumpkin, cut into chunks
1 tablespoon chicken-flavored bouillon powder
1 tablespoon finely chopped pickled jalapeno pepper
1 tablespoon onion powder
1 tablespoon garlic powder
1 cup corn
3/4 cup cooked Great Northern beans
2 tablespoons chopped cilantro, or to taste
ground black pepper to taste
Direction
In a small pot, add onion and pork loin. Pour dark ale over pork and coat with tomato sauce. Use plastic warp to cover and allow to marinate in the fridge for 8 hours to overnight.
Move the pork mixture to a slow cooker. Cook on low setting for 8 hours until an inserted instant-read thermometer into the center reaches a minimum of 63°C or 145°F.
Move the pork to cutting board and reserve the cooking liquid. Use one fork to hold the pork and another to shred the meat.
In a big pot on moderate heat, add cumin and chili powder, then toss for 1-2 minutes until aromatic. Put in garlic powder, onion powder, jalapeno pepper, chicken bouillon, pumpkin and water. Bring the mixture to a simmer and cook for 20 minutes until pumpkin is softened. Use an immersion blender to puree until the sauce is smooth.
Stir into the sauce the black pepper, cilantro, beans and corn. Put in the reserved cooking liquid as well as the shredded pork, then mix to blend. Cook for a half hour until chili reaches preferred thickness and flavors are combined.
Nutrition Information
Calories: 204 calories;;Total Fat: 5.8;Sodium: 290;Total Carbohydrate: 17.7;Cholesterol: 43;Protein: 19.1

432. Quick And Easy Clam Chowder
Serving: 10 | Prep: 10mins | Cook: 8hours | Ready in:
Ingredients
1 (10.75 ounce) can condensed cream of celery soup
1 (10.75 ounce) can condensed cream of potato soup
1 (10.75 ounce) can New England clam chowder
2 (6.5 ounce) cans minced clams
1 quart half-and-half cream
1 pint heavy whipping cream
Direction
In a slow cooker, combine cream of potato soup, a can of undrained clams, a can of drained clams, whipped cream, cream of celery soup, clam chowder, and half-and-half cream.
Cook on low with cover on for 6 to 8 hours.
Nutrition Information
Calories: 425 calories;;Total Fat: 32.5;Sodium: 740;Total Carbohydrate: 17.6;Cholesterol: 134;Protein: 16.1

433. Red Chicken Chili
Serving: 6 | Prep: 10mins | Cook: 6hours20mins | Ready in:
Ingredients
2 pounds chicken thighs, cut into pieces
salt and ground black pepper to taste
1/4 cup vegetable oil
2 (14.5 ounce) cans fire-roasted diced tomatoes with garlic
2 cups chicken stock
1 (15 ounce) can kidney beans, rinsed and drained
1 small onion, chopped
1 jalapeno pepper, seeded and chopped
2 tablespoons chili powder
Direction
Flavor chicken with black pepper and salt.
In a heavy skillet, heat vegetable oil over medium-high heat. Let the chicken cook for about 8 minutes until it becomes brown and no longer pink in the center on each side; stir. In a slow cooker, place the cooked chicken then discard extra oil. Mix in the slow cooker, chili powder, chicken stock, tomatoes, onion, kidney beans, and jalapeno pepper.
Let it cook over low heat for 6 to 8 hours or over high heat for 4 hours.
Nutrition Information
Calories: 395 calories;;Sodium: 942;Total Carbohydrate: 21.6;Cholesterol: 93;Protein: 31;Total Fat: 19.9

434. Rustic Slow Cooker Stew
Serving: 12 | Prep: 15mins | Cook: 6hours | Ready in:
Ingredients
3 pounds beef stew meat
salt and pepper to taste
2 (14 ounce) cans beef broth
1 (10.5 ounce) can condensed beef consomme
2 cups Burgundy wine
1 cup water
1 teaspoon ground mustard seed
1 teaspoon dried thyme
5 red potatoes, cut into chunks
1/2 pound baby carrots
1/2 pound pearl onions, peeled
2 tablespoons cornstarch (optional)

1 tablespoon water (optional)
Direction
Taste the beef with pepper and salt; put in to a frying pan over medium heat. Cook till it evenly turns brown; strain.
In a slow cooker, combine together thyme, mustard, water, wine, condensed beef consommé and beef broth. Add the prepared beef into the liquid; mix in onions, carrots and potatoes.
Cook with a cover for 4 hours on high heat or 6 hours on low heat. For a thicker stew, combine water and cornstarch; mix into the slow cooker about 30 minutes before done; mix occasionally until thickened.
Nutrition Information
Calories: 349 calories;;Total Fat: 15.7;Sodium: 415;Total Carbohydrate: 21.2;Cholesterol: 63;Protein: 22.4

435. Sauerkraut Soup II

Serving: 6 | Prep: 15mins | Cook: 4hours | Ready in:
Ingredients
1 (10.75 ounce) can condensed cream of mushroom soup
1 (10.75 ounce) can condensed cream of chicken soup
2 1/2 cups water
4 cups chicken broth
1/2 pound sauerkraut
1 onion, finely diced
1 (15 ounce) can carrots, drained
1 (15 ounce) can sliced potatoes, drained
1 pound smoked sausage of your choice, sliced
1 teaspoon dried dill weed
1 teaspoon minced garlic (optional)
salt and pepper to taste
Direction
In the 4-6 qt. slow cooker, puree chicken broth, water, cream of the chicken soup, and cream of the mushroom soup. Mix in the sausage, potatoes, carrots, onion and sauerkraut. Season with garlic and dill. Keep covered, and cook over Low heat for 8 hours, or High heat for 4 hours. Taste it, and use pepper and salt to season to taste.
Nutrition Information
Calories: 387 calories;;Total Fat: 23.4;Sodium: 2557;Total Carbohydrate: 26.4;Cholesterol: 53;Protein: 17.7

436. Sausage Barley Soup

Serving: 4 | Prep: 15mins | Cook: 4hours | Ready in:
Ingredients
1 pound Italian sausage
1/2 cup diced onion
1 tablespoon minced garlic
1/2 teaspoon Italian seasoning
1 (48 fluid ounce) can chicken broth
1 large carrot, sliced
1 (10 ounce) package frozen chopped spinach
1/4 cup uncooked pearl barley
Direction
Cook the garlic, onion, and the sausage in a skillet on medium heat until the sausage turns brown evenly. Use Italian seasoning to season. Take away from the heat and strain.
Combine the barley, spinach, carrot, chicken broth, and sausage mixture in a slow cooker.
Cook, covered, on Low for 6-8 hours or on High for 4 hours.
Nutrition Information
Calories: 382 calories;;Total Fat: 22.9;Sodium: 2722;Total Carbohydrate: 23.2;Cholesterol: 54;Protein: 20.7

437. Savory Pork Stew

Serving: 8 | Prep: 15mins | Cook: 2hours | Ready in:
Ingredients
1 tablespoon extra virgin olive oil
2 pounds cubed pork stew meat
salt to taste
ground black pepper to taste
garlic powder to taste
2 tablespoons cornstarch, or as needed
8 red potatoes
1 green bell pepper, chopped
1 red bell pepper, chopped
1 sweet onion, diced
1 (11 ounce) can whole kernel corn
1 (14 ounce) can stewed tomatoes
1 (10.75 ounce) can cream of mushroom soup
1 1/4 cups milk
1 (14 ounce) can beef broth
1 tablespoon Italian seasoning
Direction
Heat olive oil over medium heat in a skillet. Season all sides of pork with garlic powder, pepper, and salt, and coat lightly with cornstarch. Transfer pork to the skillet, and cook until browned lightly, but not done. Transfer pork to a slow cooker; add corn, onion, red bell pepper, green bell pepper, and potatoes to the slow cooker.
Combine Italian seasoning, broth, milk, cream of mushroom soup, and tomatoes in a bowl. Pour the mixture into the slow cooker.
Cook, covered, on High setting for 60 minutes. Turn heat to low, and keep on cooking for at least 60 minutes.
Nutrition Information
Calories: 526 calories;;Cholesterol: 71;Protein: 30;Total Fat: 22.5;Sodium: 707;Total Carbohydrate: 52.9

438. Scallop And Shrimp Chowder

Serving: 8 | Prep: 15mins | Cook: 6hours35mins | Ready in:
Ingredients
4 cups chicken broth
4 potatoes, cut into cubes
1 (14 ounce) can whole kernel corn, drained
1 onion, chopped
1/4 cup flour
1 cup heavy whipping cream
1/2 pound sea scallops
1/2 pound peeled, deveined, and cooked shrimp
1/4 cup dry potato flakes
1/4 teaspoon garlic pepper
1 pinch salt, to taste
Direction
Pour broth, corn, potatoes, onion, and flour in a 3 1/2 quart slow cooker container. Cook on low setting, about 6 hours or until potatoes are tender. Add in potato flakes, shrimp, cream, scallops, and garlic pepper into the broth. Cook the mixture over high setting about 35-45 minutes or until the soup slightly thickens. Add salt to taste.
Nutrition Information

Calories: 332 calories;;Total Fat: 14.4;Sodium: 369;Total Carbohydrate: 37.9;Cholesterol: 110;Protein: 14.8

439. Shipwreck Stew

Serving: 10 | Prep: 20mins | Cook: 5hours | Ready in:

Ingredients
2 pounds ground beef
2 (10.75 ounce) cans condensed tomato soup
2 medium onions, chopped
5 large potatoes, cubed
2 (15.25 ounce) cans kidney beans, undrained

Direction
Break up the ground beef into the big skillet on medium high heat. Cook and stir till browned. Drain off the grease and move the beef into the slow cooker. Stir in beans, potatoes, onions and the tomato soups (which are undiluted).
Keep it covered and cooked on Low setting for 4 - 5 hours or till stew thickens and potatoes become soft.

Nutrition Information
Calories: 425 calories;;Total Fat: 12.1;Sodium: 586;Total Carbohydrate: 55.3;Cholesterol: 55;Protein: 24.8

440. Short Rib Tsimmes

Serving: 6 | Prep: 20mins | Cook: 8hours10mins | Ready in:

Ingredients
4 pounds beef short ribs
1 teaspoon garlic powder
1 teaspoon salt
1/2 teaspoon ground black pepper
2 tablespoons olive oil, or as needed
4 large sweet potatoes, peeled and chopped
4 large carrots, peeled and chopped
2 large onions, chopped
1 1/2 pounds pitted prunes
3/4 cup honey
5 whole cloves

Direction
Use pepper, salt and garlic powder to season the short ribs.
Heat 1 tbsp. of the olive oil on medium high heat in the big skillet. Sauté the onions in hot oil for 7-10 minutes or till becoming tender and translucent; move into the bowl.
Lower the heat to medium and put in the rest tbsp. of the oil to skillet. Cook the short ribs in hot oil for 2-4 minutes on each side or till turning brown on all of the sides; move into the slow cooker.
Whisk together cloves, honey, prunes, onions, carrots, and sweet potatoes in the big bowl. Add the onion mixture on top of the short ribs into the slow cooker.
Cook over Low heat for 8 hours.

Nutrition Information
Calories: 1363 calories;;Total Fat: 60.9;Sodium: 664;Total Carbohydrate: 176.3;Cholesterol: 124;Protein: 37.5

441. Simple Slow Cooker Jambalaya

Serving: 12 | Prep: 19mins | Cook: 4hours30mins | Ready in:

Ingredients
2 pounds chicken thighs, cut into bite-size pieces
1 pound andouille sausage, sliced
1 (12 ounce) package mirepoix (diced celery, carrots and onions)
2 (14.5 ounce) cans diced tomatoes, undrained
1/2 cup chopped green bell pepper
3 cloves garlic, minced
2 cups Swanson® Chicken Broth
1 tablespoon Cajun seasoning
1 teaspoon dried thyme
1 teaspoon dried oregano
1 pound uncooked medium shrimp, peeled and deveined
2 cups converted long-grain white rice
1 tablespoon chopped fresh parsley (optional)

Direction
In a slow cooker, mix oregano, thyme, Cajun seasoning, Swanson Chicken Broth, garlic, bell pepper, diced tomatoes, mirepoix mix, sausage, and chicken. Cook on High and stir occasionally for 4 to 5 hours until chicken is soft. In the last half an hour, stir in shrimp and rice until well mixed. Shut slow cooker down.
Let stand with a lid for 15 minutes or more to let rice absorb most of the rest of liquid. Sprinkle if desired with fresh parsley.

Nutrition Information
Calories: 404 calories;Protein: 26.3;Total Fat: 19.1;Sodium: 843;Total Carbohydrate: 31.9;Cholesterol: 123

442. Slow Cooked Beef Stew

Serving: 6 | Prep: 25mins | Cook: 8hours5mins | Ready in:

Ingredients
2 pints water
3 carrots, cut into chunks
3 cups mushrooms, halved or quartered
1/2 rutabaga, peeled and cut into small chunks
1 1/2 pounds cubed beef stew meat
2 tablespoons vegetable oil, or more if needed
3/4 cup all-purpose flour
2 teaspoons dried parsley
2 teaspoons dried thyme
3 cubes beef bouillon, crumbled
5 grinds freshly ground black pepper
1 teaspoon yeast extract spread (such as Marmite®)
2 teaspoons tomato paste (optional)
2 dashes Worcestershire sauce

Direction
Put kettle on in order to have the boiled water ready. Into the slow cooker, mix rutabaga, mushrooms and carrots.
In the big bowl, mix vegetable oil and beef. Turn beef in oil till well-coated with your hands or wooden spoon.
In the second big bowl, stir pepper, beef bouillon cubes, thyme, parsley and flour together. Put in beef, reserving oil for another use, and coat using seasoned flour.
Heat reserved oil to the big skillet or wok and heat on medium low heat. Put in beef, shaking off the excess flour and saving for later use. If meat sticks to pan, put in additional oil; stir in Worcestershire sauce, tomato paste, and yeast extract spread. Cook 5-10 minutes or till beef is not pink in the middle anymore.
Drizzle the reserved flour on top of vegetables in slow cooker. Add the boiling water, small amount at a time, onto the vegetables and whisk to mix in the flour. Put in beef along with the cooking juices.
Cook on Low setting for 8-10 hours or till meat becomes soft and flavors become well-combined.

Nutrition Information

Calories: 471 calories;;Cholesterol: 99;Protein: 34.5;Total Fat: 27.5;Sodium: 586;Total Carbohydrate: 20.7

443. Slow Cooked Chicken Stew

Serving: 8 | Prep: 20mins | Cook: 7hours5mins | Ready in:
Ingredients
1 teaspoon olive oil
1 onion, chopped
3 cloves garlic, minced
4 skinless, boneless chicken breasts
1 (32 fluid ounce) container vegetable broth
1 (14.5 ounce) can diced tomatoes
2 sweet potatoes, diced
1 cup uncooked quinoa
1 teaspoon ground black pepper
5 mushrooms, chopped
2 teaspoons dried oregano
2 teaspoons curry powder
5 green onions, chopped
1 bay leaf
Direction
Over medium heat, heat oil in a skillet; stir in garlic and onion. Cook and stir for 5 minutes until garlic and onion have turned translucent and soft.
In the bottom of a slow cooker, place breasts of chicken; add bay leaf, pepper, oregano, curry powder, mushrooms, green onions, quinoa, sweet potatoes, diced tomatoes, vegetable broth, garlic and onion and combine well. Cook on Low for 7 to 8 hours until chicken is softened.
Discard bay leaf. Take chicken out; use 2 forks to shred and return to the stew, mixing well prior to serving.
Nutrition Information
Calories: 210 calories;;Sodium: 356;Total Carbohydrate: 27.8;Cholesterol: 29;Protein: 16.3;Total Fat: 3.5

444. Slow Cooked Ham And Potato Chowder

Serving: 8 | Prep: 20mins | Cook: 4hours | Ready in:
Ingredients
3 cups warm water
2 tablespoons chicken soup base
1 (10.75 ounce) can condensed cream of chicken soup
4 potatoes, peeled and cut into 1 inch cubes
1 cup cubed cooked ham
1 cup corn kernels
1 small yellow onion, diced
2 tablespoons butter
1/4 cup all-purpose flour
1/2 cup warm water
1 tablespoon dried parsley
1 teaspoon dried dill weed
1 teaspoon celery seed
salt and ground black pepper to taste
Direction
Put 3 cups of warm water that has chicken soup base in the slow cooker and whisk until the soup base has dissolved. Pour in the cream of chicken soup and stir until it's almost smooth.
Add the potatoes, corn, ham, butter and yellow onion, stirring them in into the soup mixture.
In a small container with a lid, put 1/2 cup water and flour then shake the container well to create a smooth mixture then pour in this mixture into the soup. Add parsley, celery seed, and dill then season soup with salt and black pepper.
Leave the chowder to cook on Low for 8 hours or High for 4 hours stirring once or twice while cooking.
Nutrition Information
Calories: 222 calories;;Total Fat: 8.4;Sodium: 1003;Total Carbohydrate: 30.3;Cholesterol: 20;Protein: 7.5

445. Slow Cooker 5 Mushroom Barley Soup

Serving: 6 | Prep: 20mins | Cook: 8hours | Ready in:
Ingredients
3 cups water
1 cup barley
4 cups beef broth
1 cup milk
2 tablespoons olive oil
1 cup diced onion
1/2 cup diced celery
1/2 cup diced carrot
1 tablespoon finely chopped garlic
1 (6 ounce) package sliced white mushrooms
1/2 cup chopped brown beech mushrooms
1/2 cup chopped oyster mushrooms
1/4 cup dried shiitake mushrooms
1/4 cup dried black mushrooms, broken into small pieces
1 (10.75 ounce) can condensed cream of mushroom soup (optional)
1/2 teaspoon salt
1/2 teaspoon ground mixed peppercorns
Direction
Set the heat to high, and use a slow cooker to heat some water. Pour the barley, milk, beef broth, olive oil, celery, onion, garlic, carrot, white mushrooms, brown beech mushrooms, shiitake mushrooms, black mushrooms, oyster mushrooms, cream of mushroom soup, salt, and ground mixed peppercorns into the slow cooker.
Set it to high. Put on the cover and let it cook for an hour.
Use a slotted spoon to take the shiitake mushrooms and cut them into 1/2-inch pieces. Adjust the heat to Low and let it cook for another 7 hours.
Nutrition Information
Calories: 271 calories;;Cholesterol: 3;Protein: 10.3;Total Fat: 9.6;Sodium: 1092;Total Carbohydrate: 38.5

446. Slow Cooker BBQ Chicken Pizza Soup

Serving: 6 | Prep: 15mins | Cook: 5hours | Ready in:
Ingredients
8 cups chicken broth
4 skinless, boneless chicken breast halves
1 (24 ounce) package frozen corn
1 red onion, diced
1 1/4 cups barbeque sauce
4 cloves garlic, minced
1 1/2 teaspoons salt
1/2 teaspoon ground black pepper
1/2 teaspoon garlic salt
1/2 cup shredded mozzarella cheese, or to taste
1/2 cup chopped fresh cilantro, or to taste
Direction
In the slow cooker, whisk garlic salt, black pepper, salt, garlic, barbeque sauce, onion, corn, chicken and chicken broth.

Cook over Low heat for 5 hours. Take the chicken out of the slow cooker and chop into the bite-sized pieces; bring back to the slow cooker and mix.
Pour the soup to the serving bowls and add the cilantro and mozzarella cheese on top of each serving.
Nutrition Information
Calories: 292 calories;;Sodium: 1413;Total Carbohydrate: 45.1;Cholesterol: 47;Protein: 21.4;Total Fat: 4.2

447. Slow Cooker Beef Barley Soup

Serving: 10 | Prep: 10mins | Cook: 8hours | Ready in:
Ingredients
1 1/2 pounds boneless lean beef, cubed
3 tablespoons vegetable oil
1 teaspoon salt
1 teaspoon ground black pepper
2 teaspoons garlic powder
3 (10.5 ounce) cans beef broth
6 cups water
4 stalks celery, chopped
6 carrots, chopped
6 green onions, chopped
1/2 cup chopped fresh parsley
1 cup barley
1 teaspoon dried thyme
Direction
Sauté beef with oil in a frying pan over medium heat until turning brown, about 5 minutes. Mix in garlic powder, pepper, and salt; and put the seasoned meat in a slow cooker. Pour a small amount of water into the frying pan and whisk to loosen the browned bits. Add to the slow cooker.
Add barley, parsley, green onions, carrots, celery, water, and broth. Put a cover on and cook on Low until the barley and vegetables are soft, about 6-8 hours. Add thyme right before eating.
Nutrition Information
Calories: 306 calories;;Cholesterol: 46;Protein: 16.6;Total Fat: 18;Sodium: 615;Total Carbohydrate: 19.7

448. Slow Cooker Beef Neck Bones And Gravy

Serving: 6 | Prep: 10mins | Cook: 5hours20mins | Ready in:
Ingredients
1 1/2 pounds beef neck bones, or more to taste
1 teaspoon ground cumin
1 teaspoon ground allspice
1 teaspoon ground black pepper
1/2 teaspoon red pepper flakes
1/2 teaspoon salt
1/2 cup all-purpose flour, divided
3 tablespoons olive oil
3 cloves garlic, minced
2 cups beef broth
1 onion, sliced into long pieces
Direction
Start preheating a slow cooker to high.
Wash neck bones and discard any extra fat. Use salt, red pepper flakes, black pepper, allspice, and cumin to season the bones; and 1/4 cup of flour to dust.
In a big frying pan, heat olive oil over medium heat, cook while stirring garlic for 1-2 minutes, or until it has fragrant smell. Rise the heat to medium-high and put in the seasoned neck bones; cook for 1 minute each side, or until the bones start to turn brown.

Move the drippings and neck bones to the preheated slow cooker; add onion and beef broth.
Cook for 1 hour on high. Lower the heat to low and cook for 4-6 hours.
Move the neck bones to a dish. Sprinkle into the slow cooker with the leftover flour and stir thoroughly. Put the neck bones back to the slow cooker. Allow to sit for 15-20 minutes, or until the gravy has thickened.
Nutrition Information
Calories: 124 calories;Protein: 2.7;Total Fat: 7.2;Sodium: 460;Total Carbohydrate: 12.8;Cholesterol: 0

449. Slow Cooker Beef Stew

Serving: 5 | Prep: 20mins | Cook: | Ready in:
Ingredients
2 pounds beef stew meat, diced into 1 inch pieces
1 tablespoon Worcestershire sauce
1 teaspoon no salt herb seasoning
5 potatoes
4 carrots
1 yellow onion
3/4 cup tomato juice
1 (14.5 ounce) can stewed tomatoes
2 fresh jalapeno peppers, sliced into rings
Direction
On the night before cooking, slice the onions and cut up the carrots and potatoes. Fill a plastic container with water before placing all the vegetables in to be stored overnight.
Similarly, marinate the stew meat with herb seasoning and Worcestershire sauce by placing everything into a plastic storage bag and refrigerating it the night before.
The next morning, place the raw beef at the bottom of the slow cooker. Drain vegetables and layer it over the beef. Pour the tomato juice and stewed tomatoes in. Add a chopped jalapeno pepper or two for a little spiciness, if desired.
Adjust the setting on the slow cooker to high and cook for 1 hour. Turn the heat to low and let it cook for another 6 to 8 hours. By the end of it, the beef should be completely cooked and extremely tender.
Nutrition Information
Calories: 684 calories;;Total Fat: 35.5;Sodium: 466;Total Carbohydrate: 52.4;Cholesterol: 122;Protein: 39.3

450. Slow Cooker Beef Stew Al La Catherine

Serving: 6 | Prep: 20mins | Cook: 8hours | Ready in:
Ingredients
1 1/2 pounds cubed beef stew meat
2 tablespoons butter
1 large onion, cut into 1-inch cubes
1 1/2 cups baby carrots
1 1/2 cups diced potatoes
3 bay leaves
1 (10.75 ounce) can tomato soup
1 1/2 (10.75 ounce) cans water
1 tablespoon steak sauce (such as A1®)
1 (1 ounce) package dry onion soup mix (such as Lipton®)
1/2 teaspoon lemon pepper seasoning
Direction
In the bottom of a slow cooker, arrange butter and beef stew meat. Top the beef with bay leaves, potatoes, baby carrots, and onion.

In a bowl, stir together onion soup mix, steak sauce, water, and tomato soup; pour the mixture over the vegetables and beef in the slow cooker. Dust the mixture with the lemon pepper seasoning.
Cook for 8-10 hours on Low.
Nutrition Information
Calories: 282 calories;;Total Fat: 11.3;Sodium: 875;Total Carbohydrate: 22;Cholesterol: 70;Protein: 23.3

451. Slow Cooker Beef Stew I
Serving: 6 | Prep: 20mins | Cook: 12hours | Ready in:
Ingredients
2 pounds beef stew meat, cut into 1-inch pieces
1/4 cup all-purpose flour
1/2 teaspoon salt
1/2 teaspoon ground black pepper
1 clove garlic, minced
1 bay leaf
1 teaspoon paprika
1 teaspoon Worcestershire sauce
1 onion, chopped
1 1/2 cups beef broth
3 potatoes, diced
4 carrots, sliced
1 stalk celery, chopped
Direction
Place meat in slow cooker. Mix together in a small bowl the salt, pepper, and flour; sprinkle flour mixture on meat, then mix to coat. Stir in the Worcestershire sauce, garlic, beef broth, bay leaf, onion, potatoes, carrots, paprika, and celery.
Cook while covered for 4 to 6 hours on High setting, or for 10 to 12 hours on Low setting.
Nutrition Information
Calories: 576 calories;;Sodium: 541;Total Carbohydrate: 29.8;Cholesterol: 132;Protein: 44.1;Total Fat: 30.3

452. Slow Cooker Beef Stew III
Serving: 6 | Prep: 10mins | Cook: 1Day | Ready in:
Ingredients
4 carrots, chopped
2 potatoes, peeled and cubed
1 cup sliced fresh mushrooms
1 onion, chopped
3 stalks celery, chopped
3 pounds cubed beef stew meat
1 packet dry onion soup mix
1 (10.75 ounce) can condensed golden mushroom soup
1 3/4 cups water
Direction
In the slow cooker, put celery, onion, mushrooms, potatoes and carrots. Top the vegetables with the stew meat.
Mix the can of soup with the soup mix in a medium bowl. Include in water, stir properly. Transfer the mixture over the meat and vegetables in the slow cooker.
Put in water if necessary; let the liquid just reach the bottom of the meat.
Cook overnight on low heat; include in more water in the morning as needed. Let it cook all day.
Nutrition Information
Calories: 581 calories;;Cholesterol: 149;Protein: 47.1;Total Fat: 32.1;Sodium: 682;Total Carbohydrate: 23.8

453. Slow Cooker Beef Stew IV
Serving: 12 | Prep: 15mins | Cook: 7hours | Ready in:
Ingredients
3 pounds cubed beef stew meat
1/4 cup all-purpose flour
1/2 teaspoon salt, or to taste
3 tablespoons olive oil
1 cup baby carrots
4 large potatoes, cubed
1 tablespoon dried parsley
1 teaspoon ground black pepper
2 cups boiling water
1 (1 ounce) package dry onion soup mix
3 tablespoons butter
3 onions, sliced
1/4 cup red wine
1/4 cup warm water
2 tablespoons all-purpose flour
Direction
Put meat into a large plastic bag. Mix together 1/2 teaspoon salt and 1/4 cup flour; pour the mixture into the bag with the meat, and shake to cover.
Place a large skillet over medium-high heat, heat olive oil. Put in stew meat, and cook until equally browned on the outside. Move to a slow cooker along with pepper, parsley, potatoes and carrots. Stir together dry soup mix and 2 cups of boiling water in a small bowl; pour into the slow cooker.
In that skillet, melt butter and sauté onions till softened; pour into the slow cooker. Put red wine into the skillet, and toss to loosen browned small pieces of food on the bottom. Take away from heat, and put into the slow cooker.
Cook on High with a cover for half an hour. Take down the heat to Low, and cook for 6 hours, or till meat is fork tender. Combine 1/4 cup warm water with 2 tablespoons flour in a small cup or bowl. Blend into stew, cook for 15 minutes without a cover, or till thickened.
Nutrition Information
Calories: 492 calories;;Sodium: 410;Total Carbohydrate: 25.7;Cholesterol: 106;Protein: 33.5;Total Fat: 27.5

454. Slow Cooker Beef Vegetable Soup
Serving: 6 | Prep: 10mins | Cook: 6hours | Ready in:
Ingredients
1 pound cubed beef stew meat
1 (15.25 ounce) can whole kernel corn, undrained
1 (15 ounce) can green beans
1 (15 ounce) can carrots with juice
1 (15 ounce) can sliced potatoes with juice
1 (28 ounce) can crushed tomatoes
1 (1.25 ounce) package beef with onion soup mix
salt and pepper to taste
Direction
Add pepper and salt to taste, soup mix, tomatoes, potatoes, carrots, green beans, corn and meat into the slow cooker; combine by stirring.
Cook over Low heat for no less than 6 hours. Pour in water as needed.
Nutrition Information
Calories: 364 calories;Protein: 20;Total Fat: 16.2;Sodium: 1252;Total Carbohydrate: 38.8;Cholesterol: 51

455. Slow Cooker Belgian Chicken Booyah
Serving: 20 | Prep: 25mins | Cook: 6hours | Ready in:

Ingredients
4 pounds skinless, boneless chicken thighs, cut into 1-inch pieces
2 pounds red potatoes, cut in 1-inch pieces
1 pound beef stew meat, cut into bite-size pieces (optional)
1 (16 ounce) package frozen whole kernel corn
1 (16 ounce) package frozen cut carrots
1 (15 ounce) can cut green beans, drained
1 (14.5 ounce) can chicken broth
8 ounces diced celery
1 (14.5 ounce) can beef broth
1 (14.5 ounce) can petite diced tomatoes
8 ounces diced onion
8 ounces diced green bell pepper
8 ounces cabbage, shredded
1/4 cup salt, or to taste
2 tablespoons dried basil
2 tablespoons dried oregano
2 tablespoons celery salt
1 tablespoon ground black pepper
1 0.42 oz packet concentrated vegetable base (such as Swanson® Vegetable Flavor Boost®) (optional)
Direction
In a slow cooker, mix vegetable base, black pepper, celery salt, oregano, basil, salt, cabbage, bell pepper, celery, onion, diced tomatoes, beef broth, chicken broth, green beans, carrots, corn, beef, potatoes and chicken.
Cook for 6 hours on low.
Nutrition Information
Calories: 248 calories;;Total Fat: 9.6;Sodium: 1918;Total Carbohydrate: 18.6;Cholesterol: 68;Protein: 21.9

456. Slow Cooker Black Eyed Pea And Sausage Soup

Serving: 8 | Prep: 15mins | Cook: 8hours10mins | Ready in:
Ingredients
10 cups water
1 (1 pound) package smoked sausage, sliced
1 1/2 cups chopped carrot
1 cup chopped celery
1 onion, chopped
5 cubes chicken bouillon
2 bay leaves
1/2 teaspoon garlic powder
1/2 teaspoon dried oregano
1 pound dried black-eyed peas
Direction
In a slow cooker crock of 5 quarts, pour 10 cups water; add carrot, sausage, celery, chicken bouillon, onion, oregano, garlic powder, and bay leaves.
In a saucepan, pour black-eyed peas; add water to cover by several inches. Bring water to a boil, remove saucepan from heat, drain and add peas to the slow cooker.
Cook on Low setting for 8 hours. Before serving, remove and throw away bay leaves.
Nutrition Information
Calories: 303 calories;;Sodium: 1614;Total Carbohydrate: 18.3;Cholesterol: 39;Protein: 15.4;Total Fat: 18.5

457. Slow Cooker Bone Broth

Serving: 8 | Prep: 25mins | Cook: 8hours25mins | Ready in:
Ingredients
3 pounds beef bones, or more to taste
3 carrots, chopped
2 stalks celery, chopped
1 onion, chopped
5 cloves garlic, smashed
1 teaspoon whole black peppercorns
2 bay leaves
cold water to cover
2 tablespoons apple cider vinegar
kosher salt to taste
Direction
Set an oven to 190°C (375°F) and start preheating.
Use aluminum foil to line a baking sheet. On the prepared baking sheet, spread the beef bones.
In the prepared oven, roast the bones for 25-30 minutes until browned.
In a slow cooker, add bay leaves, peppercorn, garlic, onion, celery, and carrots. Put the roasted bones over vegetables; cover the bones by adding in enough cold water. Add in kosher salt and apple cider vinegar.
Cook on low heat for 8 hours. Pass the broth into a bowl through a fine-mesh strainer and discard all strained solids.
Nutrition Information
Calories: 27 calories;;Total Fat: 0.1;Sodium: 77;Total Carbohydrate: 6;Cholesterol: 0;Protein: 0.7

458. Slow Cooker Borscht

Serving: 8 | Prep: 30mins | Cook: 9hours | Ready in:
Ingredients
1 pound beef stew meat, cut into 1/2 inch pieces
4 beets, peeled and chopped
1 (28 ounce) can diced tomatoes
2 potatoes, peeled and chopped
1 cup baby carrots, cut into 1/2 inch pieces
1 onion, chopped
3 cloves garlic, minced
2 cups beef broth, or more
1 (6 ounce) can tomato paste
6 tablespoons red wine vinegar
3 tablespoons brown sugar
1 1/2 teaspoons dried dill weed
1 tablespoon dried parsley
1 bay leaf
1 teaspoon salt
1/2 teaspoon ground black pepper
3 cups shredded green cabbage
1 cup sour cream, as garnish
Direction
Prepare your slow cooker and add in garlic, onion, carrots, potatoes, tomatoes, beets and beef. Whisk together pepper, salt, bay leaf, parsley, dill weed, brown sugar, vinegar, tomato paste and beef broth. Pour mixture into the slow cooker over the vegetables and beef. Add more broth to cover if necessary.
Cover the slow cooker and cook for 8 hours and 30 minutes on Low, or 4 hours on High.
Turn heat to high and stir in shredded cabbage, then place the lid back on. Keep on cooking for about 30 minutes, until the shredded cabbage is tender.
Remove the bay leaf. Serve in a bowl and add a dollop of sour cream.
Nutrition Information
Calories: 345 calories;;Total Carbohydrate: 33.2;Cholesterol: 51;Protein: 16.2;Total Fat: 17.5;Sodium: 897

459. Slow Cooker Buffalo Chicken Wing Soup

Serving: 8 | Prep: 20mins | Cook: 6hours30mins | Ready in:

Ingredients
6 cups half-and-half
3 (10.75 ounce) cans condensed cream of chicken soup
4 cups shredded cooked chicken breast
1 cup sour cream
1 cup hot pepper sauce, or to taste
4 carrots, diced
3 celery stalks, diced
3 potatoes, peeled and cubed
5 ounces crumbled blue cheese

Direction
In a slow cooker, mix together potatoes, celery, carrots, hot pepper sauce, sour cream, chicken breast meat, cream of chicken soup, and half-and-half. Put the lid on and cook for 6 1/2 hours on low, mixing sometimes. Mix in blue cheese once the soup has cooked for 5 hours.

Nutrition Information
Calories: 634 calories;;Cholesterol: 137;Protein: 27.9;Total Fat: 42.4;Sodium: 1909;Total Carbohydrate: 36.5

460. Slow Cooker Butternut Squash Soup With Sausage

Serving: 6 | Prep: | Cook: | Ready in:

Ingredients
PAM® Original No-Stick Cooking Spray
2 (8 count) cans Hunt's® Tomato Sauce with Basil, Garlic and Oregano
2 cups water
1 (12 ounce) package refrigerated butternut squash pieces
1/2 teaspoon garlic powder
1 pound bulk Italian pork sausage
1/2 cup dry ditalini pasta, uncooked
1 (6 ounce) package baby spinach leaves

Direction
Use the cooking spray to spray inside of 4-qt. slow cooker. Put the garlic powder, squash, water and tomato sauce into the slow cooker; combine by stirring. Pinch the sausage into bite-sized pieces and add into the slow cooker.
Keep covered; cook over Low heat for 7.5 hours or over High heat for 3.5 hours.
Mix in the spinach and pasta; keep covered and cook over High heat till the pasta softens or for half an hour longer.

Nutrition Information
Calories: 271 calories;;Cholesterol: 30;Protein: 13.1;Total Fat: 14.6;Sodium: 1096;Total Carbohydrate: 21.9

461. Slow Cooker Cactus Chili

Serving: 10 | Prep: 10mins | Cook: 4hours5mins | Ready in:

Ingredients
2 pounds ground beef
1 large onion, chopped
2 (28 ounce) cans diced tomatoes
2 (15.25 ounce) cans black beans, drained
2 (15.25 ounce) cans yellow corn, drained
1 (30 ounce) jar diced nopales (cactus)
1 (8 ounce) can tomato paste
3 tablespoons chili powder
2 tablespoons white sugar
1 chipotle pepper, chopped
2 teaspoons garlic powder
1 teaspoon ground cumin
1 teaspoon salt
1 teaspoon ground black pepper

Direction
In a big skillet, mix together onion and ground beef on moderate heat, then cook and stir for 5 minutes until beef is browned.
Put onion and beef to a slow cooker. Stir in pepper, salt, cumin, garlic powder, chipotle pepper, sugar, chili powder, tomato paste, nopales, corn, black beans and diced tomatoes.
Cook on low setting for 4 hours until flavors blend.

Nutrition Information
Calories: 400 calories;;Total Fat: 12.4;Sodium: 1347;Total Carbohydrate: 48.7;Cholesterol: 55;Protein: 26.6

462. Slow Cooker Cassoulet

Serving: 6 | Prep: 20mins | Cook: 5hours | Ready in:

Ingredients
2 pounds skinless, boneless chicken breast halves, cut into chunks
1 onion, quartered and thinly sliced
2 large cloves garlic, minced
1/4 cup chopped fresh parsley
1/2 teaspoon salt
1/4 teaspoon black pepper
2 (15 ounce) cans cannellini beans, drained and rinsed
1 pound turkey kielbasa, cut into 1/2-inch slices
1/3 cup dry white wine

Direction
In bottom of slow cooker, put chicken. In a big bowl, mix turkey kielbasa, cannellini beans, pepper, salt, parsley, garlic and onion. Put mixture on chicken in slow cooker. Put wine over all the ingredients. Cover. Put cooker on low. Cook for 5-6 hours till cassoulet is thick and chicken is very tender.

Nutrition Information
Calories: 417 calories;;Sodium: 1253;Total Carbohydrate: 24.9;Cholesterol: 135;Protein: 51.4;Total Fat: 9.1

463. Slow Cooker Chicken Chili With Greens And Beans

Serving: 8 | Prep: 15mins | Cook: 6hours | Ready in:

Ingredients
2 cups canned black beans, rinsed and drained
2 cups canned white beans, rinsed and drained
2 (14.5 ounce) cans petite diced tomatoes
1 1/2 cups frozen cooked kale
1 tablespoon butter
1/2 cup diced onion
2 tablespoons chili powder, or more to taste
1 tablespoon garlic and herb seasoning, or more to taste
1 1/2 teaspoons salt
2 large skinless, boneless chicken breast halves
4 cups chicken broth
1 cup heavy cream

Direction
In a slow cooker, put kale, tomatoes, white beans and black beans.

In a large skillet, melt butter over medium heat. Mix in the onion; cook and mix for 5 minutes till translucent and softened.
To the slow cooker, place the onion.
Dust with salt, garlic and herb seasoning and chili powder.
Put halves of chicken breast on top, then into the slow cooker, add the chicken broth.
For 6 hours, cook on Low. Take the chicken breasts out and cut or shred the chicken into bite-size pieces. Return the shredded chicken into the chili.
Mix in the heavy cream, let it heat for a several minutes then serve.

Nutrition Information
Calories: 344 calories;Protein: 22.4;Total Fat: 14.8;Sodium: 1364;Total Carbohydrate: 32.5;Cholesterol: 76

464. Slow Cooker Chicken Enchilada Soup

Serving: 8 | Prep: 15mins | Cook: 6hours15mins | Ready in:

Ingredients
4 cups chicken broth
2 (15 ounce) cans black beans, drained
2 (10 ounce) cans diced tomatoes with green chile peppers
1 (12 fluid ounce) can pale ale
1 (10 ounce) package frozen corn
1 (8 ounce) package red enchilada sauce (such as Frontera®)
1 onion, diced
1 (1.25 ounce) package taco seasoning
1 jalapeno pepper, seeded and diced
1 pound frozen chicken breasts
1 bunch cilantro, chopped

Direction
Whisk together jalapeno pepper, taco seasoning, onion, red enchilada sauce, corn, pale ale, diced tomatoes, black beans and chicken broth in the slow cooker. Put in the whole chicken breasts.
Cook over Low heat till the instant-read thermometer inserted to chicken's middle reaches no less than 74 degrees C (165 degrees F), 5 - 6 hours.
Take out the chicken and shred with 2 forks; mix back to the slow cooker. Keep on cooking, 1 - 2 hours longer.
Mix the cilantro into the slow cooker. Cook over Low heat for roughly 15 minutes or till combining the flavors.

Nutrition Information
Calories: 267 calories;;Total Fat: 2.7;Sodium: 1595;Total Carbohydrate: 37.4;Cholesterol: 32;Protein: 20.6

465. Slow Cooker Chicken Gumbo With Shrimp

Serving: 8 | Prep: 15mins | Cook: 6hours | Ready in:

Ingredients
1 Reynolds® Slow Cooker Liner
2 (14.5 ounce) cans stewed tomatoes, undrained
1 pound skinless, boneless chicken thighs, cut up
1 (14.5 ounce) can reduced-sodium chicken broth
1 green sweet pepper, chopped
1 large onion, chopped
2 stalks celery, chopped
1 tablespoon Cajun seasoning
3 cloves garlic, minced
1/4 teaspoon ground black pepper
1/4 teaspoon cayenne pepper
1 pound fresh or frozen medium shrimp (thawed if frozen), peeled and deveined
4 cups hot cooked white or brown rice

Direction
Use a Reynolds(R) Slow Cooker Liner to line a 5-to-6-qt slow cooker.
In the prepared cooker, place cayenne pepper, black pepper, garlic, Cajun seasoning, celery, onion, green pepper, broth, chicken, and tomatoes. Take a rubber scraper or wooden spoon and stir gently to combine. Cover and cook for 6 hours over low heat.
Take out the lid and gently stir in shrimp with rubber scraper or a wooden spoon. Cover and cook until the shrimp is opaque, or for about 3 more minutes. Serve on cooked rice.

Nutrition Information
Calories: 282 calories;Protein: 22.4;Total Fat: 6.7;Sodium: 562;Total Carbohydrate: 32.3;Cholesterol: 119

466. Slow Cooker Chicken Pot Pie Stew

Serving: 16 | Prep: 20mins | Cook: 6hours | Ready in:

Ingredients
4 large skinless, boneless chicken breast halves, cut into cubes
10 medium red potatoes, quartered
1 (8 ounce) package baby carrots
1 cup chopped celery
2 (26 ounce) cans condensed cream of chicken soup
6 cubes chicken bouillon
2 teaspoons garlic salt
1 teaspoon celery salt
1 tablespoon ground black pepper
1 (16 ounce) bag frozen mixed vegetables

Direction
In a slow cooker, combine black pepper, celery salt, garlic salt, chicken bouillon, chicken soup, celery, carrots, potatoes and chicken; cook for 5 hours on high.
Stir in the frozen mixed vegetables and cook for another 1 hour.

Nutrition Information
Calories: 263 calories;;Total Carbohydrate: 33.7;Cholesterol: 37;Protein: 17.1;Total Fat: 6.9;Sodium: 1416

467. Slow Cooker Chicken Pozole Blanco

Serving: 8 | Prep: 20mins | Cook: 3hours | Ready in:

Ingredients
2 pounds boneless, skinless chicken breasts, cut into 1 1/2- to 2-inch pieces
1/4 cup Mazola® Corn Oil
1 medium onion, diced
1 tablespoon minced garlic
1 small jalapeno or serrano chili pepper, seeded and minced
2 tablespoons Mazola® Chicken Flavor Bouillon Powder
2 quarts water
1 (28 ounce) can white or yellow hominy, drained
2 teaspoons Spice Islands® Oregano
1 Spice Islands® Bay Leaves
1/4 cup fresh lime juice
Traditional garnishes:
Lime wedges, diced avocado, cilantro, radish slices, finely shredded cabbage, minced chiles, fried corn tortilla strips or tostadas, sour cream and crumbled or shredded Mexican cheese

Direction

Using paper towels, tap chicken dry, and use pepper and salt to season if you want. In a big frying pan, heat oil over medium-high heat. Put in chicken and brown a bit, approximately 2 minutes each side. Move the chicken to 6-qt. slow cooker. Lower the heat to medium and add onions to the frying pan. Cook until the onions start to tender, about 2-3 minutes. Mix in bouillon powder, minced chile, and garlic; keeping cooking for 1 minute. Add 1 cup of water and whisk thoroughly. Take away from heat and add to a slow cooker. Pour in lime juice, bay leaf, oregano, hominy, and the rest of the water.
Put a cover on and cook on high for 3-4 minutes or on low for 4-6 minutes. Once the chicken is crumbly and soft, then you can serve the soup. With 2 forks, shred the chicken. Pour the soup into bowls and allow your guests to garnish the soup if wanted.
Nutrition Information
Calories: 264 calories;;Total Fat: 10.3;Sodium: 909;Total Carbohydrate: 17.5;Cholesterol: 59;Protein: 23.8

468. Slow Cooker Chicken Thai Ramen Noodles

Serving: 6 | Prep: 20mins | Cook: 4hours15mins | Ready in:
Ingredients
3 cups water
1 tablespoon soy sauce
1 (13.5 ounce) can light coconut milk
1 tablespoon Thai garlic chile paste
1/2 cup peanut butter
1 onion, chopped
2 cloves garlic, minced
1 inch piece fresh ginger, grated
2 green bell peppers, diced
2 pounds skinless, boneless chicken thighs, diced
2 (3 ounce) packages ramen noodles
1/2 cup diced cucumber
2 green onions, chopped
1/2 cup chopped fresh cilantro
1/2 cup chopped fresh basil
Direction
In slow cooker crock, mix peanut butter, chile pasta, coconut milk, soy sauce and water. Mix diced chicken, green pepper, ginger, garlic and onion in. Cook for 4 hours on high till chicken isn't pink.
Mix ramen noodles into crock; put seasoning packets aside. Cook for 15-20 minutes on high till noodles soften. Season with ramen seasoning packets to taste. Before serving, garnish soup with basil, cilantro, green onions and cucumbers.
Nutrition Information
Calories: 479 calories;;Total Fat: 32.5;Sodium: 458;Total Carbohydrate: 16.3;Cholesterol: 85;Protein: 31.3

469. Slow Cooker Chicken And Corn Congee

Serving: 4 | Prep: 5mins | Cook: 8hours | Ready in:
Ingredients
5 cups water
1 (15 ounce) can whole kernel corn, drained
1 (14 ounce) can chicken broth
1 cup jasmine rice
1 skinless, boneless chicken breast, cubed
salt and ground white pepper to taste
2 tablespoons sesame oil, or to taste
Direction
Mix chicken broth, chicken breast, water, jasmine rice, and corn in a slow cooker.
Cook mixture on Low for 8 hours until the rice is creamy and the chicken is tender. Add salt and white pepper to taste. Pour sesame oil on top of each serving.
Nutrition Information
Calories: 352 calories;;Cholesterol: 17;Protein: 12;Total Fat: 8.6;Sodium: 842;Total Carbohydrate: 58.6

470. Slow Cooker Chicken And Mushroom Stew

Serving: 6 | Prep: 20mins | Cook: 6hours15mins | Ready in:
Ingredients
1/2 cup all-purpose flour
1 teaspoon dried basil
1 teaspoon dried thyme
1 teaspoon dried rubbed sage
1 teaspoon ground black pepper
5 chicken thighs, quartered
1 tablespoon olive oil, or as needed
1 large yellow onion, diced
1 large bell pepper, diced
8 ounces chorizo sausage, thinly sliced
2 cloves garlic, crushed
1 (8 ounce) package sliced fresh mushrooms
1 cup chicken stock
1 (10.75 ounce) can cream of mushroom soup
1 (10.75 ounce) can cream of celery soup
1 cup sour cream
2 teaspoons Cajun seasoning
1 teaspoon cayenne pepper
Direction
In a large resealable bag, combine black pepper, sage, thyme, basil, and flour; put chicken in bag and seal, shake to evenly coat the chicken.
In a large skillet placed over medium heat, heat olive oil. Cook and stir onion and bell pepper for 5 to 10 minutes until lightly soft. Add garlic and chorizo sausage; cook and stir until sausage is done, approximately 5 minutes. Remove mixture to a slow cooker and throw mushrooms on top.
In the same skillet, cook and stir coated chicken (with all the flour included), adding more oil if required, 5 to 10 minutes until chicken is browned. Transfer to the slow cooker.
In the same skillet, pour chicken stock and heat to a boil, while scraping with a wooden spoon to remove the browned bits of food from the bottom of the skillet. Pour all brown bits and liquid into slow cooker.
In a bowl, combine cayenne pepper, Cajun seasoning, sour cream, cream of celery soup and cream of mushroom soup; scoop into slow cooker.
Cook on High for 2 hours; lower setting to Low and continue to cook for 4 more hours.
Nutrition Information
Calories: 554 calories;;Total Fat: 37.3;Sodium: 1577;Total Carbohydrate: 23.7;Cholesterol: 115;Protein: 31

471. Slow Cooker Chicken And Sausage Gumbo

Serving: 6 | Prep: 20mins | Cook: 6hours20mins | Ready in:

Ingredients
1/3 cup vegetable oil
1/3 cup all-purpose flour
3 cups water
3/4 pound smoked sausage, quartered lengthwise and sliced
1 1/2 cups cubed cooked chicken
2 cups sliced okra
1 cup chopped onion
1/2 cup chopped green bell pepper
1/2 cup chopped celery
4 cloves garlic, minced
1/2 teaspoon salt
1/2 teaspoon ground black pepper
1/4 teaspoon cayenne pepper
Direction
Heat vegetable oil in saucepan on medium high heat. Whisk flour in to make a thick paste for about 3 minutes till smooth.
Lower heat to medium. Cook, constantly whisking, for about 15 minutes till flour is dark reddish-brown roux. Put aside; cool.
Put water in slow cooker.
Mix cayenne pepper, black pepper, salt, garlic, celery, bell pepper, onion, okra, chicken, sausage and roux in. Cover. Cook for 6-7 hours on low.
Use a spoon to skim off fat.
Nutrition Information
Calories: 447 calories;;Sodium: 1083;Total Carbohydrate: 13;Cholesterol: 65;Protein: 24.2;Total Fat: 33

472. Slow Cooker Chili

Serving: 7 | Prep: 15mins | Cook: 4hours | Ready in:
Ingredients
1 pound ground beef
1 onion, chopped
2 green bell peppers, chopped
5 (15 ounce) cans kidney beans with liquid
1 (28 ounce) can whole peeled tomatoes, with liquid
1/4 teaspoon chili powder
Direction
Sauté ground beef in a big skillet over medium high heat for 5 to 10 minutes until it becomes brown. Place it in a slow cooker. Mix into the slow cooker, tomatoes, beans, green bell peppers and onions.
Spice with chili powder to taste. Let it cook on high setting for 4 hours until vegetables become tender.
Nutrition Information
Calories: 487 calories;;Cholesterol: 55;Protein: 28.3;Total Fat: 18.6;Sodium: 853;Total Carbohydrate: 53.7

473. Slow Cooker Chili II

Serving: 8 | Prep: 15mins | Cook: 8hours | Ready in:
Ingredients
1 pound ground beef
3/4 cup diced onion
3/4 cup diced celery
3/4 cup diced green bell pepper
2 cloves garlic, minced
2 (10.75 ounce) cans tomato puree
1 (15 ounce) can kidney beans with liquid
1 (15 ounce) can kidney beans, drained
1 (15 ounce) can cannellini beans with liquid
1/2 tablespoon chili powder
1/2 teaspoon dried parsley
1 teaspoon salt
3/4 teaspoon dried basil
3/4 teaspoon dried oregano
1/4 teaspoon ground black pepper
1/8 teaspoon hot pepper sauce
Direction
Cook and evenly brown beef in a skillet over medium heat. Drain excess grease.
Put the beef into a slow cooker, mix in celery, green pepper, onion, garlic, tomato puree, kidney beans, and cannellini beans. Season with oregano, parsley, salt, basil, black pepper, hot pepper sauce and chili powder.
Cover and cook on low for 8 hours.
Nutrition Information
Calories: 273 calories;;Total Fat: 7.6;Sodium: 975;Total Carbohydrate: 33.4;Cholesterol: 34;Protein: 18.9

474. Slow Cooker Chipotle Chili

Serving: 12 | Prep: 25mins | Cook: 6hours10mins | Ready in:
Ingredients
2 pounds ground beef
1 pound bulk Italian sausage
1 large onion, diced
1 tablespoon minced garlic
2 (16 ounce) cans kidney beans, rinsed and drained
2 (16 ounce) cans chili beans, undrained
2 (14.5 ounce) cans diced tomatoes
2 (14.5 ounce) cans crushed tomatoes
2 ribs celery, chopped
1 green bell pepper, coarsely chopped
1/2 red bell pepper, chopped
1/2 (7 ounce) can chipotle chiles in adobo sauce, finely chopped
1/2 (3 ounce) package bacon bits
1 tablespoon chili sauce
1 tablespoon hot pepper sauce (such as Frank's RedHot®)
1 tablespoon chili powder
2 teaspoons brown sugar
1/4 teaspoon ground cumin
1/4 teaspoon salt
Direction
Over medium-high heat, heat a big skillet. In the hot skillet, cook and mix sausage for 2 to 3 minutes and beef till some fat has been released; put garlic and onion and keep cooking and mixing for 5 to 7 minutes longer till meats are crumbly and browned.
To a slow cooker, put the beef mixture.
Mix salt, cumin, brown sugar, chili powder, hot pepper sauce, chili sauce, bacon bits, chipotle chiles, red bell pepper, green bell pepper, celery, crushed tomatoes, diced tomatoes, chili beans and kidney beans with the beef mixture.
Allow to cook on Low till vegetables are entirely soft yet celery remains a little bit of firmness for 6 to 8 hours or 3 to 4 hours on High.
Nutrition Information
Calories: 402 calories;;Total Fat: 18.3;Sodium: 1257;Total Carbohydrate: 33.7;Cholesterol: 65;Protein: 28.1

475. Slow Cooker Clam Chowder

Serving: 6 | Prep: 15mins | Cook: 6hours | Ready in:
Ingredients
1 (6 ounce) can minced clams
4 slices bacon, cut into small pieces
3 potatoes, peeled and cubed
1 cup chopped onion

1 carrot, grated
1 (10.75 ounce) can condensed cream of mushroom soup
1/4 teaspoon ground black pepper
2 (12 fluid ounce) cans evaporated milk
Direction
Drain the clams in a small container and reserve the juice. Adjust the juice to reach 1 3/4 cups of liquid by adding water. Leave the clams covered in the refrigerator for later use.
Mix the water and reserved clam juice mixture, ground black pepper, onions, soup, bacon, potatoes, carrots, and evaporated milk in a slow cooker. Cook in the covered cooker on high setting for 4 to 5 hours or on low setting for 9 to 11 hours. Add in the clams and allow to cook for another hour on high setting.
Nutrition Information
Calories: 407 calories;Protein: 16;Total Fat: 21.1;Sodium: 748;Total Carbohydrate: 39.4;Cholesterol: 54

476. Slow Cooker Corn Chowder

Serving: 9 | Prep: 20mins | Cook: 8hours30mins | Ready in:
Ingredients
5 potatoes, peeled and cubed
2 onions, chopped
2 cups diced ham
3 stalks celery, chopped
1 (15.25 ounce) can whole kernel corn, undrained
2 tablespoons margarine
salt and pepper to taste
2 cubes chicken bouillon
1 (12 fluid ounce) can evaporated milk
Direction
Add the potatoes, onions, ham, corn, celery, and margarine or butter into a slow cooker. Add a dash of salt and pepper. Pour in enough water to cover with two bouillon cubes.
Set the cooker to low and wait for 8 to 9 hours. Mix the evaporated milk in. Let it cook for 30 minutes.
Nutrition Information
Calories: 266 calories;;Cholesterol: 27;Protein: 11.2;Total Fat: 8.8;Sodium: 823;Total Carbohydrate: 37.8

477. Slow Cooker Cream Of Broccoli Soup

Serving: 6 | Prep: 10mins | Cook: 3hours5mins | Ready in:
Ingredients
1 tablespoon vegetable oil
1 small onion, chopped
2 (10 ounce) packages frozen chopped broccoli, thawed
2 (10.75 ounce) cans cream of celery soup
1 (10.75 ounce) can condensed cream of mushroom soup
1 cup shredded American cheese
2 (10.75 ounce) cans milk
Direction
In a large pot, heat vegetable oil over medium heat; sauté onion in heated oil for 5 to 7 minutes until tender.
Drain liquid from the onion as much as you can. Place drained onion into a slow cooker. Add milk, American cheese, cream of mushroom soup, cream of celery soup, and broccoli into the slow cooker.
Cook for 3 to 4 hours on low setting until flavors blend and broccoli is softened.

Nutrition Information
Calories: 289 calories;;Sodium: 1456;Total Carbohydrate: 21.2;Cholesterol: 39;Protein: 12.3;Total Fat: 18.1

478. Slow Cooker Cream Of Potato Soup

Serving: 8 | Prep: 20mins | Cook: 4hours | Ready in:
Ingredients
8 potatoes, chopped
3 leeks, white and light green parts only, cut into 1/4-inch rounds
1 onion, diced
3 tablespoons margarine
2 chicken bouillon cubes
1 tablespoon salt
1/2 teaspoon ground black pepper
1 (12 ounce) can evaporated milk
Direction
In a slow cooker, put pepper, salt, chicken bouillon, margarine, onion, leeks, and potatoes. Add enough water atop to cover the mixture. Cook for 4 hours on High setting.
Mix in the evaporated milk. Ladle soup into a blender and process until smooth. Serve while hot.
Nutrition Information
Calories: 285 calories;;Total Fat: 7.6;Sodium: 1272;Total Carbohydrate: 47.9;Cholesterol: 12;Protein: 8.1

479. Slow Cooker Creamy Chicken And Dumplings

Serving: 8 | Prep: 15mins | Cook: 5hours | Ready in:
Ingredients
4 skinless, boneless chicken breast halves
2 (10.75 ounce) cans condensed cream of mushroom soup
1 onion, minced
2 tablespoons butter
2 tablespoons rosemary
ground black pepper to taste
1 cup vegetable broth, or as needed
2 (10 ounce) packages refrigerated biscuit dough, torn into pieces
Direction
In a slow cooker, combine black pepper, rosemary, butter, onion, cream of mushroom soup, and chicken. Fully cover the ingredients with sufficient vegetable broth.
Choose High setting and cook for 4 1/2 - 5 1/2 hours
Place torn biscuit dough atop chicken mixture; keep cooking about 30 minutes longer till the dough is cooked through.
Nutrition Information
Calories: 385 calories;;Sodium: 1294;Total Carbohydrate: 37.9;Cholesterol: 38;Protein: 17.3;Total Fat: 18.3

480. Slow Cooker Creamy Potato Soup

Serving: 6 | Prep: 30mins | Cook: 6hours30mins | Ready in:
Ingredients
6 slices bacon, cut into 1/2 inch pieces
1 onion, finely chopped
2 (10.5 ounce) cans condensed chicken broth
2 cups water
5 large potatoes, diced
1/2 teaspoon salt
1/2 teaspoon dried dill weed
1/2 teaspoon ground white pepper

1/2 cup all-purpose flour
2 cups half-and-half cream
1 (12 fluid ounce) can evaporated milk
Direction
Put onion and bacon in a large, deep skillet. Sauté over medium-high heat until onions are tender and bacon is browned evenly. Drain off excess drippings. Pour onion and bacon into a slow cooker, and mix in white pepper, dill weed, salt, potatoes, water, and chicken broth. Cook, covered on low setting, stirring sometimes, for 6 to 7 hours.
Combine flour and half-and-half in a small bowl. Mix into the soup along with evaporated milk. Cook, covered for 30 minutes longer until done.
Nutrition Information
Calories: 553 calories;;Cholesterol: 59;Protein: 22;Total Fat: 19.3;Sodium: 1151;Total Carbohydrate: 74.2

481. Slow Cooker French Onion Soup

Serving: 8 | Prep: 30mins | Cook: 4hours35mins | Ready in:
Ingredients
6 tablespoons butter
4 large yellow onions, sliced and separated into rings
1 tablespoon white sugar
2 cloves garlic, minced
1/2 cup cooking sherry
7 cups reduced-sodium beef broth
1 teaspoon sea salt, or to taste
1/4 teaspoon dried thyme
1 bay leaf
8 slices of French bread
1/2 cup shredded Gruyere cheese
1/3 cup shredded Emmental cheese
1/4 cup freshly shredded Parmesan cheese
2 tablespoons shredded mozzarella cheese
Direction
In a big, heavy pot, heat butter over medium-high heat; stir and cook onions for 10 minutes until they are translucent. Sprinkle sugar over the onions, lower the heat to medium. Cook for a minimum of 30 minutes until the onions are brown and tender, tossing continuously. Mix in garlic and cook for 1 minute until aromatic.
Mix into onion mixture with sherry and scrape the pot's bottom to dissolve the small browned food bits from the pot. Move the onions to a slow cooker and add beef broth. Use sea salt to season, mix in thyme and thyme. Put a cover on the cooker, cook on high heat for 4-6 hours. If you want, cook on low for 8-10 hours.
Approximately 10 minutes before eating, put the oven rack about 8-in. from the heat source and start preheating the oven's broiler. Put slices of bread on a baking sheet.
Broil the slices of bread for 1-2 minutes each side until toasted.
In a bowl, mix together mozzarella cheeses, Parmesan, Emmental, and Gruyere; stirring gently. Fill the onion soup into oven-safe soup crocks until 3/4 full and float a slice of bread in each bowl. Put 2 tablespoons of the cheese mixture on top of each serving.
On a baking sheet, put the filled bowls and broil for 2 minutes until the cheese topping is bubbly and light brown.
Nutrition Information
Calories: 250 calories;;Sodium: 596;Total Carbohydrate: 17.5;Cholesterol: 38;Protein: 11;Total Fat: 14.7

482. Slow Cooker Fresh Vegetable Beef Barley Soup

Serving: 10 | Prep: 20mins | Cook: 8hours | Ready in:
Ingredients
1 1/2 pounds cubed beef stew meat
2 (14.5 ounce) cans diced tomatoes with garlic
1 (12 ounce) can tomato-vegetable juice cocktail (such as V8®)
2 large potatoes, diced
1 (8 ounce) can tomato sauce
1 cup sliced carrot
3/4 cup barley
3/4 cup chopped onion
3/4 cup frozen green beans, cut into 1-inch pieces
2/3 cup frozen whole kernel corn
1/2 cup chopped bell pepper
1/2 cup chopped celery
1 tablespoon Worcestershire sauce
1/2 teaspoon dried parsley
1/4 teaspoon ground thyme
1/4 teaspoon dried oregano
1/4 teaspoon dried marjoram
1/4 teaspoon dried basil
2 beef bouillon cubes
2 bay leaves
sea salt and ground black pepper to taste
2 cups sliced fresh mushrooms
Direction
In the crock of a large slow cooker, mix together diced tomatoes with garlic, beef, potatoes, tomato-vegetable juice cocktail, carrot, tomato sauce, onion, barley, corn, celery, bell pepper, green beans, Worcestershire sauce, thyme, parsley, black pepper, marjoram, oregano, basil, beef bouillon cubes, sea salt, and bay leaves.
Cook on Low setting for 7 to 8 hours until the beef is tender. Add mushrooms and cook for an addition of 1 hour.
Nutrition Information
Calories: 264 calories;;Total Fat: 5.2;Sodium: 880;Total Carbohydrate: 37.7;Cholesterol: 36;Protein: 19

483. Slow Cooker Game Day Chili

Serving: 4 | Prep: 30mins | Cook: 6hours | Ready in:
Ingredients
1 Reynolds® Slow Cooker Liner
1 pound lean ground beef
1 medium green bell pepper, chopped
1 small onion, chopped
2 (15 ounce) cans red kidney beans, undrained
2 (1.25 ounce) packages chili seasoning mix
1 (15 ounce) can tomato sauce
1 (10 ounce) can diced tomatoes and green chiles
Shredded cheese (optional)
Sour cream (optional)
Direction
In a 5-6 1/2-quart slow cooker, fit the Reynolds® Slow Cooker Liner inside, positioning it tightly against the bottom and sides of the bowl. Pull the liner upward until it reaches the rim of the bowl.
In a large skillet, cook the ground beef, onion, and bell pepper over medium-high heat, stirring it occasionally until the beef is no longer pink. Drain and remove excess fats.

Pour the beef mixture into the slow cooker liner. In a medium bowl, combine all the remaining ingredients and pour the mixture over the beef mixture. Use a plastic or wooden spoon to stir the mixture. Cover the slow cooker with its lid.

Allow it to cook on Low setting for 6-7 hours, or on High setting for 3-3 1/2 hours until cooked through. Slowly remove the lid and step back, allowing the steam to escape from the cooker. Do not remove or lift the liner with the food inside. You can serve the chili directly from the slow cooker, or you can cool the slow cooker before removing the liner and toss it in a container to serve.

Nutrition Information
Calories: 497 calories;;Sodium: 3025;Total Carbohydrate: 52.3;Cholesterol: 81;Protein: 38.9;Total Fat: 17

484. Slow Cooker Ground Beef Stew

Serving: 6 | Prep: 25mins | Cook: 8hours10mins | Ready in:

Ingredients
1 pound lean ground beef
1 small onion, chopped
2 cloves garlic, minced
1 (10.75 ounce) can condensed cream of mushroom soup
1 cup vegetable broth
1/2 cup tomato-vegetable juice cocktail
2 tablespoons sherry wine (optional)
2 teaspoons Worcestershire sauce
4 potatoes, peeled and diced
1 (8 ounce) can whole kernel corn, drained
1 cup frozen green peas, thawed
1 cup diced carrots
1 (4.5 ounce) can mushroom pieces and stems, drained
1 teaspoon dried celery flakes
1 teaspoon salt
1/2 teaspoon ground black pepper
1/2 teaspoon dried marjoram
1/2 teaspoon dried thyme

Direction
Place a frying pan over medium heat to cook while stirring ground beef with garlic and onion until the meat is extremely browned, about 10 minutes. Drain off excess grease.

In a slow cooker, mix Worcestershire sauce, sherry, vegetable juice cocktail, vegetable broth and cream of mushroom soup together. Put in beef mixture; mix in thyme, marjoram, black pepper, salt, celery flakes, mushroom pieces, carrots, peas, corn and potatoes. Set the cooker to Low with a cover, and cook for about 8 hours, till vegetables are tender and sauce has thickened. If preferred, set slow cooker on High heat and cook for 4 hours.

Nutrition Information
Calories: 384 calories;;Total Carbohydrate: 46.7;Cholesterol: 50;Protein: 21.5;Total Fat: 13;Sodium: 1200

485. Slow Cooker Ham And Bean Soup

Serving: 8 | Prep: 15mins | Cook: 8mins | Ready in:

Ingredients
1 (8 ounce) package 15-bean soup mix
1 ham bone
3 cups cubed fully cooked ham
2 cups chicken broth
2 cups water
1 onion, chopped
3 carrots, chopped
1 (15.5 ounce) can great Northern beans, drained and rinsed
2 cloves garlic, finely chopped
1 teaspoon freshly ground black pepper
1/2 teaspoon salt
1 bay leaf

Direction
In a large bowl, put the 15-bean soup mix and pour several inches of cool water to cover; put in the fridge and soak for 8 hours to overnight. Drain and wash.

In a slow cooker, put bay leaf, salt, black pepper, garlic, great Northern beans, carrots, onion, water, chicken broth, cooked ham, ham bone, and 15-bean soup mix; mix to blend. Allow to cook on low for 8-10 hours.

Nutrition Information
Calories: 305 calories;;Total Carbohydrate: 32;Cholesterol: 30;Protein: 20.5;Total Fat: 10.2;Sodium: 1114

486. Slow Cooker Ham And Bean Stew

Serving: 8 | Prep: 20mins | Cook: 5hours | Ready in:

Ingredients
1 (15 ounce) can black-eyed peas, undrained
1 (15 ounce) can black beans, undrained
1 (15 ounce) can garbanzo beans, drained
1 (16 ounce) can chili beans in sauce
1 large onion, chopped
1 pound cooked ham, cubed
1 clove garlic, minced, or to taste
1 tablespoon sour cream

Direction
In a slow cooker, cook garlic, black-eyed peas, ham, black beans, onion, chili beans, and garbanzo beans together for 5 hours on Low. Add sour cream on top to serve.

Nutrition Information
Calories: 281 calories;Protein: 18;Total Fat: 12;Sodium: 1244;Total Carbohydrate: 27;Cholesterol: 33

487. Slow Cooker Hearty Mixed Bean Stew With Sausage

Serving: 8 | Prep: 15mins | Cook: | Ready in:

Ingredients
3/4 pound sweet Italian pork sausage, casing removed
10 cups Swanson® Chicken Broth or Swanson® Chicken Stock
1/4 teaspoon ground black pepper
2 medium carrots, peeled and chopped
1 stalk celery, chopped
4 ounces dried pinto beans
4 ounces dried navy beans
4 ounces dried kidney beans
6 sun-dried tomatoes in oil, drained and thinly sliced
1 tablespoon grated Parmesan cheese

Direction
In a 10-inch skillet cook sausage over medium-high heat until well browned, stirring often to separate meat. Discard any fat.

In a 5-quart slow cooker add the sausage, broth, carrots, beans, celery and black pepper and cook with the lid on for 7 to 8 hours in low heat.

Add and stir in tomatoes. Cook and cover for 1hour or until the beans have softened. Top with cheese.

Nutrition Information
Calories: 319 calories;;Total Fat: 15;Sodium: 1550;Total Carbohydrate: 29.8;Cholesterol: 39;Protein: 17.2

488. Slow Cooker Hoppin John

Serving: 6 | Prep: 15mins | Cook: 5hours | Ready in:
Ingredients
1 pound dry black-eyed peas
6 cups water
1 large ham hock
12 ounces andouille sausage, sliced
1 onion, chopped
2 stalks celery, chopped
4 cloves garlic, minced
2 bay leaves
1 teaspoon ground cumin
1/2 teaspoon salt
1 pinch red pepper flakes, or to taste
Direction
Into a large container, add black-eyed peas and cover it with a few inches of cool water; allow to rest for 8 hours to overnight. Drain and wash.
Add 6 cups of water to the pot; put in ham hock. Boil, lower the heat to medium low, and let simmer for roughly 60 minutes or till meat becomes soft. Move the ham hock into a dish to cool down, reserve 4 cups cooking liquid.
Layer soaked peas, Andouille sausage, onion, celery, and garlic in the slow cooker's bottom. Take the meat off the ham hock and put meat into the slow cooker. Drizzle red pepper flakes, salt cumin and bay leaves on top. Add reserved cooking water on top of the pea's mixture.
Cook on High heat for no less than 4 hours or till peas become soft.
Nutrition Information
Calories: 543 calories;;Sodium: 755;Total Carbohydrate: 51.7;Cholesterol: 55;Protein: 30.9;Total Fat: 24.2

489. Slow Cooker Hoppin' John Chowder

Serving: 6 | Prep: 30mins | Cook: 6hours | Ready in:
Ingredients
1 1/2 cups instant white rice
1 pound ground beef sirloin
1/2 cup chopped green bell pepper
1 cup chopped onion
3 (15.5 ounce) cans black-eyed peas with liquid
1 (10.5 ounce) can condensed beef broth
2 (10 ounce) cans diced tomatoes and green chiles
1/2 cup water, or as needed
Direction
Follow the package instructions when preparing the rice then set it aside. Put a large pan over medium-high heat and combine in the green pepper, ground sirloin, and onion. Cook with frequent stirring and crumble the beef until it's no longer pink. Drain the grease off.
In a 5-quart slow cooker, put the rice and the beef mixture. Pour in the beef broth, black-eyed peas, cubed tomatoes with green chilies and water that is enough to cover everything.
Cover the cooker and cook for 4 to 6 hours on Low heat.
Nutrition Information
Calories: 413 calories;;Total Carbohydrate: 56.7;Cholesterol: 40;Protein: 27.8;Total Fat: 8.4;Sodium: 1314

490. Slow Cooker Island Beef

Serving: 6 | Prep: 30mins | Cook: 7hours | Ready in:
Ingredients
1 (20 ounce) can unsweetened pineapple chunks in juice, undrained
2 1/2 pounds cubed beef stew meat
2 large onions, cut into wedges
1/2 cup beef broth
3 tablespoons red wine vinegar
2 garlic cloves, crushed
3/4 teaspoon seasoned salt
3/4 teaspoon ground paprika
1/4 teaspoon ground black pepper
1 green bell pepper, diced
1 red bell pepper, diced
3 tablespoons brown sugar
1 1/2 tablespoons cornstarch
2 tablespoons soy sauce
2 tablespoons red wine vinegar
2 large tomatoes, cut into wedges
Direction
Pour pineapple juice into a slow cooker; keep the pine apple chunks. Put in black pepper, paprika, seasoned salt, garlic, 3 tablespoon of red wine vinegar, beef broth, onions and beef. Stir properly; cook on low heat with a cover for 6-6 1/2 hours, until the beef is tender.
Raise heat to High; mix in brown sugar, red bell pepper and green bell pepper. In a small bowl, combine 2 tablespoons of red wine vinegar, soy sauce and cornstarch until smooth; mix into the slow cooker; blend properly. Cook with a cover for 1 hour more. Lightly stir in the reserved pineapple chunks and tomatoes. Serve.
Nutrition Information
Calories: 387 calories;;Total Carbohydrate: 34.5;Cholesterol: 100;Protein: 37.2;Total Fat: 11.2;Sodium: 568

491. Slow Cooker Italian Beef Stew

Serving: 8 | Prep: 20mins | Cook: 4hours5mins | Ready in:
Ingredients
1/4 cup all-purpose flour, or as needed
1/4 teaspoon onion powder, or more to taste
1/4 teaspoon garlic powder, or to taste
salt and ground black pepper to taste
1 1/2 pounds cubed beef stew meat
1 tablespoon vegetable oil
1/2 (16 ounce) package baby carrots, quartered
1/2 yellow onion, quartered and sliced
4 red potatoes, quartered
2 stalks celery, roughly chopped
2 cloves garlic, chopped
3/4 cup red wine
1/4 cup beef broth
1/4 cup tomato paste
1 teaspoon dried rosemary
Direction
In a shallow bowl, blend together pepper, salt, garlic powder, onion powder and flour. Put beef to the seasoned flour mixture; toss to make an even coat; shake properly to discard any excess flour.
Place a frying pan on medium heat and heat oil. Cook in beef for 5-10 minutes, until browned on all sides. Place the beef into the slow cooker; include in garlic, celery, potatoes, onion and carrots.

In a bowl, blend together rosemary, tomato paste, beef broth and red wine until smooth; transfer over the vegetables and the beef.
Cook for 4-6 hours on Low, until the vegetables and beef become tender.
Nutrition Information
Calories: 398 calories;;Sodium: 178;Total Carbohydrate: 26.8;Cholesterol: 74;Protein: 25.9;Total Fat: 18.8

492. Slow Cooker Jambalaya

Serving: 8 | Prep: 15mins | Cook: 7hours10mins | Ready in:
Ingredients
3 cups Swanson® Chicken Broth or Swanson® Chicken Stock
1 tablespoon Creole seasoning
1 large green pepper, diced
1 large onion, diced
2 cloves garlic, minced
1/2 teaspoon ground black pepper
2 large stalks celery, diced
1 (14.5 ounce) can diced tomatoes
1 pound kielbasa, diced
3/4 pound skinless, boneless chicken thighs, cut into cubes
1 cup uncooked regular long-grain white rice
1/2 pound fresh medium shrimp, peeled and deveined
Direction
In a 6-quart slow cooker, stir the rice, chicken, kielbasa, tomatoes, celery, black pepper, garlic, onion, green pepper, Creole seasoning and broth.
Cook on LOW for 7-8 hours with a lid until the chicken is cooked through.
Put the shrimp in the cooker. Cook for 10 minutes with a lid on until the shrimp are cooked through.
Nutrition Information
Calories: 386 calories;;Total Fat: 20.7;Sodium: 1201;Total Carbohydrate: 26.7;Cholesterol: 106;Protein: 22.4

493. Slow Cooker Jambalaya (Vegan)

Serving: 6 | Prep: 25mins | Cook: 4hours30mins | Ready in:
Ingredients
1 tablespoon olive oil, or to taste
1 (28 ounce) can diced tomatoes with juice
8 ounces seitan, cut into cubes
8 ounces smoked vegan sausage, cut into 2-inch slices
1/2 large onion, chopped
1/2 large green bell pepper, seeded and chopped
3 stalks celery, chopped
1 cup vegetable broth
2 cloves garlic, minced
1 tablespoon miso paste
1 1/2 teaspoons Cajun seasoning
1/2 teaspoon dried thyme
1/2 teaspoon dried oregano
1 cup rice
1 tablespoon chopped fresh parsley, or to taste (optional)
Direction
Grease the bottom of a 4-qt. slow cooker crock with olive oil. Mix oregano, thyme, Cajun seasoning, miso paste, garlic, vegetable broth, celery, green bell pepper, onion, sausage, seitan, juice with tomatoes into crock.
Cook on Low for 4 hours. Put some rice into the crock and cook on HIGH for about 30 minutes more, till rice is cooked through. Decorate with parsley.
Nutrition Information
Calories: 334 calories;;Total Fat: 10.3;Sodium: 965;Total Carbohydrate: 40.8;Cholesterol: 0;Protein: 19.9

494. Slow Cooker Kielbasa Stew

Serving: 8 | Prep: 15mins | Cook: 4hours | Ready in:
Ingredients
2 pounds kielbasa sausage, cut into 1 inch pieces
1 1/2 pounds sauerkraut, drained and rinsed
2 Granny Smith apples - peeled, cored and sliced into rings
3/4 onion, sliced into rings
2 pounds red potatoes, quartered
1 1/2 cups chicken broth
1/2 teaspoon caraway seeds
1/2 cup shredded Swiss cheese
Direction
In slow cooker, put 1/2 sausage. Put sauerkraut on top. Use onion, apples and leftover sausage to cover. Put potatoes on top. Over all, put chicken broth. Sprinkle caraway seeds on top.
Cook on high, covered, for 4 hours till potatoes are tender. Put Swiss cheese over on each serving.
Nutrition Information
Calories: 495 calories;;Total Fat: 33.3;Sodium: 1789;Total Carbohydrate: 30.7;Cholesterol: 82;Protein: 19

495. Slow Cooker Lentil Rice Soup

Serving: 11 | Prep: 20mins | Cook: 7hours | Ready in:
Ingredients
2 cups dry lentils
2 cups uncooked long grain brown rice
1 cup chopped carrots
1/2 cup chopped celery
1/2 onion, chopped
8 cups water
1 cup vegetable broth
1 teaspoon garlic powder
1/2 teaspoon ground black pepper
1 tablespoon salt
1 cup sliced fresh mushrooms
Direction
Put salt, ground black pepper, garlic powder, broth, water, onion, celery, carrots, rice and lentils in slow cooker.
Cover; cook for 7-8 hours on low; 1 hour prior to serving, mix in mushrooms.
Nutrition Information
Calories: 261 calories;Protein: 12.2;Total Fat: 1.5;Sodium: 699;Total Carbohydrate: 49.6;Cholesterol: 0

496. Slow Cooker Lentil And Ham Soup

Serving: 6 | Prep: 20mins | Cook: 11hours | Ready in:
Ingredients
1 cup dried lentils
1 cup chopped celery
1 cup chopped carrots
1 cup chopped onion
2 cloves garlic, minced
1 1/2 cups diced cooked ham
1/2 teaspoon dried basil
1/4 teaspoon dried thyme
1/2 teaspoon dried oregano

1 bay leaf
1/4 teaspoon black pepper
32 ounces chicken broth
1 cup water
8 teaspoons tomato sauce

Direction

Mix together ham, garlic, onion, carrots, celery and lentils in a 3 1/2-qt. or bigger slow cooker; season with pepper, bay leaf, oregano, thyme and basil. Mix in tomato sauce, water and chicken broth; cover and cook for 11 hours on low; before serving, discard bay leaf.

Nutrition Information

Calories: 222 calories;Protein: 15.1;Total Fat: 6.1;Sodium: 1170;Total Carbohydrate: 26.3;Cholesterol: 20

497. Slow Cooker Low Carb Santa Fe Chicken

Serving: 8 | Prep: 10mins | Cook: 10hours | Ready in:

Ingredients

1 (15 ounce) can black beans, rinsed and drained
1 (14.5 ounce) can fat-free chicken broth
1 (14.5 ounce) can diced tomatoes with green chile peppers
1 (8 ounce) bag frozen corn
1/4 cup chopped fresh cilantro
3 scallions, chopped
1 teaspoon garlic powder
1 teaspoon onion powder
1 teaspoon ground cumin
1 teaspoon cayenne pepper, or to taste
salt to taste
1 1/2 pounds skinless, boneless chicken breast halves

Direction

In a slow cooker, put together the diced tomatoes with green chile peppers, cilantro, scallions, corn, black beans, chicken broth, onion powder, garlic powder, cayenne pepper, sale, and cumin. Place the chicken breast seasoned with salt on top of the beans mixture.
Set the slow cooker on low and leave for 9 1/2 hours. Remove the chicken from the slow cooker and shred into strands. Put the chicken strands back in the slow cooker and mix with the bean mixture.
Continue cooking for 30 minutes more on low heat.

Nutrition Information

Calories: 178 calories;;Total Fat: 2.3;Sodium: 548;Total Carbohydrate: 17.6;Cholesterol: 44;Protein: 22.5

498. Slow Cooker Manly Stew

Serving: 12 | Prep: 10mins | Cook: 8hours | Ready in:

Ingredients

1 (10.75 ounce) can condensed cream of mushroom soup
1 (10.75 ounce) can condensed Cheddar cheese soup
1 (1.25 ounce) package beef with onion soup mix
3 pounds beef stew meat

Direction

In the slow cooker, combine properly onion soup mix, cheese soup and the cream of mushroom soup.
Include in beef; cook with a cover for 4-5 hours on High, or 8 hours on Low.

Nutrition Information

Calories: 402 calories;;Total Fat: 27.5;Sodium: 642;Total Carbohydrate: 5.5;Cholesterol: 104;Protein: 31.4

499. Slow Cooker Mexican Beef Stew

Serving: 6 | Prep: 20mins | Cook: 7hours10mins | Ready in:

Ingredients

1 Reynolds® Slow Cooker Liner
1 pound beef stew meat, cut into 1-inch pieces
2 tablespoons all-purpose flour
1 tablespoon canola oil
1 (15 ounce) can black beans, rinsed and drained
2 medium carrots, peeled and chopped
1 medium onion, chopped
2 cloves garlic, minced
1 (14.5 ounce) can diced tomatoes, undrained
1 (14.5 ounce) can reduced-sodium beef broth
1 1/2 teaspoons chili powder
1 teaspoon ground cumin
1/2 teaspoon salt
1/4 teaspoon ground black pepper
1 cup frozen whole kernel corn
Chopped avocado, cilantro, and/or crushed red pepper (optional)

Direction

Line a slow cooker (5 to 6 quarts) with a Reynolds(R) Slow Cooker Liner.
Cover the beef with flour. In a large skillet, cook and stir beef over medium-high heat in hot oil until browned about 5 minutes.
In the prepared slow cooker liner, place the garlic, beans, onion, and carrots. Top with the beef. Add cumin, salt, tomatoes, chili powder, broth, and pepper.
Cook on low while covered for 7 hours until the beef is fork-tender.
Use a rubber spatula to stir in the corn gently. Cover and cook until heated through for 10 minutes more, serve with cilantro, avocado, and/or crushed red pepper if desired.

Nutrition Information

Calories: 272 calories;;Total Fat: 8.7;Sodium: 646;Total Carbohydrate: 27;Cholesterol: 40;Protein: 21.9

500. Slow Cooker Mexican Chili Bowls From Del Monte®

Serving: 8 | Prep: 5mins | Cook: | Ready in:

Ingredients

3 (14.5 ounce) cans Del Monte® Diced Tomatoes with Zesty Mild Green Chilies, undrained
1 (15.25 ounce) can Del Monte® Whole Kernel Corn, drained
1 (15 ounce) can black beans, rinsed and drained
1 (1.25 ounce) package taco seasoning mix
2 tablespoons mini chocolate chips
12 ounces boneless, skinless chicken breasts or thighs
2 tablespoons creamy peanut butter
2 (8.8 ounce) packages heat-and-serve brown rice
Topping Options:
Sour cream or plain Greek yogurt
Shredded Cheddar cheese
Sliced green onion
Chopped fresh cilantro
Lime wedges

Direction

In a 5-quart slow cooker, mix the chocolate chips, taco seasoning, beans, corn and tomatoes together.
Add chicken, press down lightly into the tomato

mixture to cover a little bit. Let cook while covered on low setting for 8 hours or on high for 4 hours. Take out the chicken, slice it into bite-size chunks then take back to the slow cooker and mix in peanut butter. Follow the package instruction to prepare rice. Add chili with optional toppings on top of rice and serve.

Nutrition Information
Calories: 246 calories;;Sodium: 1040;Total Carbohydrate: 33.8;Cholesterol: 24;Protein: 15.8;Total Fat: 5.2

501. Slow Cooker Northern White Bean Bacon Chowder

Serving: 6 | Prep: 30mins | Cook: 10hours | Ready in:

Ingredients
1 1/2 cups dried great Northern beans, rinsed
2 cups water
6 slices bacon
1 carrot, chopped
1 stalk celery, chopped
1 onion, chopped
1 potato - peeled and cubed
1 teaspoon Italian-style seasoning
1/8 teaspoon ground black pepper
3 (14.5 ounce) cans low-sodium chicken broth
1 cup milk

Direction
Soak beans overnight covered in a larger bowl of water.
Sauté the bacon in a large skillet over medium to medium-high heat until it becomes crispy. Remove the bacon fat and crush the bacon; leave aside.
Mix the crumbled bacon, reserved beans, ground black pepper, Italian-style seasoning, potato, onion, celery and carrots in a slow cooker. Spread the broth over the mixture.
Set cooker to low and let it cook while covered until the beans are crisp to soft, for 7 1/2 to 9 hours.
Blend 2 cups at once in a blender or food processor until it becomes smooth. Take it all back to the cooker, pour in the milk and heat covered on high until well heated, for 10 to 15 minutes.

Nutrition Information
Calories: 330 calories;;Total Fat: 14.3;Sodium: 365;Total Carbohydrate: 34.2;Cholesterol: 26;Protein: 17.2

502. Slow Cooker Onion Soup

Serving: 3 | Prep: 15mins | Cook: 4hours15mins | Ready in:

Ingredients
1/4 cup butter, melted
1 large sweet onion (such as Vidalia®), cut into thin slivers
1 small red onion, cut into thin slivers
2 cloves garlic, minced
4 cups beef stock
3 tablespoons brandy
2 teaspoons soy sauce
2 teaspoons Worcestershire sauce
salt and ground black pepper to taste
2 cups Italian-style seasoned croutons
3 slices provolone cheese

Direction
In a skillet, melt butter on medium heat; mix and cook red onion and sweet onion in melted butter for 10 minutes till soft. Mix and cook garlic in onion mixture for 2 minutes till fragrant. Put in a slow cooker.
Put Worcestershire sauce, soy sauce, brandy and beef stock in the slow cooker; season with black pepper and salt.
Cook soup for 4-5 hours on high.
Preheat oven's broiler; put oven rack 6-inches away from heat source.
Put soup in 3 ovenproof bowls. Put provolone slice and croutons over each bowl.
In the preheated oven, broil for 3 minutes till cheese starts to brown and melts.

Nutrition Information
Calories: 498 calories;;Total Fat: 29.3;Sodium: 1044;Total Carbohydrate: 30.6;Cholesterol: 62;Protein: 16.8

503. Slow Cooker Oxtail Soup

Serving: 8 | Prep: 20mins | Cook: 12hours10mins | Ready in:

Ingredients
2 tablespoons butter, or as needed
1 pound beef oxtail, cut into pieces
1 onion, chopped
1/2 (750 milliliter) bottle red wine, or to taste
water to cover
1 pound potatoes, peeled and cubed
2 carrots, chopped
2 ribs celery, chopped
1 cup green beans
1 (14.5 ounce) can stewed tomatoes
salt and ground black pepper to taste

Direction
In a large skillet, heat the butter over medium heat. Add the onion and oxtail and cook 5-7 minutes on each side until the oxtail gets browned. Arrange onion and oxtail into a slow cooker.
While using a wooden spoon to scrape the brown bits of food off the bottom of the skillet, add wine to the skillet and allow to boil. Pour the wine mixture in the slow cooker; cover by water.
Set slow cooker to the Low mode; cook the soup for 8 hours. Mix in green beans, celery, carrots, and potatoes; cook the soup for 4 more hours.
Slightly cool the soup; put in the fridge for around an hour until fat rises to the surface and becomes solidified. Defat with a scoop; stir in the tomatoes. On the stove, heat the soup again, then serve.

Nutrition Information
Calories: 211 calories;;Total Fat: 6.9;Sodium: 241;Total Carbohydrate: 18.7;Cholesterol: 39;Protein: 11

504. Slow Cooker Potato Broccoli Soup

Serving: 6 | Prep: 25mins | Cook: 4hours30mins | Ready in:

Ingredients
4 potatoes, peeled and cubed
2 potatoes, peeled and diced
1 head broccoli, diced
1 onion, minced
7 cups milk
2 tablespoons garlic powder
2 tablespoons minced fresh chives
2 cups instant potato flakes
1/4 cup dry bread crumbs

Direction

In a slow cooker, mix together chives, garlic powder, milk, onion, broccoli, diced potatoes, and cubed potatoes; put a cover on and cook for 4 hours on high. Mix bread crumbs and instant potato flakes into the soup. Lower the heat to low and simmer for 30 minutes more. Enjoy hot.

Nutrition Information
Calories: 415 calories;;Sodium: 194;Total Carbohydrate: 75;Cholesterol: 23;Protein: 16.7;Total Fat: 6.3

505. Slow Cooker Pumpkin Soup

Serving: 8 | Prep: 30mins | Cook: 4hours | Ready in:
Ingredients
1 tablespoon olive oil
1 medium sugar pumpkin, seeded and cubed
1 medium onion, chopped
3 cups chicken stock, or as needed
1 sprig fresh rosemary
1 sprig fresh thyme
1 sprig fresh sage
2 small cinnamon sticks
2 bay leaves
1/2 cup heavy cream
Direction
Heat olive oil on medium high heat in the big skillet. Put in the onion and pumpkin; cook and stir till becoming brown a bit. Move into the slow cooker. Add in enough chicken broth to cover the pumpkin. Tie the bay leaves, cinnamon, sage, thyme and rosemary into a piece of the cheesecloth, and add into the slow cooker. Keep covered and cook over Low heat for 4 hours.
After 4 hours, discard the herb sachet. Mix in cream, and blend the soup using the hand blender till becoming smooth. Serve.

Nutrition Information
Calories: 129 calories;;Sodium: 265;Total Carbohydrate: 15.5;Cholesterol: 21;Protein: 2.7;Total Fat: 7.7

506. Slow Cooker Pumpkin Turkey Chili

Serving: 6 | Prep: 15mins | Cook: 3hours10mins | Ready in:
Ingredients
1 tablespoon olive oil
1 pound ground turkey
1 onion, chopped
1 (28 ounce) can diced tomatoes
2 cups cubed fresh pumpkin
1 (15 ounce) can chili beans
1 (15 ounce) can seasoned black beans
3 tablespoons brown sugar
1 tablespoon pumpkin pie spice
1 tablespoon chili powder
Direction
In a big soup pot, heat olive oil on moderate heat, then brown turkey for 10 minutes while stirring frequently until it is not pink anymore and crumbly. Drain and get rid of any excess fat.
Put turkey to a slow cooker and stir in chili powder, pumpkin pie spice, brown sugar, black beans, chili beans, pumpkin, diced tomatoes and onions. Set the cooker to low setting, then cover and cook for a minimum of 3 hours until pumpkin has begun to break apart and is softened.

Nutrition Information
Calories: 338 calories;;Total Carbohydrate: 41.9;Cholesterol: 56;Protein: 25.1;Total Fat: 9.1;Sodium: 857

507. Slow Cooker Quinoa Sweet Potato Chicken

Serving: 6 | Prep: 15mins | Cook: 8hours | Ready in:
Ingredients
2 (14.5 ounce) cans chicken broth
2 1/2 cups chopped cooked chicken, or more to taste
1 (28 ounce) can petite-cut diced tomatoes with garlic and olive oil
2 (16 ounce) cans red kidney beans, drained and rinsed
1 (15 ounce) can black beans, drained and rinsed
2 large sweet potatoes, peeled and cut into cubes
1/2 cup quinoa
1 tablespoon dried minced onion
1 tablespoon chili powder
1 teaspoon minced garlic
1/4 teaspoon red pepper flakes
salt and ground black pepper to taste
Direction
In a slow cooker, mix together black pepper, salt, red pepper flakes, minced garlic, chili powder, minced onion, quinoa, sweet potatoes, black beans, kidney beans, tomatoes, chopped chicken, and chicken broth. Set the slow cooker to Low and cook about 8 hours.

Nutrition Information
Calories: 533 calories;Protein: 36.7;Total Fat: 4.9;Sodium: 1965;Total Carbohydrate: 86.8;Cholesterol: 53

508. Slow Cooker Salmon Chowder

Serving: 4 | Prep: 15mins | Cook: 4hours10mins | Ready in:
Ingredients
1 tablespoon butter
1 tablespoon coconut oil
1 potato, diced
2 carrots, diced
1 (32 ounce) carton chicken broth
1 (14.75 ounce) can salmon, drained
1 cup milk
1 cup chopped kale
1/2 cup chopped onion
1/2 cup corn
1/2 cup shredded Cheddar cheese
1 teaspoon garlic powder
1 teaspoon dill
1/2 teaspoon cayenne pepper
1/2 teaspoon salt
1/2 teaspoon ground black pepper
Direction
Place a big cooking pan on medium heat and heat the butter and coconut oil in it. Cook and stir the potato and carrots in the butter and oil for 10-15 minutes until softened.
Move the carrots and potato to the slow cooker. Pour in the chicken broth, milk, salmon, kale, corn, onion, Cheddar cheese, dill, garlic powder, cayenne pepper, pepper, and salt, stirring them all in. Cook for 4 hours on low until all the flavors have blended together completely.

Nutrition Information
Calories: 403 calories;;Total Fat: 22.4;Sodium: 2041;Total Carbohydrate: 23.2;Cholesterol: 102;Protein: 29.9

509. Slow Cooker Spanish Beef Stew

Serving: 6 | Prep: 10mins | Cook: 4hours10mins | Ready in:

Ingredients
1 pound beef stew meat
salt and ground black pepper to taste
1/2 cup chopped Spanish onion
2 cloves garlic, minced
2 cups chopped red potatoes
1 (14.5 ounce) can diced tomatoes
1 (12 ounce) jar sofrito
1/2 cup pitted and halved green olives

Direction
Place a large frying pan over medium heat. In hot skillet, cook beef till totally browned, about 5 minutes; season with pepper and salt. Move beef to a slow cooker, keep some of the beef drippings in the frying pan.
Place the frying back to heat and warm the retained drippings up. Sauté garlic and onion in hot drippings till softened, about 5 minutes; put beef into the slow cooker.
Mix olives, sofrito, diced tomatoes and potatoes into the beef combination.
Cook on Low till potatoes and beef are fork-tender, about 4-5 hours.

Nutrition Information
Calories: 241 calories;;Total Fat: 11.6;Sodium: 822;Total Carbohydrate: 13.6;Cholesterol: 40;Protein: 19.6

510. Slow Cooker Spanish Rice Chili

Serving: 6 | Prep: 10mins | Cook: 6hours12mins | Ready in:

Ingredients
2 cups water
1 (5.6 ounce) package Spanish rice mix (such as Knorr® Fiesta Sides™)
1 tablespoon vegetable oil (optional)
2 (16 ounce) cans chili beans, undrained
1 (8 ounce) package frozen chopped bell peppers and onions
1 (8 ounce) jar chunky salsa
1 tablespoon chili powder
1 teaspoon ground paprika
1 teaspoon ground cumin
salt and ground black pepper to taste

Direction
In a saucepan, mix together vegetable oil, Spanish rice mix and water, then bring to a boil. Lower heat and simmer with a cover for 7 minutes until rice is softened.
Put into a slow cooker. Mix in black pepper, salt, cumin, paprika, chili powder, salsa, frozen bell peppers and onions, and chili beans. Stir well together to mix.
Cook on low for 6-8 hours until flavors blend.

Nutrition Information
Calories: 212 calories;Protein: 10.8;Total Fat: 4.4;Sodium: 987;Total Carbohydrate: 39.7;Cholesterol: 1

511. Slow Cooker Split Pea Sausage Soup

Serving: 8 | Prep: 20mins | Cook: 5hours | Ready in:

Ingredients
1 pound dried split peas
10 cups water
1 pound smoked sausage of your choice, sliced
5 cubes chicken bouillon
1 1/2 cups chopped carrot
1 cup chopped celery
2 potatoes, peeled and chopped
1/2 teaspoon garlic powder
1/2 teaspoon dried oregano
2 bay leaves
1 onion, chopped

Direction
Mix together onion, bay leaves, oregano, garlic powder, potatoes, celery, carrot, bouillon, sausage, water and peas in a 5-quart slow cooker.
Cover; cook for 4 to 5 hours on High. Discard bay leaves before placing in bowls.

Nutrition Information
Calories: 412 calories;;Cholesterol: 37;Protein: 23.9;Total Fat: 13.1;Sodium: 1492;Total Carbohydrate: 50.8

512. Slow Cooker Split Pea Soup With Bacon And Hash Browns

Serving: 8 | Prep: 25mins | Cook: 8hours5mins | Ready in:

Ingredients
1/4 pound bacon, chopped
1 pound split peas, rinsed
1/3 (20 ounce) package frozen southern-style hash brown potatoes (such as Ore Ida®)
1 onion, chopped
3 carrots, peeled and diced
3 ribs celery, diced
2 cloves garlic, minced
1/8 teaspoon ground black pepper
1 pinch red pepper flakes, or more to taste (optional)
8 cups chicken broth

Direction
Fry the bacon in a big skillet over medium-high heat for about 5 minutes or until a little bit browned, flip the bacon from time to time. Place fried bacon on paper towels to drain excess oil.
In a slow cooker, mix the chicken broth, hash brown potatoes, bacon, red pepper flakes, black pepper, onion, garlic, celery, split peas, carrots and hash brown potatoes together until well combined.
Let it cook for 8 hours on low setting (or 6 hours for high setting).

Nutrition Information
Calories: 273 calories;;Total Fat: 3.4;Sodium: 1116;Total Carbohydrate: 44;Cholesterol: 10;Protein: 17.7

513. Slow Cooker Squirrel And Veggies

Serving: 4 | Prep: 25mins | Cook: 8hours | Ready in:

Ingredients
1 onion, cut into chunks
2 cups baby carrots
4 large potatoes, cut into small chunks
1 large green bell pepper, cut into chunks
2 cloves garlic
4 cubes chicken bouillon
salt and pepper to taste
3 squirrels - skinned, gutted, and cut into pieces
water to cover
2 tablespoons flour

Direction
In a slow cooker, put pepper, salt, chicken bouillon, garlic, bell pepper, potatoes, carrots, and onion. Top the vegetable mixture with squirrel meat. Fully cover the mixture with enough water. Put a cover on and

cook for 6 hours on high. Mix flour into the mixture and cook for 2 hours more.
Nutrition Information
Calories: 520 calories;;Total Fat: 4.9;Sodium: 1357;Total Carbohydrate: 82.7;Cholesterol: 105;Protein: 37

514. Slow Cooker Stout Stew
Serving: 8 | Prep: 15mins | Cook: 8hours10mins | Ready in:
Ingredients
3/4 cup flour
2 1/2 pounds beef stew meat, cut into 1 1/2-inch cubes
2 tablespoons vegetable oil
2 large potatoes, peeled and cut into bite-size pieces
2 carrots, peeled and cut into bite-size pieces
2 large yellow onions, quartered
1 sprig fresh thyme, or more to taste
2 cups Irish stout beer (such as Guinness®)
1 teaspoon salt
1 tablespoon chopped fresh parsley (optional)
Direction
In a plastic bag that is sealable put the flour. Put the beef, several pieces at a time, to coat shake the bag.
In a big skillet over medium-high heat, heat the vegetable oil. Mix in the beef, cook for 8 to 10 minutes till all sides are browned. To a plate lined with paper towels, put the browned beef to drain.
Into a slow cooker put the thyme, onions, carrots, potatoes and beef, and add the stout beer over. Cover, cook on Low for 8 hours till the meat is very soft. Add salt to season, then get rid of thyme. Jazz it up with parsley prior serving.
Nutrition Information
Calories: 463 calories;;Total Fat: 22.8;Sodium: 365;Total Carbohydrate: 32.3;Cholesterol: 78;Protein: 27

515. Slow Cooker Sweet Chicken Chili
Serving: 8 | Prep: 30mins | Cook: 5hours | Ready in:
Ingredients
6 skinless, boneless chicken breast halves
1 (15 ounce) can dark red kidney beans, undrained
1 (15 ounce) can pinto beans, undrained
1 (15 ounce) can black beans, undrained
2 onions, cut into chunks
1 green bell pepper, coarsely chopped
1 (6 ounce) can tomato paste
1/3 cup brown sugar
2 tablespoons seasoned rice vinegar
1 tablespoon Asian chili black bean sauce
1/2 teaspoon sea salt
1/2 cup shredded Cheddar cheese
Direction
Into a slow cooker, put the chicken breasts, and add in the sea salt, chili black bean sauce, rice vinegar, brown sugar, tomato paste, green bell pepper, onion, black beans, pinto beans and kidney beans. Mix to blend completely the ingredients, set cooker to High. Cook for an hour; mix once more, and put the cooker to Low. Cook for 4 hours longer.
Take chicken breasts off, with 2 forks, torn to pieces, and return shredded chicken into the chili, mix. Put atop the chili with Cheddar cheese, serve.
Nutrition Information
Calories: 262 calories;;Sodium: 702;Total Carbohydrate: 30.5;Cholesterol: 53;Protein: 25.3;Total Fat: 4.8

516. Slow Cooker Sweet Potato Soup
Serving: 6 | Prep: 15mins | Cook: 6hours | Ready in:
Ingredients
4 sweet potatoes, sliced
2 (16 ounce) cans coconut milk
1 onion, sliced
1 tablespoon dried basil
1 tablespoon chili powder
1 tablespoon ground cumin
Direction
In a slow cooker, mix cumin, chili powder, basil, onion, coconut milk and sweet potatoes.
Cook for 8 hours on low or 6 hours on high.
Put soup in a blender, no more than 1/2 full. Cover then hold lid down and pulse several times then leave on to blend. In batches, puree till smooth.
Nutrition Information
Calories: 467 calories;;Total Fat: 30.8;Sodium: 139;Total Carbohydrate: 47;Cholesterol: 0;Protein: 6.7

517. Slow Cooker Taco Bean Soup
Serving: 10 | Prep: 15mins | Cook: 4hours10mins | Ready in:
Ingredients
1 pound ground beef
1 onion, chopped
1 (1.25 ounce) package taco seasoning mix
1 (15 ounce) can white beans, undrained
1 (15 ounce) can red kidney beans, undrained
1 (15 ounce) can white kidney beans, undrained
1 (15 ounce) can ranch-style beans, undrained
1 (15 ounce) can pinto beans, undrained
1 (15 ounce) can black beans, undrained
1 (15 ounce) can white hominy, drained
1 (10 ounce) can diced tomatoes with green chile peppers
Direction
Cook and stir ground beef over medium high heat in a skillet for 5 to 10 minutes until browned and crumbly; drain fat. Remove beef to a slow cooker and sprinkle with taco seasoning mix and onion.
In the beef mixture, mix red kidney beans, white beans, ranch-style beans, white kidney beans, black beans, tomatoes with green chile peppers, hominy, and pinto beans.
Cook in the slow cooker on Low setting for 4 to 5 hours until cooked through and flavors blend.
Nutrition Information
Calories: 352 calories;;Sodium: 1123;Total Carbohydrate: 50.1;Cholesterol: 28;Protein: 22.5;Total Fat: 6.7

518. Slow Cooker Tofu Chili
Serving: 8 | Prep: 35mins | Cook: 10hours5mins | Ready in:
Ingredients
1 (1 pound) package tofu, cubed
1 (29 ounce) can tomato puree
2 cups cooked kidney beans
2 sweet peppers, chopped
1 green bell pepper, seeded and chopped
1 red bell pepper, seeded and chopped
2 green onions, chopped
2 jalapeno peppers, chopped
2 habanero peppers, chopped
2 serrano peppers, chopped
2 tablespoons chili powder, or more to taste

1 teaspoon ground black pepper
1 teaspoon ground cumin
salt to taste
Direction
Heat a big, nonstick saucepan on medium heat. Add tofu. Cook for 5-7 minutes until it turns brown in color. Put the cooked tofu in a 3 1/2 - 4-qt. slow cooker. Add salt, cumin, black pepper, chili powder, serrano peppers, habanero peppers, jalapeno peppers, green onions, green and red bell peppers, sweet peppers, kidney beans, and tomato puree. Mix well.
Cover slow cooker. Cook for 10-12 hours on low until veggies are soft and heated through.
Nutrition Information
Calories: 163 calories;;Sodium: 589;Total Carbohydrate: 25.6;Cholesterol: 0;Protein: 10.8;Total Fat: 3.8

519. Slow Cooker Tomato Soup
Serving: 6 | Prep: 10mins | Cook: 1hours | Ready in:
Ingredients
1 (46 fluid ounce) bottle low-sodium vegetable juice (such as V8®)
3 (15 ounce) cans tomato puree
3 cups low-sodium chicken broth
1 pint heavy whipping cream
3 tablespoons extra-virgin olive oil
1/2 cup unsalted butter, softened
1/4 cup onion powder
2 tablespoons ground black pepper
2 tablespoons grated Parmesan cheese
6 bay leaves
1 teaspoon white sugar
Direction
In a slow cooker, add olive oil, heavy cream, chicken broth, tomato puree, and vegetable juice. Mix sugar, bay leaves, Parmesan cheese, pepper, onion powder, and butter into the juice mixture.
Cook for 1 hour on High. Discard the bay leaves and enjoy.
Nutrition Information
Calories: 637 calories;;Sodium: 1092;Total Carbohydrate: 36.4;Cholesterol: 153;Protein: 10;Total Fat: 52.7

520. Slow Cooker Tortellini
Serving: 12 | Prep: 35mins | Cook: 10mins | Ready in:
Ingredients
1 Reynolds® Slow Cooker Liner
1 (15 ounce) jar roasted red peppers, drained and chopped
1 (32 ounce) container chicken broth
2 (15.5 ounce) cans white (cannelloni) beans, rinsed and drained
1 (28 ounce) can Italian-style diced tomatoes, drained
1 (14 ounce) can artichoke hearts, rinsed, drained, and quartered
4 stalks celery, chopped
2 medium onions, chopped
1 tablespoon olive oil
4 cloves garlic, minced
8 cups Swiss chard, chopped
20 ounces fresh or frozen cheese tortellini, uncooked
1/4 cup finely shredded Parmesan cheese
Parmesan Crisps:
1 1/2 cups finely shredded Parmesan cheese
1 teaspoon snipped fresh thyme or rosemary
1/2 teaspoon coarsely ground black pepper
Direction
Line a Reynolds ® Slow Cooker Liner in a 5-6-qt. slow cooker. Put aside.
In lined-slow cooker, put garlic, olive oil, onions, celery, artichoke hearts, tomatoes, beans, broth and roasted peppers. Use a rubber scrapper/wooden spoon to mix gently to combine.
Cook, covered, for 5 hours on high.
Use a rubber spatula to mix tortellini and Swiss chard in. Cook till pasta is just al dente for 7-9 more minutes. Serve with parmesan crisps (optional) and parmesan cheese.
Parmesan crisps. Preheat the oven to 375°F. Line Reynolds ® Parchment Paper on 2 big baking sheets. Mix black pepper, fresh rosemary/thyme and parmesan cheese in a small bowl. On prepped baking sheets, spoon cheese mixture to 12 portions, 4-in. apart. Pat every cheese portion to 5-in. circle. Bake till golden brown and bubbly for 4-6 minutes. Let stand on the baking sheet till cooled completely. Remove crisps carefully from parchment paper.
Nutrition Information
Calories: 315 calories;;Total Fat: 9.1;Sodium: 1482;Total Carbohydrate: 42.8;Cholesterol: 30;Protein: 16.4

521. Slow Cooker Turkey Soup With Dumplings
Serving: 6 | Prep: 30mins | Cook: 6hours15mins | Ready in:
Ingredients
2 cups chopped cooked turkey
1 onion, chopped
2 stalks celery, chopped
3 potatoes, peeled and cubed
1 cup carrots, chopped
1 cup corn kernels
2 tablespoons poultry seasoning
1 teaspoon onion powder
1 teaspoon garlic powder
1 (32 fluid ounce) container chicken stock
salt and ground black pepper to taste
1 cup all purpose flour
2 teaspoons baking powder
1 teaspoon salt
2 tablespoons butter, melted
Direction
In a slow cooker, combine the carrots, garlic powder, onion powder, corn, celery, onion, poultry seasoning, potatoes, and turkey. Pour in chicken stock and mix well. Season the mixture with salt and black pepper to taste. Set the setting of the slow cooker to Low. Cover the cooker and cook for 6 hours until the vegetables are tender.
In a bowl, mix 1 tsp. of salt, flour, and baking powder. Stir in melted butter. Add the dumpling dough and mix for 1-2 minutes until it starts to firm up. In a simmering soup, drop the dough in by tablespoon. Replace the lid of the cooker and simmer the mixture for 15 minutes.
Nutrition Information
Calories: 336 calories;;Total Fat: 7.3;Sodium: 1099;Total Carbohydrate: 48.7;Cholesterol: 46;Protein: 20.2

522. Slow Cooker Turkey Stew
Serving: 8 | Prep: 10mins | Cook: 8hours | Ready in:
Ingredients

1 (28 ounce) can canned stewed tomatoes
1/4 cup white wine
6 cubes chicken bouillon
1/4 cup dried onion flakes
1/2 teaspoon lemon pepper seasoning
1/2 teaspoon dried Italian seasoning
1/4 teaspoon garlic powder
1/4 teaspoon dried thyme leaves
3 pounds turkey thigh meat, cubed
Direction
Put wine and tomatoes into a slow cooker. Mix in thyme, garlic powder, Italian seasoning, lemon pepper, onion flakes and bouillon cubes; include in turkey.
Cook with a cover on Low until the turkey meat becomes easily pulled apart, 8-10 hours.
Nutrition Information
Calories: 317 calories;Protein: 51.3;Total Fat: 6.8;Sodium: 1248;Total Carbohydrate: 8.8;Cholesterol: 203

523. Slow Cooker Turkey And Dumplings

Serving: 4 | Prep: 10mins | Cook: 4hours | Ready in:
Ingredients
2 (10.75 ounce) cans condensed cream of chicken soup
1 (15 ounce) can chicken broth
1 1/2 cups chopped cooked turkey, or more to taste
1 cup chopped potatoes, or more to taste
1 cup chopped carrots, or more to taste
1/2 onion, chopped
2 tablespoons butter
1 pinch garlic powder
1 pinch poultry seasoning
1/2 (10 ounce) can refrigerated buttermilk biscuit dough (such as Pillsbury Grands!®), cut into squares
Direction
In a slow cooker, combine poultry seasoning, garlic powder, butter, onion, carrots, potatoes, turkey, chicken broth, and cream of chicken soup.
Cook for 3 hours on high, mix. Put biscuits on top of the turkey mixture and cook for another 1 hour until the biscuits have fully cooked.
Nutrition Information
Calories: 449 calories;;Sodium: 1961;Total Carbohydrate: 38.2;Cholesterol: 70;Protein: 23.3;Total Fat: 22.4

524. Slow Cooker Turkey And White Bean Chili

Serving: 8 | Prep: 20mins | Cook: 4hours25mins | Ready in:
Ingredients
1 tablespoon vegetable oil
2 pounds boneless turkey breast
2 onions, chopped
4 cloves garlic, minced
1 (15 ounce) can cannellini (white) beans, drained
1 (29 ounce) can white hominy, drained
3 (14 ounce) cans low-sodium chicken broth
3 (15 ounce) cans cannellini (white) beans, drained
1/4 cup chopped fresh cilantro
1 1/2 tablespoons ground cumin
1 teaspoon Cajun seasoning
3 serrano chile peppers
Direction
In a big skillet, heat vegetable oil on medium heat. Pan-fry turkey breast, 10 minutes per side, till meat isn't pink. Into a bowl, put turkey breast; cool. Use 2 forks to shred turkey. Put aside turkey meat. Cook garlic and onion in the same skillet on medium heat for 5 minutes till onion is translucent. Scrape garlic, onions and any drippings into bowl with turkey.
Into slow cooker, put chicken broth, hominy and 1 can cannellini beans. Blend mixture with an immersion blender till smooth. Put Cajun seasoning, cumin, cilantro, 3 more cans of cannellini beans, garlic, onions and shredded turkey into slow cooker. Mix to combine. Cut off serrano chili stems, wearing gloves. Split chiles. Use a spoon to scrape membranes and seeds from 2 chiles. Mince all 3 chiles. Remove membranes and seeds from all chiles for milder chili flavor. Mix serrano chiles into soup.
Cover cooker. Cook for 4-6 hours on low setting or 2-3 hours on high setting.
Nutrition Information
Calories: 427 calories;;Total Fat: 4.7;Sodium: 838;Total Carbohydrate: 50.9;Cholesterol: 84;Protein: 42.3

525. Slow Cooker Vegan Sweet Potato Chili

Serving: 4 | Prep: 10mins | Cook: 3mins | Ready in:
Ingredients
2 sweet potatoes, peeled and chopped into 2-inch pieces
1 (15 ounce) can kidney beans, rinsed and drained
1 (14.5 ounce) can diced tomatoes
1 yellow onion, diced
1 red bell pepper, seeded and chopped
2 cloves garlic, minced
1 tablespoon chili powder
1 teaspoon smoked paprika
1/2 teaspoon Kosher salt
1 cup water
1/2 cup orange juice
Direction
In a 6-qt. slow cooker, put sweet potatoes. Add salt, paprika, chili powder, garlic, bell pepper, onion, diced tomatoes, and kidney beans. Put in orange juice and water. Cover.
Cook for 3-4 hours on high or 6-8 hours on low until sweet potatoes are easily cut with a fork.
Nutrition Information
Calories: 276 calories;;Sodium: 729;Total Carbohydrate: 57.6;Cholesterol: 0;Protein: 10;Total Fat: 1.1

526. Slow Cooker Vegetable Soup With Ground Beef

Serving: 4 | Prep: 10mins | Cook: 8hours5mins | Ready in:
Ingredients
1 pound ground beef
4 (14 ounce) cans mixed vegetables, drained
1 (15 ounce) can garbanzo beans, drained
1 (10.75 ounce) can tomato soup
1 small zucchini, chopped
1 tablespoon Italian seasoning
2 cups water
Direction
Place a frying pan on medium-high heat. Stir and cook beef in the heated frying pan for 5-7 minutes until turning brown. Strain.
In a slow cooker, mix together Italian seasoning, zucchini, tomato soup, garbanzo beans, and vegetables. Add water and the cooked beef; stir together. Put a cover on and cook for 8 hours on Low for the flavors to blend.

Nutrition Information
Calories: 438 calories;Protein: 28.6;Total Fat: 15.3;Sodium: 1191;Total Carbohydrate: 46.4;Cholesterol: 69

527. Slow Cooker Vegetarian Minestrone

Serving: 8 | Prep: 20mins | Cook: 6hours15mins | Ready in:
Ingredients
6 cups vegetable broth
1 (28 ounce) can crushed tomatoes
1 (15 ounce) can kidney beans, drained
1 large onion, chopped
2 ribs celery, diced
2 large carrots, diced
1 cup green beans
1 small zucchini
3 cloves garlic, minced
1 tablespoon minced fresh parsley
1 1/2 teaspoons dried oregano
1 teaspoon salt
3/4 teaspoon dried thyme
1/4 teaspoon freshly ground black pepper
1/2 cup elbow macaroni
4 cups chopped fresh spinach
1/4 cup finely grated Parmesan cheese, or more to taste
Direction
In a 6-qt. slow cooker, mix black pepper, thyme, salt, oregano, parsley, garlic, zucchini, green beans, carrots, celery, onion, kidney beans, tomatoes, and vegetable broth.
Set on low and cook for 6-8 hours.
Add the lightly salted water in a large pot and let it boil. Add elbow macaroni in the boiling water and cook for 8 minutes, whisking occasionally until cooked through yet firm to the bite; strain.
Add macaroni and spinach into minestrone and cook for 15 more minutes. Sprinkle Parmesan cheese on top.
Nutrition Information
Calories: 138 calories;;Total Fat: 1.7;Sodium: 941;Total Carbohydrate: 25.2;Cholesterol: 2;Protein: 6.9

528. Slow Cooker Veggie Beef Soup With Okra

Serving: 4 | Prep: 20mins | Cook: 4hours | Ready in:
Ingredients
1 pound ground beef
1/4 cup onion, chopped
1 (14.5 ounce) can diced tomatoes, drained
1 (14.5 ounce) can Italian diced tomatoes, drained
1 (16 ounce) package frozen mixed vegetables
1 cup sliced fresh or frozen okra
2 potatoes, peeled and chopped
1 tablespoon ketchup
salt and pepper to taste
Direction
Cook onion and ground beef in skillet on medium heat till onion is tender and beef is evenly brown. Drain grease.
Mix pepper, salt, ketchup, potatoes, okra, veggies, Italian diced tomatoes, diced tomatoes, onion and beef in a slow cooker. Cover with enough water. Cover slow cooker. Cook on low for 4 hours.
Nutrition Information
Calories: 413 calories;;Total Fat: 14;Sodium: 488;Total Carbohydrate: 44.2;Cholesterol: 69;Protein: 27.3

529. Slow Cooker Venison Stew

Serving: 6 | Prep: 30mins | Cook: 7hours15mins | Ready in:
Ingredients
3 stalks celery, diced
1/2 cup chopped onion
2 cloves garlic, minced
1 tablespoon chopped fresh parsley
2 tablespoons vegetable oil
2 pounds venison stew meat
salt and pepper to taste
dried oregano to taste
dried basil to taste
1 cup tomato sauce
1/2 cup dry red wine
1/2 cup water
Direction
In the bottom of the slow cooker, put parsley, garlic, onion and celery. Turn the heat to medium-high and place over a large skillet; heat in oil. Cook in venison in two batches until well browned; transfer to the slow cooker.
Season with basil, oregano, pepper and salt. Pour in water, red wine and tomato sauce. Cook for 7-10 hours on Low.
Nutrition Information
Calories: 239 calories;;Total Fat: 7.9;Sodium: 657;Total Carbohydrate: 5.1;Cholesterol: 114;Protein: 31.8

530. Slow Cooker White Chili

Serving: 12 | Prep: 10mins | Cook: 1hours | Ready in:
Ingredients
2 cups chopped, cooked chicken breast
1 (15.5 ounce) can white beans, drained
1 (14.5 ounce) can chicken broth
1 (15.25 ounce) can white corn, drained
1 (7 ounce) can green salsa
1 (4 ounce) can chopped green chilies
1 large tomato, chopped
1/4 cup chopped fresh cilantro
2 green onions, chopped
1 tablespoon lemon juice
1 tablespoon lime juice
Direction
Stir lime juice, lemon juice, green onion, cilantro, tomato, green chilies, green salsa, white corn, chicken broth, white beans and chicken into the crock of a slow cooker.
Cook on low setting for an hour until hot.
Nutrition Information
Calories: 126 calories;;Total Fat: 4.7;Sodium: 395;Total Carbohydrate: 15.9;Cholesterol: 9;Protein: 5.8

531. Slow Cooker White Chili With Chicken

Serving: 4 | Prep: 15mins | Cook: 4hours | Ready in:
Ingredients
1/2 pound dried Great Northern beans
1 pound skinless, boneless chicken breast halves
1 small onion, chopped
3 cups chicken broth
1 tablespoon chopped jalapeno pepper
1 teaspoon ground cumin

1/2 teaspoon ground oregano
1/2 teaspoon garlic powder
1 tomato, chopped (optional)
4 ounces shredded Mexican cheese blend (optional)
1/4 cup chopped fresh cilantro, or to taste (optional)
Direction
In a big container, add Great Northern beans and a few inches of cool water to cover, then allow to stand for about 8 hours to overnight. Drain and rinse beans.
In a slow cooker, add garlic powder, oregano, cumin, jalapeno pepper, chicken broth, onion, chicken and beans.
Cook on low setting for 8 hours or high setting for about 4 hours. Take the chicken breasts out to a work surface and use a fork to shred the meat, then stir back into the chili in the slow cooker.
Scoop chili into four bowls and put 1 tbsp. chopped cilantro, 1 ounce Mexican cheese blend and 1/4 of the chopped tomato on top of each serving.
Nutrition Information
Calories: 416 calories;;Sodium: 1000;Total Carbohydrate: 32.8;Cholesterol: 95;Protein: 42.2;Total Fat: 12.9

532. Slow Cooker Zucchini Soup

Serving: 6 | Prep: 30mins | Cook: 4hours15mins | Ready in:
Ingredients
1 1/2 pounds sweet Italian sausage
2 cups 1/2-inch pieces celery
2 pounds zucchini, cut into 1/2-inch slices
2 (28 ounce) cans diced tomatoes
2 green bell peppers, cut into 1/2-inch slices
1 cup chopped onion
2 teaspoons salt
1 teaspoon white sugar
1 teaspoon dried oregano
1 teaspoon Italian seasoning
1 teaspoon dried basil
1/4 teaspoon garlic powder
6 tablespoons grated Parmesan cheese, or to taste
Direction
Heat a big pan over medium-high heat. Cook while stirring the sausage in hot pan until crumbly and brown, around 5-7 minutes. Drain and throw away the grease. Mix in the celery and cook, stirring, until the celery becomes soft, roughly 10 minutes.
In a slow cooker, combine garlic powder, basil, Italian seasoning, oregano, sugar, salt, onion, bell peppers, tomatoes, zucchini, and the sausage mixture. Cook this on a low setting for around 4-6 hours. Garnish each of the servings with 1 tablespoon of Parmesan cheese.
Nutrition Information
Calories: 389 calories;;Cholesterol: 49;Protein: 21.8;Total Fat: 23.6;Sodium: 2218;Total Carbohydrate: 25.8

533. Slow Cooker Zuppa Toscana

Serving: 8 | Prep: 15mins | Cook: 5hours38mins | Ready in:
Ingredients
1 pound bulk pork sausage
1 large yellow onion, chopped
2 tablespoons minced garlic
4 large russet potatoes, chopped
1/2 teaspoon salt
1/4 teaspoon ground black pepper
1 pinch red pepper flakes
1 (32 ounce) container chicken broth
2 cups water, or as needed
1 cup heavy whipping cream
1 bunch kale, stems removed and discarded, leaves torn into bite-size pieces
1/4 cup shredded Parmesan cheese (optional)
Direction
Prepare a big skillet over medium-high heat. Add sausage in hot skillet, cook and stir for 5-7 minutes till browned. Put in garlic and onion, then sauté for 3-5 minutes till the onion becomes translucent. Drain; remove grease.
Prepare a slow cooker such as Crock Pot® and put in potatoes. Put in onion mixture and cooked sausage. Season with red pepper flakes, salt and black pepper. Pour chicken broth atop the mixture. Cover potatoes fully with 2 cups of water. Lightly stir the soup. Cook, covered, for 5-6 hours on Low till the potatoes are fork-tender.
Add heavy cream to the soup. Put kale into the soup and stir to mix. Cover and cook for another 30 minutes on High till flavors become incorporated. Decorate with Parmesan cheese.
Nutrition Information
Calories: 447 calories;;Sodium: 1275;Total Carbohydrate: 42.3;Cholesterol: 78;Protein: 15.8;Total Fat: 24.8

534. Slow Cooker, Easy Baked Potato Soup

Serving: 4 | Prep: 15mins | Cook: 7hours15mins | Ready in:
Ingredients
10 red potatoes, cut into cubes
3 tablespoons all-purpose flour
3/4 cup real bacon bits
1 small red onion, chopped
1 clove garlic, minced
2 tablespoons chicken bouillon granules
1 tablespoon ranch dressing mix
2 teaspoons dried parsley
1 teaspoon seasoned salt
1/2 teaspoon ground black pepper
3 cups water
1 cup half-and-half
1/2 cup shredded Cheddar cheese, or to taste
1/4 cup chopped green onion, or to taste
Direction
In the bottom of a slow cooker crock, put potatoes. Scatter over the potatoes with flour, toss to blend. Scatter black pepper, seasoned salt, parsley, ranch dressing mix, chicken bouillon, garlic, red onion, and bacon bits over the potatoes.
Add water to the slow cooker.
Cook for 7-9 hours on Low.
Add to the soup with half-and-half, cook for 15 minutes more.
Use green onion and Cheddar cheese to garnish and enjoy.
Nutrition Information
Calories: 336 calories;;Sodium: 1720;Total Carbohydrate: 26.6;Cholesterol: 56;Protein: 18.4;Total Fat: 17.9

535. Slow Cooked Chicken And Sausage Gumbo

Serving: 8 | Prep: 35mins | Cook: 6hours23mins | Ready in:
Ingredients
1/3 cup vegetable oil

1/3 cup all-purpose flour
1 (19 ounce) package mild Italian sausage, cut into bite-size pieces
4 chicken thighs, cut into bite-size pieces
1 (14 ounce) can diced tomatoes
1 onion, diced
1 yellow bell pepper, diced
2 stalks celery, diced
1 jalapeno pepper, finely chopped
4 cloves garlic, minced
1 teaspoon garlic powder
1 teaspoon ground paprika
1 teaspoon onion powder
1 teaspoon ground black pepper
1 teaspoon dried oregano
2 cups chicken broth

Direction

Place a large saucepan over medium heat and heat oil. Add flour; cook and toss until getting a golden brown paste, about 10 minutes.
Place a large frying pan over medium heat. Put in sausage; cook and stir till golden brown, about 8-10 minutes. Move to a slow cooker.
Put chicken thighs into the same frying pan; cook and toss until no longer pink, about 5 minutes. Move chicken thighs to the slow cooker.
In the slow cooker, mix minced garlic, jalapeno pepper, celery, yellow bell pepper, onion and diced tomatoes. Pour in oregano, pepper, onion powder, paprika, garlic powder and flour paste. Mix in chicken broth.
Cook on Low till flavors mix together, 6-8 hours.

Nutrition Information

Calories: 375 calories;;Total Fat: 27.7;Sodium: 914;Total Carbohydrate: 10.9;Cholesterol: 60;Protein: 19.4

536. Slow Cooked Chili

Serving: 10 | Prep: 15mins | Cook: 8hours | Ready in:

Ingredients

2 pounds ground beef
2 (16 ounce) cans kidney beans, rinsed and drained
2 (14.5 ounce) cans diced tomatoes, undrained
1 onion, chopped
2 green bell peppers, chopped, divided
1 red bell pepper, chopped, divided
2 tablespoons chili powder
2 cloves garlic, minced
2 teaspoons salt
1 teaspoon ground black pepper
10 tablespoons shredded Cheddar cheese for garnish (optional)

Direction

In a skillet, cook and stir the ground beef over medium heat for 10 minutes, until the beef is no longer pink. Let it drain and transfer them to a slow cooker.
Add diced tomatoes, half of the red bell peppers, salt, garlic, onion, kidney beans, half of the green bell peppers, ground black pepper, and chili powder, and combine well into the beef.
Top the mixture with the remaining green and red bell pepper.
Cover the cooker with its lid and set it on High setting. Allow it to cook for about 2 hours until the flavors are well-blended and the vegetables are already tender.
Stir the chili. Set the cooker again into Low setting and cook for 6 more hours.
Distribute them in bowls. Top each bowl with 1 tbsp. of shredded Cheddar cheese.

Nutrition Information

Calories: 333 calories;;Total Fat: 17.7;Sodium: 896;Total Carbohydrate: 21;Cholesterol: 64;Protein: 23.2

537. Slow Cooked White Chili

Serving: 8 | Prep: 10mins | Cook: 8hours10mins | Ready in:

Ingredients

2 pounds skinless, boneless chicken breast halves, cubed
1 (14.5 ounce) can chicken broth
5 (14 ounce) cans navy beans, rinsed and drained
2 (14 ounce) cans white corn, drained
2 (4 ounce) cans chopped green chilies
1 1/2 teaspoons minced garlic
2 teaspoons ground cumin
1 1/2 teaspoons red pepper flakes
1 teaspoon dried oregano
1/2 teaspoon salt
1 tablespoon dried minced onion, or to taste

Direction

In a saucepan, boil chicken broth and chicken on medium heat. Cook for 7-10 minutes till juices are clear and chicken isn't pink.
Put broth and chicken into slow cooker. Mix onion powder, salt, oregano, red pepper flakes, cumin, garlic, green chilies, corn and navy beans in. Cook on low, covered, for 8-9 hours till flavors merge.

Nutrition Information

Calories: 474 calories;Protein: 43.3;Total Fat: 4.2;Sodium: 2063;Total Carbohydrate: 68.8;Cholesterol: 60

538. Slow Cooker Baked Bean Stew

Serving: 8 | Prep: 15mins | Cook: 4hours | Ready in:

Ingredients

1 cup chopped onion
1 cup chopped green bell pepper
1 tablespoon extra-virgin olive oil
3/4 teaspoon crumbled dried sage
3/4 teaspoon cumin seed
1 pound smoked sausage, sliced
2 (16 ounce) cans baked beans
1 (15 ounce) can garbanzo beans, drained
1 (14.5 ounce) can diced tomatoes
2 cloves garlic, minced

Direction

In the slow cooker, put cumin seed, sage, olive oil, green bell pepper and onion. Set the cooker on low heat; simmer with a cover for 2 hours. Mix in garlic, diced tomatoes, garbanzo beans, baked beans and smoked sausage; keep cooking on low heat for an extra 2-4 hours, until flavors are well blended.

Nutrition Information

Calories: 409 calories;;Total Fat: 20.6;Sodium: 1427;Total Carbohydrate: 37.9;Cholesterol: 39;Protein: 20.6

539. Slow Cooker Fish Chowder

Serving: 9 | Prep: 30mins | Cook: 4hours | Ready in:

Ingredients

4 slices bacon, chopped
1 onion, chopped
2 cloves garlic, minced

6 cups chicken stock
1 cup fresh corn kernels
2 large potatoes, diced
3 stalks celery, diced
2 large carrots, diced
ground black pepper to taste
1/2 teaspoon red pepper flakes, or to taste
1 cup scallops
1 cup uncooked medium shrimp, peeled and deveined
1/4 pound halibut, cut into bite-size pieces
1 (12 ounce) can evaporated milk

Direction

Put a pan over medium heat and cook and stir the bacon for 5 to 8 minutes, until it has browned then drain the excess oil. Add the garlic and onion to the bacon and cook and stir for about 5 minutes, until the onion is translucent. Move the mixture to a slow cooker.

Pour into the slow cooker the chicken stock, then add the potatoes, corn, carrots, and celery. Add the black pepper and red pepper flakes to season. Cover the slow cooker then cook for 3 hours on High.

Add the shrimp, scallops, and halibut into the soup, stirring them in and cook for another hour. Pour the evaporated milk into the chowder, stir, and then heat thoroughly and serve.

Nutrition Information

Calories: 235 calories;Protein: 18.4;Total Fat: 6;Sodium: 724;Total Carbohydrate: 27.9;Cholesterol: 56

540. Smashed Potato Soup

Serving: 8 | Prep: 20mins | Cook: 8hours | Ready in:

Ingredients

3 1/2 pounds potatoes, peeled and cut into 3/4-inch cubes
1/2 cup chopped yellow or red sweet pepper
1 1/2 teaspoons bottled roasted garlic
1/2 teaspoon ground black pepper
4 1/2 cups chicken broth
1/2 cup whipping cream. half-and-half or light cream
1 cup shredded Cheddar cheese
1/2 cup thinly sliced green onions
Chopped green onions, for garnish (optional)
1 Reynolds® Slow Cooker Liner

Direction

Line a Reynolds(R) Slow Cooker Liner on a 5- to 6-quart slow cooker. Open slow cooker liner and put it inside the bowl of the slow cooker. Fit liner snugly against the sides and bottoms of the bowl; pull the liners top over the rim of the bowl.

Combine black pepper, garlic, sweet pepper, and potatoes in the slow cooker. Add broth over everything in the cooker.

Cook, covered for 4 to 5 hours on high-heat setting or 8 to 10 hours on low-heat setting.

Carefully take off the lid to release the steam. Use a potato masher to mash potatoes slightly. Mix in 1/2 cup thinly sliced green onions, Cheddar cheese, and whipping cream. Garnish each serving with more sliced green onions if desired.

Do not transport or lift the liner with the food inside. Allow the slow cooker to cool entirely, scoop out the excess liquid, take out the liner and stir well.

Nutrition Information

Calories: 289 calories;;Cholesterol: 35;Protein: 10.8;Total Fat: 11.2;Sodium: 536;Total Carbohydrate: 37.2

541. Smashing Pumpkin Soup

Serving: 8 | Prep: 35mins | Cook: 5hours15mins | Ready in:

Ingredients

3 large potatoes, peeled and cubed
1 small pumpkin
1 teaspoon butter, melted
1 pinch salt and ground black pepper to taste
1 (15 ounce) can diced tomatoes
2 tablespoons chopped fresh parsley
2 teaspoons Himalayan salt
1 1/2 teaspoons dried thyme
1/2 teaspoon ground white pepper
4 cups coconut milk
4 cups milk

Direction

Preheat an oven to 175°C/350°F.

Cover potatoes in salted water in a big pot; boil. Lower the heat to medium low; simmer for 10 minutes till soft. Drain; cool.

Halve pumpkin; scoop the seeds and pulp out. Wash the seeds; dry. Put pumpkin halves in a baking pan, cut side down. Mix black pepper, butter, salt and seeds; spread on a rimmed baking sheet in 1 layer.

On the top rack of the preheated oven, bake pumpkin halves for 1 hour till liquid begins to collect in the pan. Bake pumpkin seeds on the bottom rack for 45 minutes till toasted.

For 10 minutes, cool the pumpkin halves. Peel off skin; discard. Fully cool for 15 minutes more.

Mash together white pepper, thyme, Himalayan salt, parsley, tomatoes, pumpkin and potatoes in a big bowl.

In small batches, in a blender, puree the potato mixture, putting each batch into a slow cooker then letting the blender cool between batches.

Mix milk and coconut milk into the slow cooker; cook for 4-6 hours till flavors merge on low. Serve the roasted pumpkin seeds alongside.

Nutrition Information

Calories: 473 calories;;Total Carbohydrate: 42.7;Cholesterol: 11;Protein: 10.6;Total Fat: 31.8;Sodium: 757

542. Snert (Split Pea Soup)

Serving: 8 | Prep: 30mins | Cook: 7hours | Ready in:

Ingredients

1 (14 ounce) bag dried split peas
1 ham hock
3 slices bacon, chopped
2 (14.5 ounce) cans chicken broth
3 1/2 cups water, plus more as needed
4 small potatoes, peeled and diced
2 carrots, peeled and diced
1 leek, diced
1/2 large onion, diced
2 stalks celery with leaves, stalks diced and leaves chopped
1 clove garlic, diced
1/2 teaspoon salt
1/2 teaspoon ground black pepper
1/2 teaspoon dried thyme
1/2 teaspoon ground nutmeg
1/4 teaspoon ground cloves
1 (1 pound) package smoked sausage, sliced

Direction
Put bacon, ham hock, dried split peas into the slow cooker then add 3 1/2 cups water and chicken broth. Cover cooker; cook for 3-4 hours till peas are tender and broken apart on high. To keep the soup from burning on bottom, mix in more water as needed; occasionally mix while cooking.
Mix garlic, celery, onion, leek, carrots and potatoes into the soup; if needed, stir in more water. Cover; cook the soup for another 2 hours on high.
Season with cloves, nutmeg, thyme, black pepper and salt; stir sausage slices into soup then cover and cook to blend the flavors for another 2 hours.
Nutrition Information
Calories: 487 calories;;Total Fat: 28.7;Sodium: 1566;Total Carbohydrate: 31.9;Cholesterol: 65;Protein: 25

543. Sonte's Slow Cooker Potato Soup

Serving: 6 | Prep: 30mins | Cook: 6hours | Ready in:
Ingredients
2 tablespoons olive oil
6 potatoes, scrubbed and diced, or more to taste
1 onion, diced
2 stalks celery with leaves, diced
1 carrot, grated
4 cloves garlic, minced
8 1/2 cups water
2 tablespoons vegetable stock powder
1 1/2 teaspoons salt
1 1/2 teaspoons dried sage leaves
1 teaspoon crushed thyme leaves
2 bay leaves
freshly ground black pepper to taste
Direction
Sprinkle the olive oil to the slow cooker. Put in the garlic, carrot, celery, onion and potatoes; cover with water. Mix in the vegetable stock powder till becoming dissolve. Use the pepper, bay leaves, thyme, sage and salt to season.
Keep covered and cooked over High heat for roughly 6 hour or till the potatoes soften.
Nutrition Information
Calories: 220 calories;Protein: 4.8;Total Fat: 4.8;Sodium: 625;Total Carbohydrate: 40.9;Cholesterol: 0

544. Southwest Style Creamy Corn Chowder

Serving: 8 | Prep: 10mins | Cook: 3hours30mins | Ready in:
Ingredients
1/4 cup white sugar
4 cups fresh corn kernels
1 (8 ounce) package cream cheese
1/2 cup shredded Mexican cheese blend
1/2 cup 2% low-fat milk
1 cup chicken broth
2 stalks celery, thinly sliced
1 tablespoon minced garlic
2 slices bacon, cut into 1 inch pieces
2 tablespoons ground black pepper
Direction
In a slow cooker, put sugar, milk, chicken stock, corn, cream cheese, celery, Mexican cheese, garlic, bacon, and pepper. Cook it on high heat for an hour, then lower temperature to continue cooking for another 2 1/2 hours.
Nutrition Information
Calories: 267 calories;;Sodium: 233;Total Carbohydrate: 24.3;Cholesterol: 45;Protein: 8.1;Total Fat: 16.9

545. Spaghetti Squash And Polish Sausage Slow Cooker Soup

Serving: 8 | Prep: 35mins | Cook: 9hours55mins | Ready in:
Ingredients
1 (2 pound) spaghetti squash
1/4 cup olive oil
1/2 sweet onion, chopped
6 green onions, white parts only, chopped
4 cloves garlic, chopped
1 Granny Smith apple, peeled and chopped
1/4 cup butter
14 ounces Polish sausage, sliced
6 cups no-salt-added chicken stock
1/2 cup white cooking wine
2 potatoes, peeled and diced
1/2 (5 ounce) package frozen cut spinach
1/2 cup heavy whipping cream
1/4 cup grated Parmesan cheese
2 teaspoons sea salt
1 teaspoon hot sauce (such as Cholula®)
1/2 teaspoon ground thyme
1/2 teaspoon ground black pepper
1/4 teaspoon ground sage
1/4 teaspoon red pepper flakes
Direction
Preheat an oven to 190°C/375°F.
Cut spaghetti squash ends off; use sharp knife to pierce skin in a few places. Put on glass baking dish.
In preheated oven, bake for 1 hour till interior is pierced easily with fork. Cool for 20 minutes minimum till easily handled. Cut in half. Scoop seeds out; discard. Use a fork to scrape flesh to strands.
In slow cooker, heat olive oil on high. Add garlic, green onions and onion; mix and cook in open cooker for 10 minutes till tender. Mix butter and apple in.
Add sausage; mix and cook for 5 minutes.
Put white cooking wine and chicken stock into slow cooker; cook for 20 minutes till heated through. Mix potatoes in; cook on low, covered, for 20 minutes.
Mix spinach and spaghetti squash strands into slow cooker. Mix red pepper flakes, sage, pepper, thyme, hot sauce, salt, Parmesan cheese and heavy cream in; cover. Cook for 8 hours till flavors merge on low.
Nutrition Information
Calories: 438 calories;;Cholesterol: 63;Protein: 13;Total Fat: 31.8;Sodium: 1159;Total Carbohydrate: 26

546. Spicy Beef Curry Stew For The Slow Cooker

Serving: 4 | Prep: 15mins | Cook: 8hours10mins | Ready in:
Ingredients
1 tablespoon olive oil
1 pound beef stew meat
salt and pepper to taste
2 cloves garlic, minced
1 teaspoon chopped fresh ginger
1 fresh jalapeno peppers, diced
1 tablespoon curry powder
1 (14.5 ounce) can diced tomatoes with juice
1 onion, sliced and quartered
1 cup beef broth

Direction
Put olive oil in a skillet and heat it over medium heat. Place the beef and brown it on all of its sides. Remove the beef from the skillet, reserving its juices. Season the beef with salt and pepper. Cook and stir jalapeno, garlic, and ginger into the skillet for 2 minutes until they are all tender. Season them with curry powder. Mix in juice and diced tomatoes.
Place the onion into the bottom of a slow cooker. Layer it with the browned beef. Transfer the skillet mixture into the slow cooker and stir in the beef broth.
Cover, set the setting to Low heat, and cook for 6-8 hours.
Nutrition Information
Calories: 291 calories;Protein: 20.6;Total Fat: 19.1;Sodium: 442;Total Carbohydrate: 7.6;Cholesterol: 62

547. Spicy Beef Vegetable Stew

Serving: 12 | Prep: 10mins | Cook: 8hours10mins | Ready in:
Ingredients
1 pound ground beef
1 cup chopped onion
1 (30 ounce) jar meatless spaghetti sauce
3 1/2 cups water
1 (16 ounce) package frozen mixed vegetables
1 (10 ounce) can diced tomatoes with green chile peppers
1 cup sliced celery
1 teaspoon beef bouillon granules
1 teaspoon ground black pepper
Direction
Place a large frying pan over medium-high heat and mix in onions and ground beef. Cook and toss until beef is no longer pink, crumbled and evenly browned, about 10 minutes. Drain and remove any excess grease.
Move beef mixture into a slow cooker. Mix in pepper, beef bouillon, celery, diced tomatoes, mixed vegetables, water and spaghetti sauce. Cook on Low with a cover till vegetables are tender, about 8 hours.
Nutrition Information
Calories: 164 calories;;Total Fat: 6.6;Sodium: 468;Total Carbohydrate: 17.3;Cholesterol: 24;Protein: 9.3

548. Spicy Black And Red Bean Soup

Serving: 10 | Prep: 15mins | Cook: 1hours10mins | Ready in:
Ingredients
1 tablespoon vegetable oil
1 1/2 cups chopped onion
1 1/4 cups sliced carrots
2 cloves garlic, minced
3 cups chicken broth
2 teaspoons white sugar
1 (16 ounce) package frozen shoepeg corn
1 (15 ounce) can kidney beans, drained and rinsed
1 (15 ounce) can black beans, rinsed and drained
1 (14.5 ounce) can Italian-style stewed tomatoes
1 (14.5 ounce) can diced tomatoes, drained
1 (4 ounce) can diced green chiles
Direction
Heat oil in a big Dutch oven till hot on medium high heat. Add garlic, carrot and onion; sauté for 5 minutes. Mix in chilies, tomatoes, beans, corn, sugar and broth; boil. Cover; lower the heat and let it simmer for 2 hours.
You can prep this soup in a crock pot. Mix together everything in the pot; cook the first hour on high. Put temperature down to low; cook for another 7 hours.
Nutrition Information
Calories: 172 calories;;Sodium: 775;Total Carbohydrate: 29.9;Cholesterol: 0;Protein: 8.4;Total Fat: 2.5

549. Spicy Pumpkin Chili

Serving: 10 | Prep: 15mins | Cook: 1hours15mins | Ready in:
Ingredients
1 pound ground beef
1/2 teaspoon crushed red pepper flakes, or to taste
1 teaspoon minced garlic
1/2 large onion, diced
1 green bell pepper, chopped
1 red bell pepper, chopped
1 (15 ounce) can kidney beans, rinsed and drained
1 (15 ounce) can black beans, rinsed and drained
1 (15 ounce) can Great Northern beans, drained and rinsed
1 (8 ounce) can tomato sauce
1 (4 ounce) can tomato sauce with garlic and onions
2 (14.5 ounce) cans petite diced tomatoes
1 (14.5 ounce) can fire roasted diced tomatoes
1 (15 ounce) can pumpkin puree
2 teaspoons pumpkin pie spice
2 teaspoons chili powder
1 teaspoon ground cumin
1 teaspoon salt, or to taste
Direction
Place the large skillet over moderate-high heat. Cook and stir the beef in the hot skillet for 5 minutes until the beef is no longer pink and when the meat is crumbly. Add the onion, red pepper flakes, and garlic and cook until the onion is tender and translucent and the beef is browned all over. Stir in red and green bell pepper and cook for 5 more minutes.
In a large slow cooker, mix black beans, kidney beans, Great Northern beans, petite diced tomatoes, fire roasted diced tomatoes, tomato sauce, pumpkin puree, and the tomato sauce with onions and garlic. Flavor the mixture with chili powder, salt, pumpkin pie spice, and cumin. Add the cooked ground beef mixture into the cooker.
Set the cooker to Low setting and cook for 1-2 hours until the chili is hot.
Nutrition Information
Calories: 271 calories;Protein: 18;Total Fat: 6.4;Sodium: 1041;Total Carbohydrate: 36;Cholesterol: 28

550. Spicy And Savory Slow Cooker Beef Ragout

Serving: 10 | Prep: 20mins | Cook: 6hours45mins | Ready in:
Ingredients
1/2 cup all-purpose flour
1 tablespoon Cajun seasoning blend (such as Tony Chachere's®)
1 pound cubed lean beef stew meat
2 tablespoons olive oil
1 (16 ounce) package frozen stew vegetables, thawed
4 cups beef broth
1 pound fresh morel mushrooms, sliced

1 (10 ounce) can diced tomatoes and green chiles (such as RO*TEL® Mild)
1 (8 ounce) can tomato sauce
1/2 cup chopped fresh basil
2 tablespoons garlic, minced
1 tablespoon herbes de Provence (optional)
2 bay leaves
1/2 cup Merlot wine
sea salt and ground black pepper to taste

Direction
In the resealable plastic bag, mix Cajun seasoning and flour.
Pat the stew meat pieces dry using the paper towels; add the meat, several pieces at a time, to the bag. Seal up bag and shake a few times to coat beef with the seasoned flour. Put the seasoned beef aside; repeat the process with the rest of the meat.
In the big skillet, heat the olive oil on medium heat. Cook meat in batches till browned on all sides, mixing frequently.
Into the big slow cooker set on High setting, add bay leaves, herbe de provence, garlic, basil, tomato sauce, diced tomatoes with green chilies, morel mushrooms, beef broth and stew vegetables.
Mix browned beef into stew and cook, covered, for roughly 6 hours or till beef becomes soft.
Adjust the slow cooker setting to Low and mix in the Merlot wine. Keep the cooker covered and cook for roughly half an hour longer or till wine is reduced a bit and flavors are blended. Use black pepper and sea salt to season.

Nutrition Information
Calories: 174 calories;;Sodium: 765;Total Carbohydrate: 16.3;Cholesterol: 24;Protein: 12.4;Total Fat: 5.7

551. Split Pea Smoked Turkey Soup

Serving: 8 | Prep: 25mins | Cook: 4hours | Ready in:
Ingredients
1 pound dried split peas
5 cups water, or more if needed
3 pounds smoked turkey legs
3 cups chicken broth
1 1/2 cups chopped carrot
1 cup chopped celery
2 potatoes, peeled and chopped
1 onion, chopped
1/2 teaspoon garlic powder
1/2 teaspoon dried oregano
2 bay leaves

Direction
In a slow cooker, combine bay leaves, oregano, garlic powder, onion, potatoes, celery, carrot, chicken broth, smoked turkey legs, water, and split peas. Cover and set the cooker on a high setting, then cook for 4 -5 hours until the peas become tender and the soup thickens. To serve, discard the bay leaves.

Nutrition Information
Calories: 613 calories;;Total Fat: 17.5;Sodium: 1740;Total Carbohydrate: 49.1;Cholesterol: 145;Protein: 63.1

552. Split Pea Soup With Homemade Ham Bone Stock

Serving: 8 | Prep: 30mins | Cook: 8hours12mins | Ready in:
Ingredients
Stock:
10 cups water, or more as needed
1/2 pound baby carrots
1/2 pound celery stalks, cut in thirds
1 large overripe tomato, punctured with a knife
1 large onion, peeled and quartered
1 meaty ham bone
3 cloves garlic, diced
2 bay leaves
Soup:
1 tablespoon butter
1/2 pound baby carrots, thinly sliced
1 red onion, chopped
3 cloves garlic, diced
1 cup dry white wine
1 pound split peas, picked over
2 russet potatoes, peeled and cut into 1-inch cubes
2 (1.41 ounce) packages sazon seasoning (such as Goya®)
2 teaspoons ground pepper, or more to taste
sea salt to taste

Direction
In the big stockpot, mix bay leaves, 3 cloves of garlic, ham bone, quartered onion, tomato, celery, half pound of baby carrots and water. Boil the stock.
Lower heat to medium and let simmer for 3 hours.
Take 1 1/2 - 2 cups of the ham meat out of the bone, dice, and put aside for use in the soup. Add stock through a strainer and throw away the solids. Move stock to the covered container and let chill in the refrigerator 1-3 hours till fat rises to the top and solidifies.
Skim off the fat and add the stock to the slow cooker.
In the saucepan, melt the butter and put in 3 cloves diced garlic, red onion and sliced baby carrots. Cook and stir for 7-8 minutes till turning browned. Add wine to pan and boil while scraping browned bits of food out off of pan's bottom using the wooden spoon. Pour into slow cooker.
Wash and drain the split peas and pour into the slow cooker. Put in salt, black pepper, sazon seasoning, potatoes, and reserved ham meat. Mix. Cook on High heat for 5-6 hours till soup becomes thick.
Move roughly a third of the soup into the blender.
Keep it covered and hold lid down using the potholder; process several times prior to leaving on to blend. Bring the puree back to slow cooker and mix.

Nutrition Information
Calories: 322 calories;;Cholesterol: 4;Protein: 16.5;Total Fat: 2.4;Sodium: 1637;Total Carbohydrate: 55.7

553. Spooky Slow Cooker Turkey Lentil Chili

Serving: 12 | Prep: 15mins | Cook: 6hours5mins | Ready in:
Ingredients
2 1/2 pounds lean ground turkey
2 (14.5 ounce) cans Italian-style diced tomatoes
1 pound cooked lentils
1 (14.5 ounce) can pumpkin puree
1 (14.5 ounce) can pinto beans, rinsed and drained
1 (12 ounce) package frozen pearl onions
1 (8 ounce) can chopped green chile peppers
3 cloves garlic, minced
1 cup water
1/4 cup brown sugar
1/4 cup chili powder
2 tablespoons pumpkin pie spice

1 tablespoon onion powder
salt and ground black pepper to taste
Direction
In a nonstick skillet, cook the turkey over medium heat for 5 to 8 minutes till browned. Let drain.
To a slow cooker, put the turkey. Put garlic, green chili peppers, pearl onions, pinto beans, pumpkin puree, lentils and tomatoes. Mix in pepper, salt, onion powder, pumpkin pie spice, chili powder, brown sugar and water.
Put cover and allow to cook on Low for 6 to 10 hours till flavors incorporate.
Nutrition Information
Calories: 262 calories;;Total Fat: 1.7;Sodium: 689;Total Carbohydrate: 29.9;Cholesterol: 68;Protein: 31.7

554. Sunday Brunswick Stew

Serving: 12 | Prep: 15mins | Cook: 4hours10mins | Ready in:
Ingredients
1 tablespoon olive oil
2 onions, diced
2 stalks celery, diced
2 cloves garlic, finely chopped
2 cups diced peeled butternut squash
3 cups shredded or chopped cooked pork
1 (28 ounce) can diced tomatoes
1 (28 ounce) can baked beans
1 (32 fluid ounce) container chicken stock
1 (15 ounce) can cream-style corn
1 cup frozen peas
1/4 teaspoon cayenne pepper
1/2 teaspoon ground cumin
3/4 teaspoon paprika
1 teaspoon salt
1 (18 ounce) bottle hickory-flavored barbeque sauce
Direction
In a big skillet, heat oil on medium heat. Sauté celery and onion in hot oil for 5-7 minutes until onion is translucent. Mix garlic into mixture. Sauté for another 2 minutes. Put mixture in a slow cooker.
Mix barbeque sauce, salt, paprika, cumin, cayenne pepper, peas, corn, chicken stock, baked beans, diced tomatoes, pork and butternut squash in the onion mixture inside the slow cooker.
Cook for 4 hours on high, covered.
Nutrition Information
Calories: 292 calories;;Total Fat: 3.9;Sodium: 1464;Total Carbohydrate: 48.3;Cholesterol: 35;Protein: 18.4

555. Sweet Pork Slow Cooker Chili

Serving: 10 | Prep: 30mins | Cook: 4hours10mins | Ready in:
Ingredients
2 pounds ground pork
2 vine-ripened tomatoes, diced small
1 yellow bell peppers, diced
1 (20 ounce) can pineapple chunks, drained
1 (15.5 ounce) can black beans, drained
1 (11 ounce) can whole kernel corn, drained
1 (12 ounce) can tomato paste
3/4 cup chopped green onions
1 cup chopped baby corn
1 1/4 cups hard apple cider
4 cloves garlic, minced
2 tablespoons brown sugar
2 teaspoons salt
1 tablespoon Hungarian sweet paprika
1 teaspoon ground black pepper
1 tablespoon molasses
1/4 teaspoon ground ancho chile pepper
1/4 teaspoon dried sage
3/4 teaspoon curry powder
1 pinch ground cinnamon
1 1/2 teaspoons honey
1 tablespoon white vinegar
Direction
In a skillet, cook the ground pork on moderate heat until browned fully, then drain.
Mix together vinegar, honey, cinnamon, curry powder, sage, ancho chile pepper, molasses, pepper, paprika, salt, brown sugar, garlic, cider, baby corn, onion, tomato paste, kernel corn, beans, pineapple, bell pepper, tomato and cooked pork in a big slow cooker, then stir.
Set slow cooker to High. Cook for a minimum of 4 hours.
Nutrition Information
Calories: 422 calories;;Total Fat: 20.1;Sodium: 1056;Total Carbohydrate: 39.8;Cholesterol: 65;Protein: 21.3

556. Sweet Potato Chili

Serving: 8 | Prep: 30mins | Cook: 6hours | Ready in:
Ingredients
2 sweet potatoes, diced
2 (14.5 ounce) cans diced stewed tomatoes with chili seasonings
1 (8 ounce) can tomato sauce
3/4 cup diced sweet onion
1/2 cup chopped celery
1/2 cup water
1 tablespoon chili powder
1 teaspoon ground cumin
1/2 teaspoon ground cinnamon
1 pinch salt
1 pinch ground black pepper
1 pinch cayenne pepper
1 pinch garlic powder
1 pinch onion powder
1/2 pound ground turkey
1/2 pound ground beef
1 (12 ounce) can black beans, drained and rinsed
1 cup corn
Direction
In a slow cooker, add onion powder, garlic powder, cayenne pepper, black pepper, salt, cinnamon, cumin, chili powder, water, celery, onion, tomato sauce, stewed tomatoes and sweet potatoes. Cook on high setting while stirring from time to time, about 5 hours.
Heat a big skillet on moderate high heat and stir in ground beef as well as ground turkey. Cook and stir for 10-15 minutes until meat is crumbly, not pink anymore and browned evenly. Drain and get rid of any excess grease. Put corn, black beans, cooked ground beef and cooked ground turkey into the slow cooker; cook for about 1 to 2 hours longer until flavors combined. Serve warm.
Nutrition Information
Calories: 250 calories;;Total Fat: 7.4;Sodium: 621;Total Carbohydrate: 32.5;Cholesterol: 38;Protein: 16

557. Swink's Chili

Serving: 6 | Prep: 20mins | Cook: 2hours | Ready in:

Ingredients
2 pounds ground beef
1 onion, chopped
1 (1.25 ounce) package chili seasoning mix
2 cups water
1 (6 ounce) can tomato paste
1 (16 ounce) can chili beans, undrained
1 (16 ounce) can baked beans
1 (10.75 ounce) can condensed tomato soup
1 (10 ounce) can diced tomatoes with green chile peppers
Direction
Cook onion and beef in a big skillet on moderate heat until beef is brown. Stir in water and chili seasoning. Transfer the beef mixture in a slow cooker, then stir diced tomatoes with green chiles, tomato soup, baked beans, chili beans and tomato paste into the slow cooker. Cook on low setting for about 2 hours.
Nutrition Information
Calories: 522 calories;;Sodium: 1926;Total Carbohydrate: 47.9;Cholesterol: 92;Protein: 37.6;Total Fat: 23.1

558. Swiss Steak Stew

Serving: 6 | Prep: 15mins | Cook: 8hours20mins | Ready in:
Ingredients
1/4 cup all-purpose flour
1/2 teaspoon salt
1 1/2 pounds boneless round steak, cut into bite size pieces
1 (14.5 ounce) can Italian-style diced tomatoes
3/4 cup water
3 cups peeled and quartered new red potatoes
1 onion, diced
1 cup sweet corn
Direction
In medium bowl, blend well salt and flour. Add beef and coat thoroughly.
Heat a nonstick skillet coated with cooking spray over medium heat. Add beef and cook until browned.
In a slow cooker, place onion, beef and potatoes in layers. Blend tomatoes with juice, water, and leftover flour mixture. Spread on top. Cook on Low setting while covered for about 7 - 8 hours, until the beef is softened. Add corn then cover and cook for around 25 minutes.
Nutrition Information
Calories: 349 calories;;Cholesterol: 71;Protein: 26.6;Total Fat: 14.9;Sodium: 447;Total Carbohydrate: 25.4

559. Taco Chili From Publix®

Serving: 6 | Prep: 30mins | Cook: 6hours | Ready in:
Ingredients
1 1/2 pounds ground beef
2 (10 ounce) cans diced tomatoes and green chiles, undrained
1 (15 ounce) can chili beans in sauce, undrained
1 (15 ounce) can kidney beans, undrained
1 (15.25 ounce) can southwest-style corn with peppers, drained
1 (15.5 ounce) can hominy, drained
1 (10 ounce) can mild enchilada sauce
1 (1 ounce) packet taco seasoning mix
Direction
Set a big nonstick sauté pan on moderate high heat for about 2 to 3 minutes to preheat. Put in beef (wash hands) and brown for 5 to 7 minutes until no pink remains, stirring to crumble meat. Stir in taco seasoning, then move meat out of pan.
In a slow cooker, mix the remaining ingredients and stir in meat. Cover and cook on low setting for 6 to 8 hours or on high setting for about 3 to 4 hours. Serve.
Nutrition Information
Calories: 504 calories;;Total Fat: 19.2;Sodium: 1760;Total Carbohydrate: 56.7;Cholesterol: 68;Protein: 29.7

560. Taiwanese Spicy Beef Noodle Soup

Serving: 8 | Prep: 25mins | Cook: 8hours15mins | Ready in:
Ingredients
2 pounds beef stew meat, cut into 1-inch cubes
water to cover
3 tablespoons vegetable oil, or more as needed
8 cups water, or more as needed
1 (14 ounce) can beef broth
1 cup soy sauce
1/2 cup rice wine
1 bunch green onions, cut into 2-inch pieces
1/4 cup brown sugar
10 cloves garlic, peeled, or more to taste
4 small chile peppers, halved and seeded, or more to taste
2 tablespoons chile paste
1 (1 1/2 inch) piece fresh ginger, peeled and cut into 5 pieces
3 star anise pods, or more to taste
1 teaspoon Chinese five-spice powder
4 small heads baby bok choy
1 (10 ounce) package udon noodles
1 tablespoon chopped pickled Chinese mustard greens, or to taste (optional)
Direction
Use a stockpot to place the beef inside. Pour water into the pot enough to cover the beef. Let it boil, then transfer and drain.
Using a slow cooker, pour vegetable into it then add in 8 cups of water, beef, beef broth, soy sauce, rice wine, brown sugar, green onions, chili paste, chili peppers, ginger, garlic, star anise, and Chinese five-spice powder.
Let it cook for 8 to 9 hours while set to Low.
Use a slotted spoon to remove the beef. Strain broth into a bowl, then remove the solids.
Boil a pot of water, then cook the bok choy in for 30 seconds. After removing, use cold water to run it.
In boiling water, add bok choy for 30 seconds. Remove and run under cold water. Cook the udon noodles for 4 minutes, just until it becomes tender yet firm to bite. Remove the water.
Prepare the serving bowls by portioning the noodles. Serve with broth, baby bok choy, and beef. Use Chinese pickled mustard greens to garnish.
Nutrition Information
Calories: 482 calories;;Sodium: 2366;Total Carbohydrate: 41.5;Cholesterol: 63;Protein: 27;Total Fat: 22

561. Tangy Vegan Crockpot Corn Chowder

Serving: 6 | Prep: 30mins | Cook: 8hours | Ready in:
Ingredients
2 (12 ounce) cans whole kernel corn
3 cups vegetable broth
3 potatoes, diced
1 large onion, diced
1 clove garlic, minced

2 red chile peppers, minced
1 tablespoon chili powder
2 teaspoons salt
1 tablespoon parsley flakes
black pepper to taste
1 3/4 cups soy milk
1/4 cup margarine
1 lime, juiced
Direction
Put the vegetable broth, corn, potatoes, garlic, onion, red chile peppers, salt, chili powder, black pepper, and parsley in a slow cooker then cover it. Leave it to cook on Low for 7 hours.
Fill the pitcher of the blender with the vegetable mixture no more than halfway full. Hold the lid of the blender with a folded kitchen towel. Leave it to puree once you carefully start the blender using a few quick pulses. Puree it in batches until it's smooth then transfer to a clean pot. You can also use a stick blender if you prefer, and puree the mixture in the cooking pot. After everything has been pureed, put it back to the slow cooker. Add in the margarine and soy milk into the mixture, stirring them in then cook for 1 more hour on Low. Pour in the lime juice and serve!
Nutrition Information
Calories: 320 calories;;Total Fat: 10.5;Sodium: 1493;Total Carbohydrate: 53.1;Cholesterol: 0;Protein: 9

562. Teddy's Duck Gumbo

Serving: 16 | Prep: 45mins | Cook: 8hours40mins | Ready in:
Ingredients
2 (3 to 3 1/2 pound) domestic whole ducklings, dressed
3 cups water
2 (8 ounce) cans diced tomatoes with green chilies, undrained
6 cloves garlic, minced
1 1/2 cups chopped onion
1 1/2 cups chopped celery
1 1/2 cups chopped green bell pepper
2 bay leaves
1 (4.5 ounce) package gumbo base, as in Zatarian's
2 pounds frozen sliced okra
1 (16 ounce) package frozen cooked shrimp (peeled and deveined)
1 pound smoked sausage, cut into 1/2 inch slices
Direction
Put the ducks inside a slow cooker. Add water to cover the duck. Cook on low for 8 hours, until the juices are clear. Remove from slow cooker. Set aside 3 cups of the duck broth. Remove and throw away the bones.
Pour 3 cups of the broth and water into the slow cooker. Toss in garlic, celery, onion, tomatoes, bell pepper, gumbo base mix, and bay leaves. Cook on high. Let it boil. Lower the heat. Add the okra, shrimp, sausage and duck meat. Cook for 30 more minutes until it becomes thick. Serve while hot.
Nutrition Information
Calories: 252 calories;;Total Fat: 8.1;Sodium: 857;Total Carbohydrate: 16.3;Cholesterol: 120;Protein: 27.3

563. Ten Bean Soup II

Serving: 8 | Prep: | Cook: | Ready in:
Ingredients
1 (16 ounce) package dry mixed beans
1 (15 ounce) can tomato sauce
1 (14.5 ounce) can diced tomatoes with green chile peppers
3 stalks celery, diced
4 carrots, diced
16 ounces smoked turkey sausage, diced
salt to taste
ground black pepper to taste
1/4 teaspoon poultry seasoning
1/2 teaspoon onion powder
2 1/2 teaspoons minced garlic
Direction
Steep the bean mix in the water overnight.
Add the sausage, carrots, celery, chilies and tomatoes, tomato sauce, drained steeped beans in the slow cooker. Pour in enough water to cover all of the ingredients and use garlic, onion powder, chicken seasoning, pepper, salt to season the soup to taste. Let simmer over low heat till the beans soften or for 8 - 10 hours.
Nutrition Information
Calories: 301 calories;Protein: 21.3;Total Fat: 2.5;Sodium: 1102;Total Carbohydrate: 47.1;Cholesterol: 20

564. Teriyaki Beef Bean Rice Bowls From Del Monte®

Serving: 8 | Prep: | Cook: 8hours | Ready in:
Ingredients
2 1/2 pounds lean stew beef, cut into 1 1/2-inch cubes
1 (14.5 ounce) can Del Monte® Original Recipe Stewed Tomatoes, not drained
1 (15 ounce) can kidney beans, rinsed and drained
1 (1.3 ounce) package pot roast seasoning mix for slow cookers
1 cup water
1/2 cup reduced-sodium teriyaki sauce, or more as needed
1 (14.5 ounce) can DEL MONTE® Cut Green Beans, drained
2 (8.8 ounce) packages heat-and-serve white rice
Topping Options:
Reduced-sodium soy sauce
Sliced green onions
Toasted sesame seeds
Grated orange zest
Direction
Mix together teriyaki sauce, water, seasoning mix, kidney beans, tomatoes and beef together in a 5-qt. slow cooker till well mixed. Cook it with a cover for 8 hours on LOW heat or 4 hours on HIGH heat.
Use a wooden spoon to crash large pieces of tomatoes, approximately 10 minutes before serving, and mix in green beans; cover to heat through.
At the same time, cook rice following package directions. In bowls, serve beef over rice, with toppings, as wanted.
Nutrition Information
Calories: 444 calories;;Total Carbohydrate: 33.5;Cholesterol: 78;Protein: 28.4;Total Fat: 21;Sodium: 1030

565. Texas Beef Soup

Serving: 6 | Prep: 20mins | Cook: 8hours | Ready in:
Ingredients
2 tablespoons olive oil
1 pound lean beef stew meat

1 tablespoon seasoning salt, or to taste
1/2 teaspoon ground black pepper
1 small onion, finely chopped
1/2 green bell pepper, finely chopped
2 1/2 cups beef broth
1 (15 ounce) can mixed vegetables
1 (11.5 fl oz) can spicy vegetable juice cocktail
Direction
In a large heavy skillet, cook the olive oil. Use pepper and seasoning salt to season the stew meat. Heat the meat in the oil together with bell pepper and onion until browned. Place into a slow cooker and stir the beef broth in.
Cook on Low until the meat becomes tender, 6 to 8 hours. Stir the vegetable juice cocktail and mixed vegetables in during the last 30 minutes.
Nutrition Information
Calories: 306 calories;;Sodium: 1124;Total Carbohydrate: 9.4;Cholesterol: 66;Protein: 23.4;Total Fat: 19

566. The Big Game Barbeque Meat Chili

Serving: 12 | Prep: 15mins | Cook: 10hours10mins | Ready in:
Ingredients
1 (55 ounce) can baked beans (such as Bush's Homestyle®)
1 (19 ounce) can red kidney beans
1 (19 ounce) can cannellini beans
1/4 cup barbeque sauce (such as Jack Daniel's®)
1/4 cup brown sugar
1 pound ground beef
1 pound bulk sweet Italian sausage
1 pound bulk hot Italian sausage
2 (13 ounce) packages kielbasa sausage, thinly sliced
13 slices crisply cooked bacon, chopped
Direction
In a big bowl, stir together brown sugar, barbeque sauce, cannellini beans, kidney beans and baked beans.
Heat a big skillet on moderate high heat. Cook and stir hot Italian sausage, sweet Italian sausage and beef in the hot skillet for 5-7 minutes until crumbly and browned, then transfer mixture into a slow cooker. In the same skillet, cook and stir kielbasa on moderate high heat for 5-7 minutes until browned; transfer to the slow cooker. Put chopped bacon on top of meats.
Pour bean mixture over meats, then stir well to mix. Cook on low setting for about 10-12 hours.
Nutrition Information
Calories: 824 calories;;Sodium: 1980;Total Carbohydrate: 49.2;Cholesterol: 138;Protein: 37.3;Total Fat: 54.2

567. The Ultimate Chili

Serving: 6 | Prep: 10mins | Cook: 6hours10mins | Ready in:
Ingredients
1 pound lean ground beef
salt and pepper to taste
3 (15 ounce) cans dark red kidney beans
3 (14.5 ounce) cans Mexican-style stewed tomatoes
2 stalks celery, chopped
1 red bell pepper, chopped
1/4 cup red wine vinegar
2 tablespoons chili powder
1 teaspoon ground cumin
1 teaspoon dried parsley
1 teaspoon dried basil
1 dash Worcestershire sauce
1/2 cup red wine
Direction
Heat your large skillet over medium-high heat before stirring in ground beef. Cook the ground beef until browned all over. Remove its grease and flavor them with pepper and salt to taste.
Mix the cooked beef, red bell pepper, red wine vinegar, kidney beans, celery, and tomatoes inside the slow cooker. Add cumin, Worcestershire sauce, chili powder, basil, and parsley to spice the mixture. Stir to distribute ingredients evenly.
Allow it to cook on High setting for 6 hours, or on Low setting for 8 hours. Stir in wine during the last 2 hours of cooking time.
Nutrition Information
Calories: 414 calories;;Total Fat: 11;Sodium: 1015;Total Carbohydrate: 49.5;Cholesterol: 50;Protein: 28.4

568. The Ultimate Slow Cooked Chili

Serving: 10 | Prep: 15mins | Cook: 6hours10mins | Ready in:
Ingredients
2 tablespoons olive oil, divided
2 pounds lean ground beef
1 onion, chopped
2 tablespoons chopped garlic
salt and ground black pepper to taste
2 (15 ounce) cans pinto beans
2 (15 ounce) cans ranch-style beans
2 (15 ounce) cans white kidney beans (cannellini)
1 (15 ounce) can tomato sauce
1 (14.5 ounce) can Mexican-style stewed tomatoes
1 (7.75 ounce) can Mexican-style hot tomato sauce (such as El Pato®)
1 green bell pepper, chopped
2 stalks celery, chopped
3 tablespoons chili powder
2 tablespoons Worcestershire sauce
2 tablespoons balsamic vinegar
1 tablespoon garlic powder
1 tablespoon ground cumin
1 tablespoon dried parsley
1 tablespoon dried basil
1 tablespoon brown sugar
1/2 cup red wine (optional)
Direction
In a big skillet, heat 1 tbsp. of olive oil on moderate high heat, then cook and stir garlic, onion and beef in the hot oil for 10 minutes until crumbly and browned; drain and get rid of grease. Season the beef mixture to taste with pepper and salt.
Combine together in a slow cooker the brown sugar, basil, parsley, cumin, garlic powder, balsamic vinegar, Worcestershire sauce, chili powder, celery, green bell pepper, Mexican-style hot tomato sauce, Mexican-style stewed tomatoes, tomato sauce, white kidney beans, ranch-style beans, pinto beans, leftover 1 tbsp. of olive oil and ground beef mixture.
Cook on high setting for about 4 hours, then stir in red wine and keep on cooking for 2 hours longer or cook on low setting for 8 hours.
Nutrition Information
Calories: 492 calories;;Sodium: 1125;Total Carbohydrate: 52.7;Cholesterol: 55;Protein: 31.4;Total Fat: 16.7

569. Thunderbird Stew

Serving: 8 | Prep: 10mins | Cook: 9hours | Ready in:

Ingredients
2 pounds chuck roast
1 (1 ounce) package dry onion soup mix
1 (.75 ounce) packet dry brown gravy mix
1 1/2 cups apple juice

Direction
Slow Cooker instructions: Place apple juice, stew beef, onion soup mix, and brown gravy mix into a slow cooker and cook for 5 to 8 hours on Low.
Oven instructions: Mix the apple juice, onion soup mix, and brown gravy together in a saucepan dish. Add stew beef; cook while covered in an oven at 325° (165° C) for 2.5 hours to 3 hours.

Nutrition Information
Calories: 271 calories;;Sodium: 525;Total Carbohydrate: 9.2;Cholesterol: 74;Protein: 22.4;Total Fat: 15.6

570. Traditional Irish Stew

Serving: 8 | Prep: 15mins | Cook: 8hours11mins | Ready in:

Ingredients
1 tablespoon olive oil, or to taste
2 pounds beef chuck roast, cubed
3 russet potatoes, diced
1 pound baby carrots
1 large onion, chopped
4 cloves garlic, minced
1 (16 ounce) bottle stout beer, divided
1 (6 ounce) can tomato paste
1 cup beef broth
1 tablespoon garlic powder
1 tablespoon onion powder
1 tablespoon smoked paprika
salt and ground black pepper to taste

Direction
In a skillet, heat olive oil over medium heat. Add beef; cook for 3-5 minutes each side, until it is evenly browned.
In a slow cooker, add garlic, onion, carrots and potatoes; arrange browned beef overtop.
In the same skillet, pour 1/4 cup beer and allow to a boil while using a wooden spoon to remove the browned pieces of beef to the bottom of the skillet. Mix in tomato paste; cook for 5 minutes, until thickened. Pour in beer mixture.
In the slow cooker, add pepper, salt, paprika, onion powder, garlic powder, remaining beer and beef broth.
Cook for 8 hours over low heat.

Nutrition Information
Calories: 334 calories;Protein: 17.5;Total Fat: 14.9;Sodium: 365;Total Carbohydrate: 29.8;Cholesterol: 51

571. Turkey And Okra Soup With Barley And Bacon

Serving: 15 | Prep: 35mins | Cook: 8hours | Ready in:

Ingredients
4 quarts turkey broth
3 cubes chicken bouillon
1 pound thick-cut bacon, cut into 1-inch square pieces
2 tablespoons minced garlic
1/2 teaspoon ground black pepper
1 pound cubed cooked turkey
1 red onion, sliced
1 cup barley
2 teaspoons chopped fresh rosemary
1 teaspoon salt
1 teaspoon Italian seasoning
1 pound okra, sliced
1/2 bunch fresh parsley, chopped

Direction
In a slow cooker, mix the chicken bouillon and turkey broth.
In a skillet, place the bacon over medium heat and add the black pepper and garlic. Cook and stir the mixture for 10 minutes until the bacon is crispy. Transfer the bacon mixture into the paper towel-lined plate. Blot it to remove excess fat as possible.
Mix the bacon mixture into the mixture inside the slow cooker. Add the red onion, Italian seasoning, salt, barley, turkey, and rosemary.
Cook the mixture on low heat for 7 1/2 hours or on high heat for 3 1/2 hours. Make sure to stir the mixture every half hour. Mix in parsley and okra. Cook for 30 more minutes.
Allow the soup to cool to room temperature. Refrigerate it for 8 hours to overnight. Skim off any solid fat that you see on top of the soup. Heat it on the stovetop.

Nutrition Information
Calories: 185 calories;;Cholesterol: 40;Protein: 16.3;Total Fat: 6.7;Sodium: 1849;Total Carbohydrate: 14.1

572. V Eight Vegetable Beef Soup

Serving: 6 | Prep: 10mins | Cook: 30mins | Ready in:

Ingredients
1 pound lean ground beef
48 ounces tomato-vegetable juice cocktail
2 (16 ounce) packages frozen mixed vegetables

Direction
Add the ground beef into the slow cooker or Dutch oven. Cook on medium high heat till becoming browned equally. Drain off excess fat, and break up into crumbles. Put in the mixed vegetables and juice cocktail.
In the Dutch oven, let simmer for half an hour.
In the slow cooker, cook 60 minutes on High setting. Then lower the heat to Low and let simmer 6 - 8 hours.

Nutrition Information
Calories: 343 calories;;Total Carbohydrate: 29.6;Cholesterol: 57;Protein: 20.3;Total Fat: 16.4;Sodium: 695

573. Vegetarian Bacon Chili

Serving: 10 | Prep: 25mins | Cook: 5hours | Ready in:

Ingredients
2 (15 ounce) cans red kidney beans with liquid
1 (28 ounce) can crushed tomatoes
1 (28 ounce) can diced tomatoes
1 (12 ounce) package vegetarian ground beef crumbles
4 cloves elephant garlic, crushed
6 2/3 tablespoons vegetarian bacon bits
1/2 large white onion, chopped
1 lime, peeled
1 serrano pepper, seeded and thinly sliced
5 teaspoons chili powder, or to taste
2 teaspoons cayenne pepper, or to taste
2 teaspoons ground cinnamon, or to taste
2 teaspoons dried oregano, or to taste

1 teaspoon curry powder, or to taste
1 teaspoon salt
Direction
In a slow cooker, put garlic, vegetarian beef crumbles, diced tomatoes, crushed tomatoes, and kidney beans with liquid.
Use a food processor or mortar and pestle to grind vegetarian bacon bits to a fine powder.
In a blender, blend serrano pepper, lime, and onion until you make a paste. Mix the ground bacon bits and the paste to the kidney bean mixture.
Cook for an hour on low heat until heated through.
Add salt, curry powder, oregano, cinnamon, cayenne pepper, and chili powder. Cook for 4 hours on low heat.
Nutrition Information
Calories: 196 calories;;Total Carbohydrate: 29.1;Cholesterol: 0;Protein: 15;Total Fat: 3.4;Sodium: 833

574. Vegetarian Pumpkin Spinach Chili
Serving: 9 | Prep: 25mins | Cook: 3hours20mins | Ready in:
Ingredients
1 (28 ounce) can diced tomatoes
1 (14 ounce) can 100% pure pumpkin
1 cup vegetable juice
1 cup chopped okra
1 cup chopped broccoli
1 carrot, peeled and chopped
1 small zucchini, diced
1 small onion, diced
2 tablespoons pumpkin pie spice
2 tablespoons white sugar
2 tablespoons white vinegar
1 teaspoon chili powder, or to taste
1 teaspoon salt
1/2 teaspoon ground black pepper
1 (12 ounce) package vegetarian ground beef crumbles
1 (19 ounce) can fava beans, drained
2 cups chopped spinach
Direction
In a slow cooker, mix salt, pepper, chili powder, vinegar, sugar, pumpkin pie spice, onion, zucchini, carrot, broccoli, okra, vegetable juice, pumpkin, and tomatoes. Cook for 3-4 hours on high heat until veggies are tender.
Mix spinach, fava beans, and vegetarian ground beef crumbles into the tomato mixture. Keep cooking for another 20-30 minutes until completely warmed.
Nutrition Information
Calories: 177 calories;;Total Fat: 2.4;Sodium: 854;Total Carbohydrate: 27.1;Cholesterol: 0;Protein: 12.1

575. White Chicken Chili With Salsa Verde
Serving: 10 | Prep: 30mins | Cook: 6hours | Ready in:
Ingredients
1 1/2 cups dried navy beans
2 tablespoons all-purpose flour
1 1/2 teaspoons garlic powder
1 1/4 teaspoons ground cumin
3/4 teaspoon dried oregano
3/4 teaspoon medium grind black pepper
1 1/2 pounds boneless, skinless chicken breast, cut in bite-sized pieces
1 tablespoon Mazola® Corn Oil
2 stalks celery, diced
1 carrot, diced
1 cup diced onion
4 ounces sliced mushrooms
1 (14 ounce) can reduced sodium chicken broth
1 cup salsa verde, divided
1 1/2 cups water
1 (5.3 ounce) can evaporated milk
1 cup shredded Monterey Jack cheese
1 tablespoon chopped fresh cilantro, or to taste
Sliced jalapenos and chopped cilantro (optional)
Direction
Steep beans in four cups water overnight.
In a big resealable plastic bag, mix together black pepper, oregano, cumin, garlic and flour, then set aside. Toss flour mixture and chicken together until coated thoroughly.
In a big nonstick skillet on moderate high heat, heat oil; put in chicken. Sauté chicken for 6-8 minutes until browned slightly.
Get rid of any floating beans, then drain water and put beans into slow cooker. Put water, 1/2 cup of salsa verde, chicken broth and vegetables into slow cooker.
Add chicken and stir to blend all ingredients.
Cook on low setting for about 7-9 hours or high setting for 4-6 hours until beans are softened. Stir in cilantro, cheese, evaporated milk, leftover salsa verde. Serve together with more cilantro and sliced jalapenos, if preferred.
Nutrition Information
Calories: 283 calories;;Sodium: 223;Total Carbohydrate: 26.6;Cholesterol: 54;Protein: 25.3;Total Fat: 8.3

576. White Chili V
Serving: 9 | Prep: 5mins | Cook: 8hours | Ready in:
Ingredients
2 (48 ounce) jars Great Northern white beans
1 (28 ounce) can crushed tomatoes (such as Hunt's®)
3 (4 ounce) cans chopped green chilies
2 cups diced cooked chicken
1 (32 ounce) can chicken broth
1 (1.25 ounce) package taco seasoning
1 teaspoon cayenne pepper
1 teaspoon ground cumin
1 teaspoon ground Mexican oregano
1 teaspoon ground marjoram
2 cloves garlic, minced
Direction
In a slow cooker, mix minced garlic, ground marjoram, ground Mexican oregano, ground cumin, cayenne pepper, taco seasoning, chicken broth, cooked chicken, green chilies, crushed tomatoes and Great North white beans.
On Low, cook for about 8 hours till the flavors are well incorporated.
Nutrition Information
Calories: 438 calories;;Sodium: 1345;Total Carbohydrate: 75.7;Cholesterol: 18;Protein: 29.8;Total Fat: 3.1

577. White Chili VI
Serving: 8 | Prep: 5mins | Cook: 4hours | Ready in:
Ingredients
1 (48 ounce) jar great Northern beans
1 (16 ounce) jar salsa
1/2 pound pepperjack cheese, cut into chunks
1 (8 ounce) can white meat chicken, shredded
Direction

In a slow cooker, mix together chicken, pepperjack cheese, salsa and the great Northern beans.
Cook on low setting for 4-5 hours until cheese is melted totally into the chili and the flavors are blended.
Nutrition Information
Calories: 368 calories;;Total Fat: 12.1;Sodium: 658;Total Carbohydrate: 40.3;Cholesterol: 48;Protein: 25.7

578. White Chili VII

Serving: 10 | Prep: 25mins | Cook: 8hours | Ready in:
Ingredients
2 tablespoons olive oil
4 skinless, boneless chicken breasts, cut into bite-size pieces
1 onion, chopped
3 large stalks celery, chopped
1 teaspoon garlic powder
1 teaspoon ground cumin
1 bay leaf
1 teaspoon salt
1/2 teaspoon ground black pepper
1/2 teaspoon ground oregano
1/8 teaspoon cayenne pepper
1/2 (4 ounce) can chopped jalapeno peppers
1 (6 ounce) can chopped green chilies
2 1/2 cups chicken stock
1 cup water
3 (14.5 ounce) cans great Northern beans
12 ounces sour cream
1/2 cup heavy cream
Direction
In a big skillet over medium heat, heat the olive oil. In hot oil, cook the chicken for 5 to 7 minutes till browned fully.
Put the celery and onion to the skillet; cook and mix for 2 to 3 minutes till the vegetables are slightly softened.
Move the chicken mixture to a slow cooker.
Add in the great Northern beans, water, chicken stock, green chilies, jalapeno peppers, cayenne pepper, oregano, black pepper, salt, bay leaf, cumin and garlic powder.
Cook 8 to 10 hours on Low, or 4 to 5 hours on High.
Take the bay leaf out of the mixture. Mix the heavy cream and sour cream through the chili, serve.
Nutrition Information
Calories: 349 calories;;Sodium: 764;Total Carbohydrate: 31.9;Cholesterol: 57;Protein: 20.6;Total Fat: 16.1

579. White Chili With Chicken Corn

Serving: 4 | Prep: 10mins | Cook: 4hours | Ready in:
Ingredients
1 pound boneless, skinless chicken breast halves, cut into 1-inch cubes
1 (15 ounce) can white beans, drained
1 (15.25 ounce) can Del Monte® Whole Kernel Corn, drained
1 (7 ounce) can fire-roasted diced green chiles
1 cup diced onion
1 tablespoon finely chopped garlic
1/4 cup cornmeal
1 tablespoon ground cumin
1 teaspoon chili powder
2 cups College Inn® Chicken Broth
1/4 cup chopped cilantro
Optional Toppings:
Sour cream
Lime wedges
Diced tomatoes
Tortilla chips
Shredded cheese
Direction
In slow cooker, put together initial 9 ingredients; mix.
Put chicken broth. Cover and cook on LOW 8 hours or on HIGH 4 hours.
Mix in cilantro. As wished, serve chili with chosen toppings.
Nutrition Information
Calories: 373 calories;;Sodium: 1173;Total Carbohydrate: 42.4;Cholesterol: 69;Protein: 37.6;Total Fat: 5.9

580. Wild Turkey Gumbo

Serving: 20 | Prep: 20mins | Cook: 1hours45mins | Ready in:
Ingredients
1 cup wild rice
water to cover
2 teaspoons Celtic sea salt, divided
3 quarts chicken broth, divided
2 tablespoons coconut oil
3 cups cubed wild turkey breast, or more to taste
1 large onion, chopped
2 large carrots, quartered lengthwise and sliced
4 stalks celery, chopped
1 pound bag frozen okra
1 teaspoon white pepper
3/4 teaspoon freshly ground black pepper
3 tablespoons chopped jarred jalapeno peppers
1 teaspoon hot sauce (such as Texas Pete®)
Direction
In a bowl put wild rice and enough water to cover it; soak for 4 hours to overnight. Drain the rice.
In a stockpot mix together 1 teaspoon of salt and wild rice, add about 3 cups of chicken broth. Bring to a boil, set heat to medium-low, cover and let it simmer for about 30 to 40 minutes until rice is soft. In a big skillet over medium heat, heat coconut oil. In the hot oil cook and mix celery, carrots, onion, and turkey for 10 to 15 minutes until vegetables are slightly soft and turkey is cooked through. Add okra into turkey mixture and cook for 5 to 7 minutes until okra is thawed. Season with black pepper, white pepper, and 1 teaspoon of salt.
In a slow cooker combine the remaining chicken stock, hot sauce, jalapeno peppers, turkey mixture, and wild rice. Set to high and cook for 1 hour.
Nutrition Information
Calories: 482 calories;;Total Fat: 10.6;Sodium: 939;Total Carbohydrate: 10;Cholesterol: 248;Protein: 81.7

581. Winter Lentil Vegetable Soup

Serving: 6 | Prep: 20mins | Cook: 1hours30mins | Ready in:
Ingredients
1/2 cup red or green lentils
1 cup chopped onion
1 stalk celery, chopped
2 cups shredded cabbage
1 (28 ounce) can whole peeled tomatoes, chopped
2 cups chicken broth
3 carrots, chopped
1 clove garlic, crushed
1 teaspoon salt

1/2 teaspoon ground black pepper
1/4 teaspoon white sugar
1/2 teaspoon dried basil
1/2 teaspoon dried thyme
1/4 teaspoon curry powder

Direction

In a Dutch oven or stockpot, put lentils and cover twice the depth of the lentils with water. Boil it, lower the heat and allow it to simmer, about 15 minutes. Strain the rinse the lentils, put back into the pot.

Add garlic, carrots, chicken broth, tomatoes, cabbage, celery, and onion to the pot, and use curry, thyme, basil, sugar, pepper, and salt to season. Cook, simmering until reaching the softness you want, about 1 1/2-2 hours.

Nutrition Information

Calories: 112 calories;;Total Fat: 0.6;Sodium: 938;Total Carbohydrate: 21.9;Cholesterol: 2;Protein: 6.4

Chapter 6: Steak Slow Cooker Recipes

582. All Day Soup

Serving: 8 servings. | Prep: 25mins | Cook: 08hours00mins | Ready in:

Ingredients
1 beef flank steak (1-1/2 pounds), cut into 1/2-inch cubes
1 medium onion, chopped
1 tablespoon olive oil
5 medium carrots, thinly sliced
4 cups shredded cabbage
4 medium red potatoes, diced
2 celery ribs, diced
2 cans (14-1/2 ounces each) diced tomatoes, undrained
2 cans (14-1/2 ounces each) beef broth
1 can (10-3/4 ounces) condensed tomato soup, undiluted
1 tablespoon sugar
2 teaspoons Italian seasoning
1 teaspoon dried parsley flakes

Direction
Start browning onion and steak in oil in a large skillet; drain. Arrange into a 5-quart slow cooker. Stir the remaining ingredients in. Place a cover on and cook on low heat until the meat becomes tender, 8-10 hours.

Nutrition Information
Calories: 274 calories;Protein: 21g protein. Diabetic Exchanges: 2 starch;Total Fat: 8g fat (3g saturated fat);Sodium: 679mg sodium
Fiber: 5g fiber);Total Carbohydrate: 29g carbohydrate (12g sugars;Cholesterol: 41mg cholesterol

583. Asian Style Round Steak

Serving: 8 servings. | Prep: 20mins | Cook: 07hours00mins | Ready in:

Ingredients
2 pounds beef top round steak, cut into 3-inch strips
2 tablespoons canola oil
3 celery ribs, chopped
1 cup chopped onion
1/4 cup reduced-sodium soy sauce
1 teaspoon sugar
1/2 teaspoon minced garlic
1/4 teaspoon ground ginger
1/4 teaspoon pepper
2 medium green peppers, julienned
1 can (15 ounces) tomato sauce
1 can (14 ounces) bean sprouts, rinsed and drained
1 can (8 ounces) sliced water chestnuts, drained
1 jar (4-1/2 ounces) sliced mushrooms, drained
1 tablespoon cornstarch
1/2 cup cold water
Hot cooked rice
Minced chives, optional

Direction
Brown meat on all sides in oil in a big skillet. Put drippings and meat into 5-qt. slow cooker. Mix pepper, ginger, garlic, sugar, soy sauce, onion and celery; put on meat. Cover; cook till meat is tender for 5 1/2-6 hours on low.
Add mushrooms, water chestnuts, bean sprouts, tomato sauce and green peppers; cover. Cook for 1 hour on low.
Mix water and cornstarch till smooth; mix into beef mixture. Cover; cook till sauce is thick for 30 minutes on high. Serve with rice; sprinkle chives, if desired.

Nutrition Information
Calories: 237 calories;Total Carbohydrate: 14g carbohydrate (4g sugars;Cholesterol: 63mg cholesterol;Protein: 29g protein. Diabetic Exchanges: 3 meat;Total Fat: 8g fat (2g saturated fat);Sodium: 659mg sodium
Fiber: 4g fiber)

584. Barbecues For The Bunch

Serving: 16 servings. | Prep: 25mins | Cook: 06hours00mins | Ready in:

Ingredients
2 pounds beef top sirloin steak, cubed
1-1/2 pounds boneless pork loin roast, cubed
2 large onions, chopped
3/4 cup chopped celery
1 can (6 ounces) tomato paste
1/2 cup packed brown sugar
1/4 cup cider vinegar
1/4 cup chili sauce
2 tablespoons Worcestershire sauce
1 tablespoon ground mustard
16 hamburger buns, split

Direction
Mix together celery, onions, pork and beef in a 5-quart slow cooker. Mix together mustard, Worcestershire sauce, chili sauce, vinegar, brown sugar and tomato paste in a small bowl, then drizzle this mixture over meat mixture.
Place a cover and cook on high setting until meat is extremely tender, about 6 to 8 hours. Use 2 forks to shred the meat directly in the slow cooker. Serve each bun with 1/2 cup of the meat mixture, using a slotted spoon.

Nutrition Information
Calories: 297 calories
Fiber: 2g fiber);Total Carbohydrate: 34g carbohydrate (13g sugars;Cholesterol: 53mg cholesterol;Protein: 24g protein. Diabetic Exchanges: 3 lean meat;Total Fat: 7g fat (2g saturated fat);Sodium: 336mg sodium

585. Beef Braciole

Serving: 6 servings. | Prep: 30mins | Cook: 06hours00mins | Ready in:

Ingredients
2 jars (24 ounces each) tomato basil pasta sauce
1 teaspoon crushed red pepper flakes
1 beef flank steak (1-1/2 pounds)
1/2 teaspoon salt
1/2 teaspoon pepper
2 large eggs, beaten
1/2 cup seasoned bread crumbs
8 thin slices prosciutto or deli ham
1 cup shredded Italian cheese blend
2 tablespoons olive oil

Direction
Mix pepper flakes and pasta sauce in oval 5-6-qt. slow cooker. Pound steak to 1/2-in. thick using a meat mallet; sprinkle pepper and salt.
Mix breadcrumbs and eggs in a small bowl. Within 1-in. from edges, put on beef; press onto meat. Layer using cheese and prosciutto. Roll up, starting at a

long side, jellyroll style; tie with kitchen string in 2-in. intervals.
Brown meat on all sides in oil in a Dutch oven. Put into slow cooker; put sauce on meat. Cover; cook till beef is tender for 6-8 hours on low.
Take meat from sauce; discard string. Cut to slices then serve with sauce.
Nutrition Information
Calories: 515 calories;Sodium: 1881mg sodium Fiber: 6g fiber);Total Carbohydrate: 31g carbohydrate (17g sugars;Cholesterol: 155mg cholesterol;Protein: 38g protein.;Total Fat: 25g fat (8g saturated fat)

586. Beef And Beans
Serving: 8 servings. | Prep: 10mins | Cook: 06hours30mins | Ready in:
Ingredients
1-1/2 pounds boneless round steak
1 tablespoon prepared mustard
1 tablespoon chili powder
1/2 teaspoon salt
1/4 teaspoon pepper
1 garlic clove, minced
2 cans (14-1/2 ounces each) diced tomatoes, undrained
1 medium onion, chopped
1 teaspoon beef bouillon granules
1 can (16 ounces) kidney beans, rinsed and drained
Hot cooked rice
Direction
Take the steak and cut it into long thin strips. In separate bowl, mix garlic, salt, mustard, pepper, and chili powder. Put the steak in the bowl with seasonings, coat well. Put the coated strips of steak in a 3-qt. slow cooker. Dump in bouillon, tomatoes, and onion. Set to low, cover, and cook for 6-8 hours. Mix in the beans and cook for 30 more minutes. Eat over rice.
Nutrition Information
Calories: 185 calories
Fiber: 5g fiber);Total Carbohydrate: 16g carbohydrate (5g sugars;Cholesterol: 47mg cholesterol;Protein: 24g protein. Diabetic Exchanges: 2 lean meat;Total Fat: 3g fat (1g saturated fat);Sodium: 584mg sodium

587. Beef Wrapped Stuffed Peppers
Serving: 4 servings. | Prep: 40mins | Cook: 06hours00mins | Ready in:
Ingredients
1 beef flank steak (1 pound)
1 teaspoon olive oil
1 small onion, chopped
3 ounces fully cooked chorizo chicken sausage links or flavor of your choice, chopped
2 garlic cloves, minced
5 ounces fat-free cream cheese
3 tablespoons minced fresh cilantro
1 tablespoon lime juice
1/2 teaspoon pepper
4 poblano peppers
1/4 cup shredded pepper jack cheese
1 cup salsa verde
Direction
Cut steak to 4 serving-sized pieces; pound to 1/4-in. thick with a meat mallet.
Heat oil on medium high heat in a big skillet. Add onion; mix and cook till tender for 2-3 minutes. Add sausage; mix and cook till brown for 3-4 minutes. Add garlic; cook for 1 minute. Take off heat. Mix in pepper, lime juice, cilantro and cream cheese.
Cut tops from peppers then discard; remove seeds. Use 1/3 cup filling and 1 tbsp. pepper jack cheese to fill each pepper. Wrap steak piece around pepper; tie using kitchen string.
Put into 4-qt. slow cooker that's coated in cooking spray; put salsa over. Cook till meat is tender for 6-8 hours on low, covered.
Nutrition Information
Calories: 324 calories;Total Carbohydrate: 14g carbohydrate (6g sugars;Cholesterol: 81mg cholesterol;Protein: 35g protein.;Total Fat: 14g fat (6g saturated fat);Sodium: 795mg sodium Fiber: 3g fiber)

588. Burgundy Beef Stew
Serving: 6 servings. | Prep: 25mins | Cook: 08hours00mins | Ready in:
Ingredients
1/2 cup all-purpose flour
1 pound beef top sirloin steak, cut into 1/2-inch pieces
3 turkey bacon strips, diced
8 small red potatoes, halved
2 medium carrots, cut into 1-inch pieces
1 cup sliced fresh mushrooms
3/4 cup frozen pearl onions, thawed
3 garlic cloves, minced
1 bay leaf
1 teaspoon dried marjoram
1/2 teaspoon salt
1/2 teaspoon dried thyme
1/4 teaspoon pepper
1/2 cup reduced-sodium beef broth
1 cup Burgundy wine or additional reduced-sodium beef broth
6 cups hot cooked egg noodles
Direction
In a big resealable plastic bag, put flour. Add beef, several pieces each time, and shake to coat. In a big grease-coated frying pan, brown bacon and beef on all sides in batches.
In a 5-qt. slow cooker, put bacon and beef. Mix in wine, broth, seasonings, garlic, and vegetables.
Put a cover on and cook on low until the meat is soft, or for about 8-9 hours. Remove the bay leaf. Thicken the cooking juices if you want. Enjoy with noodles.
Nutrition Information
Calories: 388 calories;Sodium: 434mg sodium Fiber: 4g fiber);Total Carbohydrate: 49g carbohydrate (4g sugars;Cholesterol: 70mg cholesterol;Protein: 26g protein. Diabetic Exchanges: 3 starch;Total Fat: 7g fat (2g saturated fat)

589. Chipotle Beef Chili
Serving: 8 servings (about 2-1/2 quarts). | Prep: 15mins | Cook: 06hours00mins | Ready in:
Ingredients
2 pounds beef flank steak, cut into 1-inch pieces
2 to 4 chipotle peppers in adobo sauce, chopped
1/4 cup chopped onion
1 tablespoon chili powder
2 garlic cloves, minced
1 teaspoon salt
1/2 teaspoon ground cumin
3 cans (15 ounces each) tomato puree
1 can (14-1/2 ounces) beef broth

1/4 cup minced fresh cilantro
Direction
Mix the first 9 ingredients together in a 4- or 5-quart slow cooker. Cover and cook on low setting until meat is tender, about 6 to 8 hours. Stir in cilantro.
Freeze option: Freeze cooled chili in freezer containers. To use, thaw partly in the fridge overnight. In a saucepan, heat through while stirring from time to time and putting in a little broth or water, if needed.
Nutrition Information
Calories: 230 calories;Protein: 25g protein. Diabetic Exchanges: 3 lean meat;Total Fat: 9g fat (4g saturated fat);Sodium: 668mg sodium Fiber: 2g fiber);Total Carbohydrate: 12g carbohydrate (3g sugars;Cholesterol: 54mg cholesterol

590. Colony Mountain Chili

Serving: 10 servings. | Prep: 25mins | Cook: 06hours00mins | Ready in:
Ingredients
1 pound beef top sirloin steak, cut into 3/4-inch cubes
4 Johnsonville® Mild Italian Sausage Links, casings removed and cut into 3/4-inch slices
2 tablespoons olive oil, divided
1 medium onion, chopped
2 green onions, thinly sliced
3 garlic cloves, minced
2 teaspoons beef bouillon granules
1 cup boiling water
1 can (6 ounces) tomato paste
3 tablespoons chili powder
2 tablespoons brown sugar
2 tablespoons Worcestershire sauce
2 teaspoons ground cumin
1 to 2 teaspoons crushed red pepper flakes
1 teaspoon salt
1/2 teaspoon pepper
3 cans (14-1/2 ounces each) stewed tomatoes, cut up
2 cans (15 ounces each) pinto beans, rinsed and drained
Shredded cheddar cheese
Direction
Brown sausage and beef in 1 tbsp. of oil in a big skillet, then drain. Move the meat to a 5-quart slow cooker. Sauté green onions and onion in the remaining oil in the same skillet until softened. Put in garlic and cook for 1 minute more. Move to a slow cooker.
Dissolve bouillon in a small bowl with water. Stir in seasonings, Worcestershire sauce, brown sugar, chili powder and tomato paste until combined, then put into slow cooker. Stir in beans and tomatoes. Cover and cook on high setting until the meat is tender, about 6 to 8 hours. Serve together with cheese, if wanted.
Nutrition Information
Calories:;Total Carbohydrate:;Cholesterol:;Protein:;Total Fat:;Sodium: Fiber:

591. Cuban Ropa Vieja

Serving: 6 | Prep: 15mins | Cook: 4hours | Ready in:
Ingredients
1 tablespoon vegetable oil
2 pounds beef flank steak
1 cup beef broth
1 (8 ounce) can tomato sauce
1 small onion, sliced
1 green bell pepper, seeded and sliced into strips
2 cloves garlic, chopped
1 (6 ounce) can tomato paste
1 teaspoon ground cumin
1 teaspoon chopped fresh cilantro
1 tablespoon olive oil
1 tablespoon white vinegar
Direction
Over medium-high heat, heat vegetable oil in a large skillet and then brown flank steak per side for about 4 minutes on each side.
Place the beef into a slow cooker. Add in the tomato sauce and beef broth. Then add the vinegar, onion, tomato paste, bell pepper, olive oil, cilantro, garlic, and cumin. Mix until blended well. Cover the cooker and let to cook on Low heat for up to 10 hours or on High heat for 4 hours. To serve, shred the meat and then serve together with rice or tortillas.
Nutrition Information
Calories: 261 calories;;Sodium: 599;Total Carbohydrate: 9.9;Cholesterol: 48;Protein: 20.5;Total Fat: 15.8

592. Easy Ham With Cherry Sauce

Serving: 10-12 servings. | Prep: 20mins | Cook: 04hours00mins | Ready in:
Ingredients
1 boneless fully cooked ham (3 to 4 pounds)
1/2 cup apple jelly
2 teaspoons prepared mustard
2/3 cup ginger ale, divided
1 can (21 ounces) cherry pie filling
2 tablespoons cornstarch
Direction
Score the outside of ham, creating half-inch deep diamond shapes. Combine 1 tablespoon ginger ale, mustard and jelly in a small bowl; spread over the ham's scored surface. Halve the ham; move into a 5-quart slow cooker. Cook while covered on low for 4-5 hours or till a thermometer reaches 140°; when the cooking time is almost over, baste with cooking juices.
For the sauce: In a saucepan, pour pie filling. Combine the leftover ginger ale and cornstarch together; mix into pie filling until blended. Set to a boil; cook and mix for 2 minutes or till thickened. Serve over ham.
Nutrition Information
Calories: 284 calories;Protein: 21g protein.;Total Fat: 10g fat (3g saturated fat);Sodium: 1469mg sodium Fiber: 0 fiber);Total Carbohydrate: 28g carbohydrate (21g sugars;Cholesterol: 60mg cholesterol

593. Easy Slow Cooked Swiss Steak

Serving: 2 servings. | Prep: 10mins | Cook: 06hours00mins | Ready in:
Ingredients
1 tablespoon all-purpose flour
1/4 teaspoon salt
1/8 teaspoon pepper
3/4 pound beef top round steak
1/2 medium onion, cut into 1/4-inch slices
1/3 cup chopped celery
1 can (8 ounces) tomato sauce
Direction

Mix pepper, salt and flour in a big resealable plastic bag. Split beef into 2 portions, put into bag and shake to coat well.

Put onion into a 3-quart slow cooker covered with cooking spray, layer with tomato sauce, celery and beef. Cover and cook on low setting until meat is softened, about 6 to 8 hours.

Nutrition Information
Calories: 272 calories;Cholesterol: 96mg cholesterol;Protein: 41g protein.;Total Fat: 5g fat (2g saturated fat);Sodium: 882mg sodium Fiber: 2g fiber);Total Carbohydrate: 13g carbohydrate (4g sugars

594. Fabulous Fajitas

Serving: 10 | Prep: 15mins | Cook: 15mins | Ready in:
Ingredients
2 green bell peppers, sliced
1 red bell pepper, sliced
1 onion, thinly sliced
1 cup fresh sliced mushrooms
2 cups diced, cooked chicken meat
1 (.7 ounce) package dry Italian-style salad dressing mix
10 (12 inch) flour tortillas

Direction
Slice onion and peppers into thin slices. Do not dice; keep the slices thin and long.

Sauté onion and peppers with a little oil until soft. Add chicken and mushrooms. Keep cooking over low heat until fully heated. Mix in dry salad dressing mix and mix well.

Warm the tortillas and roll the mixture inside. Put shredded cheddar cheese, diced tomato and shredded lettuce on top if you want.

Nutrition Information
Calories: 427 calories;;Total Fat: 10.3;Sodium: 1078;Total Carbohydrate: 64.2;Cholesterol: 21;Protein: 18

595. Fiesta Beef Bowls

Serving: 6 servings. | Prep: 25mins | Cook: 08hours30mins | Ready in:
Ingredients
1-1/2 pounds boneless beef top round steak
1 can (10 ounces) diced tomatoes and green chilies
1 medium onion, chopped
2 garlic cloves, minced
1 teaspoon dried oregano
1 teaspoon chili powder
1 teaspoon ground cumin
1/4 teaspoon salt
1/4 teaspoon pepper
2 cans (15 ounces each) pinto beans, rinsed and drained
3 cups hot cooked rice
1/2 cup shredded cheddar cheese
6 tablespoons sliced ripe olives
6 tablespoons thinly sliced green onions
6 tablespoons guacamole

Direction
In 3-qt. slow cooker, put round steak. Mix seasonings, garlic, onion and tomatoes in a small bowl; put on steak. Cover; cook till meat is tender for 8-9 hours on low.

Take meat from slow cooker. Put beans in tomato mixture; cover. Cook for 30 minutes on high heat till beans heat through. Slice meat when cool to handle.

Layer bean mixture, meat and rice in individual bowls; top with guacamole, onions, olives and cheese.

Nutrition Information
Calories: 460 calories;Total Fat: 11g fat (4g saturated fat);Sodium: 720mg sodium Fiber: 9g fiber);Total Carbohydrate: 52g carbohydrate (4g sugars;Cholesterol: 74mg cholesterol;Protein: 38g protein.

596. Flank Steak Fajitas

Serving: 8-10 servings. | Prep: 10mins | Cook: 08hours00mins | Ready in:
Ingredients
1-1/2 to 2 pounds beef flank steak, cut into thin strips
1 can (10 ounces) diced tomatoes and green chilies, undrained
2 garlic cloves, minced
1 jalapeno pepper, seeded and chopped
1 tablespoon minced fresh cilantro or parsley
1 teaspoon chili powder
1/2 teaspoon ground cumin
1/4 teaspoon salt
1 medium sweet red pepper, julienned
1 medium green pepper, julienned
8 to 10 flour tortillas (7 to 8 inches)
Sour cream, salsa and shredded cheddar cheese, optional

Direction
In a 3-quart slow cooker, put the beef. Mix salt, cumin, chili powder, cilantro, jalapeno, garlic, and tomatoes together in a small bowl; add to the beef. Put the lid on and cook for 7-8 hours on low.

Mix in green peppers and red peppers. Cook until the peppers and meat are soft, about another 60 minutes. If you want, thicken the juices.

Down the middle of each tortilla, put approximately 1/2 cup beef mixture with a slotted spoon; fold over the filling with the sides. Enjoy with cheese, salsa, and sour cream if you like.

Nutrition Information
Calories: 231 calories;Protein: 17g protein.;Total Fat: 8g fat (2g saturated fat);Sodium: 416mg sodium Fiber: 1g fiber);Total Carbohydrate: 23g carbohydrate (1g sugars;Cholesterol: 33mg cholesterol

597. Game Stopper Chili

Serving: 12 servings (4 quarts). | Prep: 25mins | Cook: 06hours00mins | Ready in:
Ingredients
1 can (28 ounces) diced tomatoes, undrained
1 can (15 ounces) black beans, rinsed and drained
1 can (15 ounces) kidney beans, rinsed and drained
1 pound boneless beef chuck steak, cut into 1-inch cubes
1 pound Jones No Sugar Pork Sausage Roll, cooked and drained
2 medium onions, chopped
1 medium sweet red pepper, chopped
1 medium green pepper, chopped
1 cup hot chunky salsa
1/3 cup medium pearl barley
2 tablespoons chili powder
2 teaspoons jarred roasted minced garlic
1 teaspoon salt
1 teaspoon ground cumin
4 cups beef stock
2 cups shredded Mexican cheese blend

Corn chips
Direction
In a 6-quart slow cooker, add all the ingredients but not chips and cheese. Cover and cook on low for 6 to 8 hours until beef is softened.
Stir in cheese until melted. Serve together with chips.
Freeze option: Freeze cooled chili in freezer containers. To use, thaw partly in the fridge overnight. In a saucepan, heat through while stirring from time to time.
Nutrition Information
Calories: 359 calories;Cholesterol: 62mg cholesterol;Protein: 23g protein.;Total Fat: 18g fat (7g saturated fat);Sodium: 1062mg sodium
Fiber: 6g fiber);Total Carbohydrate: 26g carbohydrate (6g sugars

598. Garlic Beef Stroganoff

Serving: 6-8 servings. | Prep: 20mins | Cook: 07hours00mins | Ready in:
Ingredients
2 teaspoons beef bouillon granules
1 cup boiling water
1 can (10-3/4 ounces) condensed cream of mushroom soup, undiluted
2 jars (4-1/2 ounces each) sliced mushrooms, drained
1 large onion, chopped
3 garlic cloves, minced
1 tablespoon Worcestershire sauce
1-1/2 to 2 pounds beef top round steak, cut into thin strips
2 tablespoons canola oil
1 package (8 ounces) cream cheese, cubed
Hot cooked noodles
Direction
Dissolve bouillon in water in a 3-quart slow cooker. Put in Worcestershire sauce, garlic, onion, mushrooms and soup. Brown beef in oil in a skillet. Move to the slow cooker. Cover and cook for 7 to 8 hours at low, until the meat is soft. Mix in cream cheese until smooth. Enjoy with noodles.
Nutrition Information
Calories: 281 calories;Sodium: 661mg sodium
Fiber: 1g fiber);Total Carbohydrate: 7g carbohydrate (2g sugars;Cholesterol: 81mg cholesterol;Protein: 23g protein.;Total Fat: 18g fat (8g saturated fat)

599. Gone All Day Casserole

Serving: 12 servings. | Prep: 15mins | Cook: 06hours00mins | Ready in:
Ingredients
1 cup uncooked wild rice, rinsed and drained
1 cup chopped celery
1 cup chopped carrots
2 cans (4 ounces each) mushroom stems and pieces, drained
1 large onion, chopped
1 garlic clove, minced
1/2 cup slivered almonds
3 beef bouillon cubes
2-1/2 teaspoons seasoned salt
2 pounds boneless round steak, cut into 1-inch cubes
3 cups water
Direction
In order listed, put ingredients into 3-qt. slow cooker; don't mix. Cover; cook till rice is tender for 6-8 hours on low; before serving, mix.
Nutrition Information
Calories: 192 calories
Fiber: 2g fiber);Total Carbohydrate: 16g carbohydrate (2g sugars;Cholesterol: 42mg cholesterol;Protein: 21g protein.;Total Fat: 5g fat (1g saturated fat);Sodium: 601mg sodium

600. Grandma Schwartz's Rouladen

Serving: 6 servings. | Prep: 35mins | Cook: 06hours00mins | Ready in:
Ingredients
3 bacon strips, chopped
1-1/2 pounds beef top round steak
2 tablespoons Dijon mustard
3 medium carrots, quartered lengthwise
6 dill pickle spears
1/4 cup finely chopped onion
1 cup sliced fresh mushrooms
1 small parsnip, peeled and chopped
1 celery rib, chopped
1 can (10-3/4 ounces) condensed golden cream of mushroom soup, undiluted
1/3 cup dry red wine
2 tablespoons Worcestershire sauce
2 tablespoons minced fresh parsley
Direction
In a big skillet, cook the bacon on medium heat till crisp. Take out the paper towels using a slotted spoon; drain, save the drippings.
At the same time, slice the steak into 6 serving-sized pieces; pound using a meat mallet to a-quarter-inch in thickness. Spread over the tops with the mustard. Add 2 carrot pieces and 1 pickle spear on top of each; drizzle with the onion. Roll up from a short side and use the toothpicks to secure.
In a big skillet, brown the roll-ups in the bacon drippings on medium high heat. Add the roll-ups into the 4-quart slow cooker. Add the cooked bacon, celery, parsnip and mushrooms on top.
In a small-sized bowl, stir Worcestershire sauce, wine and soup. Add onto the top. Keep covered and cook over low heat till the beef softens or for 6 to 8 hours. Drizzle with the parsley.
Nutrition Information
Calories: 288 calories;Protein: 28g protein.;Total Fat: 11g fat (3g saturated fat);Sodium: 1030mg sodium
Fiber: 3g fiber);Total Carbohydrate: 14g carbohydrate (4g sugars;Cholesterol: 74mg cholesterol

601. Herbed Beef With Noodles

Serving: 8 servings. | Prep: 25mins | Cook: 05hours00mins | Ready in:
Ingredients
2 pounds beef top round steak
1/2 teaspoon salt
1/2 teaspoon pepper, divided
2 teaspoons canola oil
1 can (10-3/4 ounces) reduced-fat reduced-sodium condensed cream of celery soup, undiluted
1 medium onion, chopped
1 tablespoon fat-free milk
1 teaspoon dried oregano
1/2 teaspoon dried thyme
6 cups cooked wide egg noodles
Chopped celery leaves, optional
Direction
Cut steak to serving-sized pieces; sprinkle 1/4 tsp. pepper and salt. Brown meat on both sides in oil in a

big nonstick skillet coated in cooking spray; put into 3-qt. slow cooker.
Mix leftover pepper, thyme, oregano, milk, onion and soup in a small bowl; put on meat. Cover; cook till meat is tender for 5-6 hours on low.
Serve with noodles; if desired, sprinkle celery leaves.
Nutrition Information
Calories: 290 calories;Sodium: 334mg sodium Fiber: 2g fiber);Total Carbohydrate: 26g carbohydrate (3g sugars;Cholesterol: 92mg cholesterol;Protein: 30g protein. Diabetic Exchanges: 3 lean meat;Total Fat: 7g fat (2g saturated fat)

602. Hunter's Delight

Serving: 8 servings. | Prep: 15mins | Cook: 06hours00mins | Ready in:
Ingredients
1/2 pound sliced bacon, diced
2-1/2 pounds red potatoes, thinly sliced
2 medium onions, sliced
1-1/2 pounds boneless venison steak, cubed
2 cans (14-3/4 ounces each) cream-style corn
3 tablespoons Worcestershire sauce
1 teaspoon sugar
1/2 to 1 teaspoon seasoned salt
Direction
Place a big skillet over a medium heat, crisp some bacon on it and drain excess oil afterwards. In a 5-quart slow cooker place onions and potatoes. Place the crisp bacon and the venison on top.
Mix together sugar, seasoned salt, corn, and Worcestershire sauce; drizzle this over the venison mixture. Cook on low flame for 6 to 8 hours until the potatoes and meat are soft.
Nutrition Information
Calories: 355 calories;Cholesterol: 80mg cholesterol;Protein: 27g protein.;Total Fat: 7g fat (3g saturated fat);Sodium: 658mg sodium
Fiber: 4g fiber);Total Carbohydrate: 47g carbohydrate (8g sugars

603. Louisiana Round Steak

Serving: 6 servings. | Prep: 20mins | Cook: 07hours00mins | Ready in:
Ingredients
2 pounds sweet potatoes, peeled and cut into 1-inch pieces
1 large onion, chopped
1 medium green pepper, sliced
2 beef top round steaks (3/4 inch thick and 1 pound each)
1 teaspoon salt, divided
2 tablespoons olive oil
1 garlic clove, minced
3 tablespoons all-purpose flour
1 can (28 ounces) diced tomatoes, undrained
1/2 cup beef broth
1 teaspoon sugar
1/2 teaspoon dried thyme
1/2 teaspoon pepper
1/4 teaspoon hot pepper sauce
Direction
In 6-qt. slow cooker, put green pepper, onion and sweet potatoes. Cut every steak to 3 serving-sized pieces; sprinkle 1/2 tsp. salt. Brown steaks in batches in oil on both sides in a big skillet on medium heat. Put steaks on veggies; keep drippings in the pan.
Put garlic in drippings; mix and cook for 1 minute.
Mix in flour till blended; mix in leftover salt and leftover ingredients. Boil, constantly mixing; mix and cook till thick for 4-5 minutes. Put on meat; cover. Cook till beef is tender for 7-9 hours on low.
Nutrition Information
Calories: 576 calories;Total Fat: 14g fat (4g saturated fat);Sodium: 1031mg sodium
Fiber: 5g fiber);Total Carbohydrate: 37g carbohydrate (16g sugars;Cholesterol: 170mg cholesterol;Protein: 71g protein.

604. Mushroom 'n' Steak Stroganoff

Serving: 6 servings. | Prep: 15mins | Cook: 06hours15mins | Ready in:
Ingredients
2 tablespoons all-purpose flour
1/2 teaspoon garlic powder
1/2 teaspoon pepper
1/4 teaspoon paprika
1-3/4 pounds beef top round steak, cut into 1-1/2-inch strips
1 can (10-3/4 ounces) condensed cream of mushroom soup, undiluted
1/2 cup water
1/4 cup Lipton onion mushroom soup mix
2 jars (4-1/2 ounces each) sliced mushrooms, drained
1/2 cup sour cream
1 tablespoon minced fresh parsley
Hot cooked egg noodles, optional
Direction
Mix paprika together with pepper, garlic powder and flour in a big resealable plastic bag. Put in beef strips then shake to coat.
Shift to a slow cooker of 3 quart. Mix soup mix, water and soup; add on beef. Cover and cook for 6 to 7 hours at low, until meat is soft.
Mix in parsley, sour cream and mushrooms. Cover and cook for another 15 minutes, until sauce thickens. If required, serve with noodles.
Nutrition Information
Calories: 281 calories;Sodium: 853mg sodium
Fiber: 2g fiber);Total Carbohydrate: 11g carbohydrate (2g sugars;Cholesterol: 90mg cholesterol;Protein: 32g protein.;Total Fat: 11g fat (4g saturated fat)

605. Mushroom Round Steak

Serving: 6 servings. | Prep: 25mins | Cook: 08hours00mins | Ready in:
Ingredients
1/2 cup all-purpose flour
1 teaspoon salt
1/4 teaspoon pepper
2 to 2-1/2 pounds boneless beef round steak (1/2 inch thick), cut into serving-size pieces
2 tablespoons vegetable oil
1 can (10-1/2 ounces) condensed French onion soup, undiluted
1 can (8 ounces) mushroom stems and pieces, drained
3/4 cup water
1/4 cup ketchup
1 tablespoon Worcestershire sauce
2 tablespoons cornstarch
1/4 cup cold water
1 cup (8 ounces) sour cream
Direction
Combine pepper, salt and flour in a big resealable plastic bag. Put in beef, a few wedges at a time; coat

by shaking. Working in batches, brown the beef in oil in a big skillet. Use a slotted spoon to move the meat to a 3-quart slow cooker.
Combine Worcestershire sauce, ketchup, water, mushrooms and soup in a bowl. Pour the mixture over the meat. Cook, covered, on low until the meat becomes tender, about 8 hours.
Use a slotted spoon, take beef out and keep warm. Pour the cooking liquid into saucepan. Mix together cold water and cornstarch until they become smooth; then stir gradually into the cooking liquid. Boil; cook while stirring until thickened, about 1 to 2 mins. Stir a little hot liquid into the sour cream. Put all back to pan. Then cook on low until they are heated through. Pour over meat to serve.
Nutrition Information
Calories: 405 calories;Sodium: 1127mg sodium Fiber: 1g fiber);Total Carbohydrate: 20g carbohydrate (5g sugars;Cholesterol: 114mg cholesterol;Protein: 38g protein.;Total Fat: 17g fat (7g saturated fat)

606. Mushroom Steak
Serving: 6 servings. | Prep: 20mins | Cook: 07hours00mins | Ready in:
Ingredients
1/3 cup all-purpose flour
1/2 teaspoon salt
1/2 teaspoon pepper, divided
1 beef top round steak (2 pounds), cut into 1-1/2-inch strips
2 cups sliced fresh mushrooms
1 small onion, cut into thin wedges
1 can (10-3/4 ounces) condensed golden mushroom soup, undiluted
1/4 cup sherry or beef broth
1/2 teaspoon dried oregano
1/4 teaspoon dried thyme
Hot cooked egg noodles
Direction
Mix 1/4 teaspoon pepper, flour, and salt together in a big resealable plastic bag. Add in beef, several pieces each time, and shake to coat.
Combine the mushrooms, onion, and beef in a 3-qt slow cooker. Mix the leftover pepper, thyme, oregano, sherry, and soup together; pour over the top. Put the lid on and cook on low until the beef is soft, about 7-9 hours. Enjoy with noodles.
Nutrition Information
Calories: 265 calories;Sodium: 612mg sodium Fiber: 1g fiber);Total Carbohydrate: 12g carbohydrate (1g sugars;Cholesterol: 87mg cholesterol;Protein: 36g protein. Diabetic Exchanges: 5 lean meat;Total Fat: 6g fat (2g saturated fat)

607. No Fuss Swiss Steak
Serving: 8-10 servings. | Prep: 10mins | Cook: 06hours00mins | Ready in:
Ingredients
3 pounds beef top round steak, cut into serving-size pieces
2 tablespoons canola oil
2 medium carrots, sliced
2 celery ribs, sliced
1-3/4 cups water
1 can (11 ounces) condensed tomato rice soup, undiluted
1 can (10-1/2 ounces) condensed French onion soup, undiluted
1/2 teaspoon pepper
1 bay leaf
Direction
Brown beef in oil on medium high heat in a big skillet; drain. Put into 5-qt. slow cooker then add celery and carrots. Mix leftover ingredients; put on veggies and meat.
Cover; cook till meat is tender for 6-8 hours on low. Discard bay leaf. If desired, thicken cooking juices.
Nutrition Information
Calories: 246 calories;Sodium: 477mg sodium Fiber: 1g fiber);Total Carbohydrate: 10g carbohydrate (5g sugars;Cholesterol: 79mg cholesterol;Protein: 32g protein.;Total Fat: 8g fat (2g saturated fat)

608. Pepper Steaks
Serving: 8 servings. | Prep: 15mins | Cook: 06hours15mins | Ready in:
Ingredients
2 pounds beef top round steak
2 cups each sliced green, sweet red and yellow peppers (1/2-inch strips)
1 can (7 ounces) mushroom stems and pieces, drained
2 medium onions, quartered and sliced
1/2 cup water
1 teaspoon salt
1/2 teaspoon pepper
1 can (15 ounces) tomato sauce
1/4 cup cornstarch
1/4 cup cold water
Hot mashed potatoes
Direction
Cut steak to serving-sized pieces; put into 5-qt. slow cooker. Add pepper, salt, water, onions, peppers and mushrooms; put tomato sauce on top.
Cover; cook till meat is tender for 6-6 1/2 hours on low.
Remove veggies and beef using slotted spoon; keep warm. Mix cold water and cornstarch till smooth in a small bowl. Mix into cooking juices slowly; cover. Cook till thick for 15 minutes on high. Serve with mashed potatoes, veggies and beef.
Nutrition Information
Calories:;Total Carbohydrate:;Cholesterol:;Protein:;Total Fat:;Sodium: Fiber:

609. Portobello Beef Burgundy
Serving: 6 servings. | Prep: 30mins | Cook: 07hours30mins | Ready in:
Ingredients
1/4 cup all-purpose flour
1/2 teaspoon salt
1/2 teaspoon seasoned salt
1-1/2 teaspoons minced fresh thyme or 1/2 teaspoon dried thyme
3/4 teaspoon minced fresh marjoram or 1/4 teaspoon dried thyme
1/2 teaspoon pepper
2 pounds beef sirloin tip steak, cubed
2 bacon strips, diced
3 tablespoons canola oil
1 garlic clove, minced
1 cup Burgundy wine or beef broth
1 teaspoon beef bouillon granules
1 pound sliced baby portobello mushrooms

Hot cooked noodles, optional
Direction
Combine the first 6 ingredients in a large resealable plastic bag. Add a few pieces of beef at a time until finish, and shake to coat.
Cook bacon in a large skillet over medium heat until it's crispy. Transfer to paper towels to drain using a slotted spoon. Cook beef in batches in hot oil until browned in the same skillet, adding garlic to the last batch; cook for 1 to 2 minutes longer. Drain well. Transfer to a 4-quart slow cooker. Pour in wine into the skillet, stirring to loosen browned bits from the pan. Add bouillon; bring to a boil. Mix into slow cooker. Mix in bacon. Cook, covered on low setting until meat is tender, or for 7 to 9 hours.
Mix in mushrooms. Cook, covered on high setting until sauce thickens slightly and mushrooms are tender, or for 30 to 45 minutes longer. Enjoy with noodles if desired.
Nutrition Information
Calories: 321 calories
Fiber: 1g fiber);Total Carbohydrate: 8g carbohydrate (2g sugars;Cholesterol: 100mg cholesterol;Protein: 34g protein.;Total Fat: 15g fat (3g saturated fat);Sodium: 552mg sodium

610. Pumpkin Harvest Beef Stew

Serving: 6 servings. | Prep: 25mins | Cook: 06hours30mins | Ready in:
Ingredients
1 tablespoon canola oil
1 beef top round steak (1-1/2 pounds), cut into 1-inch cubes
1-1/2 cups cubed peeled pie pumpkin or sweet potatoes
3 small red potatoes, peeled and cubed
1 cup cubed acorn squash
1 medium onion, chopped
2 cans (14-1/2 ounces each) reduced-sodium beef broth
1 can (14-1/2 ounces) diced tomatoes, undrained
2 bay leaves
2 garlic cloves, minced
2 teaspoons reduced-sodium beef bouillon granules
1/2 teaspoon chili powder
1/2 teaspoon pepper
1/4 teaspoon ground allspice
1/4 teaspoon ground cloves
1/4 cup water
3 tablespoons all-purpose flour
Direction
Heat oil in big skillet on medium high heat; in batches, brown beef. Use slotted spoon to put into 4-5-qt. slow cooker. Add onion, squash, potatoes and pumpkin; mix seasonings, tomatoes and broth in. Cover; cook for 6-8 hours on low till meat is tender. Discard bay leaves. Mix flour and water till smooth in small bowl; mix into stew slowly. Cover; cook for 30 minutes on high till liquid is thick.
Nutrition Information
Calories: 258 calories;Total Fat: 6g fat (1g saturated fat);Sodium: 479mg sodium
Fiber: 4g fiber);Total Carbohydrate: 21g carbohydrate (6g sugars;Cholesterol: 67mg cholesterol;Protein: 29g protein. Diabetic Exchanges: 3 lean meat

611. Round Steak Italiano

Serving: 8 servings. | Prep: 15mins | Cook: 07hours00mins | Ready in:
Ingredients
2 pounds beef top round steak
1 can (8 ounces) tomato sauce
2 tablespoons onion soup mix
2 tablespoons canola oil
2 tablespoons red wine vinegar
1 teaspoon ground oregano
1/2 teaspoon garlic powder
1/4 teaspoon pepper
8 medium potatoes (7 to 8 ounces each)
1 tablespoon cornstarch
1 tablespoon cold water
Direction
Cut steak to serving-sized pieces; put into 5-qt. slow cooker. Mix pepper, garlic powder, oregano, oil, vinegar, soup mix and tomato sauce in a big bowl; put on meat. Scrub then pierce potatoes; put on meat. Cover; cook till potatoes and meat are tender for 7-8 hours on low.
Remove potatoes and meat; keep warm. Gravy: Put cooking juices in a small saucepan and skim fat. Mix water and cornstarch till smooth; mix into juices slowly. Boil; mix and cook till thick for 2 minutes. Serve with potatoes and meat.
Nutrition Information
Calories: 357 calories;Total Fat: 7g fat (2g saturated fat);Sodium: 329mg sodium
Fiber: 4g fiber);Total Carbohydrate: 42g carbohydrate (4g sugars;Cholesterol: 64mg cholesterol;Protein: 31g protein. Diabetic Exchanges: 3 lean meat

612. Round Steak Roll Ups

Serving: 6 servings. | Prep: 20mins | Cook: 06hours00mins | Ready in:
Ingredients
2 pounds beef top round steak
1/2 cup grated carrot
1/3 cup chopped zucchini
1/4 cup chopped sweet red pepper
1/4 cup chopped green pepper
1/4 cup sliced green onions
2 tablespoons grated Parmesan cheese
1 tablespoon minced fresh parsley or 1 teaspoon dried parsley flakes
1 garlic clove, minced
1/4 teaspoon salt
1/4 teaspoon pepper
2 tablespoons canola oil
1 jar (14 ounces) meatless spaghetti sauce
Hot cooked spaghetti
Additional Parmesan cheese, optional
Direction
Cut meat to 6 serving-sized pieces and pound to 1/4-in. thick. Mix seasonings, cheese and veggies; put 1/3 cup in middle of every piece. Roll up meat around filling; use toothpicks to secure.
Brown roll-ups in the oil in a big skillet on medium high heat; put into 5-qt. slow cooker. Put spaghetti sauce over; cover. Cook till meat is tender for 6-8 hours on low.
Discard toothpicks; serve sauce and roll-ups with spaghetti. If desired, sprinkle extra cheese.
Nutrition Information

Calories: 289 calories;Protein: 38g protein. Diabetic Exchanges: 4 lean meat;Total Fat: 11g fat (3g saturated fat);Sodium: 500mg sodium Fiber: 2g fiber);Total Carbohydrate: 9g carbohydrate (0 sugars;Cholesterol: 96mg cholesterol

613. Round Steak Sauerbraten

Serving: 4 | Prep: 15mins | Cook: 1hours | Ready in:
Ingredients
1 1/2 pounds top round steak, trimmed and sliced thin
1 tablespoon vegetable oil
1 (.75 ounce) packet dry brown gravy mix
2 cups water
1 tablespoon onion powder
1 tablespoon brown sugar
2 tablespoons red wine vinegar
1 teaspoon Worcestershire sauce
1/4 teaspoon ground ginger
1 bay leaf
1/2 teaspoon salt
ground black pepper to taste
Direction
Heat the oil over medium heat in a big saucepan. Put in the sliced meat and brown well. Take out the meat.
Put in the gravy mix and water, and boil, mixing constantly.
Mix in the ground black pepper, salt, bay leaf, ginger, Worcestershire sauce, vinegar, brown sugar and onion powder to taste. Bring the meat back to the pan, lower heat to low, cover, then simmer until the meat is soft, about an hour. Discard the bay leaf.
Note: It is also possible to move to a casserole dish, then bake with a cover for 1 1/2 hours at 175°C (350°F).
Nutrition Information
Calories: 440 calories;;Total Fat: 29.6;Sodium: 655;Total Carbohydrate: 8.2;Cholesterol: 114;Protein: 33.3

614. Roundup Chili

Serving: 12 servings (3 quarts). | Prep: 35mins | Cook: 06hours00mins | Ready in:
Ingredients
2 pounds lean ground beef (90% lean)
1 beef flank steak (1-1/2 pounds), cubed
1 medium onion, chopped
1 celery rib, chopped
1 can (29 ounces) tomato sauce
2 cans (14-1/2 ounces each) diced tomatoes, undrained
1 can (16 ounces) kidney beans, rinsed and drained
1 can (15 ounces) pinto beans, rinsed and drained
1 can (4 ounces) chopped green chilies
2 to 3 tablespoons chili powder
3 teaspoons ground cumin
2 teaspoons salt
2 teaspoons pepper
1/2 teaspoon ground mustard
1/2 teaspoon paprika
1/2 teaspoon cayenne pepper
1/4 teaspoon garlic powder
Hot pepper sauce, shredded cheddar cheese and additional chopped onion, optional
Direction
Cook celery, onion, flank steak and ground beef in a big skillet on medium heat until the meat is not pink anymore, then drain.
Move to a 6-quart slow cooker. Stir in seasonings, chilies, beans, tomatoes and tomato sauce. Cover and cook on low setting until steak is tender, about 6 to 8 hours.
Serve together with cheese, hot pepper sauce and onion, if wanted.
Nutrition Information
Calories: 309 calories;Cholesterol: 64mg cholesterol;Protein: 31g protein.;Total Fat: 10g fat (4g saturated fat);Sodium: 1187mg sodium Fiber: 6g fiber);Total Carbohydrate: 22g carbohydrate (5g sugars

615. Sausage Stuffed Flank Steak

Serving: 4 servings. | Prep: 35mins | Cook: 06hours00mins | Ready in:
Ingredients
1/4 cup dried cherries
3/4 cup dry red wine or beef broth, divided
1 beef flank steak (1-1/2 pounds)
3/4 teaspoon salt, divided
1/2 teaspoon pepper, divided
1 medium onion, finely chopped
3 tablespoons olive oil, divided
4 garlic cloves, minced
1/2 cup seasoned bread crumbs
1/4 cup pitted Greek olives, halved
1/4 cup grated Parmesan cheese
1/4 cup minced fresh basil
1/2 pound Johnsonville® Ground Hot Italian sausage
1 jar (24 ounces) marinara sauce
Hot cooked pasta
Direction
Mix 1/4 cup wine and cherries in a small bowl; stand for 10 minutes. Meanwhile, slice steak to 4 serving-sized pieces then flatten to 1/4-in. thick. Sprinkle 1/4 tsp. pepper and 1/2 tsp. salt on both sides.
Sauté onion in 1 tbsp. oil till tender in a big skillet. Add garlic; cook for 1 minute. Put into big bowl; mix in leftover pepper and salt, cherry mixture, basil, cheese, olives and breadcrumbs. Crumble sausage on mixture; stir well.
On each steak piece, spread 1/2 cup of sausage mixture; roll up, starting at long side, jellyroll style; use kitchen string to tie.
Brown meat on all sides in leftover oil in same skillet; put into 3-qt. greased slow cooker. Put leftover wine and marinara sauce over; cover. Cook till beef is tender for 6-8 hours on low; serve with pasta.
Nutrition Information
Calories: 815 calories;Protein: 49g protein.;Total Fat: 45g fat (14g saturated fat);Sodium: 1687mg sodium Fiber: 4g fiber);Total Carbohydrate: 44g carbohydrate (22g sugars;Cholesterol: 129mg cholesterol

616. Savory Beef Fajitas

Serving: 12 servings. | Prep: 10mins | Cook: 07hours00mins | Ready in:
Ingredients
1 beef flank steak (2 pounds), thinly sliced
1 cup tomato juice
2 garlic cloves, minced
1 tablespoon minced fresh cilantro
1 teaspoon chili powder
1 teaspoon ground cumin
1/2 teaspoon salt
1/2 teaspoon ground coriander
1 medium onion, sliced

1 medium green pepper, julienned
1 medium sweet red pepper, julienned
1 medium jalapeno, cut into thin strips
12 flour tortillas (6 inches)
Sour cream, guacamole, salsa or shredded cheddar cheese, optional
Direction
In 3-qt. slow cooker, put beef. Mix next 7 ingredients; put on beef. Cover; cook for 6-7 hours on low.
Add jalapeno, peppers and onion; cover. Cook till veggies and meat are tender for 1 hour.
On each tortilla, put 1/2 cup meat-veggie mixture using a slotted spoon. Add preferred toppings; roll up.
Nutrition Information
Calories: 225 calories;Cholesterol: 39mg cholesterol;Protein: 20g protein. Diabetic Exchanges: 2 lean meat;Total Fat: 7g fat (3g saturated fat);Sodium: 264mg sodium
Fiber: 2g fiber);Total Carbohydrate: 19g carbohydrate (0 sugars

617. Shredded Steak Sandwiches

Serving: 12-14 servings. | Prep: 15mins | Cook: 06hours00mins | Ready in:
Ingredients
3 pounds beef top round steak, cut into large pieces
2 large onions, chopped
3/4 cup thinly sliced celery
1-1/2 cups ketchup
1/2 to 3/4 cup water
1/3 cup lemon juice
1/3 cup Worcestershire sauce
3 tablespoons brown sugar
3 tablespoons cider vinegar
2 to 3 teaspoons salt
2 teaspoons prepared mustard
1-1/2 teaspoons paprika
1 teaspoon chili powder
1/2 teaspoon pepper
1/8 to 1/4 teaspoon hot pepper sauce
12 to 14 sandwich rolls, split
Direction
In a 5-quart slow cooker, add meat. Put in celery and onions. Mix together hot pepper sauce, pepper, chili powder, paprika, mustard, salt, vinegar, brown sugar, Worcestershire sauce, lemon juice, water and ketchup in a bowl. Drizzle the mixture over meat. Place a cover on slow cooker and cook on high setting about 6 to 8 hours. Take the meat out of cooker and allow to cool a bit. Use 2 forks to shred the meat and turn back to the slow cooker to heat through. Serve meat on rolls.
Nutrition Information
Calories: 321 calories;Sodium: 1029mg sodium
Fiber: 2g fiber);Total Carbohydrate: 40g carbohydrate (10g sugars;Cholesterol: 54mg cholesterol;Protein: 24g protein.;Total Fat: 7g fat (2g saturated fat)

618. Skillet Steak Fajitas

Serving: 6-8 servings. | Prep: 20mins | Cook: 03hours30mins | Ready in:
Ingredients
1-1/2 pounds beef top sirloin steak, cut into thin strips
2 tablespoons vegetable oil
2 tablespoons lemon juice
1 garlic clove, minced
1-1/2 teaspoons ground cumin
1 teaspoon salt-free seasoning blend
1/2 teaspoon chili powder
1/4 to 1/2 teaspoon crushed red pepper flakes
1 large green pepper, julienned
1 large onion, julienned
6 to 8 flour tortillas (8 inches)
Shredded cheddar cheese, salsa, sour cream, lettuce and tomatoes, optional
Direction
Brown steak on medium heat in an oiled skillet. Bring drippings and steak into a 3-quart slow cooker. Mix in red pepper flakes, chili powder, seasoning blend, cumin, garlic and lemon juice. Cook, covered, for 2 1/2-3 hours over high heat or until meat is softened. Put in onion and green pepper; cook vegetables, covered, until tender or for 60 minutes.
Follow package instructions to warm the tortillas; scoop vegetables and beef in the middle of tortillas. Add on top the tomatoes (optional), lettuce, sour cream, salsa and cheese. Fold in the sides of tortillas and serve on the spot.
Nutrition Information
Calories: 313 calories
Fiber: 2g fiber);Total Carbohydrate: 31g carbohydrate (0 sugars;Cholesterol: 50mg cholesterol;Protein: 23g protein.;Total Fat: 10g fat (0 saturated fat);Sodium: 286mg sodium

619. Slow Cook Beef Stew

Serving: 6 servings. | Prep: 20mins | Cook: 06hours00mins | Ready in:
Ingredients
2 pounds beef top round steak, cut into 1-inch cubes
8 medium carrots, cut into 1-inch pieces
1 pound small red potatoes, quartered
1/2 pound sliced fresh mushrooms
1 medium sweet red pepper, chopped
1 can (14-1/2 ounces) diced tomatoes, undrained
1/4 cup all-purpose flour
1 can (6 ounces) tomato paste
3/4 cup beef broth
1/3 cup dry red wine or additional beef broth
1-1/2 teaspoons salt
1 teaspoon minced garlic
1 teaspoon pepper
1/2 teaspoon dried thyme
Direction
Cook beef in a large skillet until all sides are browned. Combine red pepper, mushrooms, potatoes, and carrots in a 5-quart slow cooker. Add tomatoes on top.
Combine broth, tomato paste, and flour in a small bowl until no lumps remain. Mix in thyme, pepper, garlic, salt, and wine; transfer into the slow cooker. Top with beef.
Cook, covered on low setting until beef is tender, or for 6 to 8 hours.
Nutrition Information
Calories:;Total Fat:;Sodium:
Fiber:;Total Carbohydrate:;Cholesterol:;Protein:

620. Slow Cooker Beef Stroganoff

Serving: 7 servings. | Prep: 20mins | Cook: 04hours00mins | Ready in:
Ingredients
2 pounds beef top sirloin steak, cut into thin strips
3 tablespoons olive oil
1 cup water

1 envelope (1-1/2 ounces) beef Stroganoff seasoning for the slow cooker
1 pound sliced baby portobello mushrooms
1 small onion, chopped
3 tablespoons butter
1/4 cup port wine or beef broth
2 teaspoons ground mustard
1 teaspoon sugar
1-1/2 cups (12 ounces) sour cream
Hot cooked egg noodles
Minced fresh parsley, optional

Direction

Brown the meat in oil in a big frying pan. Add seasoning mix and water, whisking to loosen the browned pieces from the pan. Remove the drippings and meat to a 3-quart slow cooker.
Sauté onion and mushrooms in butter in the same frying pan until soft. Stir together sugar, mustard, and wine; mix into the mushroom mixture. Pour into the slow cooker, mix to blend. Put the lid on and cook on low until the meat is soft, about 3-4 hours. Mix in sour cream. Serve together with noodles. Sprinkle parsley on top if you want.

Nutrition Information

Calories: 418 calories;Protein: 32g protein.;Total Fat: 25g fat (12g saturated fat);Sodium: 812mg sodium Fiber: 1g fiber);Total Carbohydrate: 10g carbohydrate (4g sugars;Cholesterol: 100mg cholesterol

621. Slow Cooker Beef Tostadas

Serving: 6 servings. | Prep: 20mins | Cook: 06hours00mins | Ready in:

Ingredients

1 large onion, chopped
1/4 cup lime juice
1 jalapeno pepper, seeded and minced
1 serrano pepper, seeded and minced
1 tablespoon chili powder
3 garlic cloves, minced
1/2 teaspoon ground cumin
1 beef top round steak (about 1-1/2 pounds)
1 teaspoon salt
1/2 teaspoon pepper
1/4 cup chopped fresh cilantro
12 corn tortillas (6 inches)
Cooking spray
TOPPINGS:
1-1/2 cups shredded lettuce
1 medium tomato, finely chopped
3/4 cup shredded sharp cheddar cheese
3/4 cup reduced-fat sour cream, optional

Direction

In 3-4-qt. slow cooker, put initial 7 ingredients. Halve steak; sprinkle pepper and salt. Put in slow cooker; cook on low for 6-8 hours till meat is tender, covered. Remove meat; slightly cool. Use 2 forks to shred meat; put beef in slow cooker. Mix in cilantro then heat through. Spritz cooking spray on both sides of tortillas. Put on baking sheets in 1 layer; broil till crisp for 1-2 minutes per side. Put beef mixture on tortillas; top with sour cream (optional), cheese, tomato and lettuce.

Nutrition Information

Calories: 372 calories
Fiber: 5g fiber);Total Carbohydrate: 30g carbohydrate (5g sugars;Cholesterol: 88mg cholesterol;Protein: 35g protein. Diabetic Exchanges:

4 lean meat;Total Fat: 13g fat (6g saturated fat);Sodium: 602mg sodium

622. Slow Cooker Burgundy Beef

Serving: 10 servings. | Prep: 10mins | Cook: 08hours15mins | Ready in:

Ingredients

4 pounds beef top sirloin steak, cut into 1-inch cubes
3 large onions, sliced
1 cup water
1 cup burgundy wine or beef broth
1 cup ketchup
1/4 cup quick-cooking tapioca
1/4 cup packed brown sugar
1/4 cup Worcestershire sauce
4 teaspoons paprika
1-1/2 teaspoons salt
1 teaspoon minced garlic
1 teaspoon ground mustard
2 tablespoons cornstarch
3 tablespoons cold water
Hot cooked noodles

Direction

Mix the first 12 ingredients in a 5-quarter slow cooker. Cook with a cover on low until the meat becomes tender, 8 to 9 hours.
Mix water and cornstarch until smooth; stir this mixture into pan juices. Cook with a cover on high until the gravy is thickened, approximately 15 minutes. Serve this with noodles.

Nutrition Information

Calories: 347 calories;Cholesterol: 74mg cholesterol;Protein: 40g protein.;Total Fat: 8g fat (3g saturated fat);Sodium: 811mg sodium Fiber: 1g fiber);Total Carbohydrate: 24g carbohydrate (15g sugars

623. Slow Cooker Fajitas

Serving: 8 servings. | Prep: 25mins | Cook: 08hours00mins | Ready in:

Ingredients

1 each medium green, sweet red and yellow peppers, cut into 1/2-inch strips
1 sweet onion, cut into 1/2-inch strips
2 pounds beef top sirloin steaks, cut into thin strips
3/4 cup water
2 tablespoons red wine vinegar
1 tablespoon lime juice
1 teaspoon ground cumin
1 teaspoon chili powder
1/2 teaspoon salt
1/2 teaspoon garlic powder
1/2 teaspoon pepper
1/2 teaspoon cayenne pepper
8 flour tortillas (8 inches), warmed
1/2 cup salsa
1/2 cup shredded reduced-fat cheddar cheese
8 teaspoons minced fresh cilantro

Direction

In 5-qt. slow cooker, put onion and peppers; put beef over. Mix seasonings, lime juice, vinegar and water; put on meat. Cover; cook till meat is tender for 8-10 hours on low.
Down the middle of every tortilla, put 3/4 cup meat mixture using slotted spoon. Put cilantro, cheese and salsa over; roll up.

Nutrition Information

Calories: 335 calories;Sodium: 564mg sodium

Fiber: 2g fiber);Total Carbohydrate: 32g carbohydrate (3g sugars;Cholesterol: 69mg cholesterol;Protein: 29g protein. Diabetic Exchanges: 3 lean meat;Total Fat: 10g fat (3g saturated fat)

624. Slow Cooker Flank Steak Fajitas

Serving: 8 servings. | Prep: 10mins | Cook: 08hours00mins | Ready in:
Ingredients
1 beef flank steak (2 pounds), halved crosswise
1 medium green pepper, cut into strips
1 medium sweet red pepper, cut into strips
1 medium onion, halved and sliced
1 envelope fajita seasoning mix
1/2 cup beer or reduced-sodium beef broth
8 flour tortillas (8 inches), warmed
1 cup pico de gallo
Chopped fresh cilantro
Direction
In 5-qt. slow cooker, put initial 5 ingredients; put beer over. Cook for 6-8 hours on low till meat is tender, covered.
Take beef from slow cooker. Strain veggie mixture; put veggies in slow cooker. Throw/keep cooking juices for another time. Use 2 forks to shred beef. Put into veggies; heat through. In tortillas, serve with cilantro and pico de gallo.
Nutrition Information
Calories: 361 calories;Protein: 27g protein. Diabetic Exchanges: 2 starch;Total Fat: 12g fat (4g saturated fat);Sodium: 668mg sodium
Fiber: 3g fiber);Total Carbohydrate: 34g carbohydrate (2g sugars;Cholesterol: 54mg cholesterol

625. Slow Cooker Mushroom Beef Stroganoff

Serving: 8 servings. | Prep: 15mins | Cook: 06hours00mins | Ready in:
Ingredients
2 pounds boneless beef chuck steak
1 pound sliced fresh mushrooms
2 medium onions, chopped
1 can (10-3/4 ounces) condensed golden mushroom soup, undiluted
2 tablespoons reduced-sodium soy sauce
2 tablespoons Dijon mustard
1 tablespoon Worcestershire sauce
3 garlic cloves, minced
3/4 teaspoon salt
1/2 teaspoon pepper
2 tablespoons cornstarch
2 tablespoons water
1 cup (8 ounces) sour cream
Hot cooked egg noodles
Minced fresh parsley, optional
Direction
Slice steak into strips, 3x1/2-inch each strip. Mix the next 9 ingredients together in a 5- or 6-quart slow cooker. Mix in the steak strips. Cover and cook on low for 6-8 hours, or until the meat is soft.
Remove the steak to a serving plate and keep warm. Remove the fat from the cooking juices. Stir together water and cornstarch until smooth, mix into the cooking juices. Cover and cook on high for 10-15 minutes, or until thickened. Mix in sour cream; spread over the beef. Serve together with noodles and if you want, minced parsley.
Nutrition Information
Calories:;Total Carbohydrate:;Cholesterol:;Protein:;Total Fat:;Sodium:
Fiber:

626. Slow Cooker Steak 'n' Gravy

Serving: 4 servings. | Prep: 15mins | Cook: 04hours30mins | Ready in:
Ingredients
1 pound beef top round steak
1 tablespoon vegetable oil
1-1/2 cups water
1 can (8 ounces) no-salt-added tomato sauce
1 teaspoon ground cumin
1 teaspoon garlic powder
1/2 teaspoon salt-free seasoning blend
1/4 teaspoon pepper
2 tablespoons all-purpose flour
1/4 cup cold water
2 cups mashed potatoes
Direction
Cut beef to 1-in. cubes; in oil, brown in a skillet. Put into 3-qt. slow cooker then cover in water; add seasonings and tomato sauce. Cover; cook till meat is tender for 4 hours on high/8 hours on low.
Mix cold water and flour in a small bowl; mix into liquid in the slow cooker. Cover; cook till gravy is thick for 30 minutes on high; serve with potatoes.
Nutrition Information
Calories: 361 calories;Protein: 28g protein. Diabetic Exchanges: 3-1/2 lean meat;Total Fat: 16g fat (0 saturated fat);Sodium: 336mg sodium
Fiber: 1g fiber);Total Carbohydrate: 26g carbohydrate (0 sugars;Cholesterol: 72mg cholesterol

627. Slow Cooker Swiss Steak

Serving: 6 | Prep: 15mins | Cook: 10hours15mins | Ready in:
Ingredients
1/4 cup all-purpose flour
salt and pepper to taste
1 1/2 pounds round steak, cut into small pieces
3 tablespoons vegetable oil
3 stalks celery, chopped
1 onion, chopped
3 carrots, shredded
2 (14.5 ounce) cans diced tomatoes with juice
1 tablespoon Worcestershire sauce
2 tablespoons brown sugar, or to taste
Direction
Combine the pepper, flour and salt in a shallow bowl. Slightly coat the round steak slices in the flour mixture.
Warm the oil in a frying pan over medium heat, and sauté the carrots, celery and onion, for about 5 minutes until soft. Take out from heat and reserve.
Add in the round steak slices and cook until slightly browned.
Put the steak and vegetables in a slow cooker. Add in the Worcestershire sauce, tomatoes with juice and brown sugar.
Cover with lid and cook 8-10 hours on Low heat until the round steak is very soft.
Nutrition Information
Calories: 246 calories;;Total Carbohydrate: 19.2;Cholesterol: 39;Protein: 16.8;Total Fat: 10.6;Sodium: 315

628. Slow Cooker Swiss Steak Supper

Serving: 6 servings. | Prep: 20mins | Cook: 05hours00mins | Ready in:
Ingredients
1-1/2 pounds beef top round steak
1/2 teaspoon seasoned salt
1/4 teaspoon coarsely ground pepper
1 tablespoon canola oil
3 medium potatoes
1-1/2 cups fresh baby carrots
1 medium onion, sliced
1 can (14-1/2 ounces) Italian diced tomatoes
1 jar (12 ounces) home-style beef gravy
1 tablespoon minced fresh parsley
Direction
Take the steak and cut into serving-size pieces, six chucks; flatten to 1/4-in. thick. Rub on pepper and seasoned salt. Put oil in a big frying pan and brown meat on both sides; drain excess grease. Take the potatoes and cut each one into eight wedges. In a 5-qt. slow cooker, layer with potatoes, carrots, then meat and onion. In a separate bowl, mix gravy and tomatoes; dump on top. Cover; set to low and cook until veggies and meat are tender, 5-6 hours. Sprinkle on parsley.
Nutrition Information
Calories: 402 calories;Total Carbohydrate: 53g carbohydrate (10g sugars;Cholesterol: 67mg cholesterol;Protein: 33g protein.;Total Fat: 6g fat (2g saturated fat);Sodium: 822mg sodium
Fiber: 5g fiber)

629. Slow Cooker Vegetable Beef Soup

Serving: 8 | Prep: 15mins | Cook: 7hours10mins | Ready in:
Ingredients
1 pound ground beef
2 cloves garlic, minced
1 small onion, diced
1 green bell pepper, diced
3 stalks celery, diced
1 (29 ounce) can Italian-style stewed tomatoes, drained
1 (15 ounce) can mixed vegetables, drained
2 quarts beef broth
3 tablespoons soy sauce
2 tablespoons Worcestershire sauce
3/4 teaspoon paprika
salt and pepper to taste
6 ounces dry fusilli pasta
Direction
In a skillet over medium heat, put the beef. Add in green bell pepper, onion, and garlic. Cook and stir till the vegetables are soft and the beef is evenly browned. Drain fat, remove to a slow cooker.
Into the slow cooker, combine Italian-style stewed tomatoes, celery, and mixed vegetables. Pour in beef broth, Worcestershire sauce, and soy sauce. Use pepper, salt, and paprika to season.
Cover the lid, cook on high heat for about 7 hours. During the last 15 minutes of the cooking time, mix in pasta.
Nutrition Information
Calories: 264 calories;;Cholesterol: 34;Protein: 18;Total Fat: 7.9;Sodium: 1504;Total Carbohydrate: 30.5

630. Slow Cooker Vegetable Soup

Serving: 8 | Prep: 30mins | Cook: 6hours | Ready in:
Ingredients
6 cups vegetable broth
1 (16 ounce) package frozen mixed vegetables
1 (14.5 ounce) can diced tomatoes, undrained
2 potatoes, peeled and cubed
1 large onion, diced
1/2 cup barley
3 cloves garlic, minced
1 teaspoon dried parsley
1 teaspoon dried oregano
1/2 teaspoon dried basil
1/2 teaspoon salt
1/2 teaspoon ground black pepper
1 bay leaf
2 cups all-purpose flour
1/4 cup vegetable shortening (such as Crisco®)
1/4 cup vegetable broth, or more if needed
Direction
In a slow cooker, mix together bay leaf, black pepper, salt, basil, oregano, parsley, garlic, barley, onion, potatoes, tomatoes with their juice, frozen vegetables, and 6 cups of vegetable broth. Put on a cover and cook for 5-6 hours on Low.
In a bowl, put flour. Using 2 knives or a pastry blender, cut shortening into the flour until the mixture looks like coarse crumbs. Pour in 1/4 cup of vegetable broth; use a fork to stir until the dough stops sticking to the sides of the bowl. Move the dough to a surface lightly scattered with flour, roll out to 1/8-in. thick. Slice the dough into small squares or strips. Put in the slow cooker, cook for 1 hour until the dumplings have cooked in the center and are tender.
Nutrition Information
Calories: 333 calories;;Total Fat: 7.8;Sodium: 618;Total Carbohydrate: 57.2;Cholesterol: 0;Protein: 9.2

631. Slow Cooked Beef 'n' Veggies

Serving: 2 servings. | Prep: 15mins | Cook: 08hours00mins | Ready in:
Ingredients
1 boneless beef top round steak (1/2 pound), cut into two pieces
Dash seasoned salt, optional
Dash pepper
Dash garlic powder
1 cup Italian salad dressing
1/2 cup water
1 tablespoon browning sauce
2 medium carrots, cut into 2-inch pieces
2 medium red potatoes, cubed
1 small onion, sliced
1/2 small green pepper, cut into small chunks
Direction
Sprinkle seasoned salt (optional) and pepper on 1 side of steak; sprinkle garlic powder on other side. Put into a big resealable plastic bag then seal bag; refrigerate bag for 2-3 hours – overnight.
Mix browning sauce, water and salad dressing in 3-qt. slow cooker. Add potatoes and carrots; toss till coated. Add steak; coat in sauce. Put green pepper and onion over.
Cover; cook till meat is tender for 8-9 hours on low.
Nutrition Information

Calories: 372 calories;Cholesterol: 68mg cholesterol;Protein: 31g protein.;Total Fat: 5g fat (2g saturated fat);Sodium: 1795mg sodium Fiber: 6g fiber);Total Carbohydrate: 48g carbohydrate (20g sugars

632. Slow Cooked Mushroom Swiss Steak

Serving: 6 servings. | Prep: 15mins | Cook: 08hours00mins | Ready in:

Ingredients
3/4 cup all-purpose flour
1 teaspoon pepper
1/4 teaspoon salt
2 to 2-1/2 pounds beef top round steak
1 to 2 tablespoons butter
1 can (10-3/4 ounces) condensed cream of mushroom soup, undiluted
1-1/3 cups water
1 cup sliced celery, optional
1/2 cup chopped onion
1 to 3 teaspoons beef bouillon granules
1/2 teaspoon minced garlic

Direction
Mix salt, pepper, and flour together in a shallow bowl. Slice steak into 6 pieces with serving-size; dredge the steak in flour mixture.
Brown the steak in butter in a big frying pan. Remove to 3-quart slow cooker. Mix together the rest of the ingredients, spread over the steak. Put the lid on and cook on low until the meat is soft, about 8-9 hours.

Nutrition Information
Calories: 313 calories;Sodium: 666mg sodium Fiber: 2g fiber);Total Carbohydrate: 18g carbohydrate (2g sugars;Cholesterol: 92mg cholesterol;Protein: 37g protein.;Total Fat: 9g fat (4g saturated fat)

633. Slow Cooked Round Steak

Serving: 6-8 servings. | Prep: 15mins | Cook: 07hours00mins | Ready in:

Ingredients
1/4 cup all-purpose flour
1/2 teaspoon salt
1/8 teaspoon pepper
2 pounds boneless beef round steak, cut into serving-size pieces
6 teaspoons canola oil, divided
1 medium onion, thinly sliced
1 can (10-3/4 ounces) condensed cream of mushroom soup, undiluted
1/2 teaspoon dried oregano
1/4 teaspoon dried thyme

Direction
Mix pepper, salt and flour together in a large resealable plastic bag. Add in beef, several pieces at a time, and shake until coated. Brown both side of meat in 4 teaspoons of oil in a large skillet. Place into a 5-quart slow cooker.
Sauté onion in the oil remaining in the same skillet until browned a little; place on top of the beef. Mix thyme, oregano and soup together; pour onto the onion. Cook, covered for 7 to 8 hours over low heat until meat is softened.

Nutrition Information
Calories: 224 calories;Sodium: 447mg sodium Fiber: 1g fiber);Total Carbohydrate: 8g carbohydrate (1g sugars;Cholesterol: 65mg cholesterol;Protein: 27g protein.;Total Fat: 9g fat (2g saturated fat)

634. Slow Cooked Sirloin

Serving: 6 servings. | Prep: 20mins | Cook: 03hours30mins | Ready in:

Ingredients
1 beef top sirloin steak (1-1/2 pounds)
1 medium onion, cut into 1-inch chunks
1 medium green pepper, cut into 1-inch chunks
1 can (14-1/2 ounces) reduced-sodium beef broth
1/4 cup Worcestershire sauce
1/4 teaspoon dill weed
1/4 teaspoon dried thyme
1/4 teaspoon pepper
Dash crushed red pepper flakes
2 tablespoons cornstarch
2 tablespoons cold water

Direction
Brown the beef on both sides in a cooking spray-coated big nonstick frying pan. Put the green pepper and onion in a 3-quart slow cooker and put the beef on top. Mix together the pepper flakes, pepper, thyme, dill, Worcestershire sauce and broth, then pour it on top of the beef. Put a cover and let it cook for 3 to 4 hours on high or until the vegetables become crisp-tender and the meat achieves the preferred doneness.
Take out the beef and keep it warm. Mix together the water and cornstarch until it becomes smooth, then slowly stir into the cooking juices. Put cover and let it cook for 30 minutes on high or until it becomes a bit thick. Put the beef back into the slow cooker and heat it through.

Nutrition Information
Calories: 199 calories;Total Fat: 6g fat (2g saturated fat);Sodium: 305mg sodium
Fiber: 1g fiber);Total Carbohydrate: 8g carbohydrate (2g sugars;Cholesterol: 68mg cholesterol;Protein: 26g protein. Diabetic Exchanges: 3 lean meat

635. Slow Cooked Steak Fajitas

Serving: 12 servings. | Prep: 10mins | Cook: 08hours30mins | Ready in:

Ingredients
1 beef flank steak (1-1/2 pounds)
1 can (14-1/2 ounces) diced tomatoes with garlic and onion, undrained
1 jalapeno pepper, seeded and chopped
2 garlic cloves, minced
1 teaspoon ground coriander
1 teaspoon ground cumin
1 teaspoon chili powder
1/2 teaspoon salt
1 medium onion, sliced
1 medium green pepper, julienned
1 medium sweet red pepper, julienned
1 tablespoon minced fresh cilantro
2 teaspoons cornstarch
1 tablespoon water
12 flour tortillas (6 inches), warmed
3/4 cup fat-free sour cream
3/4 cup salsa

Direction
Slice the steak into thin strips across the grain; put in a 5-qt. slow cooker. Add the chili powder, jalapeno, salt, cumin, tomatoes, coriander, and garlic. Cover; set to low and cook for 7 hours. Add cilantro, onion, and peppers. Cover; cook until beef is tender, 1-2 hours. Mix water and cornstarch until smooth; slowly stir into slow cooker. Cover; set to high and cook

until slightly thick, 30 minutes. Use a slotted spoon to put a 1/2 cup of meat mixture in the middle of each tortilla. Fold the tortilla bottom over filling and roll it up. Serve with salsa and sour cream.
Nutrition Information
Calories: 273 calories;Total Carbohydrate: 35g carbohydrate (0 sugars;Cholesterol: 23mg cholesterol;Protein: 21g protein. Diabetic Exchanges: 2 starch;Total Fat: 11g fat (3g saturated fat);Sodium: 494mg sodium
Fiber: 2g fiber)

636. Slow Cooked Stroganoff

Serving: 8-10 servings. | Prep: 20mins | Cook: 05hours00mins | Ready in:
Ingredients
3 pounds beef top round steaks
1/2 cup all-purpose flour
1-1/2 teaspoons salt
1/2 teaspoon ground mustard
1/8 teaspoon pepper
1 medium onion, sliced and separated into rings
1 can (8 ounces) mushroom stems and pieces, drained
1 can (10-1/2 ounces) condensed beef broth, undiluted
1-1/2 cups (12 ounces) sour cream
Hot cooked noodles
Direction
Cut beef to thin strips. Mix pepper, mustard, salt and flour in a shallow bowl. In batches, add beef; toss till coated.
Layer beef, mushrooms and onion in 5-qt. slow cooker; put broth over. Cook till meat is tender for 5-7 minutes on low, covered. Mix in sour cream just before serving; serve with noodles.
Nutrition Information
Calories: 275 calories;Sodium: 680mg sodium
Fiber: 1g fiber);Total Carbohydrate: 8g carbohydrate (2g sugars;Cholesterol: 99mg cholesterol;Protein: 34g protein.;Total Fat: 10g fat (5g saturated fat)

637. Slow Cooked Stuffed Flank Steak

Serving: 8 servings. | Prep: 20mins | Cook: 08hours10mins | Ready in:
Ingredients
1 beef flank steak (2 pounds)
1 medium onion, chopped
1 garlic clove, minced
1 tablespoon butter
1-1/2 cups soft bread crumbs (about 3 slices)
1/2 cup chopped fresh mushrooms
1/4 cup minced fresh parsley
1/4 cup egg substitute
3/4 teaspoon poultry seasoning
1/2 teaspoon salt
1/8 teaspoon pepper
1/2 cup beef broth
2 teaspoons cornstarch
4 teaspoons water
Direction
Flatten steak to 1/2-in. thickness; put aside.
Sauté garlic and onion in butter in a nonstick skillet until tender. Add pepper, salt, poultry seasoning, egg substitute, parsley, mushrooms, and the bread crumbs; combine well.
Pour the mixture over steak to within 1 in. of edge. Starting with a long side, roll it up like jelly; use kitchen string to tie. Transfer to a 5-qt. slow cooker; add broth. Cook, covered, for 8-10 hours on low.
Transfer the meat to a serving platter, and keep it warm. Skim fat from the cooking juices; keep in a small saucepan.
Combine water and cornstarch until the mixture becomes smooth; and stir into juices. Bring to a boil; cook while stirring until thickened, about 1-2 minutes. Get rid of the string before cutting steak into slices; serve with gravy.
Nutrition Information
Calories: 230 calories
Fiber: 1g fiber);Total Carbohydrate: 6g carbohydrate (0 sugars;Cholesterol: 62mg cholesterol;Protein: 26g protein. Diabetic Exchanges: 3 lean meat;Total Fat: 11g fat (5g saturated fat);Sodium: 348mg sodium

638. Slow Cooked Swiss Steak

Serving: 6 servings. | Prep: 10mins | Cook: 06hours00mins | Ready in:
Ingredients
2 tablespoons all-purpose flour
1/2 teaspoon salt
1/4 teaspoon pepper
1-1/2 pounds beef round steak, cut into six pieces
1 medium onion, cut into 1/4-inch slices
1 celery rib, cut into 1/2-inch slices
2 cans (8 ounces each) tomato sauce
Direction
Mix pepper, salt and flour in a big resealable plastic bag. Add steak; seal bag. Shake till coated.
Put onion into 3-qt. greased slow cooker. Put tomato sauce, celery and steak over; cover. Cook till meat is tender for 6-8 hours on low.
Nutrition Information
Calories: 171 calories;Protein: 27g protein. Diabetic Exchanges: 3 lean meat;Total Fat: 4g fat (1g saturated fat);Sodium: 409mg sodium
Fiber: 1g fiber);Total Carbohydrate: 6g carbohydrate (2g sugars;Cholesterol: 64mg cholesterol

639. Smothered Round Steak

Serving: 4 servings. | Prep: 15mins | Cook: 06hours00mins | Ready in:
Ingredients
1/3 cup all-purpose flour
1/2 teaspoon salt
1/4 teaspoon pepper
1-1/2 pounds beef top round steak, cut into strips
1 large onion, sliced
1 large green pepper, sliced
1 can (14-1/2 ounces) diced tomatoes, undrained
1 jar (4 ounces) sliced mushrooms, drained
3 tablespoons reduced-sodium soy sauce
2 tablespoons molasses
Hot cooked egg noodles, optional
Direction
Mix beef together with pepper, salt, and flour in a 3-quart slow cooker. Mix in all the rest of the ingredients, apart from the noodles.
Cover and cook on low for 6-8 hours, or until the meat is soft. Serve together with noodles if you like.
Nutrition Information
Calories: 335 calories;Protein: 42g protein.;Total Fat: 6g fat (2g saturated fat);Sodium: 1064mg sodium
Fiber: 4g fiber);Total Carbohydrate: 28g carbohydrate (14g sugars;Cholesterol: 95mg cholesterol

640. Steak 'n' Gravy

Serving: 4 servings. | Prep: 15mins | Cook: 04hours30mins | Ready in:

Ingredients
1 pound beef top round steak, trimmed
1 tablespoon canola oil
1-1/2 cups water
1 can (8 ounces) tomato sauce
1 teaspoon garlic powder
1 teaspoon ground cumin
1/2 teaspoon salt
1/4 teaspoon pepper
2 tablespoons all-purpose flour
1/4 cup cold water
Hot cooked rice or mashed potatoes

Direction
Cut beef to bite-sized pieces; in oil, brown in a skillet. Put into 1 1/2-qt. slow cooker and cover in water; add seasonings and tomato sauce. Cover; cook till meat is tender for 4 hours on high/8 hours on low. Mix cold water and flour till smooth in a small bowl; mix into liquid in the slow cooker. Cover; cook till gravy is thick for 30 minutes on high. Serve with potatoes or rice.

Nutrition Information
Calories: 204 calories;Total Fat: 7g fat (2g saturated fat);Sodium: 588mg sodium
Fiber: 1g fiber);Total Carbohydrate: 7g carbohydrate (1g sugars;Cholesterol: 64mg cholesterol;Protein: 27g protein.

641. Steak Strips With Dumplings

Serving: 2 servings. | Prep: 25mins | Cook: 05hours00mins | Ready in:

Ingredients
3/4 pound beef top round steak, cut into 1/2-inch strips
1/4 teaspoon pepper
2 teaspoons canola oil
2/3 cup condensed cream of chicken soup, undiluted
1/2 cup beef broth
4 large fresh mushrooms, sliced
1/4 cup each chopped onion, green pepper and celery
DUMPLINGS:
1/2 cup all-purpose flour
3/4 teaspoon baking powder
1/4 teaspoon salt
2 tablespoons beaten egg
3 tablespoons 2% milk
1/2 teaspoon dried parsley flakes

Direction
Sprinkle pepper to steak. Brown steak in a small skillet with oil on moderate high, then turn to a 1 1/2-quart slow cooker. Mix together vegetables, broth and soup, then drizzle over steak. Cover and cook on low setting about 4 to 5 hours.
To make dumplings, mix together salt, baking powder and flour in a small bowl. Stir in milk and egg just until combined. Drop onto meat mixture by tablespoonfuls, then sprinkle over with parsley. Cover and cook on high until toothpick tucked in a dumpling comes out clean without lifting the cover in the cooking process, about an hour.

Nutrition Information
Calories: 506 calories;Total Carbohydrate: 36g carbohydrate (5g sugars;Cholesterol: 168mg cholesterol;Protein: 49g protein.;Total Fat: 17g fat (4g saturated fat);Sodium: 1372mg sodium
Fiber: 3g fiber)

642. Steak Stroganoff

Serving: 16 servings. | Prep: 25mins | Cook: 07hours00mins | Ready in:

Ingredients
3 to 4 pounds beef top sirloin steak, cubed
2 cans (14-1/2 ounces each) chicken broth
1 pound sliced fresh mushrooms
1 can (12 ounces) regular cola
1/2 cup chopped onion
1 envelope onion soup mix
1 to 2 teaspoons garlic powder
2 teaspoons dried parsley flakes
1/2 teaspoon pepper
2 envelopes country gravy mix
2 cups (16 ounces) sour cream
Hot cooked noodles

Direction
Mix the first 9 ingredients in a 5 quarts slow cooker. Cook on low for 7 to 8 hours while covered, until meat is tender.
Take out mushrooms and beef using a slotted spoon. Put gravy mix in a big saucepan; whip in cooking liquid slowly. Heat to a boil; cook and mix for two minutes or until thickened. Take away from the heat; mix in sour cream. Put mushrooms and beef into the gravy. Serve together with noodles.

Nutrition Information
Calories: 262 calories;Sodium: 630mg sodium
Fiber: 1g fiber);Total Carbohydrate: 9g carbohydrate (6g sugars;Cholesterol: 73mg cholesterol;Protein: 22g protein.;Total Fat: 13g fat (8g saturated fat)

643. Steak And Mushroom Sauce

Serving: 2 servings. | Prep: 20mins | Cook: 06hours00mins | Ready in:

Ingredients
1/2 medium green pepper, cut into 1/2-inch pieces
1/4 cup sliced onion
1 beef top round steak (10 ounces), cut into two pieces
2/3 cup condensed cream of mushroom soup, undiluted
1/3 cup water
1-1/2 cups uncooked egg noodles

Direction
In a 1 1/2-quart slow cooker, add onion and green pepper, then put beef on top. Mix water and soup together in a small bowl, then pour over meat. Cover and cook on low heat until meat is softened, about 6 to 7 hours.
Following package directions to cook noodles, then drain. Serve together with gravy and round steak.

Nutrition Information
Calories: 354 calories;Cholesterol: 86mg cholesterol;Protein: 38g protein.;Total Fat: 6g fat (2g saturated fat);Sodium: 378mg sodium
Fiber: 2g fiber);Total Carbohydrate: 33g carbohydrate (5g sugars

644. Stuffed Flank Steak

Serving: 4 | Prep: 10mins | Cook: 1hours | Ready in:

Ingredients
2 cups dry stuffing mix
1 cup boiling water
2 tablespoons butter or margarine

1 1/2 pounds flank steak, pounded thin for easy rolling
2 green onions, chopped
1 red bell pepper, chopped
1 (10.5 ounce) can mushroom gravy
1/4 cup red wine
1 clove garlic, minced
2 tablespoons grated Parmesan cheese
Direction
Preheat the oven to 175°C (350°F).
Mix the margarine or butter with water and stuffing mix in a medium bowl. Blend well, then allow to stand about 5 minutes. Spoon stuffing over the steak, leaving a border of 1 inch. Put in the red bell pepper and green onions.
Roll from the steak's long edge, then secure using wooden toothpicks. Put the steak seam side down into a baking dish of 9x13-inch.
Mix the cheese, garlic, apple juice OR wine and gravy in a separate small bowl. Blend well, then pour atop the steak.
Bake for an hour at 175°C (350°F), discard from the oven, then allow to stand prior to slicing.
Nutrition Information
Calories: 497 calories;;Cholesterol: 71;Protein: 25.7;Total Fat: 29.4;Sodium: 1102;Total Carbohydrate: 28.9

645. Sweet Sour Beef

Serving: 10-12 servings. | Prep: 15mins | Cook: 07hours00mins | Ready in:
Ingredients
2 pounds beef top round steak or boneless beef chuck roast, cut into 1-inch cubes
2 tablespoons canola oil
2 cans (8 ounces each) tomato sauce
2 cups sliced carrots
2 cups pearl onions or 2 small onions, cut into wedges
1 large green pepper, cut into 1-inch pieces
1/2 cup molasses
1/3 cup cider vinegar
1/4 cup sugar
2 teaspoons chili powder
2 teaspoons paprika
1 teaspoon salt
Hot cooked pasta
Direction
Brown steak in oil in a big skillet; put into 5-qt. slow cooker. Add following 10 ingredients; mix well. Cover; cook till meat is tender for 7-8 hours on low; if desired, thicken cooking liquid. Serve with pasta.
Nutrition Information
Calories: 207 calories;Total Carbohydrate: 23g carbohydrate (16g sugars;Cholesterol: 42mg cholesterol;Protein: 18g protein.;Total Fat: 5g fat (1g saturated fat);Sodium: 328mg sodium Fiber: 1g fiber)

646. Tangy Venison Stroganoff

Serving: 4 servings. | Prep: 10mins | Cook: 03hours15mins | Ready in:
Ingredients
1-1/2 pounds boneless venison steak, cubed
1 medium onion, sliced
1 can (10-1/2 ounces) condensed beef broth, undiluted
1 tablespoon Worcestershire sauce
1 tablespoon ketchup
1 teaspoon curry powder
1/2 teaspoon ground ginger
1/2 teaspoon salt
1/4 teaspoon pepper
4-1/2 teaspoons cornstarch
1/2 cup sour cream
2 tablespoons prepared horseradish
Hot cooked noodles
Direction
In a 3-quart slow cooker, add onion and venison. Mix the next 7 ingredients together and drizzle over venison. Cook, covered, on high setting until meat becomes tender, about 3 to 3 1/2 hours.
Mix together horseradish, sour cream and cornstarch in a small bowl, then stir into the venison mixture gradually. Place a cover and cook until sauce is thickened, about 15 more minutes. Serve together with noodles.
Nutrition Information
Calories: 317 calories;Total Fat: 10g fat (5g saturated fat);Sodium: 1081mg sodium
Fiber: 1g fiber);Total Carbohydrate: 10g carbohydrate (4g sugars;Cholesterol: 165mg cholesterol;Protein: 43g protein.

647. Tomato Basil Steak

Serving: 4 servings. | Prep: 15mins | Cook: 06hours00mins | Ready in:
Ingredients
1-1/4 pounds boneless beef shoulder top blade or flat iron steaks
1/2 pound whole fresh mushrooms, quartered
1 medium sweet yellow pepper, julienned
1 can (14-1/2 ounces) stewed tomatoes, undrained
1 can (8 ounces) tomato sauce
1 envelope onion soup mix
2 tablespoons minced fresh basil
Hot cooked rice
Direction
Arrange the steaks into a 4-quart slow cooker. Put in the pepper and mushrooms. In a small-sized bowl, combine the basil, soup mix, tomato sauce and tomatoes; add over the top.
Cook, with a cover, over low heat till the veggies and beef soften or for 6 to 8 hours. Serve alongside the rice.
Nutrition Information
Calories: 324 calories;Protein: 32g protein.;Total Fat: 14g fat (5g saturated fat);Sodium: 1116mg sodium
Fiber: 3g fiber);Total Carbohydrate: 19g carbohydrate (8g sugars;Cholesterol: 92mg cholesterol

648. Veggie Topped Swiss Steak

Serving: 6 servings. | Prep: 35mins | Cook: 06hours00mins | Ready in:
Ingredients
1-1/2 pounds beef top round steak
1/4 cup all-purpose flour
2 teaspoons ground mustard
3/4 teaspoon salt
1/4 teaspoon pepper
2 tablespoons canola oil
2 tablespoons butter
1 can (14-1/2 ounces) diced tomatoes
2 celery ribs, finely chopped
2 medium carrots, grated
1 medium onion, finely chopped
2 tablespoons Worcestershire sauce

1 tablespoon brown sugar
Direction
Cut steak to serving-sized pieces. Mix pepper, salt, mustard and flour in a big resealable plastic bag. Few pieces at 1 time, add beef; shake till coated.
Brown meat in butter and oil on both sides in a big skillet. Put meat in 3-qt. slow cooker. Mix brown sugar, Worcestershire sauce, onion, carrots, celery and tomatoes; put on meat,
Cover; cook till meat is tender for 6-8 hours on low.
Nutrition Information
Calories: 287 calories;Total Carbohydrate: 16g carbohydrate (8g sugars;Cholesterol: 74mg cholesterol;Protein: 28g protein. Diabetic Exchanges: 4 lean meat;Total Fat: 12g fat (4g saturated fat);Sodium: 524mg sodium
Fiber: 3g fiber)

649. Zesty Orange Beef

Serving: 5 servings. | Prep: 15mins | Cook: 05hours00mins | Ready in:
Ingredients
1 beef top sirloin steak (1-1/2 pounds), cut into 1/4-inch strips
2-1/2 cups sliced fresh shiitake mushrooms
1 medium onion, cut into wedges
3 dried hot chilies
1/4 cup packed brown sugar
1/4 cup orange juice
1/4 cup reduced-sodium soy sauce
3 tablespoons cider vinegar
1 tablespoon cornstarch
1 tablespoon minced fresh gingerroot
1 tablespoon sesame oil
2 garlic cloves, minced
1-3/4 cups fresh snow peas
1 tablespoon grated orange zest
Hot cooked rice
Direction
Place beef in a 4-quart slow cooker. Add chilies, onion, and mushrooms. Combine garlic, oil, ginger, cornstarch, vinegar, soy sauce, orange juice, and brown sugar in a small mixing bowl. Pour the cornstarch mixture over the beef.
Cook, covered, for 5 to 6 hours on high power until meat is tender, adding snow peas during the last 30 minutes of cooking process. Add orange zest and mix well. Serve over rice.
Nutrition Information
Calories: 310 calories;Protein: 33g protein. Diabetic Exchanges: 4 lean meat;Total Fat: 8g fat (3g saturated fat);Sodium: 554mg sodium
Fiber: 3g fiber);Total Carbohydrate: 24g carbohydrate (16g sugars;Cholesterol: 55mg cholesterol

650. Zippy Beef Fajitas

Serving: 6 servings. | Prep: 20mins | Cook: 06hours00mins | Ready in:
Ingredients
1 beef flank steak (1-1/2 pounds)
2 teaspoons ground ginger
2 teaspoons crushed red pepper flakes
3/4 teaspoon garlic powder
1/4 teaspoon pepper
1 medium sweet red pepper, cut into strips
1 medium green pepper, cut into strips
1 can (12 ounces) cola
5 green onions, chopped
1/3 cup soy sauce
2 tablespoons minced fresh gingerroot
2 tablespoons tomato paste
1 garlic clove, minced
6 flour tortillas (8 inches), warmed
Direction
Cut steak lengthwise in half. In a small bowl, combine the pepper flakes, ground ginger, pepper and garlic powder; rub over steak. Place to a slow cooker of 3-quart; put in green and red peppers. Combine the green onions, cola, gingerroot, soy sauce, garlic and tomato paste; pour over top.
Cover and cook on low for around 6 to 7 hours till meat is tender. Shred meat using two forks; return to the slow cooker and heat through. On tortillas, spoon beef mixture by using a slotted spoon.
Nutrition Information
Calories: 365 calories;Protein: 26g protein.;Total Fat: 12g fat (4g saturated fat);Sodium: 1125mg sodium
Fiber: 2g fiber);Total Carbohydrate: 37g carbohydrate (9g sugars;Cholesterol: 48mg cholesterol

651. Zippy Steak Chili

Serving: 5 servings. | Prep: 15mins | Cook: 06hours00mins | Ready in:
Ingredients
1 pound beef top sirloin steak, cut into 1/2-inch cubes
1/2 cup chopped onion
2 tablespoons canola oil
2 tablespoons chili powder
1 teaspoon garlic powder
1 teaspoon ground cumin
1 teaspoon dried oregano
1 teaspoon pepper
2 cans (10 ounces each) diced tomatoes and green chilies, undrained
1 can (15-1/2 ounces) chili starter
Shredded cheddar cheese, chopped onion and sour cream, optional
Direction
Cook onion and steak in a big skillet with oil on moderate heat until meat is browned. Sprinkle with seasonings.
Mix together chili starter and tomatoes in a 3-quart slow cooker. Stir in beef mixture. Cover and cook until meat is softened for about 6 to 8 hours on low. Serve together onion, cheese and sour cream, if wanted.
Nutrition Information
Calories: 275 calories;Protein: 22g protein. Diabetic Exchanges: 3 lean meat;Total Fat: 11g fat (3g saturated fat);Sodium: 1127mg sodium
Fiber: 6g fiber);Total Carbohydrate: 21g carbohydrate (3g sugars;Cholesterol: 50mg cholesterol

Chapter 7: Bean Slow Cooker Recipes

652. Apple Sausage Beans

Serving: 12 servings. | Prep: 30mins | Cook: 05hours00mins | Ready in:

Ingredients
1 package (12 ounces) Johnsonville® Original Breakfast Sausage Links
1/2 cup finely chopped onion
1 garlic clove, minced
1/2 cup unsweetened apple juice
2 tablespoons brown sugar
2 tablespoons maple syrup
2 tablespoons molasses
1/2 teaspoon apple pie spice
1/4 teaspoon ground nutmeg
2 cans (28 ounces each) baked beans
1 large red apple, cubed

Direction
Slice the sausage links into 1/2-inch pieces. Cook the garlic, onion, and sausage in a large skillet on medium until the vegetables become tender and the meat is not pink anymore; if needed, let them drain. Place into a 3- or 4-quart slow cooker.
Mix the nutmeg, pie spice, molasses, maple syrup, brown sugar, and apple juice in a small bowl. Put into the same skillet and stir to scrape the browned bits in the pan. Stir and cook until the sugar has dissolved. Put the apple juice mixture, apple, and beans into the slow cooker. Put a cover on and cook on low heat until the apple becomes tender, 5-6 hours.

Nutrition Information
Calories: 257 calories;Protein: 11g protein.;Total Fat: 8g fat (3g saturated fat);Sodium: 816mg sodium Fiber: 8g fiber);Total Carbohydrate: 39g carbohydrate (9g sugars;Cholesterol: 24mg cholesterol

653. Bacon Lima Beans

Serving: 8 servings. | Prep: 15mins | Cook: 06hours00mins | Ready in:

Ingredients
1 pound dried lima beans
1/2 pound bacon strips, cooked and crumbled
1 can (10-3/4 ounces) condensed tomato soup, undiluted
1-1/3 cups water
1 cup packed brown sugar
1 garlic clove, minced
1 teaspoon salt
1 teaspoon paprika
1/2 teaspoon ground mustard

Direction
Sort the beans and wash; let soak following the package instructions. Let drain and wash the beans, then discard the liquid. Blend the remaining ingredients and beans in a 3-quart slow cooker. Cover and cook on low heat for 6-8 hours until the beans become tender.

Nutrition Information
Calories:
Fiber:;Total Carbohydrate:;Cholesterol:;Protein:;Total Fat:;Sodium:

654. Baked Beans With Bacon

Serving: 8 servings. | Prep: 15mins | Cook: 06hours00mins | Ready in:

Ingredients
3 cans (15 ounces each) pork and beans
1/2 cup finely chopped onion
1/2 cup chopped green pepper
1/2 cup ketchup
1/2 cup maple syrup
2 tablespoons finely chopped seeded jalapeno pepper
1/2 cup crumbled cooked bacon

Direction
Blend the first 6 ingredients in a 3-quart slow cooker. Cook, covered, on low heat until the vegetables become tender, or for 6-8 hours. Add in the bacon and stir just before serving.

Nutrition Information
Calories: 232 calories;Total Fat: 3g fat (0 saturated fat);Sodium: 932mg sodium
Fiber: 8g fiber);Total Carbohydrate: 47g carbohydrate (25g sugars;Cholesterol: 5mg cholesterol;Protein: 10g protein.

655. Barbecued Beans

Serving: 12-15 servings. | Prep: 5mins | Cook: 10hours00mins | Ready in:

Ingredients
1 pound dried navy beans
1 pound bacon strips, cooked and crumbled
1 bottle (32 ounces) tomato juice
1 can (8 ounces) tomato sauce
2 cups chopped onions
2/3 cup packed brown sugar
1 tablespoon reduced-sodium soy sauce
2 teaspoons garlic salt
1 teaspoon ground mustard
1 teaspoon Worcestershire sauce

Direction
Put beans into a large saucepan. Pour water over beans to cover by 2 inches, bring to a boil for 2 minutes. Turn off the heat; allow to stand for 60 minutes. Drain beans and pour off cooking liquid. Combine remaining ingredients in a 5-quart slow cooker. Add beans, cook, covered for 2 hours on high setting. Turn heat to low and cook until beans are tender, or for 8 to 10 hours more.

Nutrition Information
Calories: 220 calories;Protein: 11g protein.;Total Fat: 5g fat (2g saturated fat);Sodium: 762mg sodium Fiber: 8g fiber);Total Carbohydrate: 33g carbohydrate (15g sugars;Cholesterol: 8mg cholesterol

656. Black Eyed Peas Ham

Serving: 12 servings (3/4 cup each). | Prep: 20mins | Cook: 05hours00mins | Ready in:

Ingredients
1 package (16 ounces) dried black-eyed peas, rinsed and sorted
1/2 pound fully cooked boneless ham, finely chopped
1 medium onion, finely chopped
1 medium sweet red pepper, finely chopped
5 bacon strips, cooked and crumbled
1 large jalapeno pepper, seeded and finely chopped
2 garlic cloves, minced
1-1/2 teaspoons ground cumin
1 teaspoon reduced-sodium chicken bouillon granules
1/2 teaspoon salt
1/2 teaspoon cayenne pepper

1/4 teaspoon pepper
6 cups water
Minced fresh cilantro, optional
Hot cooked rice
Direction
Soak peas following the instructions of the package. Transfer peas to a slow cooker of 6-qt.; add in the next 12 components. Cover, cook until peas are soft on low setting or for 5-7 hours. If desired, dust with cilantro. Serving with rice.
Nutrition Information
Calories: 170 calories;Total Fat: 3g fat (1g saturated fat);Sodium: 386mg sodium
Fiber: 7g fiber);Total Carbohydrate: 24g carbohydrate (5g sugars;Cholesterol: 13mg cholesterol;Protein: 13g protein. Diabetic Exchanges: 1-1/2 starch

657. Boston Baked Beans

Serving: 6 | Prep: 30mins | Cook: 4hours | Ready in:
Ingredients
2 cups navy beans
1/2 pound bacon
1 onion, finely diced
3 tablespoons molasses
2 teaspoons salt
1/4 teaspoon ground black pepper
1/4 teaspoon dry mustard
1/2 cup ketchup
1 tablespoon Worcestershire sauce
1/4 cup brown sugar
Direction
Start by soaking the beans in cold water overnight. Let the beans simmer in the same water for about 1 to 2 hours until tender. Drain off the water and save the liquid.
Preheat the oven to 165 degrees C (325 degrees F). Spread beans on a two quart bean pot or casserole dish by putting some beans in the bottom of the dish and layering them with onion and bacon.
Mix together Worcestershire sauce, molasses, brown sugar, salt, dry mustard, pepper and ketchup in a saucepan. Heat the mixture to boil and then spread on top of the beans. Add enough reserved bean water just to cover beans. Use aluminum foil or a lid to cover the dish.
Bake in the preheated oven for about 3 to 4 hours until the beans become tender. Take out the lid when about halfway through the cooking process and pour in extra liquid if need be to stop beans from becoming too dry.
Nutrition Information
Calories: 382 calories;;Sodium: 1320;Total Carbohydrate: 63.1;Cholesterol: 14;Protein: 20.7;Total Fat: 6.3

658. Chuck Wagon Beans With Sausage

Serving: 24 servings (2/3 cup each). | Prep: 15mins | Cook: 08hours00mins | Ready in:
Ingredients
2 cans (28 ounces each) baked beans
3 cans (16 ounces each) kidney beans, rinsed and drained
2 cans (15 ounces each) pinto beans, rinsed and drained
1 pound Johnsonville® Fully Cooked Polish Kielbasa Sausage Rope, sliced
1 jar (12 ounces) pickled jalapeno slices, drained
1 medium onion, chopped

1 cup barbecue sauce
1/2 cup spicy brown mustard
1/4 cup steak seasoning
Direction
Mix the entire ingredients together in a greased 6-quart slow cooker, then cover and cook on low until heated through, or for about 8 to 10 hours.
Nutrition Information
Calories: 229 calories;Cholesterol: 17mg cholesterol;Protein: 11g protein.;Total Fat: 7g fat (2g saturated fat);Sodium: 1299mg sodium
Fiber: 8g fiber);Total Carbohydrate: 32g carbohydrate (3g sugars

659. Cowboy Calico Beans

Serving: 8 servings. | Prep: 30mins | Cook: 04hours00mins | Ready in:
Ingredients
1 pound lean ground beef (90% lean)
1 large sweet onion, chopped
1/2 cup packed brown sugar
1/4 cup ketchup
3 tablespoons cider vinegar
2 tablespoons yellow mustard
1 can (16 ounces) butter beans, drained
1 can (16 ounces) kidney beans, rinsed and drained
1 can (15 ounces) pork and beans
1 can (15-1/4 ounces) lima beans, rinsed and drained
Direction
Cook onion and beef in a big frying pan over medium heat until the meat is not pink anymore; strain. Remove into a 3-quart slow cooker. Stir together mustard, vinegar, ketchup, and brown sugar; put on the meat mixture. Mix in the beans. Put a cover on and cook on low until heated through, or about 4-5 hours.
Nutrition Information
Calories: 326 calories;Sodium: 808mg sodium
Fiber: 10g fiber);Total Carbohydrate: 52g carbohydrate (22g sugars;Cholesterol: 35mg cholesterol;Protein: 22g protein.;Total Fat: 5g fat (2g saturated fat)

660. Fiesta Corn And Beans

Serving: 10 servings. | Prep: 25mins | Cook: 03hours00mins | Ready in:
Ingredients
1 large onion, chopped
1 medium green pepper, cut into 1-inch pieces
1 to 2 jalapeno peppers, seeded and sliced
1 tablespoon olive oil
1 garlic clove, minced
2 cans (16 ounces each) kidney beans, rinsed and drained
1 package (16 ounces) frozen corn
1 can (14-1/2 ounces) diced tomatoes, undrained
1 teaspoon chili powder
3/4 teaspoon salt
1/2 teaspoon ground cumin
1/2 teaspoon pepper
Optional toppings: plain yogurt and sliced ripe olives
Direction
Sauté peppers and onion in oil in a large skillet until softened. Add garlic; sauté for another minute. Pour onion mixture into a 4-quart slow cooker. Mix in seasonings, tomatoes, corn, and beans.

Cook, covered for 3 to 4 hours on low setting until thoroughly heated. Serve with olives and yogurt if desired.
Nutrition Information
Calories: 149 calories;Sodium: 380mg sodium Fiber: 7g fiber);Total Carbohydrate: 28g carbohydrate (5g sugars;Cholesterol: 0 cholesterol;Protein: 8g protein. Diabetic Exchanges: 1 starch;Total Fat: 2g fat (0 saturated fat)

661. Four Bean Medley

Serving: 8-10 servings. | Prep: 40mins | Cook: 06hours00mins | Ready in:
Ingredients
8 bacon strips, diced
2 medium onions, quartered and sliced
3/4 cup packed brown sugar
1/2 cup cider vinegar
1 teaspoon salt
1 teaspoon ground mustard
1/2 teaspoon garlic powder
1 can (16 ounces) baked beans, undrained
1 can (16 ounces) kidney beans, rinsed and drained
1 can (16 ounces) butter beans, rinsed and drained
1 can (14-1/2 ounces) cut green beans, drained
Direction
Cook the bacon in a large skillet until getting crisp. Let drain and retain 2 tablespoons of drippings; put the bacon aside. Allow to sauté onions in the drippings until getting tender. Stir in garlic powder, mustard, salt, vinegar, and brown sugar.
Uncover and allow to simmer until the onions turn golden brown, or for 15 minutes. In a 3-quart slow cooker, arrange the beans. Add in the bacon and the onion mixture; blend by stirring. Cook, covered, on low heat until heated through, or for 6-7 hours. Use a slotted spoon to serve.
Nutrition Information
Calories: 297 calories;Protein: 10g protein.;Total Fat: 11g fat (4g saturated fat);Sodium: 920mg sodium Fiber: 8g fiber);Total Carbohydrate: 43g carbohydrate (23g sugars;Cholesterol: 15mg cholesterol

662. Georgian Bay Baked Beans

Serving: 12 servings. | Prep: 30mins | Cook: 10hours00mins | Ready in:
Ingredients
1 pound dried navy beans
1 pound thick-sliced bacon strips, chopped
6 medium onions, chopped
2 medium tomatoes, chopped
3 garlic cloves, minced
1 cup packed brown sugar
1 cup beef stock
1 cup strong brewed coffee
3/4 cup chili sauce
1/2 cup tomato paste
1/4 cup molasses
1 tablespoon white vinegar
1 tablespoon ground mustard
3 bay leaves
1/2 teaspoon salt
1/2 teaspoon ground cinnamon
1/2 teaspoon ground cumin
1/2 teaspoon pepper
1/4 teaspoon ground cloves
1/4 teaspoon cayenne pepper
1 smoked ham hock
Direction
Sort and wash the beans under cold water. In a large bowl, arrange the beans; pour in water to cover by 2 inches. Allow to stand, covered, overnight. Let the beans drain and wash, discard the liquid. Place into a greased 5-quart slow cooker.
Cook the bacon over medium heat in a large skillet until getting crisp. Using a slotted spoon, transfer to paper towels; let drain and retain 3 tablespoons of drippings. Let the onions brown in drippings. Add garlic and tomatoes and cook for 2 more minutes. Add to the slow cooker with the retained bacon and stir.
Blend the seasonings, bay leaves, mustard, vinegar, molasses, tomato paste, chili sauce, coffee, stock, and brown sugar. Add to the slow cooker and stir. Add ham hock. Cook, covered, on low heat setting until the beans become tender, about 10-12 hours. Discard the bay leaves. Remove the fat. Put the ham hock aside until it is cool enough to handle. Debone and discard the bone. Slice the meat into small cubes; bring back to the slow cooker. Heat through.
Nutrition Information
Calories: 399 calories;Sodium: 654mg sodium Fiber: 8g fiber);Total Carbohydrate: 62g carbohydrate (32g sugars;Cholesterol: 21mg cholesterol;Protein: 16g protein.;Total Fat: 11g fat (3g saturated fat)

663. Hawaiian Barbecue Beans

Serving: 9 servings. | Prep: 10mins | Cook: 05hours00mins | Ready in:
Ingredients
4 cans (15 ounces each) black beans, rinsed and drained
1 can (20 ounces) crushed pineapple, drained
1 bottle (18 ounces) barbecue sauce
1-1/2 teaspoons minced fresh gingerroot
1/2 pound bacon strips, cooked and crumbled
Direction
Combine ginger, barbecue sauce, pineapple, and beans in a 4-quart slow cooker. Cook, covered for 5 to 6 hours on low setting. Mix in bacon just before serving.
Nutrition Information
Calories: 286 calories;Sodium: 981mg sodium Fiber: 9g fiber);Total Carbohydrate: 47g carbohydrate (20g sugars;Cholesterol: 9mg cholesterol;Protein: 13g protein.;Total Fat: 5g fat (1g saturated fat)

664. Hearty Pork N Beans

Serving: 8 main-dish servings or 12 side-dish servings. | Prep: 15mins | Cook: 04hours00mins | Ready in:
Ingredients
1 pound ground beef
1 medium green pepper, chopped
1 small onion, chopped
1 package (16 ounces) Johnsonville® Fully Cooked Smoked Sausage Rope, halved lengthwise and thinly sliced
1 can (16 ounces) pork and beans, undrained
1 can (15-1/4 ounces) lima beans, rinsed and drained
1 can (15 ounces) pinto beans, rinsed and drained
1 cup ketchup
1/2 cup packed brown sugar
1 teaspoon salt

1/2 teaspoon garlic powder
1/4 teaspoon pepper
Direction
Cook onion, green pepper, and beef in a big frying pan over medium heat until the meat is not pink anymore; strain.
Mix the rest of the ingredients together in a 5-quart slow cooker. Mix in the beef mixture. Put the lid on and cook on high until very heated, about 4-5 hours.
Nutrition Information
Calories: 485 calories;Protein: 26g protein.;Total Fat: 21g fat (9g saturated fat);Sodium: 1757mg sodium Fiber: 7g fiber);Total Carbohydrate: 50g carbohydrate (23g sugars;Cholesterol: 66mg cholesterol

665. Partytime Beans

Serving: 16 servings (1/2 cup each). | Prep: 10mins | Cook: 05hours00mins | Ready in:
Ingredients
1-1/2 cups ketchup
1 medium onion, chopped
1 medium green pepper, chopped
1 medium sweet red pepper, chopped
1/2 cup water
1/2 cup packed brown sugar
2 bay leaves
2 to 3 teaspoons cider vinegar
1 teaspoon ground mustard
1/8 teaspoon pepper
1 can (16 ounces) kidney beans, rinsed and drained
1 can (15-1/2 ounces) great northern beans, rinsed and drained
1 can (15-1/4 ounces) lima beans
1 can (15 ounces) black beans, rinsed and drained
1 can (15-1/2 ounces) black-eyed peas, rinsed and drained
Direction
Mix the first 10 ingredients in a 5-qt. slow cooker. Add peas and beans then stir. Put a lid on and cook on low for 5 to 7 hours or till peppers and onion are soft. Remove bay leaves.
Nutrition Information
Calories: 166 calories;Total Carbohydrate: 34g carbohydrate (15g sugars;Cholesterol: 0 cholesterol;Protein: 6g protein. Diabetic Exchanges: 2 starch.;Total Fat: 0 fat (0 saturated fat);Sodium: 528mg sodium
Fiber: 7g fiber)

666. Pineapple Baked Beans

Serving: 8 servings. | Prep: 15mins | Cook: 06hours00mins | Ready in:
Ingredients
1 pound ground beef
1 can (28 ounces) baked beans
3/4 cup pineapple tidbits, drained
1 jar (4-1/2 ounces) sliced mushrooms, drained
1 large onion, chopped
1 large green pepper, chopped
1/2 cup barbecue sauce
2 tablespoons reduced-sodium soy sauce
1 garlic clove, minced
1/2 teaspoon salt
1/4 teaspoon pepper
Direction
In a large skillet over medium heat, cook beef until no longer pink inside; drain. Put cooked beef into a 5-quart slow cooker. Put the remaining ingredients into the cooker and stir to combine with beef. Cook, covered for 6 to 8 hours on low setting until bubbly.
Nutrition Information
Calories: 249 calories
Fiber: 7g fiber);Total Carbohydrate: 28g carbohydrate (6g sugars;Cholesterol: 42mg cholesterol;Protein: 17g protein.;Total Fat: 9g fat (3g saturated fat);Sodium: 1032mg sodium

667. Root Beer Apple Baked Beans

Serving: 12 servings. | Prep: 20mins | Cook: 45mins | Ready in:
Ingredients
6 thick-sliced bacon strips, chopped
4 cans (16 ounces each) baked beans
1 can (21 ounces) apple pie filling
1 can (12 ounces) root beer
1 teaspoon ground ancho chili pepper, optional
1 cup shredded smoked cheddar cheese, optional
Direction
Use 32 to 36 charcoal briquettes or large wood chips to make campfire or bring grill to medium heat. Cook bacon in 10-inch Dutch oven over the campfire until crisp. Take bacon out and discard bacon grease. Put bacon back into the pan; mix in ancho chili pepper (if using), root beer, pie filling, and baked beans; put the lid on. Once wood chips or briquettes are covered with ash, position the Dutch oven atop 16 to 18 briquettes. Arrange the remaining 16 to 18 briquettes over the lid.
Cook until flavors blend, for 30 to 40 minutes. Sprinkle with cheese before serving, if desired.
Nutrition Information
Calories: 255 calories
Fiber: 9g fiber);Total Carbohydrate: 47g carbohydrate (11g sugars;Cholesterol: 16mg cholesterol;Protein: 10g protein.;Total Fat: 5g fat (2g saturated fat);Sodium: 778mg sodium

668. Simple Vegetarian Slow Cooked Beans

Serving: 8 servings. | Prep: 15mins | Cook: 04hours00mins | Ready in:
Ingredients
4 cans (15-1/2 ounces each) great northern beans, rinsed and drained
4 medium carrots, finely chopped (about 2 cups)
1 cup vegetable stock
6 garlic cloves, minced
2 teaspoons ground cumin
3/4 teaspoon salt
1/8 teaspoon chili powder
4 cups fresh baby spinach, coarsely chopped
1 cup oil-packed sun-dried tomatoes, patted dry and chopped
1/3 cup minced fresh cilantro
1/3 cup minced fresh parsley
Direction
Mix together the first 7 ingredients in a 3-quart slow cooker. Cook on low setting with a cover until carrots are softened, or for about 4 to 5 hours while putting in tomatoes as well as spinach during the last ten minutes of cooking process. Stir in parsley and cilantro.
Nutrition Information
Calories: 229 calories;Total Carbohydrate: 40g carbohydrate (2g sugars;Cholesterol: 0

cholesterol;Protein: 12g protein.;Total Fat: 3g fat (0 saturated fat);Sodium: 672mg sodium
Fiber: 13g fiber)

669. Slow Cooker BBQ Baked Beans

Serving: 12 servings (1/2 cup each). | Prep: 10mins | Cook: 08hours30mins | Ready in:
Ingredients
1 package (16 ounces) dried great northern beans
2 smoked ham hocks (about 1/2 pound each)
2 cups water
1 medium onion, chopped
2 teaspoons garlic powder, divided
2 teaspoons onion powder, divided
1 cup barbecue sauce
3/4 cup packed brown sugar
1/2 teaspoon ground nutmeg
1/4 teaspoon ground cloves
2 teaspoons hot pepper sauce, optional
Direction
Wash and sort beans; soak following the instructions on the package. Drain and wash beans, pouring off liquid.
Combine 1 teaspoon onion powder, 1 teaspoon garlic powder, onion, water, ham hocks, and beans in a 4-quart slow cooker. Cover and cook for 8 to 10 hours on low setting until beans are tender.
Take ham hocks out of the cooker; allow to cool a bit. Dice meat into small cubes and discard bones; put meat back into the slow cooker. Mix in pepper sauce (if using), remaining onion powder, remaining garlic powder, cloves, nutmeg, brown sugar, and barbecue sauce. Cover and cook for about half an hour on high setting until thoroughly heated.
Nutrition Information
Calories: 238 calories;Total Fat: 1g fat (0 saturated fat);Sodium: 347mg sodium
Fiber: 8g fiber);Total Carbohydrate: 48g carbohydrate (22g sugars;Cholesterol: 4mg cholesterol;Protein: 10g protein.

670. Slow Cooker Calico Beans

Serving: Serves 12-16 | Prep: | Cook: | Ready in:
Ingredients
1 pound ground beef, browned and drained
1 pound bacon, cooked and crumbled
1 large onion, chopped
1/2 cup ketchup
1/3 cup firmly packed brown sugar
1 tablespoon apple cider vinegar
1 tablespoon Worcestershire sauce
1 teaspoon yellow mustard
1 teaspoon salt
1/2 teaspoon crushed red pepper flakes
1 (15-ounce) can tomato sauce
6 cups cooked mixed beans (if you like to use dried); or 2 (15-ounce) cans white beans, drained, plus 1 (15-ounce) can kidney beans, drained
Direction
Preparation: In a large slow cooker, mix all ingredients, and toss gently until well-combined. Cook on low for a minimum of 4 hours up to 8 hours. Note: If you use dried beans, you can prepare them ahead of time and let freeze in already portioned out amounts in freezer bags, this is almost as easy as opening a can for a fraction of the cost.
Nutrition Information
Calories: 547;Total Carbohydrate: 63 g(21%);Cholesterol: 44 mg(15%);Protein: 30 g(61%);Total Fat: 20 g(31%)
Saturated Fat: 7 g(35%);Sodium: 489 mg(20%)
Fiber: 14 g(55%)

671. Slow Cooker Potluck Beans

Serving: 12 servings. | Prep: 10mins | Cook: 04hours00mins | Ready in:
Ingredients
1 cup brewed coffee
1/2 cup packed brown sugar
1/4 cup spicy brown mustard
2 tablespoons molasses
2 cans (16 ounces each) butter beans
2 cans (16 ounces each) kidney beans
2 cans (16 ounces each) navy beans
Direction
Combine the first 4 ingredients in a greased 3- or 4-quart slow cooker. Let wash and drain the beans; add into the coffee mixture and stir. Cover and cook on low heat for 4-5 hours until the flavors are mixed.
Freeze option: In the freezer containers, place the cooled beans to freeze. To use: put in the fridge overnight to thaw partially. In a covered saucepan, heat through and slowly stir, if needed, pour in a little water.
Nutrition Information
Calories: 243 calories;Protein: 14g protein.;Total Fat: 0 fat (0 saturated fat);Sodium: 538mg sodium
Fiber: 10g fiber);Total Carbohydrate: 50g carbohydrate (13g sugars;Cholesterol: 0 cholesterol

672. Slow Cooked Baked Beans

Serving: 12 | Prep: 10mins | Cook: 8hours | Ready in:
Ingredients
3 cups dried navy beans
water, to cover
1 1/2 cups ketchup
1/2 pound fully cooked ham
1 1/2 cups water
1/2 cup brown sugar
1/4 cup molasses
1 1/2 tablespoons onion powder
1 tablespoon dry mustard
1 tablespoon salt
1 tablespoon Worcestershire sauce
1/4 teaspoon ground black pepper
Direction
In a big pot, put beans, pour in much water to cover. Put on lid, soak beans 8 hours or all night. Drain, pour fresh water into the pot.
Cook beans on medium heat, about 1 hour until tender. Drain beans, saving water to use later.
In a slow cooker, add 1 cup reserved beans water, black pepper, Worcestershire sauce, salt, mustard, onion powder, molasses, brown sugar, 1 1/2 cup water, ham, ketchup, and beans. If beans are too dry, add more bean water.
Choose Low setting and cook for 7-9 hours.
Nutrition Information
Calories: 302 calories;;Total Fat: 4.7;Sodium: 1185;Total Carbohydrate: 51.3;Cholesterol: 11;Protein: 16

673. Slow Cooked Bean Medley

Serving: 12 servings (3/4 cup each). | Prep: 25mins | Cook: 05hours00mins | Ready in:
Ingredients

1-1/2 cups ketchup
2 celery ribs, chopped
1 medium onion, chopped
1 medium green pepper, chopped
1 medium sweet red pepper, chopped
1/2 cup packed brown sugar
1/2 cup water
1/2 cup Italian salad dressing
2 bay leaves
1 tablespoon cider vinegar
1 teaspoon ground mustard
1/8 teaspoon pepper
1 can (16 ounces) kidney beans, rinsed and drained
1 can (15-1/2 ounces) black-eyed peas, rinsed and drained
1 can (15-1/2 ounces) great northern beans, rinsed and drained
1 can (15-1/4 ounces) whole kernel corn, drained
1 can (15-1/4 ounces) lima beans, rinsed and drained
1 can (15 ounces) black beans, rinsed and drained
Direction
Combine into a slow cooker of 5-qt. the first 12 ingredients. Stir in the remaining ingredients. Cook covered until onion and peppers are soft on low setting or for 5-6 hours. Remove bay leaves.
Nutrition Information
Calories: 255 calories;Sodium: 942mg sodium Fiber: 7g fiber);Total Carbohydrate: 45g carbohydrate (21g sugars;Cholesterol: 0 cholesterol;Protein: 9g protein.;Total Fat: 4g fat (0 saturated fat)

674. Slow Cooked Calico Beans

Serving: 10 servings. | Prep: 30mins | Cook: 06hours00mins | Ready in:
Ingredients
1 pound ground beef
2 cans (16 ounces each) baked beans
1 can (16 ounces) kidney beans, rinsed and drained
1 can (15 ounces) white kidney or cannellini beans, rinsed and drained
1 can (20 ounces) unsweetened crushed pineapple, drained
1 medium onion, finely chopped
1/2 cup packed brown sugar
1/2 cup ketchup
2 tablespoons cider vinegar
1 tablespoon Dijon mustard
1/2 pound bacon strips, cooked and crumbled
Direction
Cook the beef over medium heat in a large skillet until no pink remains; let drain. Put into a 4-quart slow cooker. Put in the mustard, vinegar, ketchup, brown sugar, onion, pineapple, and beans.
Cook, covered, on low heat setting until heated through, about 6-8 hours. Add the bacon and stir just before serving.
Nutrition Information
Calories: 385 calories;Cholesterol: 43mg cholesterol;Protein: 20g protein.;Total Fat: 10g fat (4g saturated fat);Sodium: 863mg sodium Fiber: 9g fiber);Total Carbohydrate: 55g carbohydrate (23g sugars

675. Slow Cooked Pork Beans

Serving: 12 servings (3/4 cup each). | Prep: 25mins | Cook: 06hours00mins | Ready in:
Ingredients

1 package (1 pound) sliced bacon, chopped
1 cup chopped onion
2 cans (15 ounces each) pork and beans, undrained
1 can (16 ounces) kidney beans, rinsed and drained
1 can (16 ounces) butter beans, rinsed and drained
1 can (15-1/4 ounces) lima beans, rinsed and drained
1 can (15 ounces) black beans, rinsed and drained
1 cup packed brown sugar
1/2 cup cider vinegar
1 tablespoon molasses
2 teaspoons garlic powder
1/2 teaspoon ground mustard
Direction
Cook the onion and bacon in a large skillet on medium heat until the bacon becomes crisp. Transfer onto paper towels to drain.
Blend the remaining ingredients in a 4-quart slow cooker; add in the bacon mixture and stir. Cook, covered, on low heat until heated through, or for 6-8 hours.
Nutrition Information
Calories: 319 calories
Fiber: 9g fiber);Total Carbohydrate: 54g carbohydrate (24g sugars;Cholesterol: 11mg cholesterol;Protein: 14g protein.;Total Fat: 7g fat (2g saturated fat);Sodium: 802mg sodium

676. Smoky Baked Beans

Serving: 8 | Prep: 25mins | Cook: | Ready in:
Ingredients
6 slices bacon, chopped
¾ cup chopped green sweet pepper (1 medium)
½ cup chopped onion (1 medium)
2 cloves garlic, minced
1 (15 ounce) can no-salt-added black beans, rinsed and drained
1 (15 ounce) can no-salt-added butter beans or cannellini beans (white kidney beans), rinsed and drained
1 (15 ounce) can no-salt-added red kidney beans, rinsed and drained
1 (8 ounce) can no-salt-added tomato sauce
¼ cup orange juice
2 tablespoons packed brown sugar or sugar substitute equivalent to 2 tablespoons (see Tip)
1 tablespoon Worcestershire sauce
1 fresh jalapeño chile pepper, seeded and finely chopped (see Tip)
Crisp-cooked bacon, crumbled (optional)
Direction
Set oven to 375°F to preheat. Sauté garlic, onion, sweet pepper, and chopped bacon in a large skillet over medium heat until onion is softened and bacon is crispy, or about 10 minutes; drain off fat.
Combine chile pepper, Worcestershire sauce, brown sugar, orange juice, tomato sauce, kidney beans, butter beans, black beans, and bacon mixture in a large bowl. Ladle bean mixture into a 1 1/2-quart casserole.
Cover and bake, stirring one time halfway through baking, for 60 minutes. Garnish with crumbled bacon on top, if desired.
Nutrition Information
Calories: 218 calories;
Saturated Fat: 2;Sodium: 168
Sugar: 7;Total Fat: 6;Cholesterol: 9;Total Carbohydrate: 31;Protein: 11

Fiber: 10

677. Sweet Hot Baked Beans

Serving: 14 servings (1/2 cup each). | Prep: 20mins | Cook: 05hours00mins | Ready in:
Ingredients
4 cans (15 ounces each) white kidney or cannellini beans, rinsed and drained
2 cans (8 ounces each) crushed pineapple, undrained
2 large onions, finely chopped
1 cup packed brown sugar
1 cup ketchup
10 bacon strips, cooked and crumbled
1/2 cup molasses
1/4 cup canned diced jalapeno peppers
2 tablespoons white vinegar
4 garlic cloves, minced
4 teaspoons ground mustard
1/4 teaspoon ground cloves
Direction
Mix all of the ingredients together in a 3-4-qt. slow cooker. Put a cover on and cook on low until very heated, about 5-6 hours.
Nutrition Information
Calories: 273 calories;Total Fat: 3g fat (1g saturated fat);Sodium: 489mg sodium
Fiber: 5g fiber);Total Carbohydrate: 55g carbohydrate (35g sugars;Cholesterol: 6mg cholesterol;Protein: 7g protein.

678. Sweet Spicy Beans

Serving: 12 servings (2/3 cup each). | Prep: 10mins | Cook: 05hours00mins | Ready in:
Ingredients
1 can (16 ounces) kidney beans, rinsed and drained
1 can (15-1/4 ounces) whole kernel corn, drained
1 can (15 ounces) garbanzo beans or chickpeas, rinsed and drained
1 can (15 ounces) black beans, rinsed and drained
1 can (15 ounces) chili with beans
1 cup barbecue sauce
1 cup salsa
1/3 cup packed brown sugar
1/4 teaspoon hot pepper sauce
Chopped green onions, optional
Direction
In a 4- to 5-quart slow cooker, blend the first nine ingredients. Cook, covered, on low about 5 to 6 hours. Sprinkle with green onions if wanted.
Nutrition Information
Calories: 201 calories;Total Fat: 2g fat (0 saturated fat);Sodium: 712mg sodium
Fiber: 7g fiber);Total Carbohydrate: 36g carbohydrate (13g sugars;Cholesterol: 4mg cholesterol;Protein: 9g protein.

679. Sweet N Sour Beans

Serving: 20 servings (1/2 cup each). | Prep: 20mins | Cook: 03hours00mins | Ready in:
Ingredients
8 bacon strips, diced
2 medium onions, halved and thinly sliced
1 cup packed brown sugar
1/2 cup cider vinegar
1 teaspoon salt
1 teaspoon ground mustard
1/2 teaspoon garlic powder
1 can (28 ounces) baked beans, undrained
1 can (16 ounces) kidney beans, rinsed and drained
1 can (15 ounces) pinto beans, rinsed and drained
1 can (15 ounces) lima beans, rinsed and drained
1 can (15-1/2 ounces) black-eyed peas, rinsed and drained
Direction
In a large frying pan, cook bacon over medium heat till crisp. Use a slotted spoon to transfer to paper towels. Drain while keeping 2 tablespoons drippings. Sauté onions in the drippings until softened. Add garlic powder, mustard, salt, vinegar and brown sugar. Allow to boil.
In a 5-qt. slow cooker, mix peas and beans. Add bacon and onion mixture, then stir well. Cover and cook on High for about 3 - 4 hours, or until heated through.
Nutrition Information
Calories:;Total Fat:;Sodium:
Fiber:;Total Carbohydrate:;Cholesterol:;Protein:

680. Sweet And Tangy Ranch Beans

Serving: 8-10 servings. | Prep: 10mins | Cook: 03hours00mins | Ready in:
Ingredients
1 can (16 ounces) kidney beans, rinsed and drained
1 can (15-3/4 ounces) pork and beans, undrained
1 can (15 ounces) lima beans, rinsed and drained
1 can (14-1/2 ounces) cut green beans, drained
1 bottle (12 ounces) chili sauce
3/4 cup packed brown sugar
1 small onion, chopped
Direction
Blend all the ingredients in a 3-quart slow cooker. Cook, covered, on high heat setting until heated through, about 3-4 hours.
Nutrition Information
Calories: 264 calories;Protein: 8g protein.;Total Fat: 0 fat (0 saturated fat);Sodium: 1300mg sodium
Fiber: 8g fiber);Total Carbohydrate: 60g carbohydrate (34g sugars;Cholesterol: 0 cholesterol

681. Tangy Cranberry Beans

Serving: 10 servings. | Prep: 20mins | Cook: 06hours00mins | Ready in:
Ingredients
3 cups dried navy beans
4 cups unsweetened cranberry juice
1/2 pound bacon strips, cooked and crumbled
1 medium onion, chopped
1/2 cup ketchup
1/3 cup packed brown sugar
1/4 cup molasses
1-1/2 teaspoons salt
1-1/2 teaspoons ground mustard
1/8 teaspoon ground ginger
Direction
Wash beans and put into a saucepan. Pour in water to cover the beans by 2 inches. Bring to a boil; boil for 2 minutes. Put off the heat; cover and allow beans to steep for 1 to 4 hours. Drain off water and rinse beans; pour off cooking liquid. Pour beans into a 4-quart slow cooker. Mix in remaining ingredients. Cover and cook for 6 to 8 hours on low setting until beans are tender.
Nutrition Information
Calories: 349 calories;Sodium: 671mg sodium
Fiber: 10g fiber);Total Carbohydrate: 63g carbohydrate (23g sugars;Cholesterol: 8mg cholesterol;Protein: 17g protein.;Total Fat: 4g fat (1g saturated fat)

Chapter 8: Rib Slow Cooker Recipes

682. "Secret's In The Sauce" BBQ Ribs
Serving: 5 servings. | Prep: 10mins | Cook: 06hours00mins | Ready in:
Ingredients
4-1/2 pounds pork baby back ribs
1-1/2 teaspoons pepper
2-1/2 cups barbecue sauce
3/4 cup cherry preserves
1 tablespoon Dijon mustard
1 garlic clove, minced
Direction
Slice ribs into serving-sized pieces; sprinkle pepper over. Put into a 5- or 6-qt. slow cooker. Mix together the remaining ingredients; transfer over the ribs. Cook with a cover on low for 6-8 hours, till the meat becomes tender. Serve with the sauce.
Nutrition Information
Calories: 921 calories
Fiber: 2g fiber);Total Carbohydrate: 50g carbohydrate (45g sugars;Cholesterol: 220mg cholesterol;Protein: 48g protein.;Total Fat: 58g fat (21g saturated fat);Sodium: 1402mg sodium

683. 4Switch And Go Ribs
Serving: 4 servings. | Prep: 10mins | Cook: 06hours00mins | Ready in:
Ingredients
1-1/2 pounds boneless country-style pork ribs
1 tablespoon canola oil
1/3 cup orange marmalade
1/3 cup teriyaki sauce
1 teaspoon minced garlic
Direction
Brown the ribs on both sides in oil into a large skillet. Combine garlic, teriyaki sauce and marmalade in small bowl.
Add 1/2 sauce to a 3 quarts slow cooker. Place ribs on top. Drizzle the remaining sauce over. Cook, with cover, on low until meat becomes tender, about 6 to 8 hours.
Nutrition Information
Calories: 382 calories;Cholesterol: 98mg cholesterol;Protein: 31g protein.;Total Fat: 19g fat (6g saturated fat);Sodium: 899mg sodium
Fiber: 0 fiber);Total Carbohydrate: 21g carbohydrate (20g sugars

684. 5 Ingredient Chinese Pork Ribs
Serving: 6 servings. | Prep: 10mins | Cook: 06hours00mins | Ready in:
Ingredients
1/4 cup reduced-sodium soy sauce
1/3 cup reduced-sugar orange marmalade
3 tablespoons ketchup
2 garlic cloves, minced
3 to 4 pounds bone-in country-style pork ribs
Direction
Combine garlic, ketchup, marmalade, and soy sauce in a small bowl. Put 1/2 into a 5-qt. slow cooker. Arrange the ribs on top; scatter with the remaining sauce. Cook, covered, on low until soft, or for 6 hours. If desired, thicken the cooking juices.
Nutrition Information
Calories: 273 calories;Total Carbohydrate: 8g carbohydrate (6g sugars;Cholesterol: 86mg cholesterol;Protein: 27g protein.;Total Fat: 14g fat (5g saturated fat);Sodium: 562mg sodium
Fiber: 0 fiber)

685. BBQ Country Style Ribs
Serving: 8 servings | Prep: 25mins | Cook: | Ready in:
Ingredients
1 qt. (4 cups) water
1/2 cup KRAFT Original Barbecue Sauce
1/3 cup KOOL-AID Orange Flavor Sugar-Sweetened Drink Mix
1 Tbsp. oil
3 lb. bone-in country-style pork ribs, separated into single ribs
Direction
In large saucepan or Dutch oven, combine all the ingredients except the ribs until they are blended. Put in the ribs. Boil on medium heat. Simmer, with cover, on medium-low heat until meat is tender, about 90 minutes.
Uncover and cook until no liquid remains, about 20 minutes. Lower the heat to medium-low and cook, turning frequently until ribs brown evenly, about 10-12 minutes.
Nutrition Information
Calories: 280;Cholesterol: 75 mg;Protein: 20 g
Saturated Fat: 5 g
Fiber: 0 g
Sugar: 14 g;Total Carbohydrate: 15 g;Total Fat: 15 g;Sodium: 200 mg

686. Baby Back Ribs
Serving: 4 | Prep: 8hours | Cook: 2hours30mins | Ready in:
Ingredients
2 pounds pork baby back ribs
1 (18 ounce) bottle barbecue sauce
Direction
Prepare four big sheets of aluminum foil just enough to wrap each rib portion; grease each piece using vegetable cooking spray. Slather barbecue sauce over every portion of ribs and wrap each rib tightly with the prepared foil. Place in the refrigerator minimum of 8 hrs up to overnight.
Preheat the oven to 300°Fahrenheit or 150°Celcius
Place foiled ribs in the preheated oven and bake for 2 1/2 hrs. Take ribs out of the foil. If desired, pour in additional sauce.
Nutrition Information
Calories: 697 calories;Protein: 43.2;Total Fat: 37.4;Sodium: 1607;Total Carbohydrate: 45.7;Cholesterol: 170

687. Barbecue Country Ribs
Serving: 10 servings. | Prep: 15mins | Cook: 05hours00mins | Ready in:
Ingredients
4 pounds boneless country-style pork ribs
1 bottle (12 ounces) chili sauce
1 cup ketchup
1/2 cup packed brown sugar
1/3 cup balsamic vinegar
2 tablespoons Worcestershire sauce
2 teaspoons onion powder
1 teaspoon salt
1 teaspoon garlic powder
1 teaspoon chili powder
1 teaspoon pepper
1/2 teaspoon hot pepper sauce, optional
1/4 teaspoon Liquid Smoke, optional

Direction
Put the ribs in a slow cooker (5 quarts in size). Mix Liquid Smoke (if desired), pepper sauce, seasonings, Worcestershire sauce, vinegar, brown sugar, ketchup and chili sauce; drizzle over ribs.
Cover and cook for 5 to 6 hours on low until meat is soft.
Nutrition Information
Calories: 396 calories;Cholesterol: 104mg cholesterol;Protein: 32g protein.;Total Fat: 17g fat (6g saturated fat);Sodium: 1211mg sodium Fiber: 0 fiber);Total Carbohydrate: 29g carbohydrate (26g sugars

688. Barbecued Beef Ribs

Serving: Serves 2 | Prep: | Cook: | Ready in:
Ingredients
3 pounds beef ribs from the loin (about 7 meaty ribs)
1 large garlic clove, minced
1 tablespoon vegetable oil
1/3 cup ketchup
2 tablespoons Worcestershire sauce
1 teaspoon curry powder
Direction
Prep grill.
Steam beef ribs for 20 minutes on steamer rack set above simmering water, covered.
Cook garlic in oil in small saucepan on moderately low heat till golden, mixing, as ribs steam; mix curry powder, Worcestershire sauce and ketchup in. Simmer for 1 minute till slightly thick.
Put ribs on big plate; sprinkle pepper and salt to taste.
Grill the ribs on rack set 5-6-in. above glowing coals for 2-3 minutes, meat sides down, till golden. Grill ribs on edges for 2 minutes per edge till golden; grill for 3 minutes, bone sides down, till golden.
Brush barbecue sauce on ribs; grill for 1 minute per side till barley charred, continuing to baste.
Nutrition Information
Calories: 2409
Fiber: 1 g(3%);Total Carbohydrate: 22 g(7%);Cholesterol: 517 mg(172%);Protein: 108 g(216%);Total Fat: 211 g(324%)
Saturated Fat: 91 g(455%);Sodium: 891 mg(37%)

689. Beef Short Ribs Vindaloo

Serving: 4 servings. | Prep: 30mins | Cook: 08hours15mins | Ready in:
Ingredients
1 tablespoon cumin seeds
2 teaspoons coriander seeds
1 tablespoon butter
1 medium onion, finely chopped
8 garlic cloves, minced
1 tablespoon minced fresh gingerroot
2 teaspoons mustard seed
1/2 teaspoon ground cloves
1/4 teaspoon kosher salt
1/4 teaspoon ground cinnamon
1/4 teaspoon cayenne pepper
1/2 cup red wine vinegar
4 bay leaves
2 pounds bone-in beef short ribs
1 cup fresh sugar snap peas, halved
Hot cooked rice and plain yogurt
Direction
In a small, dry frying pan over medium heat, toast coriander seeds and cumin while stirring often, until fragrant. Let cool. Use a spice grinder, or a mortar and pestle to coarsely crush seeds.
In a big saucepan, heat butter over medium heat. Put in the ginger, garlic and onion; cook and stir for about 1 minute. Put in the crushed seeds, cayenne pepper, cinnamon, salt, cloves and mustard seed; cook and stir for 1 more minute. Allow to cool completely.
In a big resealable plastic bag, combine the onion mixture, bay leaves and vinegar. Put in ribs; seal the bag and flip to coat. Let it refrigerate overnight.
Move the rib mixture into a 4-quart slow cooker. Cook with cover on Low for 8-10 hours, or till meat becomes soft. Mix in peas; cook for 8-10 minutes more, or until peas become crisp-tender. Scoop off fat; eliminate bay leaves. Serve rib mixture along with yogurt and rice.
Nutrition Information
Calories: 266 calories;Total Carbohydrate: 13g carbohydrate (4g sugars;Cholesterol: 62mg cholesterol;Protein: 21g protein.;Total Fat: 15g fat (6g saturated fat);Sodium: 180mg sodium Fiber: 3g fiber)

690. Braised Beef Short Ribs

Serving: 10 | Prep: 15mins | Cook: 2hours40mins | Ready in:
Ingredients
1/2 cup all-purpose flour for coating
2 teaspoons salt
1 pinch ground black pepper
4 pounds beef short ribs
2 tablespoons vegetable oil
1 cup water
1 cup stewed tomatoes
1 clove garlic, minced
6 potatoes, peeled and cubed
3 onions, chopped
6 carrots, chopped
1 1/2 tablespoons all-purpose flour
4 tablespoons water
Direction
Mix ground black pepper, salt and 1/2 cup flour in a bowl. In the seasoned flour, turn the ribs.
Heat the oil and brown the all sides of ribs well in a Dutch oven or big pot. Put in garlic, tomatoes and a cup of boiling water. Turn heat to low, put cover, and let simmer for 1 1/2 hours, putting additional water if needed.
In the pot, put carrots, onions and potatoes. Keep simmering for 30 minutes to 1 hour longer, or till every vegetable are soft. Take off vegetables and meat to a serving platter.
In another small bowl, dissolve two tablespoons water and 1 1/2 tablespoons flour for each cup liquid left in pot. Put the mixture to pot and mix thoroughly till thickened. Put on top of vegetables and meat.
Nutrition Information
Calories: 889 calories;;Total Fat: 68.8;Sodium: 646;Total Carbohydrate: 36.3;Cholesterol: 138;Protein: 30.4

691. Brazilian Pork Black Bean Stew

Serving: 8 servings. | Prep: 15mins | Cook: 07hours00mins | Ready in:
Ingredients
1-1/2 cups dried black beans
1 pound Johnsonville® Fully Cooked Polish Kielbasa Sausage Rope, sliced

1 pound boneless country-style pork ribs
1 package (12 ounces) fully cooked Spanish chorizo links, sliced
1 smoked ham hock
1 large onion, chopped
3 garlic cloves, minced
2 bay leaves
3/4 teaspoon salt
1/2 teaspoon pepper
5 cups water
Hot cooked rice

Direction
Wash and sort beans; follow the directions in the package to soak properly. Strain and rinse, completely remove soaking liquid.
Mix beans together with the next 9 ingredients in a 6-qt. slow cooker. Put in water; cook on low heat with a cover for 7-9 hours, until beans and meat are tender. Discard ham hock and pork ribs. Separate meat from bones when cool enough to handle; remove the bay leaves and bones. Using 2 forks, shred meat and return to the slow cooker. Coupled with hot cooked rice. Serve.
For freezing option: Place cooled stew in freezer containers. For use, place in a refrigerator overnight to partially unfreeze. In a saucepan, heat through while occasionally stirring and including in a little water if needed.

Nutrition Information
Calories: 531 calories;Sodium: 1069mg sodium Fiber: 6g fiber);Total Carbohydrate: 27g carbohydrate (3g sugars;Cholesterol: 101mg cholesterol;Protein: 33g protein.;Total Fat: 33g fat (11g saturated fat)

692. Busy Day Barbecued Ribs

Serving: 6-8 servings. | Prep: 10mins | Cook: 05hours00mins | Ready in:

Ingredients
3-1/2 to 4 pounds bone-in country-style pork ribs
1 can (10-3/4 ounces) condensed tomato soup, undiluted
1/2 cup packed brown sugar
1/3 cup cider vinegar
1 tablespoon soy sauce
1 teaspoon celery seed
1 teaspoon chili powder

Direction
In a 5-quart slow cooker, put the ribs. Mix remaining ingredients then add over the ribs.
Cook, with cover, for 60 minutes on high. Turn the heat to low; cook longer until meat becomes tender, about 4 to 5 hours. If desired, thicken the cooking liquid.

Nutrition Information
Calories: 286 calories;Sodium: 404mg sodium Fiber: 1g fiber);Total Carbohydrate: 20g carbohydrate (17g sugars;Cholesterol: 76mg cholesterol;Protein: 24g protein.;Total Fat: 12g fat (4g saturated fat)

693. Caribbean Beef Short Ribs

Serving: 8 servings. | Prep: 30mins | Cook: 05hours30mins | Ready in:

Ingredients
3 pounds boneless beef short ribs, cut into 1-1/2-inch pieces
1/4 cup olive oil
2/3 cup thawed pineapple juice concentrate
2/3 cup reduced-sodium soy sauce
1/2 cup water
1/3 cup rum
1/3 cup honey
2 tablespoons minced fresh gingerroot
6 garlic cloves, minced
2 teaspoons pepper
1 teaspoon ground allspice
1/2 teaspoon salt
2 large sweet red peppers, chopped
2 cups cubed fresh pineapple
2 cups cubed peeled mango
6 green onions, cut into 1-inch pieces
2 tablespoons cornstarch
2 tablespoons cold water
Lettuce leaves

Direction
Brown ribs in oil in batches on all sides in a big skillet. Move to a slow cooker of 4 quart.
Put to the skillet the salt, allspice, pepper, garlic, ginger, honey, rum, water, soy sauce and pineapple juice concentrate. Take to a boil; lower the heat and simmer for 5 minutes. Drizzle over ribs.
Cover and cook for 5-6 hours at low or until meat is soft. Toss in the red peppers. Top with the onions, mango and pineapple (don't mix). Cover and cook for another 30 minutes or until heated through.
Transfer beef mixture to a big bowl; keep warm. Move cooking juices to a small saucepan. Mix cold water and cornstarch until smooth; stir in pan gradually. Take to a boil; cook and mix until thicken, about 2 minutes. Enjoy beef mixture on lettuce; pour the gravy over.

Nutrition Information
Calories: 450 calories;Protein: 26g protein.;Total Fat: 20g fat (7g saturated fat);Sodium: 1004mg sodium Fiber: 3g fiber);Total Carbohydrate: 42g carbohydrate (34g sugars;Cholesterol: 68mg cholesterol

694. Chinese Pork Ribs

Serving: 6 | Prep: 10mins | Cook: 3hours | Ready in:

Ingredients
1/4 cup soy sauce
1/3 cup orange marmalade
3 tablespoons ketchup
1 tablespoon rice wine
1 tablespoon sesame oil
4 cloves garlic, minced
3 pounds bone-in country style pork ribs

Direction
In a bowl, mix together garlic, sesame oil, rice wine, ketchup, marmalade, and soy sauce. Pour 1/2 of the sauce to a slow cooker, put the ribs on top. Drizzle the leftover sauce over.
Put the lid on and cook on low for 3 hours until the pork is soft. If you want, in a small skillet, thicken the cooking juices over medium heat.

Nutrition Information
Calories: 354 calories;;Sodium: 753;Total Carbohydrate: 15.3;Cholesterol: 102;Protein: 27.3;Total Fat: 19.9

695. Chinese Style Ribs

Serving: 6 servings. | Prep: 20mins | Cook: 06hours00mins | Ready in:

Ingredients
3 pounds boneless country-style pork ribs
6 green onions, cut into 1-inch pieces

1 can (8 ounces) sliced water chestnuts, drained
3/4 cup hoisin sauce
3 tablespoons soy sauce
2 tablespoons sherry or chicken stock
5 garlic cloves, minced
1 tablespoon minced fresh gingerroot
1 tablespoon light corn syrup
1 tablespoon orange marmalade
1 teaspoon pumpkin pie spice
1/2 teaspoon crushed red pepper flakes
2 tablespoons cornstarch
2 tablespoons water
Hot cooked rice
Additional sliced green onions, optional
Direction
In a 5-qt. slow cooker, place water chestnuts, green onions and pork. In a bowl, combine pepper flakes, pie spice, marmalade, corn syrup, gingerroot, garlic, sherry, soy sauce and hoisin sauce. Transfer over pork. Cook with a cover on low for 6-8 hours, till the meat turns tender.
Transfer onto a serving platter and keep warm. Skim off the fat from cooking juices; pour into a small saucepan. Boil the liquid. Stir water and cornstarch together till smooth. Slowly mix into the saucepan. Boil the mixture; cook while stirring for around 2 minutes, till thickened. Serve with rice, ribs and more green onions if you like.
Nutrition Information
Calories:;Protein:;Total Fat:;Sodium: Fiber:;Total Carbohydrate:;Cholesterol:

696. Coffee Braised Short Ribs

Serving: 8 servings. | Prep: 25mins | Cook: 06hours00mins | Ready in:
Ingredients
4 pounds bone-in beef short ribs
1-1/2 teaspoons salt, divided
1 teaspoon ground coriander
1/2 teaspoon pepper
2 tablespoons olive oil
1-1/2 pounds small red potatoes, cut in half
1 medium onion, chopped
1 cup reduced-sodium beef broth
1 whole garlic bulb, cloves separated, peeled and slightly crushed
4 cups strong brewed coffee
2 teaspoons red wine vinegar
3 tablespoons butter
Direction
Scatter pepper, coriander and 1 teaspoon salt on ribs. Brown ribs in oil in batches in a big skillet. Move ribs to a 6-quart slow cooker using tongs. Put in onion and potatoes.
Put broth to the skillet, stir to loosen browned bits. Take to a boil; cook until liquid is decreased by half. Toss in leftover salt and garlic; place to the slow cooker. Pour coffee on top. Cover and cook for 6-8 hours at low, until meat is soft.
Transfer potatoes and ribs to a serving plate; keep warm. In a small saucepan, strain cooking juices; skim the fat. Take to a boil; cook till liquid is decreased by half. Mix in vinegar. Take off from heat; stir in butter. Enjoy with ribs and potatoes.
Nutrition Information
Calories: 320 calories
Fiber: 2g fiber);Total Carbohydrate: 17g carbohydrate (2g sugars;Cholesterol: 66mg cholesterol;Protein: 21g protein.;Total Fat: 18g fat (8g saturated fat);Sodium: 569mg sodium

697. Cola Barbecue Ribs

Serving: 4 servings. | Prep: 10mins | Cook: 09hours00mins | Ready in:
Ingredients
1/4 cup packed brown sugar
2 garlic cloves, minced
1 teaspoon salt
1/2 teaspoon pepper
3 tablespoons liquid smoke, optional
4 pounds pork spareribs, cut into serving-size pieces
1 medium onion, sliced
1/2 cup cola
1-1/2 cups barbecue sauce
Direction
Mix pepper, salt, garlic and brown sugar and liquid smoke (if desired) in a small bowl; rub over ribs.
In a greased 5 to 6-quarts slow cooker, layer onion and ribs; drizzle cola over ribs. Cover and cook for 8 to 10 hours on low, until the ribs are soft. Drain liquid. Pour the sauce on top of ribs and cook for another hour.
Nutrition Information
Calories: 999 calories;Sodium: 1650mg sodium
Fiber: 2g fiber);Total Carbohydrate: 34g carbohydrate (31g sugars;Cholesterol: 255mg cholesterol;Protein: 64g protein.;Total Fat: 66g fat (24g saturated fat)

698. Contest Winning Braised Short Ribs

Serving: 7 servings. | Prep: 20mins | Cook: 06hours00mins | Ready in:
Ingredients
1/2 cup all-purpose flour
1-1/2 teaspoons salt
1-1/2 teaspoons paprika
1/2 teaspoon ground mustard
4 pounds bone-in beef short ribs
2 tablespoons canola oil
2 medium onions, sliced
1 cup beer or beef broth
1 garlic clove, minced
GRAVY:
2 teaspoons all-purpose flour
1 tablespoon cold water
Direction
Mix mustard, paprika, salt and flour together in a big resealable plastic bag. Put in ribs in batches then shake to coat. Brown ribs in oil in a big skillet; drain. Position onions in a slow cooker of 5 quart; put in ribs. Add garlic and beer on top. Cover and cook for 6-7 hours on low, until meat is soft.
Place onions and ribs on a serving plate; keep warm. Skim fat from cooking juices; move to a small pan. Take to a boil. Mix water and flour until smooth; stir into the pan gradually. Take to a boil; cook and stir until thickened, about 2 minutes. Enjoy with ribs.
Nutrition Information
Calories: 281 calories;Sodium: 547mg sodium
Fiber: 1g fiber);Total Carbohydrate: 12g carbohydrate (4g sugars;Cholesterol: 62mg cholesterol;Protein: 22g protein.;Total Fat: 14g fat (5g saturated fat)

699. Country Ribs Dinner

Serving: 4 servings. | Prep: 10mins | Cook: 06hours15mins | Ready in:

Ingredients
2 pounds boneless country-style pork ribs
1/2 teaspoon salt
1/4 teaspoon pepper
8 small red potatoes (about 1 pound), halved
4 medium carrots, cut into 1-inch pieces
3 celery ribs, cut into 1/2-inch pieces
1 medium onion, coarsely chopped
3/4 cup water
1 garlic clove, crushed
1 can (10-3/4 ounces) condensed cream of mushroom soup, undiluted
Direction
Season ribs with pepper and salt; remove ribs to a 4-quart slow cooker. Add garlic, water, onion, celery, carrots, and potatoes. Cover and cook for 6 to 8 hours on low setting until vegetables and meat are tender. Take vegetables and meat out of the cooker; ladle fat off cooking liquid. Stir soup into the cooking liquid; place vegetables and meat back into the cooker; cover and cook for 15 to 30 minutes more or until heated through.
Nutrition Information
Calories: 528 calories;Sodium: 1016mg sodium Fiber: 6g fiber);Total Carbohydrate: 30g carbohydrate (6g sugars;Cholesterol: 134mg cholesterol;Protein: 43g protein.;Total Fat: 25g fat (8g saturated fat)

700. Country Style Ribs
Serving: 4 servings. | Prep: 15mins | Cook: 05hours30mins | Ready in:
Ingredients
1-1/2 pounds boneless country-style pork ribs
1 medium onion, sliced
2 cups tomato juice
1/2 cup packed brown sugar
1/4 cup cider vinegar
1/4 cup ketchup
2 tablespoons Worcestershire sauce
1 teaspoon ground mustard
1/4 teaspoon chili powder
Direction
Put onion and ribs in a slow cooker of 3 quarts. Mix together the remaining ingredients in a small bowl. Drizzle over ribs. Cover and cook for 5 1/2 to 6 hours on low, until a thermometer shows 160°.
Nutrition Information
Calories: 434 calories;Total Fat: 16g fat (6g saturated fat);Sodium: 686mg sodium
Fiber: 1g fiber);Total Carbohydrate: 42g carbohydrate (38g sugars;Cholesterol: 98mg cholesterol;Protein: 31g protein.

701. Country Style Barbecue Ribs
Serving: 10 servings. | Prep: 15mins | Cook: 03hours00mins | Ready in:
Ingredients
2 tablespoons paprika
2 tablespoons brown sugar
2 teaspoons salt
2 teaspoons garlic powder
2 teaspoons chili powder
1 teaspoon onion powder
1 teaspoon ground chipotle pepper
1 teaspoon pepper
3/4 teaspoon dried thyme
4 pounds boneless country-style pork ribs
1 bottle (18 ounces) barbecue sauce
3/4 cup amber beer or reduced-sodium chicken broth
Direction
Preheat the broiler. Blend the first nine ingredients together. In a foil-lined 15x10x1-inch pan, place the pork and generously rub with seasonings. Broil 4-5 inches away from heat for 2 – 3 minutes each side until browned.
Move into a 5-quart slow cooker. Whisk beer and barbecue sauce together; spread over ribs. Cook while covered on Low for 3 – 4 hours until softened. Take the ribs out. Keep 2 cups of cooking juices and get rid of the leftover juices. Drain fat from the reserved juices. Serve with ribs.
Nutrition Information
Calories: 393 calories;Sodium: 1098mg sodium Fiber: 1g fiber);Total Carbohydrate: 26g carbohydrate (20g sugars;Cholesterol: 105mg cholesterol;Protein: 33g protein.;Total Fat: 17g fat (6g saturated fat)

702. Cranberry Ginger Pork Ribs
Serving: 8 servings. | Prep: 20mins | Cook: 05hours00mins | Ready in:
Ingredients
1 can (14 ounces) whole-berry cranberry sauce
2 habanero peppers, seeded and minced
4-1/2 teaspoons minced grated gingerroot
3 garlic cloves, minced
2-1/2 pounds boneless country-style pork ribs
1/2 teaspoon salt
1/2 teaspoon cayenne pepper
1/2 teaspoon pepper
2 tablespoons olive oil
Hot cooked rice
Direction
Mix garlic, ginger, habanero peppers and cranberry sauce together in a small bowl. Sprinkle peppers and salt onto the ribs. Brown the ribs on all sides in a large skillet with oil; strain.
Remove into a 3-qt. slow cooker; transfer the cranberry mixture over the ribs. Cook with a cover on low till the meat turns tender, or for 5-6 hours. Trim fat from cooking juices. Serve with rice and pork.
Nutrition Information
Calories: 334 calories;Protein: 25g protein.;Total Fat: 16g fat (5g saturated fat);Sodium: 220mg sodium Fiber: 1g fiber);Total Carbohydrate: 21g carbohydrate (13g sugars;Cholesterol: 81mg cholesterol

703. Crazy Delicious Baby Back Ribs
Serving: 8 servings. | Prep: 15mins | Cook: 05hours15mins | Ready in:
Ingredients
2 tablespoons smoked paprika
2 teaspoons chili powder
2 teaspoons garlic salt
1 teaspoon onion powder
1 teaspoon pepper
1/2 teaspoon cayenne pepper
4 pounds pork baby back ribs
SAUCE:
1/2 cup Worcestershire sauce
1/2 cup mayonnaise
1/2 cup yellow mustard
1/4 cup reduced-sodium soy sauce
3 tablespoons hot pepper sauce

Direction
Mix together the first 6 ingredients in a small bowl. Slice ribs into serving-sized pieces; rub with the seasoning mixture. Put the ribs into a 6-qt. slow cooker. Cook with a cover on low till the meat is tender, or for 5-6 hours.
Set the oven at 375° and start preheating. Whisk together the sauce ingredients in a small bowl. Transfer the ribs into a 15x10x1-in. baking pan lined with foil; brush with some of the sauce. Bake till browned, or for 15-20 minutes, turning once and using the sauce to brush occasionally. Serve accompanied with the remaining sauce.
Nutrition Information
Calories: 420 calories;Total Carbohydrate: 6g carbohydrate (2g sugars;Cholesterol: 86mg cholesterol;Protein: 24g protein.;Total Fat: 33g fat (9g saturated fat);Sodium: 1082mg sodium
Fiber: 2g fiber)

704. Farm Style BBQ Ribs

Serving: 4 servings. | Prep: 20mins | Cook: 06hours00mins | Ready in:
Ingredients
4 pounds bone-in beef short ribs
1 can (15 ounces) thick and zesty tomato sauce
1-1/2 cups water
1 medium onion, chopped
1 can (6 ounces) tomato paste
1/3 cup packed brown sugar
3 tablespoons cider vinegar
3 tablespoons Worcestershire sauce
2 tablespoons chili powder
4 garlic cloves, minced
2 teaspoons ground mustard
1-1/2 teaspoons salt
Direction
In a slow cooker of 5- or 6-quart, place the ribs. In a large saucepan, combine the rest of the ingredients. Allow to boil. Lessen heat; simmer with no cover for approximately 5 minutes or until slightly thick. Pour over ribs; cook with cover on low for nearly 6 to 8 hours or until tender.
Nutrition Information
Calories: 578 calories;Protein: 44g protein.;Total Fat: 24g fat (9g saturated fat);Sodium: 2503mg sodium
Fiber: 7g fiber);Total Carbohydrate: 46g carbohydrate (32g sugars;Cholesterol: 110mg cholesterol

705. German Style Short Ribs

Serving: 8 servings. | Prep: 15mins | Cook: 08hours00mins | Ready in:
Ingredients
3/4 cup dry red wine or beef broth
1/2 cup mango chutney
3 tablespoons quick-cooking tapioca
1/4 cup water
3 tablespoons brown sugar
3 tablespoons cider vinegar
1 tablespoon Worcestershire sauce
1/2 teaspoon salt
1/2 teaspoon ground mustard
1/2 teaspoon chili powder
1/2 teaspoon pepper
4 pounds bone-in beef short ribs
2 medium onions, sliced
Hot cooked egg noodles
Direction
Mix the first eleven ingredients in a 5 quarts slow cooker. Put ribs and flip to coat. Top with onions. Cook on low for 8 to 10 hours while covered, until ribs are tender. Take ribs out of cooker. Skim fat from cooking juices; serve together with noodles and ribs.
Nutrition Information
Calories: 302 calories
Fiber: 1g fiber);Total Carbohydrate: 28g carbohydrate (17g sugars;Cholesterol: 55mg cholesterol;Protein: 19g protein.;Total Fat: 11g fat (5g saturated fat);Sodium: 378mg sodium

706. Ginger Country Style Pork Ribs

Serving: 8 servings. | Prep: 15mins | Cook: 04hours15mins | Ready in:
Ingredients
4 pounds boneless country-style pork ribs
1/2 teaspoon salt
1/4 teaspoon pepper
1 cup orange juice
1/2 cup balsamic vinegar
1/4 cup reduced-sodium soy sauce
2 tablespoons minced fresh gingerroot
2 tablespoons honey
3 garlic cloves, minced
1/4 teaspoon crushed red pepper flakes
2 tablespoons cornstarch
2 tablespoons cold water
Direction
Sprinkle pepper and salt onto the ribs; put into a 5-qt. slow cooker. Whisk together pepper flakes, garlic, honey, ginger, soy sauce, vinegar and orange juice in a small bowl; transfer over the ribs. Cook with a cover on low till the meat turns tender, or for 4-5 hours.
Transfer the ribs onto a serving platter and keep warm. Pour cooking juices into a small saucepan; skim off the fat. Boil the liquid. Stir water and cornstarch together in a small bowl, till smooth; mix into the cooking juices. Boil the mixture; cook while stirring till thickened. Transfer over the ribs using a spoon.
Nutrition Information
Calories: 417 calories;Sodium: 535mg sodium
Fiber: 0g fiber);Total Carbohydrate: 15g carbohydrate (11g sugars;Cholesterol: 131mg cholesterol;Protein: 40g protein.;Total Fat: 21g fat (8g saturated fat)

707. Gingered Short Ribs

Serving: 4 servings. | Prep: 25mins | Cook: 07hours00mins | Ready in:
Ingredients
4 pounds bone-in beef short ribs
2 medium parsnips, peeled and halved widthwise
2 large carrots, halved widthwise
1/2 cup reduced-sodium soy sauce
1/3 cup packed brown sugar
1/4 cup rice vinegar
1 tablespoon minced fresh gingerroot
2 garlic cloves, minced
1/2 teaspoon crushed red pepper flakes
1 small head cabbage, quartered
2 tablespoons cornstarch
2 tablespoons cold water
2 teaspoons sesame oil
4 green onions, thinly sliced
Hot cooked couscous, optional
Direction

Add carrots, parsnips and ribs into a 5-6-quart slow cooker. In the small-sized bowl, mix pepper flakes, garlic, ginger, vinegar, brown sugar and soy sauce; add on top of the ribs. Add the cabbage on top. Cook with cover on low till the meat softens or for 7 to 8 hours.

Transfer the veggies and meat out onto the serving platter; keep them warm. Skim the fat off the cooking juices; move into the small-sized sauce pan. Boil the liquid. Mix water and cornstarch till smooth. Slowly whisk into pan. Boil; cook and stir till thicken or for 2 minutes.

Whisk in the sesame oil. Serve along with the veggies and meat. Scatter with the green onions. Serve along with the couscous if you want.

Nutrition Information
Calories: 603 calories;Protein: 42g protein.;Total Fat: 24g fat (10g saturated fat);Sodium: 1354mg sodium Fiber: 9g fiber);Total Carbohydrate: 55g carbohydrate (30g sugars;Cholesterol: 109mg cholesterol

708. Gingered Short Ribs With Green Rice

Serving: 6 servings. | Prep: 35mins | Cook: 08hours00mins | Ready in:

Ingredients
1/2 cup reduced-sodium beef broth
1/3 cup sherry or additional reduced-sodium beef broth
1/4 cup reduced-sodium soy sauce
3 tablespoons honey
1 tablespoon rice vinegar
1 tablespoon minced fresh gingerroot
3 garlic cloves, minced
4 medium carrots, chopped
2 medium onions, chopped
3 pounds bone-in beef short ribs
1/2 teaspoon salt
1/2 teaspoon pepper
3 cups uncooked instant brown rice
3 green onions, thinly sliced
3 tablespoons minced fresh cilantro
2 tablespoons chopped pickled jalapenos
3/4 teaspoon grated lime zest
1 tablespoon cornstarch
1 tablespoon cold water

Direction
Stir the first 7 ingredients in a small bowl until mixed. Put onions and carrots in a slow cooker of 5 quart. Dust ribs with pepper and salt; position over the vegetables. Drizzle broth blend on top.
Cook, covered, for 8 to 10 hours on low, until meat is soft.
Prepare rice according to package instructions just prior serving. Mix in lime zest, jalapenos, cilantro and green onions.
Transfer ribs to a serving dish; keep warm. Shift cooking juices to a small saucepan; skim fat. Take juices to a boil. Stir water and cornstarch in a small bowl until smooth; mix into cooking juices. Bring back to a boil; cook and mix for 2 minutes, until thickened. Serve with rice and ribs.

Nutrition Information
Calories: 444 calories;Protein: 24g protein.;Total Fat: 12g fat (5g saturated fat);Sodium: 714mg sodium Fiber: 5g fiber);Total Carbohydrate: 56g carbohydrate (14g sugars;Cholesterol: 55mg cholesterol

709. Green Chili Ribs

Serving: 8 servings. | Prep: 20mins | Cook: 05hours00mins | Ready in:

Ingredients
4 pounds pork baby back ribs
2 tablespoons ground cumin, divided
2 tablespoons olive oil
1 small onion, finely chopped
1 jar (16 ounces) salsa verde
3 cans (4 ounces each) chopped green chilies
2 cups beef broth
1/4 cup minced fresh cilantro
1 tablespoon all-purpose flour
3 garlic cloves, minced
1/4 teaspoon cayenne pepper
Additional minced fresh cilantro

Direction
Cut the ribs into serving-size pieces; then rub one tablespoon of the cumin over. Heat oil in large skillet over medium-high heat. Working in batches, brown the ribs. Put ribs into a 6 quarts slow cooker.
Put onion into the same pan; cook while stirring until onion soften, about 2 to 3 minutes. Put remaining cumin, cayenne, garlic, flour, a quarter cup cilantro, broth, green chilies and salsa verde into slow cooker. Cover and cook on low until meat soften, about 5 to 6 hours. Sprinkle with more cilantro.

Nutrition Information
Calories: 349 calories
Fiber: 1g fiber);Total Carbohydrate: 8g carbohydrate (2g sugars;Cholesterol: 81mg cholesterol;Protein: 24g protein.;Total Fat: 25g fat (8g saturated fat);Sodium: 797mg sodium

710. Hearty Short Ribs

Serving: 6 servings. | Prep: 15mins | Cook: 06hours00mins | Ready in:

Ingredients
1 large onion, sliced
4 pounds bone-in beef short ribs
1/2 pound sliced fresh mushrooms
1 can (10-3/4 ounces) condensed cream of mushroom soup, undiluted
1/2 cup water
1 envelope brown gravy mix
1 teaspoon minced garlic
1/2 teaspoon dried thyme
1 tablespoon cornstarch
2 tablespoons cold water
Hot mashed potatoes

Direction
In a 5-quart slow cooker, add onion then top with ribs. Mix the thyme, garlic, gravy mix, a half cup of water, soup and mushrooms; spread over ribs. Cook on low with cover for 6 to 6 and a half hours, or till meat becomes tender.
Transfer meat to a serving platter; keep warm. Scoop off fat from cooking juices; move to a small saucepan. Let it boil.
Stir cold water and cornstarch until smooth. Slowly mix into pan. Allow it to boil. Cook and mix for about 2 minutes, or until thick. Serve with mashed potatoes and meat.

Nutrition Information
Calories: 317 calories;Sodium: 769mg sodium
Fiber: 1g fiber);Total Carbohydrate: 12g carbohydrate (3g sugars;Cholesterol: 75mg

cholesterol;Protein: 27g protein.;Total Fat: 18g fat (7g saturated fat)

711. Home Style Ribs

Serving: 8 servings | Prep: 10mins | Cook: | Ready in:
Ingredients
4 lb. pork baby back ribs
1 Tbsp. HEINZ Yellow Mustard
1 cup KRAFT Original Barbecue Sauce
1/2 cup maple-flavored or pancake syrup
Direction
Smear mustard on both sides of ribs; arrange in single layer in foil-lined 15x10x1-inch pan.
Combine syrup and barbecue sauce; scoop on top of ribs. Cover.
Bake until ribs are tender, about 2 hours. Pour any leftover sauce in pan on top and serve.
Nutrition Information
Calories: 510;Sodium: 580 mg;Total Carbohydrate: 25 g;Cholesterol: 130 mg;Protein: 27 g;Total Fat: 33 g Saturated Fat: 12 g
Fiber: 0 g
Sugar: 23 g

712. Lazy Man's Ribs

Serving: 4 servings. | Prep: 20mins | Cook: 05hours00mins | Ready in:
Ingredients
2-1/2 pounds pork baby back ribs, cut into eight pieces
2 teaspoons Cajun seasoning
1 medium onion, sliced
1 cup ketchup
1/2 cup packed brown sugar
1/3 cup orange juice
1/3 cup cider vinegar
1/4 cup molasses
2 tablespoons Worcestershire sauce
1 tablespoon barbecue sauce
1 teaspoon stone-ground mustard
1 teaspoon paprika
1/2 teaspoon garlic powder
1/2 teaspoon liquid smoke, optional
Dash salt
5 teaspoons cornstarch
1 tablespoon cold water
Direction
Use Cajun seasoning to rub over ribs. In a 5-qt. slow cooker, place a layer of ribs then onion. In a small bowl, mix the salt, liquid smoke if wanted, garlic powder, paprika, mustard, barbecue sauce, Worcestershire sauce, molasses, vinegar, orange juice, brown sugar, and ketchup. Spread over ribs. Cook with a cover on low until meat is soft, about 5-6 hours.
Take out ribs and keep warm. Strain cooking liquid and discard fat; pour into a small saucepan. Mix water and cornstarch until smooth; mix into juices. Bring it to a boil; cook while stirring until thick, about 2 minutes. Enjoy with ribs.
Nutrition Information
Calories: 753 calories;Sodium: 1335mg sodium Fiber: 2g fiber);Total Carbohydrate: 70g carbohydrate (52g sugars;Cholesterol: 153mg cholesterol;Protein: 33g protein.;Total Fat: 39g fat (14g saturated fat)

713. Lip Smackin' Ribs

Serving: 8 servings. | Prep: 20mins | Cook: 06hours00mins | Ready in:
Ingredients
3 tablespoons butter
3 pounds boneless country-style pork ribs
1 can (15 ounces) tomato sauce
1 cup packed brown sugar
1 cup ketchup
1/4 cup prepared mustard
2 tablespoons honey
3 teaspoons pepper
2 teaspoons dried savory
1 teaspoon salt
Direction
Place a large skillet on medium heat; heat butter. Brown ribs, working in batches; move to a 5-qt slow cooker. Put in the remaining ingredients. Cook with a cover on low till the meat is tender, or for 6-8 hours.
Nutrition Information
Calories: 474 calories;Total Carbohydrate: 43g carbohydrate (40g sugars;Cholesterol: 109mg cholesterol;Protein: 31g protein.;Total Fat: 20g fat (8g saturated fat);Sodium: 1117mg sodium Fiber: 1g fiber)

714. Maple Pork Ribs

Serving: 2 servings. | Prep: 10mins | Cook: 05hours00mins | Ready in:
Ingredients
1 pound boneless country-style pork ribs, trimmed and cut into 3-inch pieces
2 teaspoons canola oil
1 medium onion, sliced and separated into rings
3 tablespoons maple syrup
2 tablespoons spicy brown or Dijon mustard
Direction
Brown ribs in oil on all sides in a big skillet; drain. In a 1 1/2-quart slow cooker, add onion and ribs. Mix mustard together with syrup; pour over the ribs. Cover and cook for 5 to 6 hours at low, or until meat is soft.
Nutrition Information
Calories: 428 calories;Total Fat: 20g fat (6g saturated fat);Sodium: 272mg sodium
Fiber: 2g fiber);Total Carbohydrate: 27g carbohydrate (24g sugars;Cholesterol: 98mg cholesterol;Protein: 31g protein.

715. My Brazilian Feijoada

Serving: 10 servings. | Prep: 20mins | Cook: 07hours00mins | Ready in:
Ingredients
8 ounces dried black beans (about 1 cup)
2 pounds boneless pork shoulder butt roast, trimmed and cut into 1-inch cubes
3 bone-in beef short ribs (about 1-1/2 pounds)
4 bacon strips, cooked and crumbled
1-1/4 cups diced onion
3 garlic cloves, minced
1 bay leaf
3/4 teaspoon salt
3/4 teaspoon pepper
1-1/2 cups chicken broth
1 cup water
1/2 cup beef broth
8 ounces Johnsonville® Fully Cooked Smoked Sausage Rope, cut into 1/2-inch slices
Orange sections
Hot cooked rice, optional

Direction
Wash and sort the beans; steep following the instructions on package. At the same time, add bacon, short ribs and pork roast into a 6-quart slow cooker. Put in the seasonings, bay leaf, garlic and onion; add the beef broth, water and chicken broth on top of the meat. Cook, with cover, on high for 2 hours. Whisk in the sausage and beans. Cook, with cover, on low for 5 to 6 hours or till the beans and meat soften. Get rid of the bay leaf. Take the short ribs out. Once cool enough to handle, debone the meat; get rid of the bones. Shred the meat using two forks; bring back to the slow cooker. Add the orange sections on top of servings. If you want, serve along with the hot cooked rice.
Nutrition Information
Calories: 481 calories;Protein: 41g protein.;Total Fat: 27g fat (11g saturated fat);Sodium: 772mg sodium Fiber: 4g fiber);Total Carbohydrate: 17g carbohydrate (2g sugars;Cholesterol: 123mg cholesterol

716. Peachy Baby Back Ribs

Serving: 6 servings. | Prep: 15mins | Cook: 06hours00mins | Ready in:
Ingredients
2 bottles (18 ounces each) hickory smoke-flavored barbecue sauce
1 can (15 ounces) sliced peaches, drained and halved crosswise
1 medium onion, chopped
3/4 cup jalapeno pepper jelly
1/2 cup pickled hot jalapeno slices
6 pounds pork baby back ribs, well-trimmed
1 teaspoon salt
1/2 teaspoon pepper
Thinly sliced green onions
Direction
Combine the first 5 ingredients in a big bowl. Slice the ribs into thirds and sprinkle pepper and salt on top. Arrange 1/2 of the ribs in a 6 quart slow cooker and pour 1/2 of the sauce over the ribs. Repeat the process with other layers. Cook while covering for 6-8 hrs on low until the meat is softened.
Take the ribs away from the slow cooker and keep warm. Drain the cooking juices and serve the vegetables and peaches. Skim fat from cooking juices and you can thicken it if you want. Whisk in the reserved vegetables and peaches, then serve with the ribs. Sprinkle green onions on top.
Nutrition Information
Calories: 1019 calories;Cholesterol: 163mg cholesterol;Protein: 46g protein.;Total Fat: 43g fat (15g saturated fat);Sodium: 2466mg sodium Fiber: 3g fiber);Total Carbohydrate: 110g carbohydrate (87g sugars

717. Pork Baby Back Ribs

Serving: 5 servings. | Prep: 10mins | Cook: 06hours00mins | Ready in:
Ingredients
2-1/2 pounds pork baby back ribs
2 tablespoons canola oil
1 medium onion, thinly sliced
1/2 cup apricot preserves
1/3 cup beef broth
3 tablespoons white vinegar
2 tablespoons Worcestershire sauce
1 tablespoon brown sugar

Direction
Slice ribs into serving-sized pieces. Brown the ribs in a large skillet with oil, working in batches. Put onion into a 5-qt. slow cooker; transfer the ribs over. Mix together the remaining ingredients in a small bowl. Transfer over the ribs.
Cook with a cover on low till the meat is tender, or for 6-7 hours.
Nutrition Information
Calories: 539 calories
Fiber: 1g fiber);Total Carbohydrate: 27g carbohydrate (17g sugars;Cholesterol: 122mg cholesterol;Protein: 26g protein.;Total Fat: 36g fat (12g saturated fat);Sodium: 246mg sodium

718. Pork Ribs Lo Mein

Serving: 6 servings. | Prep: 25mins | Cook: 06hours30mins | Ready in:
Ingredients
1-1/2 pounds boneless country-style pork ribs
3 medium carrots, chopped
1 small onion, sliced
3/4 cup packed brown sugar
1/2 cup reduced-sodium soy sauce
1/2 cup ketchup
1/4 cup honey
2 tablespoons cider vinegar
2 garlic cloves, minced
1/2 teaspoon ground ginger
1/4 to 1/2 teaspoon crushed red pepper flakes
1 cup fresh broccoli florets, chopped
1 can (8 ounces) sliced water chestnuts, drained
1 pound uncooked spaghetti
4 green onions, sliced
Direction
Combine onion, carrots and ribs in a 3 quarts slow cooker. Combine pepper flakes, ginger, garlic, vinegar, honey, ketchup, soy sauce and brown sugar in small bowl. Add over ribs. Cook, with cover, on low until pork is tender, about 6 to 8 hours. Transfer to a plate; use 2 forks to shred then put back to the slow cooker. Mix in water chestnuts and broccoli. Cook, with cover, or until the broccoli becomes crisp-tender, about 30 more minutes. In the meantime, cook spaghetti following the package instructions; drain. Combine pork mixture and spaghetti in large bowl. Sprinkle green onions over.
Nutrition Information
Calories: 684 calories
Fiber: 5g fiber);Total Carbohydrate: 112g carbohydrate (49g sugars;Cholesterol: 65mg cholesterol;Protein: 32g protein.;Total Fat: 12g fat (4g saturated fat);Sodium: 1153mg sodium

719. Pork Ribs With Apple Mustard Glaze

Serving: 5 servings. | Prep: 30mins | Cook: 06hours00mins | Ready in:
Ingredients
2 racks pork baby back ribs (about 4-1/2 pounds)
1 teaspoon salt
1/2 teaspoon pepper
1 large onion, chopped
1 cup picante sauce
3/4 cup thawed apple juice concentrate
1/2 cup ketchup
1/3 cup packed brown sugar
2 tablespoons Dijon mustard
1 tablespoon soy sauce
2 teaspoons hot pepper sauce

Direction

Cut ribs into pieces, about serving size; sprinkle with salt and pepper. On a broiler pan, place ribs with meat side up. Broil for 5-7 minutes, about 4-in. from the heat, until browned.

In a 5- or 6-qt. slow cooker, add onions; put ribs on top. In a small bowl, mix the rest of ingredients; spread over ribs. Cook with a cover on low until meat is soft, about 6-8 hours.

Transfer meat to a serving platter; keep warm. Remove fat from cooking liquid; bring to a small saucepan. Boil. Cook until liquid is reduced by 1/2. Enjoy with ribs.

Nutrition Information
Calories: 877 calories;Protein: 46g protein.;Total Fat: 55g fat (21g saturated fat);Sodium: 1690mg sodium Fiber: 1g fiber);Total Carbohydrate: 45g carbohydrate (40g sugars;Cholesterol: 220mg cholesterol

720. Pork Spareribs

Serving: 6 servings. | Prep: 5mins | Cook: 06hours00mins | Ready in:
Ingredients
3 pounds pork spareribs
2 cans (28 ounces each) diced tomatoes, undrained
2 cups barbecue sauce
1/4 cup packed brown sugar
1/4 cup white wine vinegar
Direction
In a 4- or 5-qt. slow cooker, add ribs. Mix the rest of ingredients; spread over ribs. Cook with a cover on low until meat is soft, about 6-8 hours. Serve along with a slotted spoon.
Nutrition Information
Calories: 579 calories;Sodium: 1198mg sodium Fiber: 5g fiber);Total Carbohydrate: 34g carbohydrate (28g sugars;Cholesterol: 128mg cholesterol;Protein: 34g protein.;Total Fat: 34g fat (12g saturated fat)

721. Root Beer BBQ Ribs

Serving: 5 servings. | Prep: 25mins | Cook: 06hours00mins | Ready in:
Ingredients
1 cup root beer
1 cup ketchup
1/4 cup orange juice
3 tablespoons Worcestershire sauce
2 tablespoons molasses
1 teaspoon onion powder
1 teaspoon garlic powder
1/2 teaspoon ground ginger
1/2 teaspoon paprika
1/4 teaspoon crushed red pepper flakes
4-1/2 pounds pork baby back ribs
1 teaspoon salt
1/2 teaspoon pepper
Direction
Mix the first 10 ingredients in a small saucepan. Boil over medium heat. Lower heat; simmer without a cover, until sauce reduces to 2 cups, about 10 minutes. Put aside.
Cut ribs into five pieces, about serving size; scatter with pepper and salt. Put in a 5- or 6-qt. slow cooker. Spread sauce over ribs. Cook with a cover on low until meat is soft, about 6-8 hours. Enjoy with sauce.
Nutrition Information
Calories: 804 calories

Fiber: 0 fiber);Total Carbohydrate: 29g carbohydrate (26g sugars;Cholesterol: 220mg cholesterol;Protein: 46g protein.;Total Fat: 55g fat (21g saturated fat);Sodium: 1378mg sodium

722. Seasoned Short Ribs

Serving: 4 servings. | Prep: 25mins | Cook: 06hours00mins | Ready in:
Ingredients
1-1/2 cups tomato juice
1/2 cup maple syrup
1/4 cup chopped onion
3 tablespoons cider vinegar
1 tablespoon Worcestershire sauce
1 tablespoon Dijon mustard
2 teaspoons minced garlic
1/4 teaspoon ground cinnamon
1/4 teaspoon ground cloves
4 pounds bone-in beef short ribs
1 teaspoon pepper
1 tablespoon cornstarch
2 tablespoons cold water
Direction
Mix the initial 9 ingredients in a small bowl; put aside. Chop ribs into serving-size pieces; put on a broiler pan. Dust with pepper. Broil 4-6 inch from heat until browned, about 3 to 5 minutes on every side; drain on paper towels.
Place ribs in a slow cooker of 5-quart; add a tomato juice mixture over. Cover and cook on low until meat soften, about 6 to 7 hours.
Mix cold water with cornstarch in a small bowl until smooth. Pour in a small saucepan 1 cup of cooking liquid; skim off fat. Take to a boil; mix in a cornstarch blend. Bring back to a boil; cook and blend until thick, about 2 minutes. Pour over ribs to serve.
Nutrition Information
Calories: 1169 calories;Cholesterol: 206mg cholesterol;Protein: 48g protein.;Total Fat: 92g fat (39g saturated fat);Sodium: 538mg sodium Fiber: 1g fiber);Total Carbohydrate: 34g carbohydrate (29g sugars

723. Sesame Pork Ribs

Serving: 5 servings. | Prep: 15mins | Cook: 05hours00mins | Ready in:
Ingredients
3/4 cup packed brown sugar
1/2 cup reduced-sodium soy sauce
1/2 cup ketchup
1/4 cup honey
2 tablespoons white wine vinegar
3 garlic cloves, minced
1 teaspoon salt
1 teaspoon ground ginger
1/4 to 1/2 teaspoon crushed red pepper flakes
5 pounds bone-in country-style pork ribs
1 medium onion, sliced
2 tablespoons sesame seeds, toasted
2 tablespoons chopped green onions
Direction
Mix the first nine ingredients in a large bowl. Place in ribs and flip to cover. Add the onion to a 5-qt. slow cooker; place ribs then sauce on top. Cook with a cover on low until meat is soft, about 5-6 hours. Put ribs on a serving platter; sprinkle green onions and sesame seeds on top.
Nutrition Information

Calories: 603 calories;Total Carbohydrate: 48g carbohydrate (45g sugars;Cholesterol: 144mg cholesterol;Protein: 47g protein.;Total Fat: 24g fat (8g saturated fat);Sodium: 2007mg sodium Fiber: 1g fiber)

724. Short Rib Poutine

Serving: 4 servings. | Prep: 45mins | Cook: 06hours00mins | Ready in:
Ingredients
1 pound well-trimmed boneless beef short ribs
3 tablespoons all-purpose flour
1/2 teaspoon pepper
2 tablespoons olive oil
1 medium onion, coarsely chopped
4 garlic cloves, minced
1-1/2 cups beef stock, divided
1/4 cup Sriracha Asian hot chili sauce
3 tablespoons ketchup
2 tablespoons Worcestershire sauce
1 tablespoon packed brown sugar
3 cups frozen french-fried potatoes (about 11 ounces)
1 cup cheese curds or 4 ounces white cheddar cheese, broken into small chunks
Direction
Toss short ribs with pepper and flour and then shake off the excess. Save the remaining flour mixture. Over medium-high heat, heat oil in a large skillet and then brown the ribs on all sides. Place into a 3-qt. slow cooker and set aside the drippings.
Over medium heat, sauté onion in the drippings in the same skillet for 2 to 3 minutes until tender. Place in garlic. Cook while stirring for one minute. Mix in one cup of stock and then heat to boil while stirring to loosen any browned bits from the pan.
Whisk remaining stock, brown sugar, Worcestershire sauce, ketchup, chili sauce and reserved flour mixture in a small bowl until smooth. Mix into the onion mixture. Pour on top of ribs.
Cook while covered on low for 6 to 8 hours until the ribs are tender. Take out the ribs, then shred with 2 forks and keep them warm. Skim off fat from the onion mixture and then puree with an immersion blender. (Alternatively, cool a bit and then puree in a blender. Place back into a slow cooker to heat through). Cook the potatoes as directed on the package. Serve the beef atop potatoes, then top with cheese and gravy.
Nutrition Information
Calories: 560 calories;Cholesterol: 80mg cholesterol;Protein: 28g protein.;Total Fat: 31g fat (12g saturated fat);Sodium: 1453mg sodium Fiber: 3g fiber);Total Carbohydrate: 39g carbohydrate (15g sugars

725. Simple Sparerib Sauerkraut Supper

Serving: 6 servings. | Prep: 30mins | Cook: 06hours00mins | Ready in:
Ingredients
1 pound fingerling potatoes
1 medium onion, chopped
1 medium Granny Smith apple, peeled and chopped
3 slices thick-sliced bacon strips, cooked and crumbled
1 jar (16 ounces) sauerkraut, undrained
2 pounds pork spareribs
1/2 teaspoon salt
1/4 teaspoon pepper
1 tablespoon vegetable oil
3 tablespoons brown sugar
1/4 teaspoon caraway seeds
1/2 pound smoked Polish sausage, cut into 1-inch slices
1 cup beer
Direction
In a 6-qt. slow cooker, place bacon, apple, onion and potatoes. Strain the sauerkraut; reserve 1/3 cup of the liquid; put the reserved liquid and sauerkraut into the slow cooker.
Slice spareribs into serving-sized portions; sprinkle with pepper and salt. Place a large skillet on medium-high heat; heat oil; brown in ribs, working in batches. Remove into the slow cooker; sprinkle caraway seeds and brown sugar over.
Put in sausage; transfer in beer. Cook with a cover on low till the ribs turn tender, or for 6-7 hours.
Nutrition Information
Calories: 590 calories
Fiber: 4g fiber);Total Carbohydrate: 32g carbohydrate (13g sugars;Cholesterol: 118mg cholesterol;Protein: 30g protein.;Total Fat: 37g fat (13g saturated fat);Sodium: 1285mg sodium

726. Slow Easy Baby Back Ribs

Serving: 4 servings. | Prep: 20mins | Cook: 05hours00mins | Ready in:
Ingredients
4 pounds pork baby back ribs, cut into 2-rib portions
1 medium onion, chopped
1/2 cup ketchup
1/4 cup packed brown sugar
1/4 cup cider vinegar
1/4 cup tomato paste or tomato sauce
2 tablespoons paprika
2 tablespoons Worcestershire sauce
1 tablespoon prepared mustard
1 teaspoon salt
1/4 teaspoon pepper
2 tablespoons cornstarch
2 tablespoons cold water
Direction
Put ribs into a 5-qt. slow cooker. Combine pepper, salt, mustard, Worcestershire, paprika, tomato paste, vinegar, brown sugar, ketchup and onion in a small bowl; transfer over the ribs. Cook with a cover on low till the meat is tender, or for 5-6 hours.
Transfer the ribs to a serving platter; keep warm. Skim fat from the cooking juices; pour the juices into a small saucepan. Allow to boil.
Mix water with cornstarch till smooth. Gradually mix into the pan. Allow to boil; cook while stirring till thickened, or for 2 minutes. Serve with the ribs.
Nutrition Information
Calories: 916 calories
Fiber: 3g fiber);Total Carbohydrate: 35g carbohydrate (26g sugars;Cholesterol: 245mg cholesterol;Protein: 52g protein.;Total Fat: 62g fat (23g saturated fat);Sodium: 1324mg sodium

727. Slow Cooked BBQ Pork Ribs

Serving: 8 servings. | Prep: 20mins | Cook: 07hours00mins | Ready in:
Ingredients
4 pounds boneless country-style pork ribs
2 cups ketchup
1/4 cup packed brown sugar
1/4 cup maple syrup
1/4 cup prepared mustard

1/4 cup reduced-sodium soy sauce
2 tablespoons lemon juice
2 teaspoons dried minced garlic
1/8 teaspoon pepper
Direction
In a 5- or 6-qt. slow cooker, place ribs. Mix the rest of ingredients; spread over top. Cook with a cover on low until meat is tender, about 7-9 hours.
Take out ribs and keep warm. Discard fat from sauce; serve along with ribs.
Nutrition Information
Calories: 480 calories
Fiber: 0 fiber);Total Carbohydrate: 31g carbohydrate (29g sugars;Cholesterol: 130mg cholesterol;Protein: 40g protein.;Total Fat: 21g fat (8g saturated fat);Sodium: 1247mg sodium

728. Slow Cooker Jerked Short Ribs

Serving: 10 servings. | Prep: 15mins | Cook: 06hours00mins | Ready in:
Ingredients
1 tablespoon ground coriander
2 teaspoons ground ginger
2 teaspoons onion powder
2 teaspoons garlic powder
1 teaspoon salt
1 teaspoon pepper
1 teaspoon dried thyme
3/4 teaspoon ground allspice
3/4 teaspoon ground nutmeg
1/2 teaspoon ground cinnamon
10 bone-in beef short ribs (about 5 pounds)
1 large sweet onion, chopped
1/2 cup beef broth
1 jar (10 ounces) apricot preserves
3 tablespoons cider vinegar
3 garlic cloves, minced
Direction
Mix the first 10 ingredients, put aside 2 tablespoons. Rub the leftover seasoning mixture over ribs. In a 6-quart slow cooker, add broth and onion; cover with ribs. Cook with cover on Low for 6 - 8 hours, till ribs soften.
Meanwhile, whisk reserved seasoning mixture, garlic, vinegar and preserves. Serve along with ribs.
Nutrition Information
Calories: 265 calories;Sodium: 330mg sodium
Fiber: 1g fiber);Total Carbohydrate: 23g carbohydrate (14g sugars;Cholesterol: 55mg cholesterol;Protein: 19g protein.;Total Fat: 11g fat (5g saturated fat)

729. Slow Cooker Memphis Style Ribs

Serving: 6 servings. | Prep: 15mins | Cook: 05hours00mins | Ready in:
Ingredients
1/2 cup white vinegar
1/2 cup water
2 racks pork baby back ribs (about 5 pounds)
3 tablespoons smoked paprika
2 tablespoons brown sugar
2 teaspoons salt
2 teaspoons coarsely ground pepper
1 teaspoon garlic powder
1 teaspoon onion powder
1 teaspoon ground cumin
1 teaspoon ground mustard
1 teaspoon dried thyme
1 teaspoon dried oregano
1 teaspoon celery salt
3/4 teaspoon cayenne pepper
Direction
Mix the water and vinegar; brush over the ribs. Pour the rest of vinegar mixture into a slow cooker of 6-quart in size. Stir the remaining ingredients together and reserve half. Scatter ribs with the remaining seasoning blend. Chop into serving-size pieces; move to the slow cooker.
Cook, covered for 5 to 6 hours on low until soft. Discard the ribs; skim the fat from cooking juices. Brush ribs generously with skimmed cooking juices using a clean brush; scatter with saved seasoning. Enjoy the ribs with the leftover juices.
Nutrition Information
Calories:;Total Carbohydrate:;Cholesterol:;Protein:;Total Fat:;Sodium: Fiber:

730. Slow Cooker Peach BBQ Ribs

Serving: 8 servings (3 cups sauce). | Prep: 10mins | Cook: 05hours00mins | Ready in:
Ingredients
2 tablespoons chili powder
1 tablespoon brown sugar
2 teaspoons ground cumin
2 teaspoons smoked paprika
2 teaspoons garlic salt
1/2 teaspoon cayenne pepper
4 pounds pork baby back ribs, cut into serving-size pieces
SAUCE:
3 medium ripe peaches, peeled and chopped
1 bottle (18 ounces) barbecue sauce
1/4 cup water
1 jalapeno pepper, thinly sliced
Direction
Combine seasonings in a small bowl; rub over meaty side of ribs. Put in a slow cooker of 6 quart in size. Cook, covered on low for 5 to 6 hours, or until meat is soft.
Mix water together with barbecue sauce and peaches in a saucepan prior to serving; Boil. Lower the heat; simmer, covered until peaches are tender, or for 15 to 20 minutes, mixing occasionally. Thin with extra water if desired. Mix in jalapeno. Enjoy with ribs.
Nutrition Information
Calories: 431 calories;Total Carbohydrate: 35g carbohydrate (28g sugars;Cholesterol: 81mg cholesterol;Protein: 24g protein.;Total Fat: 22g fat (8g saturated fat);Sodium: 1048mg sodium
Fiber: 3g fiber)

731. Slow Cooker Ribs

Serving: 6 | Prep: 10mins | Cook: 8hours | Ready in:
Ingredients
1 pinch steak seasoning, or to taste
1 pinch garlic salt, or to taste
1 pinch ground black pepper, or to taste
1 pinch chili powder, or to taste
1 (4 pound) package boneless country-style pork ribs
1 cup barbecue sauce
1/4 cup Worcestershire sauce
1/4 cup soy sauce
1/4 cup teriyaki sauce
1/4 cup orange juice
2 dashes hot pepper sauce, or to taste
Direction
In a small bowl, combine chili powder, black pepper, garlic salt and steak seasoning. Massage the entire ribs with seasoning mix, and set into the base of a slow cooker. Add in the hot pepper sauce, orange juice, teriyaki sauce, soy sauce, Worcestershire sauce

and barbecue sauce. Liquid must not submerge the whole ribs.
Turn the cooker to Low, and allow to cook for 8 hours till ribs are soft.
Nutrition Information
Calories: 455 calories;;Total Fat: 23.6;Sodium: 1819;Total Carbohydrate: 21.3;Cholesterol: 136;Protein: 36.6

732. Slow Cooker Short Ribs

Serving: 8 | Prep: 15mins | Cook: 5hours | Ready in:
Ingredients
cooking spray
3 ribs celery, sliced
2 carrots, sliced
1 onion, chopped
3 cloves garlic, smashed
5 pounds beef short ribs
salt and ground black pepper to taste
1 (10.5 ounce) can condensed beef consomme (such as Campbell's ®)
1/2 (10.5 ounce) can water
Direction
Coat the slow cooker crock with cooking spray.
At the bottom of the crock, spread the garlic, carrots, celery, and onion. Season the short ribs with salt and pepper; place the short ribs on top of the vegetables. Pour in water and beef consommé.
Cook the ribs on high setting for 5-7 hours until fork-tender.
Transfer the ribs from the slow cooker into the platter. Strain the broth, discarding the vegetables. Get the meat from the bones of the ribs. Discard the bones; place the meat in a bowl. Shred it using the 2 forks; serve the meat together with the strained broth.
Nutrition Information
Calories: 618 calories;;Cholesterol: 117;Protein: 29.1;Total Fat: 52.2;Sodium: 289;Total Carbohydrate: 6

733. Slow And Easy BBQ Ribs

Serving: 4 servings. | Prep: 15mins | Cook: 05hours30mins | Ready in:
Ingredients
2 pounds boneless country-style pork ribs
1 can (6 ounces) unsweetened pineapple juice
1 medium onion, thinly sliced
1 garlic clove, minced
2/3 cup barbecue sauce
1/3 cup plum jam
Direction
Coat a large skillet with cooking spray, brown all sides of ribs. Bring to a 3-qt. slow cooker; add garlic, onion and pineapple juice on top. Cook with a cover on low until meat is soft, about 5-6 hours.
Take out ribs; drain and remove onion and cooking juices. Bring ribs back to the slow cooker. Mix jam and barbecue sauce; pour over ribs. Cook with a cover on high heat setting for 30 minutes.
Nutrition Information
Calories: 495 calories;Sodium: 478mg sodium Fiber: 1g fiber);Total Carbohydrate: 33g carbohydrate (28g sugars;Cholesterol: 130mg cholesterol;Protein: 41g protein.;Total Fat: 21g fat (8g saturated fat)

734. Slow Cooked Country Ribs In Gravy

Serving: 6 servings. | Prep: 10mins | Cook: 04hours00mins | Ready in:
Ingredients
3 pounds country-style pork ribs
1 cup water
1/2 cup ketchup
1 medium onion, chopped
2 tablespoons white vinegar
1 tablespoon sugar
4 teaspoons Worcestershire sauce
1 teaspoon salt
1 teaspoon ground mustard
1 beef bouillon cube
1/4 teaspoon paprika
1/4 teaspoon pepper
Direction
In a 5-quart slow cooker, put the ribs. Mix the remaining ingredients; add over the ribs. Cook, with cover, for 60 minutes on high. Turn the heat to low, ten cook for 3 to 4 more hours. Move the ribs to the serving platter; keep them warm. For gravy, thicken the cooking liquid.
Nutrition Information
Calories: 280 calories;Sodium: 876mg sodium Fiber: 1g fiber);Total Carbohydrate: 11g carbohydrate (6g sugars;Cholesterol: 86mg cholesterol;Protein: 27g protein.;Total Fat: 14g fat (5g saturated fat)

735. Slow Cooked Mesquite Ribs

Serving: 8 servings | Prep: 10mins | Cook: 06hours30mins | Ready in:
Ingredients
1 cup water
2 tablespoons cider vinegar
1 tablespoon soy sauce
2 tablespoons mesquite seasoning
4 pounds pork baby back ribs, cut into serving-size portions
1/2 cup barbecue sauce
Direction
Combine soy sauce, vinegar, and water in a 6-quart slow cooker. Rub the mesquite seasoning over the ribs, put in the slow cooker.
Put the lid on and cook on low for 6-8 hours until soft. Transfer the ribs to a dish. Brush the barbecue sauce over the ribs, put back into the slow cooker. Cook on low for 30 minutes, covered, until the ribs have glazed.
Nutrition Information
Calories: 314 calories;Protein: 23g protein.;Total Fat: 21g fat (8g saturated fat);Sodium: 591mg sodium Fiber: 0 fiber);Total Carbohydrate: 7g carbohydrate (6g sugars;Cholesterol: 81mg cholesterol

736. Slow Cooked Peachy Spareribs

Serving: 8 servings. | Prep: 10mins | Cook: 05hours30mins | Ready in:
Ingredients
4 pounds pork spareribs
1 can (15-1/4 ounces) sliced peaches, undrained
1/2 cup packed brown sugar
1/4 cup ketchup
1/4 cup white vinegar
2 tablespoons soy sauce
1 garlic clove, minced
1 teaspoon salt
1 teaspoon pepper
2 tablespoons cornstarch
2 tablespoons cold water
Hot cooked rice
Direction
Cut the ribs into the serving-size pieces. Brown all sides of the ribs in large skillet; drain.
Place into a 5 quarts slow cooker. Mix pepper, garlic salt, soy sauce, vinegar, ketchup, brown sugar and peaches; add over the ribs. Cook, with cover, on low until the meat becomes tender, about 5-1/2 - 6 hours.

Move peaches and pork onto serving platter; then keep them warm. Skim the fat from the cooking juices. Put into the small saucepan. Boil the liquid. Mix water and cornstarch until they become smooth. Stir into pan gradually. Boil and cook while stirring until thicken, about 2 minutes. Enjoy with rice and pork.

Nutrition Information
Calories: 518 calories;Sodium: 727mg sodium Fiber: 0 fiber);Total Carbohydrate: 24g carbohydrate (22g sugars;Cholesterol: 128mg cholesterol;Protein: 31g protein.;Total Fat: 32g fat (12g saturated fat)

737. Slow Cooked Ribs

Serving: 8 servings. | Prep: 15mins | Cook: 06hours00mins | Ready in:
Ingredients
4 pounds boneless country-style pork ribs
1 cup barbecue sauce
1 cup Catalina salad dressing
1/2 teaspoon minced garlic
2 tablespoons all-purpose flour
1/4 cup cold water
Direction
Cut the ribs into serving-size pieces. Put into a 5-quart slow cooker. Mix salad dressing and barbecue sauce; add over the ribs. Scatter with the garlic. Cook, with cover, on low until meat soften, about 6 to 7 hours.
Move the meat to serving platter; then keep it warm. Skim the fat from the cooking juices. Place into small saucepan. Boil the liquid. Mix water and flour until they become smooth. Stir into pan gradually. Boil and cook while stirring until thicken, about 2 minutes. Enjoy with meat.
Nutrition Information
Calories:;Sodium:
Fiber:;Total Carbohydrate:;Cholesterol:;Protein:;Total Fat:

738. Slow Cooked Short Ribs

Serving: 12 servings. | Prep: 25mins | Cook: 09hours00mins | Ready in:
Ingredients
2/3 cup all-purpose flour
2 teaspoons salt
1/2 teaspoon pepper
4 to 4-1/2 pounds boneless beef short ribs
1/4 to 1/3 cup butter
1 large onion, chopped
1-1/2 cups beef broth
3/4 cup red wine vinegar
3/4 cup packed brown sugar
1/2 cup chili sauce
1/3 cup ketchup
1/3 cup Worcestershire sauce
5 garlic cloves, minced
1-1/2 teaspoons chili powder
Direction
In a big resealable plastic bag, blend the pepper, salt and flour together. Put in batches of ribs and shake to coat. In a big frying pan over medium heat, sear ribs in butter.
Shift to a 6-quart. slow cooker. In the same pan, stir the leftover ingredients together. Cook and combine up to the mixture reaches a boil; then pour over ribs. Cook with cover on Low for 9-10 hours, or up to meat becomes soft.
Nutrition Information
Calories: 342 calories;Cholesterol: 71mg cholesterol;Protein: 22g protein.;Total Fat: 16g fat (8g saturated fat);Sodium: 899mg sodium

Fiber: 1g fiber);Total Carbohydrate: 28g carbohydrate (19g sugars

739. Slow Cooked Short Ribs With Salt Skin Potatoes

Serving: 8 servings. | Prep: 40mins | Cook: 06hours00mins | Ready in:
Ingredients
6 thick slices pancetta or thick-sliced bacon, chopped
6 pounds bone-in beef short ribs
1 teaspoon plus 1 cup kosher salt, divided
1 teaspoon pepper
1 tablespoon olive oil
3 medium carrots, chopped
1 medium red onion, chopped
1 cup beef broth
1 cup dry red wine
1/4 cup honey
1/4 cup balsamic vinegar
1 tablespoon minced fresh thyme or 1 teaspoon dried thyme
2 teaspoons minced fresh oregano or 3/4 teaspoon dried oregano
2 garlic cloves, minced
2 pounds small red potatoes
4 teaspoons cornstarch
3 tablespoons cold water
Direction
Cook pancetta over medium heat in a large skillet until crisp while stirring occasionally. Take out with a slotted spoon and drain on paper towels.
At the meantime, top ribs with 1 teaspoon salt and pepper. Heat oil over medium-high heat, in another large skillet. Brown ribs on all sides in batches; place in a 4- or 5-qt. slow cooker.
In the same skillet, add onion and carrots; cook while stirring over medium heat until crisp-tender or for 2-4 minutes. Add vinegar, honey, wine and broth; stir to loosen browned bits from pan. Place into the slow cooker; add garlic, herbs and pancetta.
Cook with a cover on low until meat becomes tender or for 6-8 hours. In the last hour of cooking, put potatoes in a 6-qt. stockpot; pour water into the stockpot to cover potatoes. Add the rest of the salt. Bring to boiling, covered, over medium-high heat; stir until salt dissolves. Cook until tender or for 15-30 minutes. Drain well
Transfer the ribs to a serving platter; keep warm. Strain cooking juices into a small saucepan; skim fat. Add pancetta and vegetables to platter. Bring juices to boiling. Mix water and cornstarch until smooth in a small bowl; stir into cooking juices. Bring back to boiling; cook while stirring until thickened or for 1-2 minutes. Serve with vegetables and ribs.
Nutrition Information
Calories: 507 calories;Protein: 33g protein.;Total Fat: 24g fat (9g saturated fat);Sodium: 859mg sodium Fiber: 3g fiber);Total Carbohydrate: 35g carbohydrate (14g sugars;Cholesterol: 96mg cholesterol

740. Stack Of Bones

Serving: 4 servings. | Prep: 15mins | Cook: 04hours00mins | Ready in:
Ingredients
1 cup chili sauce
2 green onions, chopped
2 tablespoons brown sugar
2 tablespoons balsamic vinegar
1 tablespoon Dijon mustard
1 tablespoon Worcestershire sauce
1 tablespoon soy sauce

1 teaspoon ground ginger
1/4 teaspoon crushed red pepper flakes
1/2 teaspoon liquid smoke, optional
4 pounds pork baby back ribs
Direction
In a large bowl, mix the first 10 ingredients. Cut ribs into single pieces; dip each into sauce. Bring to a 5-qt. slow cooker; add the rest of sauce on top. Cook with a cover on low until meat is soft, about 4-5 hours.
Nutrition Information
Calories: 872 calories;Protein: 51g protein.;Total Fat: 61g fat (23g saturated fat);Sodium: 1497mg sodium Fiber: 0 fiber);Total Carbohydrate: 26g carbohydrate (20g sugars;Cholesterol: 245mg cholesterol

741. Super Easy Country Style Ribs

Serving: 4 servings. | Prep: 10mins | Cook: 05hours00mins | Ready in:
Ingredients
1-1/2 cups ketchup
1/2 cup packed brown sugar
1/2 cup white vinegar
2 teaspoons seasoned salt
1/2 teaspoon liquid smoke, optional
2 pounds boneless country-style pork ribs
Direction
Mix seasoned salt, vinegar, brown sugar, ketchup and liquid smoke, if desired, in a 3-quart slow cooker. Put in ribs; coat by turning. Cover and cook on low until meat become tender, about 5 to 6 hours.
Take away pork and place onto the serving plate. Skim the fat from the cooking liquid. Place into small saucepan, if desired, to thicken. Boil; cook until the sauce is reduced to 1-1/2 cups, about 12 to 15 minutes. Enjoy with the ribs. Do ahead: Combine seasoned salt, vinegar, brown sugar, ketchup and liquid smoke, if desired, in large resealable plastic freezer bag. Put in pork. Seal the bag then freeze. Put the filled freezer bag in fridge until ribs are thawed completely, about 2 days to use. Cook as instructions.
Nutrition Information
Calories: 550 calories;Sodium: 2003mg sodium Fiber: 0 fiber);Total Carbohydrate: 51g carbohydrate (51g sugars;Cholesterol: 131mg cholesterol;Protein: 40g protein.;Total Fat: 21g fat (8g saturated fat)

742. Super Short Ribs

Serving: 8 | Prep: 30mins | Cook: 2hours | Ready in:
Ingredients
1 tablespoon olive oil
4 1/4 pounds beef short ribs
2 onions, quartered
1 (8 ounce) can pineapple chunks
1 (14 ounce) can beef broth
1/2 cup chili sauce
1/4 cup honey
3 tablespoons Worcestershire sauce
4 cloves garlic, minced
salt and pepper to taste
2 tablespoons chopped fresh parsley, for garnish
Direction
Preheat an oven to 175 °C or 350 °F.
In a Dutch oven, heat oil over moderate high heat. Put the ribs and working in small batches, brown thoroughly on every side. Reserve the ribs.
Put garlic, Worcestershire sauce, honey, chili sauce, pineapple, broth and onions. Put ribs back to the pot, covering them thoroughly with this sauce.
Allow to bake with a cover for an hour at 175 °C or 350 °F. Uncover, season to taste with pepper and salt, and let bake for an hour longer. Jazz up with parsley.
Nutrition Information
Calories: 600 calories;;Sodium: 508;Total Carbohydrate: 21.7;Cholesterol: 99;Protein: 24.3;Total Fat: 46.1

743. Sweet 'n' Sour Ribs

Serving: 8 servings. | Prep: 10mins | Cook: 08hours00mins | Ready in:
Ingredients
3 to 4 pounds boneless country-style pork ribs
1 can (20 ounces) pineapple tidbits, undrained
2 cans (8 ounces each) tomato sauce
1/2 cup thinly sliced onion
1/2 cup thinly sliced green pepper
1/2 cup packed brown sugar
1/4 cup cider vinegar
1/4 cup tomato paste
2 tablespoons Worcestershire sauce
1 garlic clove, minced
1/2 teaspoon salt
1/2 teaspoon pepper
1 tablespoon cornstarch
1 tablespoon cold water
Direction
Put the ribs into an ungreased 5-quart slow cooker. Mix next eleven ingredients; add over the ribs. Cover and cook on low for 8 to 10 hours or until meat soften.
For the sauce, put cooking juices into small saucepan. Boil. In the meantime, combine water and cornstarch in small bowl until they become smooth; then stir into the juices. Bring back to a boil, stirring constantly; then cook while stirring for 1 to 2 minutes or until thicken. Enjoy with the ribs.
Nutrition Information
Calories: 378 calories
Fiber: 2g fiber);Total Carbohydrate: 29g carbohydrate (25g sugars;Cholesterol: 98mg cholesterol;Protein: 31g protein.;Total Fat: 16g fat (6g saturated fat);Sodium: 256mg sodium

744. Sweet Chili Short Ribs

Serving: 5 servings. | Prep: 30mins | Cook: 06hours00mins | Ready in:
Ingredients
1/4 cup all-purpose flour
1/2 teaspoon salt
1/4 teaspoon pepper
1-1/2 pounds boneless beef short ribs
2 tablespoons olive oil
1/2 pound sliced fresh mushrooms
4 medium carrots, sliced
2 cups frozen pearl onions
2 celery ribs, chopped
1 can (15 ounces) tomato sauce
1 jar (12 ounces) apricot preserves
1 jar (12 ounces) pineapple preserves
2 envelopes taco seasoning
1/4 cup packed dark brown sugar
Hot cooked rice or mashed potatoes
Direction
Stir pepper with salt and flour in a big resealable plastic bag. Put in ribs, a few at a time, and shake to coat. Brown ribs in oil in batches on all sides in a big skillet. Shift to a slow cooker of 5-quart. Put in the celery, onions, carrots and mushrooms.
Mix brown sugar, taco seasoning, preserves and tomato sauce in a small bowl; pour over vegetables. Cover and cook for 6 to 8 hours on low, until meat is soft. Serve with potatoes or rice.
Nutrition Information
Calories: 770 calories;Protein: 23g protein.;Total Fat: 17g fat (5g saturated fat);Sodium: 2038mg sodium

Fiber: 3g fiber);Total Carbohydrate: 138g carbohydrate (84g sugars;Cholesterol: 55mg cholesterol

745. Sweet And Savory Ribs

Serving: 8 servings. | Prep: 10mins | Cook: 08hours00mins | Ready in:
Ingredients
1 large onion, chopped
4 pounds boneless country-style pork ribs
1 bottle (18 ounces) honey barbecue sauce
1/3 cup maple syrup
1/4 cup spicy brown mustard
1/2 teaspoon salt
1/4 teaspoon pepper
Direction
Add onion to a 5-quart slow cooker. Place ribs on top. Mix the remaining ingredients in a small bowl and pour over the ribs. Cook while covering for 8-9 hours on low until the meat becomes soft.
Nutrition Information
Calories: 509 calories;Sodium: 945mg sodium Fiber: 0 fiber);Total Carbohydrate: 34g carbohydrate (28g sugars;Cholesterol: 130mg cholesterol;Protein: 40g protein.;Total Fat: 21g fat (7g saturated fat)

746. Sweet And Spicy Jerk Ribs

Serving: 5 servings. | Prep: 10mins | Cook: 06hours00mins | Ready in:
Ingredients
4-1/2 pounds pork baby back ribs
3 tablespoons olive oil
1/3 cup Caribbean jerk seasoning
3 cups honey barbecue sauce
3 tablespoons apricot preserves
2 tablespoons honey
Direction
Divide ribs into serving-size portions; brush oil and rub jerk seasoning. Arrange in a 5- or 6-quart slow cooker. Mix together the remaining ingredients; pour over ribs.
Cook, covered, for 6 to 8 hours on low setting until meat is tender. Ladle fat off the sauce before serving.
Nutrition Information
Calories: 1082 calories;Cholesterol: 220mg cholesterol;Protein: 45g protein.;Total Fat: 61g fat (21g saturated fat);Sodium: 2498mg sodium Fiber: 0 fiber);Total Carbohydrate: 77g carbohydrate (64g sugars

747. Tasty Pork Ribs

Serving: 8 servings. | Prep: 10mins | Cook: 06hours00mins | Ready in:
Ingredients
4 pounds bone-in country-style pork ribs
1 cup ketchup
1 cup barbecue sauce
1/4 cup packed brown sugar
1/4 cup Worcestershire sauce
1 tablespoon balsamic vinegar
1 tablespoon molasses
1 garlic clove, minced
2 tablespoons dried minced onion
1 teaspoon Cajun seasoning
1 teaspoon ground mustard
1/2 teaspoon salt
1/4 teaspoon pepper
Direction
In a 5-quart slow cooker, put ribs. Mix together the rest of the ingredients, pour over the ribs.
Put the lid on and cook on low until the meat is soft, about 6-7 hours.
Nutrition Information
Calories: 371 calories;Cholesterol: 86mg cholesterol;Protein: 27g protein.;Total Fat: 14g fat (5g saturated fat);Sodium: 1076mg sodium Fiber: 1g fiber);Total Carbohydrate: 34g carbohydrate (30g sugars

748. Tender 'n' Tangy Ribs

Serving: 2-3 servings. | Prep: 15mins | Cook: 04hours00mins | Ready in:
Ingredients
3/4 to 1 cup white vinegar
1/2 cup ketchup
2 tablespoons sugar
2 tablespoons Worcestershire sauce
1 garlic clove, minced
1 teaspoon ground mustard
1 teaspoon paprika
1/2 to 1 teaspoon salt
1/8 teaspoon pepper
2 pounds pork spareribs
1 tablespoon canola oil
Direction
In a 3-qt. slow cooker, mix together the first 9 ingredients. Slice ribs into serving-sized pieces; heat oil in a skillet brown in the ribs. Remove into the slow cooker. Cook with a cover on low till tender, or for 4-6 hours.
Nutrition Information
Calories: 689 calories;Protein: 42g protein.;Total Fat: 48g fat (16g saturated fat);Sodium: 1110mg sodium Fiber: 1g fiber);Total Carbohydrate: 22g carbohydrate (13g sugars;Cholesterol: 170mg cholesterol

749. Tender Spareribs

Serving: 8 servings. | Prep: 10mins | Cook: 05hours00mins | Ready in:
Ingredients
4 pounds pork spareribs, cut into serving-size pieces
1/4 cup soy sauce
1/4 cup prepared mustard
1/4 cup molasses
3 tablespoons cider vinegar
2 tablespoons Worcestershire sauce
1 to 2 teaspoons hot pepper sauce
Direction
Put ribs into a 5-qt slow cooker. Mix together the remaining ingredients; transfer over the ribs. Cook with a cover on low till the meat is tender, or for 5-6 hours.
Nutrition Information
Calories: 460 calories;Sodium: 691mg sodium Fiber: 0 fiber);Total Carbohydrate: 9g carbohydrate (6g sugars;Cholesterol: 128mg cholesterol;Protein: 32g protein.;Total Fat: 32g fat (12g saturated fat)

Chapter 9: Mexican Slow Cooker Recipes

750. Barbacoa Style Shredded Beef

Serving: 8 | Prep: 25mins | Cook: 8hours4mins | Ready in:

Ingredients

1 (3 pound) beef chuck roast, cut into 6 to 8 chunks
salt and ground black pepper to taste
2 tablespoons vegetable oil
1/2 cup beef broth
1/4 cup apple cider vinegar
1/4 cup fresh lime juice
4 chipotle peppers in adobo sauce, chopped
5 cloves garlic, chopped
1 tablespoon ground cumin
1 tablespoon dried oregano
1/4 teaspoon ground cloves
3 bay leaves

Direction

Sprinkle salt and pepper on all sides of beef chunks for seasoning.
In a large skillet, heat oil over medium-high heat. Put in the beef in batches, sear each side about 1 minute or until browned. Remove the beef to a slow cooker.
In a mixing bowl, mix cloves, oregano, cumin, garlic, chipotle peppers, lime juice, apple cider vinegar, and beef broth together. Add pepper and salt, mix evenly. Pour the mixture over the beef. Add bay leaves and stir.
Cook on Low heat for 8-10 hours until the beef is really tender.
Remove bay leaves. Take the beef out, and use 2 forks to shred. Dip the beef into the sauce in the slow cooker for at least 10 more minutes before enjoying.

Nutrition Information

Calories: 303 calories;;Total Carbohydrate: 2.6;Cholesterol: 77;Protein: 20.3;Total Fat: 22.9;Sodium: 150

751. Bean And Beef Shaloupias

Serving: 6 | Prep: 30mins | Cook: 30mins | Ready in:

Ingredients

1 pound pinto beans, boiled according to package directions
2 cubes beef bouillon
water to cover
1 1/2 pounds ground beef
1/4 teaspoon salt
1/4 teaspoon ground black pepper
1/2 onion, diced
10 (6 inch) corn tortillas
3 cups shredded Mexican-style cheese

Direction

Mix bouillon cubes and boiled pinto beans together in a slow cooker, add enough water to nearly fill the slow cooker. Simmer it for 8 hours on Low.
Brown beef with onion, pepper, and salt in a big frying pan. Strain thoroughly and put aside.
Put together as follow: Put on top of each tortilla with beef mixture, cheese, and a spoon of beans along with the juice from the slow cooker. Put any garnishes you want on top and enjoy.

Nutrition Information

Calories: 814 calories;;Total Fat: 36;Sodium: 1509;Total Carbohydrate: 72.1;Cholesterol: 129;Protein: 54.3

752. Big Ben's Beef Machaca

Serving: 8 | Prep: 20mins | Cook: 7hours50mins | Ready in:

Ingredients

1 (4 pound) boneless beef chuck roast, trimmed and cut into 8 portions
1/2 cup olive oil
1/4 cup Worcestershire sauce
2 limes, juiced
1 (14 ounce) can diced tomatoes, undrained
1 large sweet onion, diced
1/2 green bell pepper, diced
4 cloves garlic, minced
1 jalapeno pepper, seeded and minced
1/2 cup beef broth
1 tablespoon dried oregano
1 tablespoon ground cumin
1 teaspoon chili powder
1/2 teaspoon salt, or more to taste
1/2 teaspoon ground black pepper

Direction

In the crock of a big slow cooker, put beef portions. In a bowl, combine lime juice, Worcestershire sauce and olive oil together, sprinkle on the meat. Put into the slow cooker black pepper, salt, chili powder, cumin, oregano, beef broth, jalapeno pepper, garlic, green bell pepper, sweet onion and diced tomatoes.
Cook on high heat within 1 hour. Then set to Low heat and cook until the beef is soft, for about 6 1/2 hours.
Use the tongs to place beef into a cutting board. Use a pair of forks to shred meat then put it into the slow cooker again. Cook in 20 to 30 minutes.

Nutrition Information

Calories: 503 calories;;Total Fat: 39.4;Sodium: 426;Total Carbohydrate: 8.7;Cholesterol: 103;Protein: 27.7

753. Birria De Chivo

Serving: 18 | Prep: 30mins | Cook: 8hours | Ready in:

Ingredients

8 dried ancho chiles - stemmed, seeded, and cut into strips
8 dried guajillo chiles - stemmed, seeded, and cut into strips
2 dried cascabel chiles - stemmed, seeded, and cut into strips
5 1/2 cups chicken broth
7 pounds goat meat
1 large onion, diced
12 cloves garlic, minced
4 teaspoons salt
3 teaspoons dried oregano
2 teaspoons ground thyme
1 1/2 teaspoons cumin seeds
1 teaspoon ground allspice
4 whole cloves
ground black pepper to taste
5 bay leaves
8 medium plum tomatoes, quartered
4 tablespoons apple cider vinegar
2 fluid ounces tequila (such as Sauza®)

Direction

On medium heat, heat the dry skillet. Toast chiles for roughly 20 seconds or till fragrant. Move into the heat-proof container with lid. Boil 5 cups water and add on top of chiles just till covered. Cover container and put aside for 20 minutes.

Add the chicken broth to the slow cooker set on Low heat. Put in bay leaves, black pepper, whole cloves, allspice, cumin, thyme, oregano, salt, garlic, onion and goat meat.

In the blender, mix tequila, vinegar and tomatoes and puree till smooth. Put in the drained chiles and blend till as smooth as possible. With a spoon, push the mixture through the small-holed strainer and put into slow cooker; throw anything that's left in the strainer.

Keep slow cooker covered and cook 8-10 hours till meat becomes soft. Skim off the fat and strain juices prior to serving.

Nutrition Information
Calories: 208 calories;;Sodium: 974;Total Carbohydrate: 7.8;Cholesterol: 85;Protein: 31.8;Total Fat: 4.3

754. Cabbage Tamales

Serving: 8 | Prep: 35mins | Cook: 1hours | Ready in:
Ingredients
8 cabbage leaves
1 pound ground beef
1 1/2 cups uncooked white rice
2 (6.5 ounce) cans tomato sauce
3 teaspoons New Mexico red chile powder
2 cloves garlic, minced
1/2 cup chopped onions
salt and ground black pepper to taste
2 (10 ounce) cans diced tomatoes with green chile peppers

Direction
For about 3 minutes, blanch cabbage leaves in a large pot of boiling water until it softens, or freeze them.
Prepare a bowl. Put in the ground beef, onion, tomato sauce, chili powder, rice, garlic, salt, and black pepper. Mix with hands till combined. Divide the meat mixture into 8. Arrange the meat on the softened cabbage leaves. Roll the cabbage leaves up to form logs. Insert the edges under the logs.
Prepare a pressure cooker or a slow cooker to put the tamales in. Put some diced tomatoes with green chilies over the tamales.
Using a pressure cooker: Cover the pressure cooker and adjust it up to full pressure. Lower the heat to low, maintaining full pressure. Cook for an hour. Allow the pressure to go down naturally or use the quick-release option.
Using a slow cooker: Cover the slow cooker and set it on High. For 4 hours, cook the tamales.

Nutrition Information
Calories: 341 calories;;Total Fat: 15.6;Sodium: 579;Total Carbohydrate: 36.4;Cholesterol: 48;Protein: 13.7

755. Carne Adovada

Serving: 8 | Prep: 20mins | Cook: 4hours | Ready in:
Ingredients
3/4 cup New Mexico red chile powder
1 teaspoon cornstarch
2 tablespoons fresh lemon juice
3 cups water
4 pounds beef roast, cut into cubes

Direction
Mix water, lemon juice, cornstarch and chili powder well in a medium bowl. Put meat into the resealable plastic bag with marinade; turn to thoroughly coat. Marinate for 6-16 hours in the fridge.
Put into slow cooker; cook on the high setting till meat easily shreds and is fully cooked for 4 hours.

Nutrition Information
Calories: 495 calories;;Cholesterol: 108;Protein: 34.7;Total Fat: 36.8;Sodium: 206;Total Carbohydrate: 7.1

756. Charley's Slow Cooker Mexican Style Meat

Serving: 12 | Prep: 30mins | Cook: 8hours | Ready in:
Ingredients
1 (4 pound) chuck roast
1 teaspoon salt
1 teaspoon ground black pepper
2 tablespoons olive oil
1 large onion, chopped
1 1/4 cups diced green chile pepper
1 teaspoon chili powder
1 teaspoon ground cayenne pepper
1 (5 ounce) bottle hot pepper sauce
1 teaspoon garlic powder

Direction
Clip roast of any extra fat, and put in pepper and salt to season. In big skillet, heat the olive oil on moderately-high heat. In hot skillet, put beef, and quickly brown it on every side.
Turn roast onto slow cooker and put chopped onion on top. Add garlic powder, hot pepper sauce, cayenne pepper, chili powder and chile peppers to season. Put in sufficient water to soak a third of roast.
Place cover, and cook for 6 hours on High, monitoring to ensure there is at least a bit of liquid in cooker bottom. Lower the heat to Low, and keep cooking till meat is completely soft and separates for 2 or up to 4 hours.
Turn roast onto bowl and pull it apart with 2 forks, set 2 cups cooking liquid aside, if wished. Serve in burritos or tacos.

Nutrition Information
Calories: 260 calories;;Total Fat: 19.1;Sodium: 315;Total Carbohydrate: 3.3;Cholesterol: 69;Protein: 18.4

757. Chicken Butternut Squash Posole

Serving: 8 | Prep: 15mins | Cook: 8hours | Ready in:
Ingredients
1 pound boneless chicken breasts, cut into 2-inch pieces
1 pound butternut squash, peeled and cut into 1-inch pieces
2 (15 ounce) cans red beans, drained and rinsed
1 (28 ounce) can hominy
3 cups low-sodium chicken broth
1 (16 ounce) jar salsa
1/2 (12 fluid ounce) can or bottle beer
2 teaspoons dried Mexican oregano
1/2 cup heavy whipping cream (optional)

Direction
In a slow cooker, combine Mexican oregano, beer, salsa, chicken broth, hominy, red beans, butternut squash, and chicken.
Cook for 3 hours and 30 minutes on High, or 7 hours and 30 minutes in Low. Mix cream into the soup and keep cooking for 30 more minutes.

Nutrition Information
Calories: 327 calories;;Total Fat: 8.5;Sodium: 913;Total Carbohydrate: 41.7;Cholesterol: 54;Protein: 21.3

758. Chicken Enchilada Slow Cooker Soup

Serving: 6 | Prep: 15mins | Cook: 6hours30mins | Ready in:
Ingredients
1 pound skinless, boneless chicken breast halves
1 (15.25 ounce) can whole kernel corn, drained
1 (14.5 ounce) can diced tomatoes including juice
1 (14.5 ounce) can chicken broth
1 (10 ounce) can enchilada sauce
1 (4 ounce) can diced green chiles
1 white onion, chopped
1/4 cup chopped fresh cilantro
2 bay leaves
3 cloves garlic, minced
1 teaspoon ground cumin
1 teaspoon chili powder
1 teaspoon salt
1/4 teaspoon ground black pepper, or to taste
Direction
Clean and pat dry the chicken breasts, position into the base of the rice cooker. Add the black pepper, salt, chili powder, cumin, garlic, bay leaves, cilantro, onion, green chiles, enchilada sauce, chicken broth, tomatoes, and corn.
Cook on Low setting for 6 hours. Place the chicken on a large plate, shred the meat using two forks.
Transfer the chicken back to the slow cooker and go on cooking for half an hour to 1 hour.
Nutrition Information
Calories: 186 calories;;Total Carbohydrate: 22.9;Cholesterol: 39;Protein: 18.4;Total Fat: 3.4;Sodium: 1075

759. Chicken Taco Filling

Serving: 4 | Prep: 5mins | Cook: 6hours | Ready in:
Ingredients
1 (1.25 ounce) package dry taco seasoning mix
1 cup chicken broth
1 pound skinless, boneless chicken breasts
Direction
Mix together taco seasoning and chicken broth in a bowl.
Put the chicken breasts into a slow cooker and pour over the chicken with the chicken broth mixture.
Put the lid on to cover and cook on Low setting for around 6-8 hours.
To serve, shred the chicken.
Nutrition Information
Calories: 149 calories;;Cholesterol: 60;Protein: 22.3;Total Fat: 2.4;Sodium: 935;Total Carbohydrate: 6.3

760. Chicken Verde Sandwiches

Serving: 6 | Prep: 10mins | Cook: 8hours | Ready in:
Ingredients
2 pounds frozen boneless chicken breast
10 ounces prepared pizza sauce
1 cup salsa verde (such as Herdez®)
1/2 cup sour cream
6 kaiser rolls
6 ounces shredded Cheddar cheese
6 ounces sour cream
12 dashes hot sauce, or to taste
Direction
In a slow cooker, mix salsa verde, prepared pizza sauce, and the frozen boneless chicken breast. Put a cover on, select Low and cook for 8-10 hours.
Pull the chicken meat apart with 2 forks until shredded completely. Add 1/2 cup of sour cream into the chicken mixture and stir. Pour the chicken mixture onto the rolls. To serve, put 2 dashes of hot sauce, 1 ounce of sour cream, and 1 ounce of the shredded Cheddar cheese atop each sandwich.
Nutrition Information
Calories: 523 calories;;Total Carbohydrate: 30.8;Cholesterol: 129;Protein: 42.6;Total Fat: 24.2;Sodium: 922

761. Chile Chicken Chili

Serving: 8 | Prep: 15mins | Cook: 4hours30mins | Ready in:
Ingredients
1 rotisserie chicken, skinned and boned, meat pulled into large chunks
2 (16 ounce) jars salsa verde (green salsa)
1 (28 ounce) can tomato puree
1 cup vegetable broth
2 tablespoons chili powder
1 tablespoon ground cumin
1 teaspoon cayenne pepper (optional)
salt and ground black pepper to taste
2 (15 ounce) cans cannellini beans, drained
1 (16 ounce) package frozen sweet white corn
1 (16 ounce) bag frozen bell pepper strips
1 white onion, chopped
Direction
In the slow cooker, put chicken meat; mix in black pepper, salt, cayenne pepper, cumin, chili powder, vegetable broth, tomato puree and salsa verde. Add onion, bell pepper strips, corn and cannellini beans; mix thoroughly.
Cook on High for 2 hours, mixing from time to time. Turn heat to Low and allow to simmer for a minimum of 2 hours or till serving time.
Nutrition Information
Calories: 370 calories;Protein: 28.9;Total Fat: 7;Sodium: 1125;Total Carbohydrate: 48.8;Cholesterol: 62

762. Chili Cumin Stuffed Chicken Breasts

Serving: 4 | Prep: 20mins | Cook: 3hours | Ready in:
Ingredients
1/2 cup shredded Cheddar cheese
1/4 cup chopped green bell pepper
1/4 cup chopped red bell pepper
1/4 cup minced cilantro
1/4 cup diced tomatoes
1/2 teaspoon chili powder
1/2 teaspoon ground cumin
1/8 teaspoon salt
4 skinless, boneless chicken breast halves - pounded to 1/4 inch thickness
toothpicks
Direction
Mix together tomatoes, cilantro, red pepper, green pepper and shredded cheddar cheese in a bowl. Add salt, cumin and chili powder to season. Cover and coat one side of the chicken breasts with enough cheese mixture. Roll breasts over mixture and use toothpicks to secure.
Put the chicken breasts in a slow cooker. Add remaining cheese mixture and cook, covered, for 3 hours on high.
Nutrition Information

Calories: 199 calories;;Total Fat: 8.3;Sodium: 259;Total Carbohydrate: 2.1;Cholesterol: 79;Protein: 27.6

763. Chipotle Barbacoa

Serving: 6 | Prep: 25mins | Cook: 6hours1mins | Ready in:

Ingredients
2 tablespoons vegetable oil
1 (2 pound) beef chuck roast, trimmed and cut into 4 to 6 pieces
1/3 cup apple cider
4 chipotle peppers in adobo sauce
3 tablespoons lime juice
4 cloves garlic, peeled, or more to taste
4 teaspoons cumin
1 serrano chile pepper, chopped (optional)
1 tablespoon ground cayenne pepper, or more to taste (optional)
2 1/2 teaspoons dried oregano
1 teaspoon ground black pepper
1 teaspoon garlic powder
1/2 teaspoon salt
1/2 teaspoon ground cloves
1 cup chicken broth
1 small onion, finely chopped
3 bay leaves

Direction
Use a big skillet to heat oil on low heat and slowly increasing to medium high heat. Add in beef chuck pieces and cook for about 10 seconds per side until browned. Put cooked beef into a slow cooker.
In a food processor or blender, mix ground cloves, salt, garlic powder, black pepper, oregano, cayenne pepper, Serrano pepper, cumin, garlic, lime juice, chipotle peppers and apple cider. Process until smooth and pour mixture onto beef in the slow cooker.
Stir in bay leaves, onion and chicken broth into the slow cooker.
Cook on Low for 6-8 hours until beef is fork-tender. Shred meat using two forks.

Nutrition Information
Calories: 244 calories;;Total Fat: 14.1;Sodium: 449;Total Carbohydrate: 7.3;Cholesterol: 71;Protein: 21.5

764. Cowboy Mexican Dip

Serving: 24 | Prep: 10mins | Cook: 30mins | Ready in:

Ingredients
12 beef tamales, husked and mashed
1 (15 ounce) can chili without beans
1 (14.5 ounce) can diced tomatoes and green chiles
1 (1 pound) loaf processed cheese, cubed

Direction
In a slow cooker, add processed cheese, diced tomatoes, chili and tamales, then set heat on high and cook until cheese has melted while stirring occasionally. Lower heat to low to keep the dip warm while serving. Serve together with tortilla chips or corn chips.

Nutrition Information
Calories: 117 calories;;Sodium: 447;Total Carbohydrate: 7.2;Cholesterol: 21;Protein: 5.7;Total Fat: 7.5

765. Easy Slow Cooker Chicken Fajitas

Serving: 4 | Prep: 10mins | Cook: 8hours | Ready in:

Ingredients
4 (6 ounce) chicken breasts
1 (15.25 ounce) can whole kernel corn, drained
1 (15 ounce) can black beans, drained
1 (8 ounce) jar salsa
1 (1.25 ounce) package taco seasoning

Direction
In a slow cooker, combine taco seasoning, salsa, beans, corn and chicken.
Cook for about 8 hours on low until the flavors blend and the chicken is softened.
With 2 forks, shred chicken meat.

Nutrition Information
Calories: 416 calories;;Cholesterol: 97;Protein: 45.5;Total Fat: 5.5;Sodium: 1793;Total Carbohydrate: 47.2

766. Easy Slow Cooker Enchiladas

Serving: 6 | Prep: 15mins | Cook: 5hours15mins | Ready in:

Ingredients
1 pound ground turkey
1 cup chopped onion
3/4 cup chopped green bell pepper
2 cloves garlic, minced
1 (16 ounce) can kidney beans, rinsed and drained
1 (15 ounce) can black beans, rinsed and drained
1 (10 ounce) can diced tomatoes with green chile peppers
1/3 cup water
1 1/2 teaspoons chili powder
1/2 teaspoon ground cumin
1/4 teaspoon salt
1/4 teaspoon ground black pepper
2 cups shredded Cheddar cheese
2 cups shredded Monterey Jack cheese
6 (6 inch) corn tortillas

Direction
Into big skillet, break up turkey on moderate heat. Into the turkey, mix garlic, bell pepper and onion. Cook and mix for 5 to 7 minutes till turkey is fully browned. Put in pepper, salt, cumin, chili powder, water, diced tomatoes, black beans and kidney beans; boil, lower heat to moderately-low, cover skillet, and let simmer for ten minutes.
In bowl, stir together Monterey jack cheese and Cheddar cheese.
Layer approximately 3/4 cup mixture of turkey, a tortilla, and half cup mixture of cheese in a 5-quart slow cooker base; redo piled till all ingredients are used, finishing with layer of cheese.
Cook on Low until heated through, 5 to 7 hours.

Nutrition Information
Calories: 614 calories;;Total Fat: 31.1;Sodium: 1216;Total Carbohydrate: 41.5;Cholesterol: 129;Protein: 44.3

767. Frijoles II

Serving: 4 | Prep: 15mins | Cook: 6hours | Ready in:

Ingredients
1 1/2 cups dry pinto beans
1/2 teaspoon white sugar
1 teaspoon minced garlic
2 tablespoons finely chopped onion
2 slices smoked bacon
2 cups water
salt to taste

Direction
Into a slow cooker, put the bacon, onion, garlic, sugar and beans. Add in water, put cover, and allow to cook

for 6 hours on High. Pour off 2/3 of liquid, and get rid of the bacon. Crush beans to a chunky consistency with a potato masher. Season to taste with salt, and serve while hot.

Nutrition Information
Calories: 320 calories;;Total Fat: 7.2;Sodium: 202;Total Carbohydrate: 46.6;Cholesterol: 10;Protein: 17.2

768. Frijoles A La Charra

Serving: 8 | Prep: 15mins | Cook: 5hours | Ready in:

Ingredients
1 pound dry pinto beans
5 cloves garlic, chopped
1 teaspoon salt
1/2 pound bacon, diced
1 onion, chopped
2 fresh tomatoes, diced
1 (3.5 ounce) can sliced jalapeno peppers
1 (12 fluid ounce) can beer
1/3 cup chopped fresh cilantro

Direction
In a slow cooker, put pinto beans and add water until fully covered. Stir in salt and garlic. Put a cover on, and cook on high for 1 hour.
Cook bacon on medium-high heat in a frying pan until soft and turning evenly brown. Strain approximately half of the grease. Put the onion in the frying pan, and cook until soft. Stir in jalapenos and tomatoes, and cook until cooked through. Move to the slow cooker, mixing into the beans.
Put a lid on the slow cooker, and keep cooking on Low for 4 hours. Approximately 30 minutes before the cooking time finishes, mix in cilantro and beer.

Nutrition Information
Calories: 353 calories;;Cholesterol: 19;Protein: 16;Total Fat: 13.8;Sodium: 741;Total Carbohydrate: 39.8

769. Green Chile Beef Tacos

Serving: 12 | Prep: 10mins | Cook: 4hours | Ready in:

Ingredients
5 pounds boneless beef chuck roast
1 (1 ounce) packet taco seasoning mix
1 (16 ounce) jar green salsa
2 cups beef broth, or more if needed

Direction
Prepare a slow cooker that comes with a tight-fitting lid, place the chuck roast into the bottom of the slow cooker. Put taco seasoning mix on top of the beef. Pour in the green salsa then the beef broth
Cook over low heat for 4 hours. If needed, you can add more beef broth. Remove the beef and use 2 forks to shred. Put the shredded beef back into the slow cooker, mix well with liquid. Serve when hot

Nutrition Information
Calories: 298 calories;;Cholesterol: 82;Protein: 23.1;Total Fat: 19.8;Sodium: 477;Total Carbohydrate: 4.3

770. Ground Turkey Enchilada Stew With Quinoa

Serving: 8 | Prep: 10mins | Cook: 4hours5mins | Ready in:

Ingredients
1 pound ground turkey
1 (19 ounce) can enchilada sauce
1 (15 ounce) can black beans, drained
1 1/2 cups uncooked quinoa
1 (10 ounce) can diced tomatoes and green chiles, undrained
1 cup water
1 cup frozen corn
1/2 cup salsa
1/2 cup chopped onion
1/2 cup chopped green bell pepper
1 tablespoon chili powder
1 teaspoon minced garlic
1 teaspoon ground cumin
2 cups shredded Mexican cheese blend
1/3 cup chopped fresh cilantro

Direction
Heat a large frying pan over medium-high heat. In the hot skillet, cook and mix turkey for 5 – 7 minutes until crumbly and browned. Drain and remove the grease.
In a slow cooker, blend cumin, garlic, chili powder, green bell pepper, onion, salsa, corn, water, chiles, diced tomatoes, quinoa, black beans, enchilada sauce, and browned turkey.
Cook on High for around 4 hours in the slow cooker until quinoa is softened and flavors are combined.
Fold in cilantro and Cheddar cheese.

Nutrition Information
Calories: 452 calories;Protein: 27.7;Total Fat: 19.4;Sodium: 943;Total Carbohydrate: 43.6;Cholesterol: 77

771. Kris' Amazing Shredded Mexican Beef

Serving: 12 | Prep: 25mins | Cook: 8hours20mins | Ready in:

Ingredients
1 (4 pound) beef bottom round roast or other lean roast
2 teaspoons ground black pepper
1 large onion, diced
1 (7 ounce) can chopped green chilies
2 teaspoons chili powder
1 teaspoon cayenne pepper
1 tablespoon garlic powder
2 teaspoons ground cumin
1 (7 ounce) can chipotle peppers in adobo sauce, or to taste
1 cube beef bouillon

Direction
Clip any excess fat of roast, and slice into 4 portions. Massage with black pepper, and put into slow cooker. Put the beef bouillon, chipotle peppers, cumin, garlic powder, cayenne pepper, chili powder, green chiles and onions. Add in sufficient water to submerge 1/3 of roast.
Put cover, and allow to cook on High for 8 hours till meat starts to crumble. Put water if necessary, to prevent roast from drying out.
Set slow cooker to Low, and using a slotted spoon, take off meat to a big bowl. Shred meat into bite-sized portions using two forks. Put the meat back to slow cooker; allow to cook for 20 minutes to reheat prior to serving.

Nutrition Information
Calories: 338 calories;;Sodium: 426;Total Carbohydrate: 4.3;Cholesterol: 97;Protein: 31.2;Total Fat: 20.8

772. Latin Inspired Spicy Cream Chicken Stew

Serving: 8 | Prep: 10mins | Cook: 8hours15mins | Ready in:
Ingredients
6 skinless, boneless chicken breast halves
3 (14.5 ounce) cans diced tomatoes
1 (16 ounce) jar green salsa
1 (15 ounce) can black beans, rinsed and drained
1 (15 ounce) can pinto beans, drained and rinsed
1 (15.25 ounce) can whole kernel corn, drained
1 (1.25 ounce) package taco seasoning
1 tablespoon chopped fresh cilantro
2 teaspoons ground red chile pepper, or to taste
1 teaspoon ground cumin
1/2 cup cream cheese, softened
Direction
In the bottom of a slow cooker, place the breasts of chicken, pour corn, pinto beans, black beans, green salsa and tomatoes over the chicken. Drizzle cumin, ground red chile, cilantro and taco seasoning to the mixture, combine by stirring. Put the lid on the cooker, cook on Low for 8-10 hours until the mixture has thickened and chicken is really soft.
Reserve all liquid in the cooker for soup; remove some liquid if you like the stew thicker. In a bowl, stir 1-2 tablespoons of liquid with cream cheese until smooth, pour the cream cheese into the cooker for a creamy sauce. Keep cooking for a quarter hour then serve.
Nutrition Information
Calories: 334 calories;;Sodium: 1302;Total Carbohydrate: 37.4;Cholesterol: 62;Protein: 26.1;Total Fat: 8

773. Mexican Pintos With Cactus

Serving: 10 | Prep: 10mins | Cook: 4hours | Ready in:
Ingredients
2 cups dry pinto beans, rinsed
3 tablespoons salt, divided
3 slices bacon, chopped
2 large flat cactus leaves (nopales)
1 jalapeno pepper, seeded and chopped
2 slices onion
Direction
Into a slow cooker, put pinto beans, and fill with hot water, reaching the top. Put onion, jalapeno, 2 tablespoons of salt and bacon. Place the cover, and allow to cook for 3 to 4 hours on High, putting water as necessary, till beans are soft.
Get rid of any cactus leaves thorns, and cut into small portions. Put in a saucepan with a tablespoon salt, and fill with sufficient water to submerge. Boil, and allow to cook for 15 minutes. Let drain and wash in cold water for a minute. Put to beans once tender, and allow to cook on High for 15 minutes longer.
Nutrition Information
Calories: 153 calories;Protein: 9.5;Total Fat: 1.6;Sodium: 2162;Total Carbohydrate: 25.2;Cholesterol: 3

774. Mexican Pot Roast

Serving: 12 | Prep: 15mins | Cook: 8hours10mins | Ready in:
Ingredients
2 tablespoons olive oil
1 (4 pound) beef chuck roast, trimmed
1 teaspoon salt
1 teaspoon ground black pepper
1 large onion, chopped
1 1/4 cups diced green chile pepper
1 (5 ounce) bottle hot sauce
1/4 cup taco seasoning
1 teaspoon chili powder
1 teaspoon cayenne pepper
1 teaspoon garlic powder
Direction
In a big skillet, heat the olive oil over medium-high heat. Use salt and pepper to season the beef chuck roast then cook it in hot oil for 2 to 3 minutes on each side. When it has browned entirely, move it to a slow cooker.
Sprinkle garlic powder, cayenne pepper, chilli powder, taco seasoning, hot sauce, chile pepper and onion over the roast and cook it on low. Let it cook for 8 to 10 hours until the meat is fall-apart tender.
Nutrition Information
Calories: 213 calories;;Cholesterol: 70;Protein: 21.2;Total Fat: 11.2;Sodium: 772;Total Carbohydrate: 5.4

775. Mexican Style Shredded Pork

Serving: 6 | Prep: 15mins | Cook: 7hours | Ready in:
Ingredients
1 (3 pound) boneless pork loin roast, cut into 2 inch pieces
1/2 teaspoon salt
2 (4 ounce) cans diced green chile peppers
3 cloves garlic, crushed
1/4 cup chipotle sauce
3 1/4 cups water, divided
1 1/2 cups uncooked long grain white rice
1/4 cup fresh lime juice
1/4 cup chopped cilantro
Direction
In a slow cooker, place the roast and sprinkle with salt to season. Top the roast with garlic and chile peppers. Pour in half a cup of water and chipotle sauce.
Cook with a cover on Low for 7 hours.
Bring a pot of rice and leftover 2 3/4 cups water to a boil. Whisk in the cilantro and lime juice. Turn to low heat, simmer with a cover for 20 minutes.
Take roast out of the slow cooker, and shred with two forks. Bring pork back to the slow cooker, and let it stand for 15 minutes to absorb some of the liquid. Place over the cooked rice and serve.
Nutrition Information
Calories: 520 calories;;Sodium: 802;Total Carbohydrate: 43;Cholesterol: 108;Protein: 41.1;Total Fat: 19

776. Mijo's Slow Cooker Shredded Beef

Serving: 8 | Prep: 20mins | Cook: 10hours | Ready in:
Ingredients
5 pounds chuck roast
3 cloves garlic, crushed
1 tablespoon paprika
1 tablespoon celery salt
1 tablespoon garlic powder
1 tablespoon dried parsley
1/2 tablespoon ground black pepper
1/2 tablespoon chili powder
1/2 tablespoon cayenne pepper
1/2 teaspoon seasoned salt
1/2 teaspoon mustard powder
1/2 teaspoon dried tarragon
4 fluid ounces beer
1 1/2 tablespoons Worcestershire sauce
4 tablespoons hot pepper sauce

2 teaspoons liquid smoke flavoring
1 large onion, chopped
1 green bell pepper, chopped
2 jalapeno chile peppers, chopped

Direction

Form a few 1 inch deep holes in the roast using a sharp knife. Put the garlic silvers into the holes.
Mix together dried tarragon, mustard powder, seasoned salt, cayenne pepper, chili powder, ground black pepper, parsley, garlic powder, celery salt, and paprika in a small bowl. Combined well and spread the mixture over the meat.
Combine together liquid smoke, hot pepper sauce, Worcestershire sauce, and beer or cola in a separate small bowl. Mix properly. In the slow cooker, put in the roast and place this mixture over the meat.
Put jalapeno chile peppers, green bell pepper and onion into the slow cooker.
On low setting, cook for 10 hours or more, if you want.

Nutrition Information

Calories: 621 calories;;Total Fat: 39.7;Sodium: 917;Total Carbohydrate: 6.6;Cholesterol: 184;Protein: 55.8

777. Paddy's Chile Verde

Serving: 8 | Prep: 30mins | Cook: 4hours15mins | Ready in:

Ingredients

4 pounds fresh tomatillos, husks removed
2 large onions (keep the skin on)
2 poblano peppers
1 head garlic
3 chipotle peppers in adobo sauce
2 (12 fluid ounce) cans or bottles lager-style beer
1 tablespoon ground cumin
1 tablespoon salt
1 tablespoon ground black pepper
4 tablespoons vegetable oil
4 pounds cubed lamb stew meat

Direction

Preheat oven's broiler, place the rack about 6 inches away from the heat source.
On a baking sheet, arrange garlic, poblano peppers, onions, and tomatillos.
Cook the vegetables under the broiler for 3 to 5 minutes on each side, until the skins on side near the heat source are charred; turn to cook the other side until equally charred.
Remove and discard the stems and seeds from the peppers, and the root and outer skin from the garlic and onion.
In a blender, combine pepper, salt, cumin, lager-style beer, chipotle peppers in adobo sauce, garlic, poblano peppers, onion, and some of the tomatillos in about half full; work in batches. Hold the lid down, pulse a few times, then leave the blender on to puree until mixture smoothens. Transfer into a slow cooker.
In a large saucepan, heat oil. Cook and stir cubed lamb in the hot oil for about 5 minutes, until all sides are evenly browned. Transfer into the slow cooker.
Cook for 4 hours on High.

Nutrition Information

Calories: 487 calories;Protein: 41.9;Total Fat: 22.4;Sodium: 1011;Total Carbohydrate: 24.6;Cholesterol: 124

778. Paleo Mexican Pulled Pork

Serving: 8 | Prep: 40mins | Cook: 8hours17mins | Ready in:

Ingredients

2 Anaheim chile peppers
3 pounds boneless pork shoulder
1 teaspoon sea salt
1/2 teaspoon ground black pepper
2 tablespoons bacon fat
1 cup beef broth
1 (6 ounce) can tomato paste
1 onion, halved and sliced
1 red bell pepper, seeded and sliced
1 yellow bell pepper, seeded and sliced
1 lime, juiced
4 cloves garlic, crushed
1 tablespoon ground cumin
1 tablespoon dried oregano
1/4 teaspoon chili powder
1/4 teaspoon ground cayenne pepper
1 bay leaf
Toppings:
2 ripe avocados, sliced
3 tablespoons chopped fresh cilantro
2 limes, quartered

Direction

Place oven rack about 6-inch away from the heat source and start preheating the oven's broiler. Line aluminum foil on a baking sheet.
Slice Anaheim chile peppers lengthwise into 2 slices; remove the ribs, seeds, and stem. Arrange peppers, with the cut-side down, on the prepared baking sheet. Cook in the prepared broiler until peppers seem blistery and blackened, about 5 to 8 minutes. Place to a bowl and with plastic wrap, cover tightly. Allow peppers to steam as they cool, for 20 minutes. Discard skins; chop the flesh.
Flavor pork with black pepper and salt.
In a large skillet, heat bacon fat on medium-high heat. Add in pork; cook until brown, for 3 minutes each side.
Transfer the pork to a slow cooker. Pour in beef broth and coat pork with tomato paste. Add in bay leaf, cayenne pepper, chili powder, oregano, cumin, garlic, lime juice, yellow bell pepper, red bell pepper, onion, and roasted chile pepper.
Cook on low until pork softens, for 8 hours. Using 2 forks, shred pork. Serve with lime wedges, cilantro, and avocados.

Nutrition Information

Calories: 251 calories;;Sodium: 553;Total Carbohydrate: 10.1;Cholesterol: 70;Protein: 21.1;Total Fat: 14.1

779. Pork Chalupas

Serving: 16 | Prep: 15mins | Cook: 9hours | Ready in:

Ingredients

1 (4 pound) pork shoulder roast
1 pound dried pinto beans
3 (4 ounce) cans diced green chile peppers
2 tablespoons chili powder
2 tablespoons ground cumin
2 tablespoons salt
2 tablespoons dried oregano
2 tablespoons garlic powder
16 flour tortillas

Direction

In a slow cooker grease with cooking spray, put the roast. Mix together the garlic powder, oregano, salt,

cumin, chili powder, 2 cans of the chili peppers and beans in another bowl. Add the entire mixture on the roast, and put sufficient water to soak most part of the roast. Wiggle the roast a bit to get some of the liquid beneath.
Put the cover, and allow to cook for 8 to 9 hours on Low. Monitor after 5 hours to ensure beans have not soaked in all of liquid. Put additional water if needed, a cup at a time. Put just the right amount to prevent beans from drying out.
Once roast is fork-tender, take off from the slow cooker, and put on a chopping board. Get rid of any fat and bone, then pull apart using forks. Put back to slow cooker, and mix in the rest of green chilies can. Heat completely, and serve together with flour tortillas and desire toppings.
Nutrition Information
Calories: 474 calories;;Total Fat: 14.9;Sodium: 1622;Total Carbohydrate: 57.8;Cholesterol: 45;Protein: 26.4

780. Pork Chile Rojo (Pulled Pork With Red Chile Sauce)

Serving: 8 | Prep: 15mins | Cook: 9hours | Ready in:
Ingredients
1 (4 pound) boneless pork shoulder roast, trimmed
3 tablespoons chili powder
1 cup chopped onions
4 cups water
2 (16 ounce) jars salsa
2 (10 ounce) cans diced tomatoes with green chilies, undrained
Direction
In an oven roasting bag placed in a slow cooker, put the pork roast. Sprinkle the roast with chili powder and top with onions. With a nylon tie, loosely close top of the bag. With scissors, cut 3 vents in top of the bag, 1-inch long each. Add water to bottom of the slow cooker to cover the surrounding of the bag, at least 1 inch deep.
Cover the slow cooker and cook the pork for 6-8 hours on Low.
Take onions and pork out of the bag; place in a big Dutch oven and save 3/4 cup liquid from the bag. With 2 forks, pull the pork apart to shred. Mix cooking liquid, tomatoes, and salsa into the shredded pork.
Heat to a boil on high heat. Decrease to low heat. Put on cover and simmer for 1 hour, mixing occasionally.
Nutrition Information
Calories: 291 calories;;Total Fat: 13.9;Sodium: 862;Total Carbohydrate: 13.4;Cholesterol: 99;Protein: 29.2

781. Queso Con Carne

Serving: 16 | Prep: 10mins | Cook: 1hours15mins | Ready in:
Ingredients
1 (1 pound) loaf processed cheese (such as Velveeta®), cubed
1/2 cup milk
2 pounds ground beef
4 (10 ounce) cans diced tomatoes with green chile peppers (such as RO*TEL®)
1 (1.25 ounce) package taco seasoning
Direction
In a slow cooker, add milk and processed cheese.
Heat a big skillet on moderately high heat, then cook and stir in the hot skillet with beef, until beef is crumbly, browned evenly and not pink anymore. Drain and get rid of any excess grease.
Stir into ground beef with taco seasoning and diced tomatoes, then bring the mixture to a boil.
Remove the ground beef mixture to the slow cook then stir with processed cheese and milk.
Cook on high setting for an hour, until cheese has melted.
Nutrition Information
Calories: 227 calories;;Sodium: 823;Total Carbohydrate: 6.6;Cholesterol: 57;Protein: 14.9;Total Fat: 15.4

782. Simple Slow Cooked Korean Beef Soft Tacos

Serving: 8 | Prep: 15mins | Cook: 8hours | Ready in:
Ingredients
1 (3 pound) beef chuck roast, trimmed
1/2 onion, diced
1/2 cup dark brown sugar
1/3 cup soy sauce
10 cloves garlic
1 jalapeno pepper, diced (optional)
1 (1 inch) piece fresh ginger root, peeled and grated
2 tablespoons seasoned rice vinegar
1 tablespoon sesame oil
salt and ground black pepper to taste
16 (6 inch) corn tortillas (optional)
Direction
Transfer the chuck roast into the crock of a slow cooker. Add onion, jalapeno pepper, brown sugar, sesame oil, soy sauce, rice vinegar, garlic, ginger root, pepper, and salt.
Cook on Low for 10 hours or on High for 8 hours. Use a pair of forks to shred the meat and then mix into the liquid in the slow cooker.
You can serve with toppings you like and corn tortillas.
Nutrition Information
Calories: 456 calories;;Total Carbohydrate: 40.3;Cholesterol: 77;Protein: 23.9;Total Fat: 22.4;Sodium: 697

783. Slow Cooker Beef Barbacoa

Serving: 8 | Prep: 30mins | Cook: 6hours | Ready in:
Ingredients
3 pounds boneless beef chuck roast
1 onion, chopped
3 bay leaves
1/2 teaspoon ground black pepper, or to taste
2 tablespoons garlic powder
1/4 cup distilled white vinegar
1 (14 ounce) can tomato sauce
1/4 cup chili powder
salt to taste
Direction
In slow cooker, place vinegar, garlic powder, black pepper, bay leaves, onion and the roast. Use water to completely cover the ingredients. Cover the meat and cook until it reaches full tenderness and start falling apart on high setting, for 4 hours.
Strain the liquids from the meat. Put the meat back in the slow cooker and start shredding with knife and fork. Stir the shredded meat together with salt, chili powder and tomato sauce. Cover the cooker, cook sauce together with meat for 2 more hours on high.
Nutrition Information

Calories: 292 calories;;Total Fat: 18.8;Sodium: 350;Total Carbohydrate: 9.1;Cholesterol: 77;Protein: 22

784. Slow Cooker Carnitas

Serving: 10 | Prep: 10mins | Cook: 10hours | Ready in:
Ingredients
1 teaspoon salt
1 teaspoon garlic powder
1 teaspoon ground cumin
1/2 teaspoon crumbled dried oregano
1/2 teaspoon ground coriander
1/4 teaspoon ground cinnamon
1 (4 pound) boneless pork shoulder roast
2 bay leaves
2 cups chicken broth
Direction
In a bowl, mix cinnamon, coriander, oregano, cumin, garlic powder and salt together. Add spice mixture over the pork to coat. In bottom of the slow cooker, put bay leaves; put pork on the top. Add chicken broth around the pork's' sides, being careful not to rinse the spice mixture off.
Cook, covered, on Low for 10 hours or until easily shreds the pork with a fork. After the meat has been cooked for 5 hours, flip. Take out of the slow cooker once pork is tender, then use 2 forks to shred. If needed, moisten meat with the cooking liquid.
Nutrition Information
Calories: 223 calories;;Sodium: 474;Total Carbohydrate: 0.7;Cholesterol: 73;Protein: 22.2;Total Fat: 13.8

785. Slow Cooker Cheesy Chicken And Tortillas

Serving: 6 | Prep: 10mins | Cook: 8hours | Ready in:
Ingredients
1 1/4 pounds skinless, boneless chicken breast halves
1 tablespoon chili powder
1 teaspoon ground cumin
1 3/4 cups Swanson® Natural Goodness Chicken Broth
2 (10.5 ounce) cans Campbell's® Condensed Cream of Chicken Soup or Campbell's® Condensed 98% Fat Free Cream of Chicken Soup
8 (6 inch) flour tortillas, cut into 1-inch pieces
2 cups shredded Mexican cheese blend
6 cups hot cooked long-grain white rice
Direction
In a 4-quart slow cooker, add the chicken. Dust with cumin and chili powder. Add the broth.
Cook while covered on LOW for about 8 - 9 hours or till the chicken is cooked through. Transfer the chicken to a cutting board. Use 2 forks to shred the chicken.
Keep 1 cup of liquid in the cooker; if needed, pour in extra broth to make 1 cup. Mix the soup into the cooker. Mix in chicken.
Heat the oven to 350°F. In a 13x9x2-inch baking dish, layer 1/2 the chicken mixture, tortillas and cheese. Redo the layers.
Bake for 30 minutes or till the mixture becomes bubbling and hot. Serve with the rice.
Nutrition Information
Calories: 687 calories;;Total Carbohydrate: 72.9;Cholesterol: 100;Protein: 39;Total Fat: 26.1;Sodium: 1482

786. Slow Cooker Chicken Taco Soup

Serving: 8 | Prep: 15mins | Cook: 7hours | Ready in:
Ingredients
1 onion, chopped
1 (16 ounce) can chili beans
1 (15 ounce) can black beans
1 (15 ounce) can whole kernel corn, drained
1 (8 ounce) can tomato sauce
1 (12 fluid ounce) can or bottle beer
2 (10 ounce) cans diced tomatoes with green chilies, undrained
1 (1.25 ounce) package taco seasoning
3 whole skinless, boneless chicken breasts
1 (8 ounce) package shredded Cheddar cheese (optional)
sour cream (optional)
crushed tortilla chips (optional)
Direction
Place diced tomatoes, beer, tomato sauce, corn, black beans, chili beans, and onion in a slow cooker. Add taco seasoning, stirring to blend. Lay the chicken breasts over the mixture and press them down slightly to just be covered by other ingredients. Set the slow cooker to a low heat setting and cook while covered for 5 hours.
Take out the chicken breasts and cool enough to handle. Mix the shredded chicken back into the soup and continue to cook for an additional 2 hours. If desired, you can serve with a topping of crushed tortilla chips, a dollop of sour cream, and shredded Cheddar cheese.
Nutrition Information
Calories: 434 calories;;Total Fat: 17.7;Sodium: 1597;Total Carbohydrate: 42.3;Cholesterol: 68;Protein: 27.2

787. Slow Cooker Chicken Tacos With Chipotle Cream Sauce

Serving: 10 | Prep: 15mins | Cook: 4hours5mins | Ready in:
Ingredients
4 frozen chicken thighs
2 frozen chicken breast halves
1/4 cup red wine vinegar
1/4 cup diced green onions
2 limes, juiced
6 cloves garlic, minced
Chipotle Cream Sauce:
1 cup sour cream
2 chipotle peppers in adobo sauce
1/4 teaspoon salt
salt and ground black pepper to taste
2 tablespoons minced fresh cilantro
10 flour tortillas
Direction
In a slow cooker, put the chicken breasts and chicken thighs. In a bowl, beat garlic, lime juice, green onions and red wine vinegar together; put on top of chicken. Allow to cook on High for 4 hours.
In a food processor, process 1/4 teaspoon salt, chipotle peppers in adobo sauce and sour cream together till sauce is velvety; chill till about to use.
On a work area, put the chicken and shred into bite-size pieces; put pepper and salt to season. In slow cooker, get half-cup cooking liquid and throw the remaining. To slow cooker, put back half-cup cooking liquid and shredded chicken and put cilantro; cook and mix for 5 minutes till chicken is heated through.

Into the tortillas, scoop the chicken and put chipotle cream sauce on top.
Nutrition Information
Calories: 311 calories;;Total Fat: 13.3;Sodium: 365;Total Carbohydrate: 30.3;Cholesterol: 47;Protein: 16.7

788. Slow Cooker Chicken Tinga

Serving: 18 | Prep: 15mins | Cook: 2hours45mins | Ready in:
Ingredients
4 skinless, boneless chicken breast halves
1 onion, chopped
1 (15 ounce) can tomato sauce
1 (7 ounce) can chipotle chile peppers in adobo sauce, chopped and seeded
2 fresh jalapeno peppers, seeded and chopped
2 cloves garlic, minced
1 teaspoon ground oregano
1 teaspoon ground cumin
1 teaspoon chili powder
1/4 teaspoon red pepper flakes
3/4 (1 pound) chorizo sausage
Direction
In a slow cooker, combine chipotle chile pepper, tomato sauce, onion, chicken with red pepper flakes, chili powder, cumin, oregano, garlic, jalapeno peppers, and adobo sauce.
Set the cooker to Low, cook for 2-3 hours until chicken is not pink inside anymore. Take chicken out of slow cooker, use two forks to shred then bring back to the slow cooker.
Heat a big skillet on medium-high heat, add chorizo sausage; stir and cook about 5-10 minutes until crumbly and brown. Drain then throw away grease. Put chorizo in the chicken mixture and stir.
Choose Low setting on the slow cooker, cook about 3/4 hour - 1 hour.
Nutrition Information
Calories: 131 calories;;Sodium: 418;Total Carbohydrate: 3.9;Cholesterol: 30;Protein: 10.2;Total Fat: 8.1

789. Slow Cooker Chicken Tinga Tacos

Serving: 10 | Prep: 20mins | Cook: 10hours | Ready in:
Ingredients
2 1/2 pounds boneless, skinless chicken breasts, cut into 2- to 3-inch pieces
1/4 cup Mazola® Corn Oil
3 cups roughly chopped onion
5 plum tomatoes, cored and chopped
2 individual chipotle peppers in adobo sauce (or more to taste), finely chopped (from a 7-ounce can)
2 teaspoons Spice Islands® Minced Garlic
1 1/4 cups chicken broth
Warm corn or flour tortillas or crisp 6-inch tostadas
Toppings for Tacos or Tostadas:
Shredded lettuce
Diced tomatoes
Shredded or crumbled Mexican cheese
Fresh cilantro
Avocado slices or guacamole
Direction
With paper towels, pat the chicken dry. In a big skillet, heat 2 tablespoons of the oil on moderately-high heat. To skillet, put 1/2 the chicken and cook for 3 to 4 minutes till slightly brown on a side. Turn the chicken onto 6 quarts slow cooker. Redo with the rest of chicken. To skillet, put onions and 2 tablespoons of the oil and cook till onions start to soften, for 3 to 4 minutes.
Put into slow cooker with chicken broth, garlic, chipotles and tomatoes. Combine thoroughly. Cook on HIGH for 3 hours to 4 hours, or on LOW 4 hours to 6 hours. Tinga Chicken is ready once chicken is soft and can easily be shredded. With 2 forks, pull chicken pieces apart. Serve Tinga together with crisp tostadas or warm tortillas and in small bowls, place the toppings. Top as preferred.
Nutrition Information
Calories: 258 calories;;Total Carbohydrate: 14.3;Cholesterol: 60;Protein: 24.6;Total Fat: 11.7;Sodium: 196

790. Slow Cooker Chile Verde

Serving: 8 | Prep: 20mins | Cook: 8hours | Ready in:
Ingredients
3 tablespoons olive oil
1/2 cup onion, chopped
2 cloves garlic, minced
3 pounds boneless pork shoulder, cubed
5 (7 ounce) cans green salsa
1 (4 ounce) can diced jalapeno peppers
1 (14.5 ounce) can diced tomatoes
Direction
Heat the oil over medium heat in a big skillet or Dutch oven. Put in the garlic and onion; cook and mix until fragrant. Put in cubed pork then cook until the outside is browned. Move the garlic, onions, and pork to a slow cooker and mix in the tomatoes, jalapeno peppers, and green salsa.
Cover and cook for 3 hours on High. Lower setting to low then cook for another 4 to 5 hours.
Nutrition Information
Calories: 265 calories;;Total Fat: 12.4;Sodium: 765;Total Carbohydrate: 12.1;Cholesterol: 64;Protein: 22.5

791. Slow Cooker Chile Verde (Green Chile)

Serving: 8 | Prep: 20mins | Cook: 6hours10mins | Ready in:
Ingredients
1 cup all-purpose flour, or as needed
5 pounds boneless pork shoulder, cut into cubes
3 tablespoons olive oil
1 yellow onion, chopped
2 (16 ounce) jars salsa verde (such as Herdez®)
1 (10 ounce) can diced tomatoes with green chile peppers (such as RO*TEL®)
1 (4 ounce) can diced jalapeno peppers, or to taste
1 (4 ounce) can diced green chiles
2 cloves garlic, minced
1 teaspoon dried oregano
1 teaspoon ground cumin
Direction
In a shallow bowl, spread flour. Dredge the pork cubes in flour to coat.
In a large Dutch oven over medium heat, heat olive oil. Cook and stir onion in hot oil until aromatic for 3 to 5 minutes. Put in pork; cook and stir until all sides of the pork is well-browned for 5 to 7 minutes. Pour the pork-and-onion mixture to a slow cooker. Stir cumin, oregano, garlic, diced green chiles, diced jalapeno peppers, diced tomatoes with green chile peppers, and salsa verde into the pork mixture.
Cook for 6 hours on low.
Nutrition Information

Calories: 505 calories;;Total Fat: 26.8;Sodium: 989;Total Carbohydrate: 25.5;Cholesterol: 113;Protein: 36.7

792. Slow Cooker Cilantro Lime Chicken

Serving: 6 | Prep: 10mins | Cook: 4hours | Ready in:

Ingredients
1 (16 ounce) jar salsa
1 (1.25 ounce) package dry taco seasoning mix
1 lime, juiced
3 tablespoons chopped fresh cilantro
3 pounds skinless, boneless chicken breast halves

Direction
In a slow cooker, put the cilantro, lime juice, taco seasoning and salsa, then mix to blend. Put in chicken breasts, then mix to coat with salsa mix. Cover the cooker, set to High, then cook for 4 hours until the chicken is very soft. Set the cooker to Low and cook for 6 to 8 hours, if you like. Shred chicken using 2 forks, serve.

Nutrition Information
Calories: 272 calories;;Total Fat: 4.7;Sodium: 976;Total Carbohydrate: 9.3;Cholesterol: 117;Protein: 45.3

793. Slow Cooker Enchiladas

Serving: 6 | Prep: 20mins | Cook: 45mins | Ready in:

Ingredients
1 pound lean ground beef
10 (6 inch) corn tortillas, quartered
1 (1 ounce) package taco seasoning mix
1 1/4 cups water
1 (12 ounce) jar chunky salsa
1 (10.75 ounce) can condensed cream of mushroom soup
1 (10.75 ounce) can condensed cream of chicken soup
4 cups shredded Mexican cheese blend

Direction
Into a skillet, crumble ground beef on moderately high heat. Cook and stir until browned evenly. Put in water and taco seasoning, then simmer on low heat, for 15 minutes.
Stir cream of chicken soup, cream of mushroom soup and salsa in a medium bowl. Combine in most of cheese, saving 3/4 cup for later use.
In the bottom of a slow cooker, put a layer of tortillas to cover, then spoon over that with a layer of ground beef, followed by a layer of cheese mixture. Repeat layers as above until stuff is used up, finishing with a layer of tortillas on top. Put leftover cheese on top. Place on a cover and cook on high setting about 45-60 minutes.

Nutrition Information
Calories: 712 calories;Protein: 40.9;Total Fat: 45.6;Sodium: 2089;Total Carbohydrate: 36;Cholesterol: 142

794. Slow Cooker Guisado Verde

Serving: 4 | Prep: 15mins | Cook: 7hours15mins | Ready in:

Ingredients
2 tablespoons vegetable oil
2 pounds boneless pork shoulder
1 large onion, coarsely chopped
3 cloves garlic, chopped
2 (12 ounce) cans tomatillos, drained and chopped
1 (7 ounce) can diced green chile peppers
2 fresh jalapeno peppers, sliced
1/2 cup fresh chopped cilantro
1 teaspoon dried oregano
salt and pepper to taste
1 quart water
1 cup shredded Monterey Jack cheese
1/4 cup sour cream
4 sprigs fresh cilantro, for garnish

Direction
In a large skillet, heat the oil over medium heat; add the pork and brown it on all sides. Transfer the pork to a slow cooker and reserve the juices left in skillet. Sauté garlic and onion in the skillet with pork juices for 1 minute over medium heat. Transfer the onion, garlic, and juices to the slow cooker.
Mix cilantro, jalapeno peppers, green chile peppers, and the tomatillos into the slow cooker. Add salt, pepper, and oregano to season. Pour enough water in to submerge all the ingredients, at least 1 quart of water. Cover the slow cooker and cook for 6 to 7 hours on High.
Use a fork to shred the cooked pork. Spoon the mixture from slow cooker mixture into serving bowls. Top with sour cream, Monterey Jack cheese, and fresh cilantro sprigs. Serve.

Nutrition Information
Calories: 553 calories;;Sodium: 1346;Total Carbohydrate: 17.7;Cholesterol: 122;Protein: 37.3;Total Fat: 36.9

795. Slow Cooker Mexican Style Chicken

Serving: 4 | Prep: 10mins | Cook: 4hours | Ready in:

Ingredients
1/2 cup tomato salsa
1/2 cup chipotle salsa
1/2 cup pineapple preserves
1 pound skinless, boneless chicken

Direction
In crock of a slow cooker, mix pineapple preserves, chipotle salsa, and tomato salsa together. Put in chicken, then toss to cover in salsa mixture.
Cook on Low for 3 – 4 hours until chicken is softened and can be shredded easily.
Transfer the chicken to a cutting board; use 2 forks to shred.
Put the shredded chicken back to salsa mixture, mix, and keep cooking for 1 more hour.

Nutrition Information
Calories: 238 calories;;Sodium: 436;Total Carbohydrate: 31.7;Cholesterol: 59;Protein: 23;Total Fat: 2.4

796. Slow Cooker Posole With Pork And Chicken

Serving: 6 | Prep: 20mins | Cook: 6hours | Ready in:

Ingredients
1 canned chipotle pepper in adobo sauce
1/4 cup water
1/2 pound boneless pork loin roast
1/2 pound skinless, boneless chicken breast halves
1 (15.5 ounce) can white hominy, drained
1 (4 ounce) can chopped green chilies
1 medium onion, chopped
1 clove garlic, minced
2 (14.5 ounce) cans chicken broth
1 teaspoon dried oregano
1 teaspoon ground cumin
1/4 teaspoon ground black pepper to taste
1 bay leaf

Direction

In a blender, add water and chipotle chile and puree until smooth. Put into a slow cooker and add the chicken broth, garlic, onion, green chilies, hominy, chicken, and pork. Use bay leaf, pepper, cumin, and oregano to season.
Cook, covered, on low until the meats become tender for 6-7 hours. Before serving, remove bay leaf.
Nutrition Information
Calories: 160 calories;;Sodium: 412;Total Carbohydrate: 13.8;Cholesterol: 37;Protein: 15;Total Fat: 4.7

797. Slow Cooker Salsa Chicken

Serving: 8 | Prep: 20mins | Cook: 6hours | Ready in:
Ingredients
2 pounds skinless, boneless chicken
2 tablespoons taco seasoning mix
1 cup diced tomatoes with habaneros (such as RO*TEL® Hot)
1 cup finely chopped onion
1/2 cup finely chopped celery
1/2 cup shredded carrot
1 cup prepared salsa
1/4 cup water
Direction
In the crock of a slow cooker, put the chicken. Sprinkle over the chicken with taco seasoning. On the chicken, layer diced tomatoes with the habaneros, the onion and the celery, then the carrot, separately; put the salsa on top. Pour over the whole mixture with water.
Cook for 6-8 hours on low until the chicken is easy to shred. An instant-read thermometer should display 165°F (74°C).
Use 2 forks to shred the chicken and mix with the salsa mixture.
Nutrition Information
Calories: 148 calories;;Cholesterol: 59;Protein: 23.1;Total Fat: 2.4;Sodium: 540;Total Carbohydrate: 7.5

798. Slow Cooker Shredded Beef For Tacos And Burritos

Serving: 12 | Prep: 5mins | Cook: 8hours | Ready in:
Ingredients
1 (4 pound) boneless beef chuck roast
2 (1 ounce) packages taco seasoning
1 onion, halved and sliced (optional)
1 teaspoon seasoned salt, or more to taste
Direction
In a crock or a slow cooker, put beef roast. Sprinkle over the beef with taco seasoning and add onion slices on top.
Cook for 8 to 10 hours on Low.
Transfer beef to a cutting board and use 2 forks to shred. Bring beef back to slow cooker and taste with seasoned salt.
Nutrition Information
Calories: 253 calories;;Sodium: 465;Total Carbohydrate: 5.1;Cholesterol: 69;Protein: 17.8;Total Fat: 17

799. Slow Cooker Spicy Chicken

Serving: 3 | Prep: 15mins | Cook: 4hours | Ready in:
Ingredients
3 skinless, boneless chicken breast halves
1/2 (8 ounce) jar medium salsa
1/4 cup tomato sauce
2 cloves garlic, minced
1 small red onion, chopped
1 teaspoon ground cumin
1 teaspoon chili powder
1 pinch salt and fresh ground pepper to taste
Direction
In the bottom of a slow cooker, place the chicken breast; add tomato sauce and salsa. Put in pepper, garlic, salt, onion, cumin, and chili powder. Cook chicken for 4-5 hours in a cooker set on Low. Use 2 forks to shred chicken. Serve.
Nutrition Information
Calories: 152 calories;Protein: 24.4;Total Fat: 2.8;Sodium: 392;Total Carbohydrate: 7.1;Cholesterol: 61

800. Slow Cooker Taco Soup

Serving: 8 | Prep: 10mins | Cook: 8hours | Ready in:
Ingredients
1 pound ground beef
1 onion, chopped
1 (16 ounce) can chili beans, with liquid
1 (15 ounce) can kidney beans with liquid
1 (15 ounce) can whole kernel corn, with liquid
1 (8 ounce) can tomato sauce
2 cups water
2 (14.5 ounce) cans peeled and diced tomatoes
1 (4 ounce) can diced green chile peppers
1 (1.25 ounce) package taco seasoning mix
Direction
Let ground beef cook in a medium skillet over medium heat until it becomes brown. Discard then put aside.
In a slow cooker, mix onion, green chile peppers, chili beans, corn, water, kidney beans, diced tomatoes, tomato sauce, taco seasoning and ground beef. Blend together and let it cook on low for 8 hours.
Nutrition Information
Calories: 362 calories;;Total Fat: 16.3;Sodium: 1356;Total Carbohydrate: 37.8;Cholesterol: 48;Protein: 18.2

801. Slow Cooker Tacos Al Pastor

Serving: 10 | Prep: 30mins | Cook: 7hours | Ready in:
Ingredients
Slow Cooker Ingredients:
2/3 large pineapple - peeled, cored, and chopped into small chunks
1 small white onion, quartered
1 chipotle peppers in adobo sauce, or more to taste
2 dried guajillo chiles, stemmed and seeded, or more to taste
1 dried chile de arbol pepper, stemmed and seeded, or more to taste
3 cloves garlic, halved
1 tablespoon minced fresh oregano
1/2 cup orange juice
2 tablespoons white vinegar
2 tablespoons achiote powder
2 teaspoons salt
1 teaspoon ground cumin
1 teaspoon lime zest, or to taste
1/2 teaspoon ground ancho chile powder
1/4 teaspoon freshly ground black pepper
1 (3 pound) boneless pork loin, cubed
Taco Ingredients:
1 tablespoon canola oil, or more as needed
20 (6 inch) corn tortillas
1/2 cup diced fresh pineapple
1/2 cup chopped fresh cilantro

2/3 white onion, diced
Direction
In a food processor, put oregano, garlic, chili de arbol, guajillo chilies, chipotle peppers plus 1 1/2 teaspoons of the adobo sauce, onion and pineapple. Mix till smooth. Turn onto a bowl and put in black pepper, chili powder, lime zest, cumin, salt, achiote powder, vinegar and orange juice. Stir sauce thoroughly.
In a slow cooker, put the pork and top with sauce to cover. Put on cover and cook for 7 to 9 hours on Low till pork is extremely soft. Start heating the tortillas for 35 to 40 minutes prior to pork is finish.
In a saucepan, heat the oil on high heat. Let tortillas cook, one by one till brown patches show for 30 seconds to a minute on each side. Put a pile of 2 tortillas for each taco.
With 2 forks, pull the pork apart; stir to coat in sauce. Onto the tacos, spoon the pork with slotted spoon. Put onion, cilantro and a pineapple portion on top of each.
Nutrition Information
Calories: 398 calories;;Sodium: 544;Total Carbohydrate: 43.2;Cholesterol: 65;Protein: 26;Total Fat: 14.2

802. South Of The Border Mac And Cheese

Serving: 4 | Prep: 10mins | Cook: 2hours15mins | Ready in:
Ingredients
2 1/2 cups rotini pasta
1 (12 fluid ounce) can evaporated milk
8 ounces American cheese, cut into cubes
4 ounces shredded sharp Cheddar cheese
1 (4 ounce) can diced green chile peppers, drained
2 teaspoons chili powder
2 tomatoes, seeded and chopped
5 green onions, sliced
Direction
Boil lightly salted water in a large pot. Cook the rotini at a boil for around 8 minutes till tender yet still firm to the bite; drain.
In a slow cooker, combine the evaporated milk, rotini pasta, Cheddar cheese, American cheese, chili powder, and canned green chiles.
Cook on High setting for nearly 2 hours, stirring twice.
Stir green onions and tomatoes through the pasta mixture.
Continue cooking for an addition of 5 to 10 minutes till the tomatoes are hot.
Nutrition Information
Calories: 675 calories;;Total Carbohydrate: 55.9;Cholesterol: 110;Protein: 34.2;Total Fat: 35.5;Sodium: 1472

803. Southwest Black Bean Chicken Soup

Serving: 8 | Prep: 15mins | Cook: 8hours | Ready in:
Ingredients
1 pound cooked dark meat chicken
3 (15.5 ounce) cans black beans, drained and rinsed
2 (14 ounce) cans chicken broth
2 (10 ounce) cans diced tomatoes with green chile peppers (such as RO*TEL®)
1 (15.25 ounce) can whole kernel corn
1/2 large onion, chopped
1/2 cup chopped jalapeno peppers
2 cloves garlic, chopped
2 1/2 teaspoons chili powder
2 teaspoons red pepper flakes
2 teaspoons ground cumin
1 teaspoon ground coriander
salt and ground black pepper to taste
1/2 cup sour cream, or to taste
Direction
Transfer black pepper, salt, coriander, cumin, red pepper flakes, chili powder, garlic, jalapeno peppers, onion, corn, tomatoes with green chile peppers, chicken broth, black beans and chicken in a slow cooker; cook for 8 hours on low; serve with 1 tbsp. of sour cream over each serving.
Nutrition Information
Calories: 389 calories;;Total Fat: 13.1;Sodium: 1740;Total Carbohydrate: 43.7;Cholesterol: 55;Protein: 26.6

804. Southwestern Style Chalupas

Serving: 8 | Prep: 5mins | Cook: 8hours | Ready in:
Ingredients
1 (4 pound) pork roast
1 pound dried pinto beans
1 (4 ounce) can chopped green chile peppers
2 tablespoons chili powder
2 teaspoons cumin seed
1 teaspoon dried oregano
salt and pepper to taste
1 quart water
1 (16 ounce) package corn chips
Direction
In a slow cooker, mix water, pepper, salt, oregano, cumin seed, chili powder, chili peppers, pinto beans and pork roast. Put the cover, and allow to simmer for 4 hours on Low.
Shred the meat, getting rid of any fat and bones. Put the cover, and keep cooking for 2 to 4 more hours. Put additional water if needed.
On serving plates, put corn chips. Scoop pork mixture on top of chips, and serve with preferred toppings.
Nutrition Information
Calories: 660 calories;;Total Fat: 23.5;Sodium: 891;Total Carbohydrate: 71.7;Cholesterol: 78;Protein: 42.7

805. Southwestern Style Fifteen Bean Soup

Serving: 8 | Prep: 15mins | Cook: 8hours | Ready in:
Ingredients
1 (8 ounce) package 15 bean soup mix
12 cups water
1 pound bacon
2 (4 ounce) cans canned green chile peppers, chopped
1 tablespoon chili powder
1 tablespoon crushed red pepper flakes
1 onion, chopped
2 cloves garlic, minced
Direction
Wash and sort the beans in the mix. Add them into the slow cooker over low setting along with water. Cook them overnight. In the following morning, put in garlic, onion, crushed red pepper, chili powder, chile peppers, and ham and keep on cooking over low setting for 8 hours.
Nutrition Information
Calories: 374 calories;;Total Fat: 26.4;Sodium: 878;Total Carbohydrate: 20.4;Cholesterol: 39;Protein: 13.6

806. Spicy Turkey Tacos

Serving: 6 | Prep: 10mins | Cook: 3hours10mins | Ready in:
Ingredients
1 pound shredded cooked turkey meat
1/3 cup chopped cilantro
1 large jalapeno pepper, stemmed and halved
1 (1 ounce) envelope hot taco seasoning mix
2 cups chicken broth, or as needed
6 small flour tortillas, or to taste
Direction
In a slow cooker, mix the taco seasoning mix, jalapeno pepper, cilantro, and turkey; cover mostly all ingredients with sufficient chicken broth.
Set on Low and cook for at least 3 hours.
Over medium-low heat, heat a griddle and cook tortillas for half a minute on each side until warmed.
Put the turkey mixture into the tortillas.
Nutrition Information
Calories: 251 calories;;Total Carbohydrate: 20.2;Cholesterol: 59;Protein: 25.3;Total Fat: 6.4;Sodium: 922

807. Super Easy Slow Cooker Chicken Enchilada Meat

Serving: 10 | Prep: 15mins | Cook: | Ready in:
Ingredients
2 cups chicken broth
1 (14.5 ounce) can diced tomatoes
1/3 cup chili powder
1/2 cup all-purpose flour
1 clove garlic
2 teaspoons ground cumin
1 teaspoon oregano
1 teaspoon salt, or to taste
1 pinch cayenne pepper, or more to taste (optional)
4 skinless, boneless chicken breast halves
Direction
In a blender, mix chicken cayenne pepper, salt, oregano, cumin, garlic, flour, chili powder, tomatoes, and chicken broth until smooth.
In bottom of a slow cooker, place chicken breast; pour over the chicken with blended enchilada sauce.
Cook for 4 to 6 hours on High (or 8 to 9 hours on Low). Use 2 large forks to shred the chicken and mix into the sauce.
Nutrition Information
Calories: 93 calories;;Sodium: 359;Total Carbohydrate: 8.8;Cholesterol: 23;Protein: 10.4;Total Fat: 1.8

808. Sweet Pork For Burritos

Serving: 12 | Prep: 30mins | Cook: 8hours | Ready in:
Ingredients
3 pounds pork shoulder roast
2 cups salsa
1 (12 fluid ounce) can or bottle cola-flavored carbonated beverage
2 cups brown sugar
1/2 (1.27 ounce) packet fajita seasoning
2 tablespoons taco seasoning mix
1 (7 ounce) can chopped green chilies
Direction
In the crock of a slow cooker, put pork roast, then put 4 cups of water. For 5 hours, cook on high.
Take pork out of slow cooker. Drain the liquid. Cut pork into 4 parts then set aside. In blender, puree salsa. In the crock of the slow cooker, combine green chilies, taco seasoning, fajita seasoning, brown sugar, cola and pureed salsa. Put the pork and cook for additional 3 hours on high.
Take the pork out and use 2 forks to shred. Serve.
Nutrition Information
Calories: 355 calories;;Total Carbohydrate: 32.6;Cholesterol: 73;Protein: 23;Total Fat: 14.7;Sodium: 728

809. Tex Mex Pork

Serving: 8 | Prep: 20mins | Cook: 10hours | Ready in:
Ingredients
1 (8 ounce) can tomato sauce
1 cup barbeque sauce
1 onion, chopped
2 (4 ounce) cans diced green chile peppers
1/4 cup chili powder
1 teaspoon ground cumin
1 teaspoon dried oregano
1/4 teaspoon ground cinnamon
2 1/2 pounds boneless pork loin roast, trimmed
1/2 cup chopped fresh cilantro
Direction
In a 3-qt. or bigger slow cooker, combine the cinnamon, oregano, cumin, chili powder, green chile peppers, onion, barbeque sauce, and tomato sauce. Add the pork into the slow cooker, and scoop the sauce over to coat meat.
Keep covered, and cook over Low heat till the pork softens or for 8 - 10 hours.
Transfer the pork onto the cutting board. With 2 forks, shred the meat. Add the sauce to the serving plate; whisk in the shredded pork and cilantro.
Nutrition Information
Calories: 281 calories;;Sodium: 908;Total Carbohydrate: 18.2;Cholesterol: 67;Protein: 24.3;Total Fat: 12.4

810. Texas Venison

Serving: 4 | Prep: 25mins | Cook: 15mins | Ready in:
Ingredients
2 pounds venison steaks
1 1/2 teaspoons seasoned salt, divided (see Note)
1 cup all-purpose flour
4 tablespoons vegetable oil
1/2 teaspoon ground cumin
1/2 cup onion, halved and sliced
2 beef bouillon cubes
1/2 teaspoon dried Mexican oregano
1 bay leaf
2 dried red chile peppers
2 cups water
Direction
Rub the venison steaks with 1/2 teaspoon Papa's Seasoning Salt to season it lightly then slice the steaks to bite-sized pieces. Mix 1 teaspoon of Papa's salt and flour. Set aside 1 tablespoon of flour mixture for use later then toss cubed meat with the seasoned flour.
For this step, you can use either a pressure cooker or a pan on medium-high heat. Pour oil in then fry the meat cubes by batches. Cook until all sides are browned then take the meat out of the pan and put aside.
Turn heat to medium, and mix in ground cumin and the leftover seasoned flour (1 tablespoon) with the pan drippings. Stir and cook for 5 minutes until the flour is browned lightly and doesn't smell raw. Toss

in sliced onion and continue to cook, stirring regularly, until onion is tender, 5 minutes.
Place the meat back in the pan and add Mexican oregano, bay leaf, chili peppers (take out the stems but keep them whole) and beef bouillon cubes. Pour in water and lock the pressure cooker, raising heat to high.
Place the pressure on high and turn the heat down to keep the pressure. Continue cooking at high pressure for 15 minutes. Turn off heat and release the pressure naturally.
Once pressure has dropped, remove the lid and take the bay leaf and chili peppers. Extract the pulp from peppers and place the pulp back in the pan; throw away the skins of the peppers and bay leaf. Season to taste.
Nutrition Information
Calories: 492 calories;;Total Fat: 19.4;Sodium: 869;Total Carbohydrate: 26.3;Cholesterol: 171;Protein: 50

811. Turkey Burrito

Serving: 10 | Prep: 30mins | Cook: 45mins | Ready in:
Ingredients
3 cups cooked turkey, cut into bite-size pieces
1 cup prepared stuffing
1 cup mashed potatoes
1 cup leftover gravy
2 quarts turkey broth
1 large onion, chopped
1/4 cup self-rising flour
10 (10 inch) flour tortillas
1 (8 ounce) package shredded Cheddar cheese
3 pickled jalapeno peppers, sliced
3 tablespoons pickled jalapeno pepper juice
salt and pepper to taste
1 tablespoon dried parsley
Direction
Combine onion, broth, gravy, mashed potatoes, stuffing and turkey in a big pot. Bring to a boil. Cook until onion is soft. If needed, thicken using flour.
Over medium heat, warm tortillas in a dry frying pan. On warm tortilla, spoon turkey mixture and sprinkle with cheese, then roll into burritos. Repeat process with the rest of the ingredients.
On top, spread more cheese and over the cheese, put another spoonful of the turkey mixture. Use jalapeño slices to garnish. Sprinkle with jalapeño juice and use parsley, pepper and salt to season. Serve while hot.
Nutrition Information
Calories: 516 calories;;Total Fat: 15.3;Sodium: 1501;Total Carbohydrate: 54.2;Cholesterol: 59;Protein: 27.7

812. White Chicken Enchilada Slow Cooker Casserole

Serving: 10 | Prep: 30mins | Cook: 4hours | Ready in:
Ingredients
15 boneless, skinless chicken thighs or breasts
1 (26 ounce) can condensed cream of chicken soup
2 cloves garlic, chopped (optional)
1 (16 ounce) container sour cream
1 (7 ounce) can diced green chile peppers
15 flour tortillas
3 1/2 cups shredded Monterey Jack cheese
1 (10 ounce) can sliced black olives (optional)
chives for garnish (optional)
black pepper to taste
Direction
In a pot, add the chicken and water to cover. Boil over high heat. Keep boiling for about 10 minutes until the chicken has done. Drain, let the chicken cool and slice into small chunks.
In a big bowl, add chicken chunks. Mix in green chiles, sour cream, garlic, and soup.
Lightly spray non-stick cooking spray over the inside of a slow cooker.
Shred tortillas into pieces and overlap 1/2 of the pieces across the bottom of the slow cooker in 1 layer. Top with 1/2 of the chicken, 1/2 half of the soup, and 1/2 of the cheese. Continue with the rest of the tortillas, chicken, soup and cheese. Put black olives on top.
Cook for 3-4 hours on Low setting. Put chives on top.
Nutrition Information
Calories: 824 calories;;Sodium: 1931;Total Carbohydrate: 66.4;Cholesterol: 123;Protein: 40;Total Fat: 44

813. Zesty White Chicken Chili

Serving: 8 | Prep: 15mins | Cook: 5hours | Ready in:
Ingredients
1 (8.75 ounce) jar Dickinson's® Sweet 'n' Hot Pepper Onion Relish
2 boneless skinless chicken breasts, cooked and cut into 1/2-inch pieces
1 (48 ounce) jar white beans, undrained
16 ounces chicken broth
2 cups shredded mozzarella cheese
1 cup sour cream
Direction
In slow cooker, mix all ingredients except sour cream and cheese. Cook for 5-7 hours on low heat. 20 minutes before serving, add cheese. Serve it with a dollop of sour cream.
Nutrition Information
Calories: 403 calories;;Cholesterol: 43;Protein: 24.6;Total Fat: 11.6;Sodium: 568;Total Carbohydrate: 50.5

Chapter 10: Family Slow Cooker Recipes

814. Apple Cinnamon Slow Cooker Oatmeal

Serving: 6 | Prep: 15mins | Cook: | Ready in:
Ingredients
6 medium sized apples, peeled if desired
¼ cup and 2 Tbsp Truvia® Brown Sugar Blend
1 tablespoon cinnamon
½ teaspoon nutmeg
Pinch of salt
1 tablespoon lemon juice
2 cups steel-cut oats
2 cups skim milk
2 eggs
1½ cups water
Direction
Grease a 3-quart slow cooker bowl.
Cut the apples into 1-inch pieces and toss them in a big bowl with lemon juice, salt, nutmeg, cinnamon, and Truvia Brown Sugar Blend to coat.
Stir in oats and move to the slow cooker.
Whisk together water, eggs, and milk till smooth, then pour this mixture over the apple mixture.
Cook on low setting for around 8 hours or on high setting for 4-5 hours.
Nutrition Information
Calories: 200 calories;
Saturated Fat: 0;Cholesterol: 55
Sugar: 20;Protein: 7;Sodium: 45
Fiber: 5;Total Carbohydrate: 42;Total Fat: 3

815. Brunswick Stew

Serving: 12 | Prep: 1hours | Cook: 2hours | Ready in:
Ingredients
4 ounces diced salt pork
2 pounds chicken parts
8 cups water
3 potatoes, cubed
3 onions, chopped
1 (28 ounce) can whole peeled tomatoes, chopped
2 cups canned whole kernel corn
1 (10 ounce) package frozen lima beans
1 tablespoon Worcestershire sauce
1/2 teaspoon salt
1/4 teaspoon ground black pepper
Direction
Mix and boil water, chicken and salt pork in a big pot on high heat. Lower heat to low. Cover then simmer until chicken is tender for 45 minutes.
Take out chicken. Let cool until easily handled. Take meat out. Throw out bones and skin. Chop meat to bite-sized pieces. Put back in the soup.
Add ground black pepper, salt, Worcestershire sauce, lima beans, corn, tomatoes, onions and potatoes. Mix well. Stir well and simmer for 1 hour, uncovered.
Nutrition Information
Calories: 368 calories;;Total Fat: 17.1;Sodium: 496;Total Carbohydrate: 25.9;Cholesterol: 71;Protein: 27.9

816. Cajun Style Pork And Shrimp Pasta

Serving: 8 | Prep: 30mins | Cook: | Ready in:
Ingredients
1 1½ to 2-pound pork sirloin roast
½ teaspoon salt
¼ teaspoon black pepper
Nonstick cooking spray
2 stalks celery, thinly sliced (1 cup)
1 large onion, cut into thin wedges
1 (15 ounce) can red beans, rinsed and drained
1 (14.5 ounce) can no-salt-added diced tomatoes, undrained
8 ounces dried multigrain rotini pasta (3¼ cups dried)
1½ tablespoons salt-free Cajun seasoning or Homemade Salt-Free Cajun Seasoning (see Tip)
1 medium green sweet pepper, chopped (¾ cup)
8 ounces frozen cooked peeled and deveined shrimp, thawed
Snipped fresh cilantro
Direction
Cut off fat from roast. Cut roast into 3 parts. Sprinkle black pepper and salt on top of pork pieces. Spray cooking spray on unheated large nonstick skillet to coat; heat on medium heat. In hot skillet, brown roast pieces, flipping to evenly brown all sides. In a 3 1/2- to 4-quart slow cooker mix tomatoes, beans, onion, and celery. Add browned pork pieces on top.
Cook with a cover for 6 to 7 hours on low-heat setting or for 3 to 3 1/2 hours on high-heat setting. In the meantime, follow the package directions to cook rotini pasta but a minute less than package directions; drain. Take meat out of cooker; put aside. If cooking on low-heat setting, increase to high-heat setting. Put sweet pepper, pasta and Cajun seasoning into the cooker. Cook with a cover for an addition of 15 minutes. Cut meat into cubes, about 1/2- to 3/4-inch in size; mix into pasta mixture together with thawed shrimp. Sprinkle cilantro on top of each serving.
Nutrition Information
Calories: 306 calories;;Total Fat: 5
Fiber: 6;Cholesterol: 109
Sugar: 4;Protein: 32
Saturated Fat: 1;Sodium: 370;Total Carbohydrate: 35

817. Carnitas Tacos

Serving: 8 | Prep: 30mins | Cook: | Ready in:
Ingredients
3 to 3½-pound bone-in pork shoulder roast
½ cup chopped onion
⅓ cup orange juice
1 tablespoon ground cumin
1½ teaspoons kosher salt
1 teaspoon dried oregano, crushed
¼ teaspoon cayenne pepper
1 lime
2 (5.3 ounce) containers plain low-fat Greek yogurt
1 pinch kosher salt
16 (6 inch) soft yellow corn tortillas, such as Mission® brand
4 leaves green cabbage, quartered
1 cup very thinly sliced red onion
1 cup salsa (optional)
Direction
Take off meat from the bone; throw away bone. Trim meat fat. Slice meat into 2 to 3-inch pieces; put in a slow cooker of 3 1/2 or 4-quart in size. Mix in cayenne, oregano, salt, cumin, orange juice and onion. Cover and cook for 8 to 10 hours on low or for 4 to 5 hours on high. Take out meat from the cooker. Shred meat with two forks. Mix in enough cooking liquid to moisten.

Take out 1 teaspoon zest (put aside) for lime crema, then squeeze 2 tablespoons lime juice. Mix dash salt, yogurt, and lime juice in a small bowl.

Serve lime crema, salsa (if wished), red onion and cabbage with meat in tortillas. Scatter with lime zest.

Nutrition Information
Calories: 301 calories;Protein: 29;Sodium: 329;Cholesterol: 69;Total Carbohydrate: 28 Sugar: 7;Total Fat: 8 Saturated Fat: 2 Fiber: 4

818. Chicken Pho

Serving: 24 | Prep: 30mins | Cook: 1hours30mins | Ready in:

Ingredients
10 quarts water
3 pounds chicken bones
1 whole chicken
1 medium onion
1 (1 inch) piece ginger
1 (32 fluid ounce) container chicken broth
1/4 cup rock sugar
3 teaspoons fish sauce
2 cubes pho ga soup seasoning
1 1/2 teaspoons salt
2 (16 ounce) packages rice stick noodles (banh pho)
1/2 pound bean sprouts
1 bunch green onion, chopped
1 bunch cilantro, chopped
6 sprigs Thai basil, or as needed
1 lime, cut in wedges

Direction
Fill a stockpot with water and let it boil. Meanwhile, put the chicken bones under hot water and rinse to remove impurities.

Put the bones in the pot of boiling water. Lessen the heat and simmer for about an hour until it is beginning to soften, removing any fat off the surface of the broth. Remove parboiled bones.

Put the whole chicken into the pot and make it simmer for about 30 to 40 minutes until no visible pink color in the middle. Take the chicken out from broth and set aside, allowing it to cool. An instant-read thermometer poked near the bone should register 165°F (74°C).

Mix together the ginger and onion in a skillet over medium-high heat. Sauté for about 7 minutes until both turns nicely browned and aromatic. Smash the ginger using the backside of a knife placed into a chopping board. Place the ginger and onion into the broth. Mix with rock sugar, pho ga seasoning, salt, fish sauce and chicken broth.

Fill a big pot with water and let it boil. Stir in the rice noodles and boil for about 2 to 3 minutes until soft yet firm to the bite. Drain the noodles.

Peel off the skin of the cooled chicken; get rid of the bones and skin, and set aside the meat.

Serve the noodles in bowls and put the chicken meat and broth on top. Garnish with Thai basil, bean sprouts, cilantro and green onion. Squeeze a wedge of lime in each bowl.

Nutrition Information
Calories: 324 calories;;Sodium: 520;Total Carbohydrate: 34.1;Cholesterol: 73;Protein: 19.9;Total Fat: 11.1

819. Chicken Ragout

Serving: 8 | Prep: 20mins | Cook: | Ready in:

Ingredients
8 chicken thighs (about 3½ pounds total), skinned
2 14.5-ounce can no-salt-added diced tomatoes, drained
3 cups 1-inch carrot slices or baby carrots
1 large onion, cut into wedges (1 cup)
⅓ cup reduced sodium chicken broth
2 tablespoons white wine vinegar
1 teaspoon dried rosemary, crushed
1 teaspoon dried thyme, crushed
¼ teaspoon black pepper
8 ounces fresh button mushrooms, sliced
1 teaspoon olive oil
3 cups hot cooked whole-wheat noodles
Snipped fresh parsley (optional)

Direction
Put the chicken thighs in a 3 1/2- or 4-quart slow cooker. Mix together thyme, vinegar, pepper, tomatoes, rosemary, carrots, onion, and broth in a large bowl. Spread atop the chicken in the cooker. Cover and cook on low-heat setting for 8 to 10 hours. Before you serve, over medium-high heat, cook while stirring mushrooms in hot oil in a large nonstick skillet for about 8 to 10 minutes or until golden. Take out the chicken from the cooker. Remove bones from chicken get rid of the bones. Mix the chicken and mushrooms into the mixture in the cooker. Serve the chicken mixture atop hot cooked noodles. Drizzle each serving with parsley if desired.

Nutrition Information
Calories: 234 calories;;Total Fat: 4
Saturated Fat: 1;Sodium: 163;Total Carbohydrate: 33
Fiber: 7;Cholesterol: 57
Sugar: 7;Protein: 20

820. Chicken And Vegetables With Herbs

Serving: 4 | Prep: 25mins | Cook: | Ready in:

Ingredients
8 ounces fresh button mushrooms, halved
1½ cups frozen small whole onions
½ cup reduced-sodium chicken broth
¼ cup dry red wine or reduced-sodium chicken broth
2 tablespoons tomato paste
½ teaspoon garlic salt
½ teaspoon dried rosemary, crushed
½ teaspoon dried thyme, crushed
¼ teaspoon black pepper
1 bay leaf
8 small chicken thighs and/or drumsticks (about 2 pounds total), skinned
Reduced-sodium chicken broth
¼ cup reduced-sodium chicken broth
2 tablespoons flour
3 cups hot cooked mashed potatoes (optional) (optional)
Fresh parsley sprigs (optional)

Direction
In a 4-to 5-quart slow cooker, mix the whole onions and mushrooms. Mix in bay leaf with pepper, thyme, rosemary, garlic salt, tomato paste, wine and 1/2 cup broth. Put chicken into the cooker.

Cover and cook for 7 hours on low-heat setting or for 3 1/2 hours on high-heat setting.

Move vegetables and chicken to a serving plate using a slotted spoon. Remove bay leaf. To keep warm, cover vegetables and chicken with foil.

Skim the fat from the cooking liquid for sauce. Measure 1 3/4 cups of the cooking liquid and, if desired, add extra chicken broth to equal 1 3/4 cups of the total liquid. Move liquid to a medium saucepan. Mix flour and 1/4 cup broth until smooth in a small bowl; mix into liquid in the saucepan. Cook and mix until bubbly and thickened; cook and mix for another minute. Spoon some of the sauce over the chicken. Pass the leftover sauce. Serve with mashed potatoes and decorate with parsley, if desired.

Nutrition Information
Calories: 215 calories;
Fiber: 2;Total Fat: 5
Saturated Fat: 1;Sodium: 342;Cholesterol: 107;Total Carbohydrate: 10
Sugar: 4;Protein: 29

821. Cider Pork Stew

Serving: 8 | Prep: 20mins | Cook: | Ready in:
Ingredients
2 pounds boneless pork shoulder roast
3 medium cubed potatoes (about 2- ½ cups)
3 medium carrots, cut into ½-inch pieces (about 1- ½ cups)
2 medium onions, sliced
1 cup coarsely chopped apple (1 medium)
½ cup coarsely chopped celery (1 stalk)
3 tablespoons quick-cooking tapioca
2 cups apple juice or apple cider
1 teaspoon salt
1 teaspoon caraway seeds
¼ teaspoon black pepper
Celery leaves (optional)
Direction
Chop the meat into 1-in. cubes. In the 3.5- 5.5 qt. slow cooker, mix the tapioca, celery, apple, onions, carrots, potatoes and meat. Whisk in pepper, caraway seeds, salt and apple juice.
Keep covered and cook over high heat setting for 5-6 hours or over low heat setting for 10-12 hours. If you want, use the celery leaves to decorate each of the servings.

Nutrition Information
Calories: 244 calories;;Sodium: 469
Fiber: 5;Cholesterol: 56;Total Fat: 4
Saturated Fat: 1;Total Carbohydrate: 33
Sugar: 15;Protein: 21

822. Corn Bread Topped Chicken Enchilada Casserole

Serving: 8 | Prep: 25mins | Cook: | Ready in:
Ingredients
Chicken Enchilada Casserole
Nonstick cooking spray
12 ounces skinless, boneless chicken breast half, cut into bite-size pieces
1 (10 ounce) can enchilada sauce
1 (8 ounce) can no-salt-added tomato sauce
1 cup canned black beans, rinsed and drained
1 4-ounce can diced, green chile peppers, undrained
2 ounces Monterey Jack cheese with jalapeno peppers, thinly sliced and cut into ½-inch pieces
½ teaspoon cumin
½ teaspoon dried oregano, crushed
½ teaspoon dried basil, crushed
½ teaspoon chili powder
Corn Bread Topper
¾ cup yellow cornmeal
½ cup all-purpose flour
2 tablespoons granulated sugar (see Tip)
1¾ teaspoons baking powder
¼ teaspoon salt
¾ cup fat-free milk
⅓ cup refrigerated or frozen egg product, thawed
3 tablespoons butter, melted
½ cup sliced green onions
Fat-free plain Greek yogurt (optional)
Direction
Use the cooking spray to lightly coat the inside of a 4-quart slow cooker; leave aside. Coat a large nonstick frying pan with cooking spray, then heat over medium-high heat. Put in chicken and cook for about 3 minutes just until browned.
Stir the chili powder, enchilada sauce, tomato sauce, green chile peppers, cheese, cumin, beans, oregano, basil and chicken in the prepared slow cooker. Cook while covered for 3 hours on low-heat setting or for 1 and a half hours on high-heat setting.
Meanwhile, make the corn bread topper. Stir the salt, baking powder, sugar, flour and cornmeal together in a medium bowl. Blend the melted butter, egg product and milk in a small bowl. Pour all the milk mixture at once into the cornmeal mixture; blend just until moistened (mixture will become thin).
Set cooker to high-heat if using low-heat setting. Carefully spoon cornbread topper evenly over the mixture in cooker. Cook while covered for around 50 more minutes or till a wooden toothpick pinned in the middle of corn bread comes out clean. (Avoid lifting the cover during cooking). If you like, garnish with sliced green onions, then with yogurt. Serve immediately.

Nutrition Information
Calories: 273 calories;
Sugar: 7;Protein: 16
Saturated Fat: 4;Sodium: 567;Total Carbohydrate: 31;Cholesterol: 46;Total Fat: 8
Fiber: 3

823. Creamy Turkey Soup

Serving: 8 | Prep: 30mins | Cook: | Ready in:
Ingredients
8 ounces red-skinned potatoes, cut in 1-inch pieces
8 ounces cremini mushrooms, sliced
1 cup coarsely chopped onion (1 large)
1 cup sliced celery (2 stalks)
2 turkey breast tenderloins (about 1½ pounds total)
3 (14.5 ounce) cans reduced-sodium chicken broth
1½ teaspoons dried thyme, crushed
½ teaspoon black pepper
1 (12 ounce) can (1½ cups) evaporated fat-free milk
3 tablespoons cornstarch
½ cup sliced green onions (4)
2 tablespoons lemon juice
Toasted sliced almonds or chopped pecans and/or dried cranberries (see Tip) (optional)
Direction
Combine the celery, onion, potatoes, and mushrooms in a 6-qt slow cooker. Top the mixture with turkey. Add the pepper, broth, and thyme.
Cover the slow cooker and cook the mixture on low heat setting for 9-10 hours (or on high heat setting for 4 1/2-5 hours).
Place the turkey in a cutting board. Shred the turkey using the two forks. Place it back into the cooker. Mix the cornstarch and evaporated milk in a small bowl and add it into the cooker. Set the setting into high heat if ever you're using the low heat.

Cover the cooker and cook for 45-60 more minutes until the edges are bubbly. Mix in lemon juice and green onions.
Top with nuts and/or cranberries if desired. Serve.
Nutrition Information
Calories: 186 calories;;Total Fat: 1;Sodium: 480;Cholesterol: 54;Total Carbohydrate: 18
Sugar: 8
Saturated Fat: 0
Fiber: 2;Protein: 27

824. Hearty Beef Chili

Serving: 6 | Prep: 15mins | Cook: 1hours15mins | Ready in:
Ingredients
2 tablespoons vegetable oil
2 yellow onions, diced
1 red bell pepper, diced
5 cloves garlic, minced
2 tablespoons chili powder
1 tablespoon ground cumin
2 pounds lean ground beef
1 1/2 teaspoons salt
2 (15 ounce) cans kidney beans, rinsed and drained
2 cups College Inn® Beef Broth
1 (14.5 ounce) can Contadina® Diced Tomatoes, undrained
2 teaspoons apple cider vinegar
Topping Options:
Shredded Cheddar cheese
onion, chopped
Sour cream
Sliced green onions
Cilantro leaves
Direction
In a Dutch oven or big, heavy-bottom pot, heat up oil upon medium-high heat. Place in the bell pepper and onions, cooking them until they become soft, near 8 minutes. Stir in cumin, chili powder, and garlic until they turn fragrant, 30 seconds.
Add in the salt and beef, and cook around 8 minutes until there is no longer pink throughout the meat while you break the beef up into small chunks using a wooden spoon.
Stir in tomatoes, broth, and beans, then simmer on medium heat, stirring every now and then, until flavors merge together, around 1 hour. Stir in the vinegar and if you want, you can serve the dish with toppings.
Nutrition Information
Calories: 560 calories;Protein: 42.6;Total Fat: 27.2;Sodium: 1663;Total Carbohydrate: 36.5;Cholesterol: 112

825. Hearty Vegetable Beef Stew

Serving: 6 | Prep: 30mins | Cook: | Ready in:
Ingredients
2 pounds boneless beef chuck roast, trimmed and cut into 1-inch cubes
12 ounces tiny new potatoes, quartered
4 medium carrots, cut into ½ inch pieces
1 medium onion, cut into wedges
1 (10.75 ounce) can reduced-fat, reduced-sodium cream of mushroom soup (such as Campbell's® Healthy Request)
1 cup reduced-sodium beef broth
1 teaspoon dried marjoram or dried thyme, crushed
2 cups frozen cut green beans
Direction
Spray a large skillet with cooking spray; heat over medium-high heat. Trim to remove any fat from beef cubes. Put in half of the beef cubes. Cook while stirring until brown; take out of skillet. Put in the leftover beef cubes; cook while stirring until brown. Drain off any fat.
In a 3 1/2- or 4-quart slow cooker, place the meat. Put in marjoram, broth, cream of mushroom soup, onion, carrots, and potatoes. Mix to blend.
Cook with a cover for 8-9 hours on low-heat setting or for 4 to 4 1/2 hours on high-heat setting.
If cooking on low-heat setting, increase cooker to high-heat setting. Mix in green beans. Cook with a cover for 30 more minutes, just until beans are soft.
Nutrition Information
Calories: 319 calories;;Total Fat: 9
Saturated Fat: 3
Fiber: 4
Sugar: 5;Protein: 35;Sodium: 396;Cholesterol: 92;Total Carbohydrate: 22

826. Mushroom Sauced Pork Chops

Serving: 6 | Prep: 30mins | Cook: | Ready in:
Ingredients
4 pork loin chops, cut ¾ inch thick (about 2 pounds)
1 tablespoon cooking oil
1 small onion, thinly sliced
2 tablespoons quick-cooking tapioca
1 (10.75 ounce) can reduced-fat, reduced-sodium condensed cream of mushroom soup
½ cup apple juice or apple cider
1½ teaspoons Worcestershire sauce
2 teaspoons snipped fresh thyme or ¾ teaspoon dried thyme, crushed
¼ teaspoon garlic powder
1½ cups sliced fresh mushrooms
Fresh thyme sprigs (optional)
Direction
Remove fat from the pork chops. On medium heat, heat oil in a big pan; cook chops until evenly brown then remove the excess fat. On a 3 1/2 or 4qt slow cooker, put in onion and chops. Pound the tapioca with a mortar and pestle. Mix garlic powder, tapioca, dried or snipped thyme, mushroom soup, Worcestershire sauce, and apple juice together in a medium bowl; toss in mushrooms. Pour the mixture on top of the chops in the cooker.
Cover and cook for 8-9hrs on low setting or 4-4 1/2 hrs. on high setting. Add thyme sprigs on top if desired.
Nutrition Information
Calories: 220 calories;;Total Fat: 7
Sugar: 4;Protein: 26;Total Carbohydrate: 12
Saturated Fat: 2;Sodium: 233
Fiber: 1;Cholesterol: 74

827. Pork Chops With Herb Tomato Sauce

Serving: 4 | Prep: 20mins | Cook: | Ready in:
Ingredients
4 pork rib chops (with bone), cut ¾ inch thick (about 1¾ pounds)
Nonstick cooking spray
1 small onion, chopped
2 teaspoons quick-cooking tapioca, crushed (see Tips)
1½ teaspoons bottled minced garlic (3 cloves)
1 teaspoon dried Italian seasoning, crushed
½ teaspoon ground black pepper
½ teaspoon Worcestershire sauce
¼ teaspoon salt

¼ teaspoon crushed red pepper
2 (14.5 ounce) cans no-salt-added stewed tomatoes, undrained

Direction

Shear fat from chops. Use a cooking spray to coat a 12-inch skillet; allow to heat over medium-high heat. In the hot skillet, brown both sides of chops. Leave aside.

Mix crushed red pepper, salt, Worcestershire sauce, black pepper, Italian seasoning, garlic, tapioca and onion in a 3 1/2 or 4-quart slow cooker. Put in chops. Put tomatoes over.

Cook while covered on High-heat setting for 3 and a half hours to 4 hours or on Low-heat setting for 7 - 8 hours.

Move the chops into serving platter to serve. Use a slotted spoon to spoon tomatoes atop chops. Pour some cooking liquid atop tomatoes and chops if you like.

Nutrition Information

Calories: 245 calories;;Cholesterol: 53;Total Carbohydrate: 19;Total Fat: 7
Saturated Fat: 2
Fiber: 2;Protein: 24;Sodium: 568
Sugar: 11

828. Pork Zuppa

Serving: 6 | Prep: 30mins | Cook: | Ready in:

Ingredients

1 pound ground pork
1 large onion, chopped (1 cup)
2 cloves garlic, minced
1 teaspoon dried oregano, crushed
¼ teaspoon salt
¼ to ½ teaspoon crushed red pepper
4 cups reduced-sodium chicken broth
12 ounces tiny red new potatoes, each cut into 8 pieces
1 (12 ounce) can fat-free evaporated milk
2 tablespoons cornstarch
2 cups chopped fresh kale
Crushed red pepper (optional)

Direction

Cook the garlic, onion, and pork in a big skillet over medium heat until the onion becomes soft and the pork is browned. Strain off the fat. Put the meat mixture back into the skillet and put in crushed red pepper, salt, and oregano. Cook for 1 more minute. Then put into a 3 1/2-or-4-quart slow cooker. Put in potatoes and broth.

Cook while covering for 6-8 hours on low heat or 3-4 hours on high heat. If you are using low-heat setting, then switch to high-heat setting. Mix the cornstarch and evaporated milk in a small bowl until smooth. Whisk into the cooker. Whisk in kale. Cook while covering for 30-60 minutes longer until the liquid around the cooker's edge bubbles. You can sprinkle more crushed red pepper on top if you want.

Nutrition Information

Calories: 303 calories;;Total Fat: 12;Cholesterol: 53;Total Carbohydrate: 19
Sugar: 4
Saturated Fat: 4;Sodium: 542
Fiber: 2;Protein: 20

829. Pot Roast Rigatoni Stew

Serving: 6 | Prep: 30mins | Cook: | Ready in:

Ingredients

1 2-pound boneless beef chuck arm pot roast, trimmed of fat and cut into 2-inch chunks
½ teaspoon salt
¼ teaspoon black pepper
1 tablespoon olive oil
2 cups 50% less sodium beef broth
1 (14.5 ounce) can no-salt-added stewed tomatoes
½ cup chopped onion
½ cup chopped celery
½ cup chopped carrot
½ cup chopped bottled roasted red peppers
½ cup dry red wine or cranberry juice
¼ cup fat-free half-and-half
1 tablespoon all-purpose flour
6 ounces dried rigatoni pasta
2 tablespoons freshly grated Parmesan cheese

Direction

Sprinkle quarter teaspoon each of ground pepper and salt over the beef. On medium-high heat, heat oil in a big pan. Cook beef in hot oil until all sides are brown; drain fat.

Mix the remaining quarter teaspoon of salt, beef, red wine, beef broth, roasted red peppers, undrained tomatoes, carrot, onion, and celery together in a 3 1/2 - 4qt slow cooker; cover. Cook for 10-12hrs on low setting or 4-5hrs on high setting.

Move beef to a cutting board using a slotted spoon. Remove fat on top of the cooking liquid. Shred the meat apart using 2 forks then put it back in the cooker.

Turn to high-heat setting if currently on low. Mix flour and half-and-half together in a small bowl; put the mixture and rigatoni into the cooker. Cook for half an hour while covered. Add Parmesan cheese on top of each serving.

Nutrition Information

Calories: 401 calories;Protein: 40
Saturated Fat: 3;Cholesterol: 100;Total Carbohydrate: 32
Fiber: 3
Sugar: 6;Total Fat: 10;Sodium: 509

830. Provencal Vegetable Stew

Serving: 4 | Prep: 25mins | Cook: | Ready in:

Ingredients

2 baby eggplants or 1 very small eggplant (about 8 oz.)
1 large zucchini, quartered lengthwise and cut into ½-inch slices
1 large yellow summer squash, quartered lengthwise and cut into ½-inch slices
1 15 to 19-ounce can cannellini (white kidney) beans or Great Northern beans, rinsed and drained
1 large tomato, chopped
2 teaspoons bottled minced garlic (4 cloves)
¼ teaspoon dried rosemary or thyme, crushed
¼ teaspoon ground black pepper
1 tablespoon snipped fresh basil or 1 teaspoon dried basil, crushed
1½ cups low-sodium tomato juice
1 tablespoon white or regular balsamic vinegar
4 (½ inch) slices baguette-style French bread
2 teaspoons olive oil
3 tablespoons finely shredded Romano or Parmesan cheese

Direction

Peel the eggplant if desired; slice into 3/4-in portions until you have about three cups of sliced eggplants.

Mix dried basil if using, eggplant, pepper, zucchini, rosemary, yellow squash, garlic, cannellini beans, and tomato together in a 3 1/2 or 4qt slow cooker. Pour in tomato juice.
Set cooker on low and cook for 8-10hrs, covered, or for 4-5hrs on high setting. Mix in balsamic vinegar, and fresh basil if using.
Make the croutons. Preheat the oven to 400 degrees F. Slather olive oil lightly on bread slices; top with a tablespoon of Romano cheese. Arrange the slices on a baking sheet; bake for 6-8mins until the croutons are toasted.
Before serving, scoop vegetable mixture in bowls; add croutons and the rest of the Romano cheese on top.
Nutrition Information
Calories: 227 calories;;Total Fat: 5
Saturated Fat: 1;Sodium: 424
Fiber: 10;Cholesterol: 4;Total Carbohydrate: 41
Sugar: 8;Protein: 12

831. Pulled Pork Tenderloin With Vidalia Onion BBQ Sauce

Serving: 8 | Prep: 30mins | Cook: | Ready in:
Ingredients
Vidalia Onion BBQ Sauce
1 tablespoon canola oil
2 medium sweet onions (about 1 pound), preferably Vidalia, grated
2½ cups ketchup
½ cup cider vinegar
¼ cup honey
2 tablespoons lemon juice
2 tablespoons Worcestershire sauce
2 tablespoons Dijon mustard
½ teaspoon ground pepper
Pinch of cayenne pepper, or to taste
Pulled Pork
2 medium sweet onions (about 1 pound), preferably Vidalia, sliced
2 1-pound pork tenderloins, trimmed
1 teaspoon ground pepper
2 cups Vidalia Onion BBQ Sauce or other barbecue sauce
Direction
To make the sauce: In a big saucepan, heat the oil on medium heat, then add grated onions and let it cook for 3-5 minutes, mixing frequently, until it turns translucent. Add the cayenne, pepper, mustard, Worcestershire, lemon juice, honey, vinegar and ketchup, then boil on high heat. Lower the heat to retain a low simmer and let it cook for 30 minutes, stirring from time to time. This makes 4 cups.
Preparing the pork: In a 5 to 6-quart slow cooker, put the sliced onions, then add pork and sprinkle it with pepper to season and put 2 cups of the sauce on top. Let it cook for 8 hours on Low or 4 hours on High. Shred and pull the pork into strips using 2 forks, then mix the pork into the sauce.
Nutrition Information
Calories: 223 calories;
Saturated Fat: 1;Sodium: 492;Cholesterol: 70;Total Carbohydrate: 25
Sugar: 17;Total Fat: 3
Fiber: 2;Protein: 24

832. Rosemary Chicken

Serving: 4 | Prep: | Cook: | Ready in:
Ingredients
4 skinless, boneless chicken breast halves
2 tablespoons olive oil
1 teaspoon seasoning salt
1 1/2 teaspoons salt free Cajun seasoning
1 teaspoon fresh rosemary
1 onion, finely diced
Direction
Preheat oven to 175°C (350°F).
Put chicken breasts in a glass baking dish (9x13 inches), covered. Season with Cajun seasoning, salt and oil. Stir using your hands until chicken pieces are uniformly coated. If using fresh rosemary, chop and dust atop chicken. If using dried rosemary, crush using hands and dust over chicken. Use your hands again to blend mix and coat chicken uniformly. Lay diced onions on top of the chicken. Cover the dish, then bake in the preheated oven for 25 to 35 minutes until the chicken is browned and cooked through (juices run clear) and the onions are caramelized.
Nutrition Information
Calories: 202 calories;;Cholesterol: 68;Protein: 27.6;Total Fat: 8.3;Sodium: 307;Total Carbohydrate: 3.6

833. Savory Barbecue Chicken

Serving: 4 | Prep: 15mins | Cook: | Ready in:
Ingredients
½ cup tomato sauce
2 tablespoons jalapeño pepper jelly
2 tablespoons lime or lemon juice
2 tablespoons quick-cooking tapioca
1 teaspoon brown sugar
1 teaspoon ground cumin
¼ to ½ teaspoon crushed red pepper
8 to 10 chicken thighs and/or drumsticks, skinned (2 to 2½ pounds)
4 to 5 slices whole grain bread (optional)
Direction
Mix red pepper, cumin, brown sugar, tapioca, lime/lemon juice, jelly and tomato sauce in a 3 1/2- or 4-qt. slow cooker. Put chicken pieces on sauce mixture, meaty side down.
Cover. Cook for 6-7 hours on low-heat setting or 3 – 3 1/2 hours on high-heat setting. If desired, serve with bread.
Nutrition Information
Calories: 224 calories;;Total Fat: 5;Sodium: 240
Fiber: 1;Cholesterol: 114
Sugar: 6;Protein: 28
Saturated Fat: 1;Total Carbohydrate: 15

834. Seeded Pork Roast

Serving: 8 | Prep: 20mins | Cook: | Ready in:
Ingredients
1 2½ to 3-pound boneless pork shoulder roast
1 tablespoon reduced-sodium soy sauce
2 teaspoons anise seeds, crushed
2 teaspoons fennel seeds, crushed
2 teaspoons caraway seeds, crushed
2 teaspoons dill seeds, crushed
2 teaspoons celery seeds, crushed
⅔ cup apple juice or apple cider
½ cup reduced-sodium beef broth
1 tablespoon cornstarch
Direction
Trim fat from the meat. Cut the meat to fit the 3- 1/2- to 5-quart slow cooker, if necessary. Brush soy sauce over the meat. On a large piece of foil mix celery seeds, dill seeds, caraway seeds, fennel seeds and

anise seeds. Evenly roll roast in the seeds to coat. Put the meat in slow cooker. Add broth and 1/3 cup apple juice around the meat.
Cook, covered, on high-heat for 4- 1/2 to 5- 1/2 hours or on low-heat for 9-11 hours
Place the meat on a cutting board, reserving the cooking liquid. Cut meat and put on the serving platter. Keep warm by covering.
For the gravy, strain cooking liquid and remove fat floating on the surface. Place the cooking liquid to the small saucepan. Combine the cornstarch and remaining 1/3 cup of apple juice in a small bowl. Mix into the liquid in saucepan. Cook while stirring over medium heat until bubbly and thickened. Cook while stirring for 2 mins longer. Pour gravy over the meat then, serve.

Nutrition Information
Calories: 220 calories;
Saturated Fat: 3;Total Carbohydrate: 5
Sugar: 2;Protein: 29;Total Fat: 9;Sodium: 269
Fiber: 0;Cholesterol: 92

835. Slow Cooked Ranch Chicken And Vegetables

Serving: 6 | Prep: 30mins | Cook: | Ready in:
Ingredients
2 medium onions, cut into thin wedges
1 tablespoon dried minced onion
2 teaspoons dried parsley flakes, crushed
1 teaspoon garlic powder
1 teaspoon salt
1 teaspoon black pepper
½ teaspoon dried thyme, crushed
½ teaspoon dried dill
5 pounds large chicken thighs, skinned (12 to 14 total)
2 (10.75 ounce) cans reduced-fat, reduced-sodium condensed cream of chicken soup
1 (8 ounce) carton sour cream
2 to 3 teaspoons finely chopped canned chipotle chile peppers in adobo sauce (see Tips)
2 medium red and/or green sweet peppers, cut into ½-inch-thick strips
2 medium zucchini, halved lengthwise and thinly sliced
1 3-pound spaghetti squash
¼ cup snipped fresh parsley (optional)
Direction
Transfer onion wedges into a 5- to 6-quart slow cooker. Mix dill, thyme, dried onion, black pepper, parsley flakes, salt, and garlic powder in a small bowl. Place an even layer of one-third of chicken thighs in the slow cooker on top of the onions. Drizzle the chicken with about one-third of spice mixture. Repeat layering twice with the remaining spice mixture and chicken thighs.
Mix together chile peppers, condensed soup, and sour cream in a medium bowl. Spread atop chicken in the cooker.
Cover the cooker and let to cook for about 6 to 7 hours on low-heat setting or on high-heat setting for about 3 to 3 1/2 hours. In case you are using low-heat setting, switch the cooker to high-heat setting. Add squash slices and sweet pepper strips into cooker. Cover and let to cook for 45 minutes.
In the meantime, chop spaghetti squash in half lengthwise. Remove the strings and seeds. In a microwave-safe baking dish, put one half with the cut side down. Prick the skin all over with a fork. Heat in microwave for about 10 to 12 minutes on 100% power (high) or until tender when pierced with a fork. Remove carefully from the baking dish. Repeat this with the other half of squash. Let the squash to cool slightly. Shred with a fork and separate squash pulp into strands.
Take out all the chicken thighs from slow cooker. Put six thighs onto a plate and then cover with foil to keep them warm. Let the sauce and veggies in the cooker to cool a bit (the sauce will thicken a little as it cools). As the sauce is cooling, take out meat from the remaining chicken thighs. Pull the meat apart into shreds with two forks. Get rid of the bones. In a very large bowl, put the shredded chicken and reserve.
To serve, separate the spaghetti squash into 6 serving plates. Put one of whole chicken thighs over the squash on each serving plate. Mix vegetable-sauce mixture in slow cooker. Scoop about half cup of vegetable-sauce mixture atop each serving. Drizzle with fresh parsley if desired.
Mix remaining vegetable-sauce mixture from cooker into shredded chicken in bowl. Cover the bowl and chill for up to two days. If desired, use this to make Chipotle Ranch Chicken Pasta.

Nutrition Information
Calories: 291 calories;;Cholesterol: 141
Sugar: 9;Protein: 31
Saturated Fat: 3
Fiber: 4;Sodium: 494;Total Carbohydrate: 20;Total Fat: 10

836. Slow Cooker Baby Back Ribs

Serving: 6 | Prep: 15mins | Cook: | Ready in:
Ingredients
¾ cup ketchup
1 tablespoon cider vinegar
1 tablespoon brown sugar
1½ teaspoons smoked paprika
¼- ½ teaspoon crushed red pepper
1 teaspoon garlic powder
1 teaspoon onion powder
¼ teaspoon salt
½ teaspoon ground pepper
2½-3 pounds baby back pork ribs
Direction
In a small bowl, whisk crushed red pepper, smoked paprika, brown sugar, vinegar, and ketchup together. In another small bowl, mix pepper, salt, onion powder, and garlic powder. Rub all over the ribs with garlic mixture. On the sinewy side of the ribs, spread 1 tablespoon of the ketchup mixture. Put in a 5- to 6-quart slow cooker. Distribute evenly the leftover ketchup mixture over the meaty side. Cook with a cover on Low for 8 hours or High for 4 hours.
Set broiler to high and start preheating.
Bring the ribs to a large baking sheet. Spread the sauce over the ribs and put under the broiler for 4-6 minutes until beginning to brown. Cut the rack between the bones and ready to serve.

Nutrition Information
Calories: 307 calories;;Total Carbohydrate: 13
Saturated Fat: 7;Sodium: 189
Fiber: 0;Total Fat: 19;Cholesterol: 74
Sugar: 10;Protein: 21

837. Slow Cooker Beef Stew

Serving: 8 | Prep: 40mins | Cook: | Ready in:
Ingredients

3 pounds boneless beef chuck, trimmed and cut into 1½-inch pieces
1 teaspoon salt, divided
1 teaspoon ground pepper, divided
½ cup all-purpose flour
4 tablespoons extra-virgin olive oil, divided
1 large onion, halved and sliced
1½ pounds Yukon Gold potatoes, cut into 1½ -inch pieces
1 pound carrots, cut into 2-inch lengths
¾ cup red wine
1½ cups low-sodium beef broth
1 (6 ounce) can tomato paste
1 teaspoon dried thyme
1 small bay leaf
Chopped fresh parsley for garnish
Direction
Add the beef into the big bowl and use half tsp. each of the pepper and salt to season. Put in the flour and coat by tossing. Shake off the redundant flour back into the bowl and save.
Heat 2 tbsp. of the oil on medium high heat in the big skillet. Put roughly 1/3 beef to the pan. Cook for roughly 4 minutes or till turning browned on all of the sides. Move into the 6-qt. slow cooker. Put 1 tbsp. of the oil into pan and cook the rest of the beef in 2 more batches, adjusting the heat if necessary. Move into slow cooker.
Put onion and rest 1 tbsp. of the oil into the pan. Cook over medium heat, mixing, for roughly 8 minutes or till becoming tender. Put onion into the slow cooker with the carrots and potatoes. Pour the wine into pan and scrape up any of the browned bits. Add to the slow cooker.
Combine the rest half tsp. each of the pepper and salt, bay leaf, thyme, tomato paste and broth to the remaining flour in the bowl. Add on top of stew ingredients and whisk them well.
Keep the slow cooker covered and cook over High heat for 4 hours or over Low heat for 7.5 hours. As you want, drizzle the stew with the parsley to serve.
Nutrition Information
Calories: 590 calories;;Total Fat: 20;Sodium: 624;Total Carbohydrate: 32
Saturated Fat: 6
Fiber: 5;Cholesterol: 177
Sugar: 8;Protein: 64

838. Slow Cooker Braised Beef With Carrots Turnips

Serving: 8 | Prep: 40mins | Cook: | Ready in:
Ingredients
1 tablespoon kosher salt
2 teaspoons ground cinnamon
½ teaspoon ground allspice
½ teaspoon ground pepper
¼ teaspoon ground cloves
3-3½ pounds beef chuck roast, trimmed
2 tablespoons extra-virgin olive oil
1 medium onion, chopped
3 cloves garlic, sliced
1 cup red wine
1 (28 ounce) can whole tomatoes, preferably San Marzano
5 medium carrots, cut into 1-inch pieces
2 medium turnips, peeled and cut into ½-inch pieces
Chopped fresh basil for garnish
Direction
In a small bowl, mix cloves with pepper, allspice, cinnamon and salt. Rub the blend all over the beef.
Heat oil over medium heat in a big skillet. Put in beef and cook for 4 to 5 minutes each side until browned. Move to a slow cooker (5 to 6 quarts in size).
Put onion and garlic to the pan. Cook for 2 minutes, mixing. Put in tomatoes (with their juice) and wine; boil, scraping up any browned bits and breaking up tomatoes. Put the blend together with turnips and carrots to the slow cooker.
Cover and cook for 4 hours on High or for 8 hours on Low.
Take the beef out of the slow cooker, then cut. Enjoy the beef with vegetables and sauce, decorate with basil, if you like.
Nutrition Information
Calories: 318 calories;
Saturated Fat: 3;Total Carbohydrate: 13;Protein: 35;Total Fat: 11;Sodium: 538
Fiber: 3;Cholesterol: 99
Sugar: 6

839. Slow Cooker Brisket Sandwiches With Quick Pickles

Serving: 8 | Prep: | Cook: 1hours | Ready in:
Ingredients
2 tablespoons smoked paprika
2 teaspoons kosher salt
1 teaspoon garlic powder
1 teaspoon onion powder
1 teaspoon coarsely ground pepper
3¼ pounds brisket (see Tip), trimmed
1 tablespoon extra-virgin olive oil
1 16-ounce bottle rauchbier (smoked beer) or 2 cups reduced-sodium beef broth
½ cup white vinegar
½ cup cider vinegar
2 tablespoons light brown sugar
1 teaspoon pickling spice
1 teaspoon kosher salt
2 pickling or mini cucumbers, sliced
1 medium sweet onion, thinly sliced into rings
2 cloves garlic, chopped
½ teaspoon kosher salt
½ cup low-fat mayonnaise
8 whole-wheat buns
Direction
For brisket: In a small bowl, put together the pepper, onion powder, garlic powder, salt and paprika. Massage all over the brisket. In a big, heavy skillet, heat the oil over medium heat. Put the brisket and brown each side for 3 to 5 minutes per side. Put to a 6-quart slow cooker.
Add the beer or broth to the pan together with any leftover spice blend from chopping board; set heat to high. Allow to cook for 5 minutes, scraping up browned bits using a wooden spoon. Pour on top of the brisket. Put cover and allow to cook for 6 hours on High or 9 hours on Low.
For pickles: In the meantime, in a small saucepan, mix the brown sugar, cider vinegar and white vinegar; boil over high heat and let it cook for a minute. Put pickling spice and a teaspoon of salt. Put into a big, heatproof glass bowl and add onion and cucumbers. Chill, mixing from time to time, for a minimum of 1 hour or till set to serve.
For garlic mayo: Using a mortar and pestle or with the back of a spoon, mash the garlic and half

teaspoon of salt into a paste on a chopping board. In a small bowl, put together the garlic mixture with mayonnaise. Put cover and chill till set to serve.
Once the brisket is done, move to a clean chopping board and allow to rest for 10 minutes.
Using 2 forks, shred the brisket, then coarsely chop the shredded meat. Put together the chopped brisket with liquid in the slow cooker.
To serve, let the pickled vegetables drain. Spread every bun with a tablespoon garlic mayo and top with approximately 3/4 cup brisket and half cup pickles.

Nutrition Information
Calories: 401 calories;
Fiber: 4;Cholesterol: 91;Sodium: 768;Total Carbohydrate: 34
Sugar: 7;Protein: 34;Total Fat: 13
Saturated Fat: 3

840. Slow Cooker Cassoulet

Serving: 8 | Prep: | Cook: 30mins | Ready in:
Ingredients
Cassoulet
1 pound dried great northern beans, soaked (see Tip) and drained
1 4-ounce ham hock
2 cups halved and sliced onion
3 cloves garlic, sliced
2 bay leaves
1 tablespoon dried thyme
1 teaspoon salt
1 cup low-sodium chicken broth
1 (28 ounce) can no-salt-added plum tomatoes
2 pounds pork shoulder or pork butt, trimmed and cut into 2-inch pieces
2 tablespoons tomato paste
1 cup dry white wine
Breadcrumbs
3 tablespoons extra-virgin olive oil
2½ cups coarse fresh whole-wheat breadcrumbs
2 cloves garlic, minced
2 tablespoons chopped fresh parsley
Direction
For cassoulet: In a 6- to 7- quart slow cooker, mix salt, thyme, bay leaves, sliced garlic, onion, ham hock and beans. Stir in juice from tomatoes (save the tomatoes) and broth. Nestle pork into the bean mixture.
In a small saucepan, cook tomato paste on medium high heat from 2-3 minutes while stirring continuously, until a couple spots on the bottom browned deeply. Pour wine and bring to a boil. Dissolve the tomato paste by stirring and get the browned bits out of the pan. Pour into the slow cooker. Chop the saved tomatoes roughly and drizzle over the top to cover almost the beans.
Cook on Low setting for 9 hours or High setting for 6 hours. Take the meat from the ham hock and chop. Stir back into the stew. Get rid of bay leaves.
For breadcrumbs: In a big nonstick skillet with oil in, cook breadcrumbs on medium heat for 10-15 minutes, stirring regularly, until beginning to crisp. Add minced garlic, cook and stir usually for 2 minutes. Stir in parsley after removing from heat. Sprinkle breadcrumbs on the cassoulet to serve.
Nutrition Information
Calories: 540 calories;
Saturated Fat: 5;Sodium: 625;Cholesterol: 64;Total Fat: 18
Fiber: 14;Total Carbohydrate: 54
Sugar: 6;Protein: 35

841. Slow Cooker Chicken Noodle Soup Meal Prep Freezer Pack

Serving: 8 | Prep: 25mins | Cook: | Ready in:
Ingredients
8 ounces whole-wheat egg noodles or other whole-wheat noodles
3 pounds bone-in chicken breast, skin removed
2 cups chopped onion
1 cup chopped carrot
1 cup chopped celery
2 sprigs thyme
8 cups low-sodium chicken broth
2 teaspoons kosher salt
2 cups frozen peas
¼ cup chopped fresh dill, plus more for garnish
2 tablespoons lemon juice
Direction
Cook the noodles following the package instructions. Drain and wash using cold water to cool.
In the meantime, in a sealable gallon-size freezer bag, put the thyme, celery, carrot, onion and chicken. In another sealable gallon-size freezer bag, place the cooled noodles. Freeze both of the bags until ready to use. Defrost the bags in the fridge for one day prior to cooking.
In a 6-quart slow cooker, mix together the salt, broth and chicken mixture; save the noodles. Let it cook for 8 hours on Low or for 4 hours on High, then add the peas during the final 10 minutes of cooking.
Move the chicken to a clean chopping board. Take out the meat from the bones and shred it into bite-size pieces, once the chicken is cool enough to touch. Mix the chicken into the soup together with lemon juice, dill and noodles. Put more dill to garnish, if preferred.
Nutrition Information
Calories: 327 calories;;Sodium: 678;Total Carbohydrate: 33
Saturated Fat: 1
Fiber: 5;Cholesterol: 68
Sugar: 6;Protein: 36;Total Fat: 5

842. Slow Cooker Chicken Parmesan Meatballs

Serving: 10 | Prep: 30mins | Cook: | Ready in:
Ingredients
Sauce
1 (28 ounce) can no-salt-added crushed tomatoes
½ medium onion, grated
¼ cup dry red wine
2 cloves garlic, minced
½ teaspoon dried basil
½ teaspoon dried oregano
¼ teaspoon salt
Meatballs
1 pound ground chicken or turkey
1 large egg, lightly beaten
½ cup grated Parmesan cheese
½ cup fine dry whole-wheat breadcrumbs (see Tip)
½ teaspoon dried basil
½ teaspoon dried oregano
½ teaspoon garlic powder
¼ teaspoon salt
30 pearl-size fresh mozzarella balls
Direction

To make the sauce: In a 5 to 6-quart slow cooker, mix together the salt, oregano, basil, garlic, wine, onion and tomatoes.
To make the meatballs: In a medium bowl, mix together the salt, garlic powder, oregano, basil, breadcrumbs, Parmesan, egg and ground chicken or turkey. Pat a tablespoon of seasoned meat into a disk and put mozzarella ball in the middle. Wrap the cheese with the meat and roll it into a ball. Redo the process with the leftover cheese and meat, then add the meatballs into the slow cooker.
Put cover and let it cook for 6 hours on Low or 3 hours on High.
Nutrition Information
Calories: 163 calories;
Saturated Fat: 3;Sodium: 277;Cholesterol: 69;Total Carbohydrate: 7;Total Fat: 7
Fiber: 2
Sugar: 3;Protein: 14

843. Slow Cooker Picadillo

Serving: 8 | Prep: | Cook: 40mins | Ready in:
Ingredients
1 tablespoon extra-virgin olive oil
2 pounds ground bison or lean (90% lean or leaner) ground beef
4 ounces chorizo-style cooked chicken sausage, diced
1 tablespoon chili powder
2 teaspoons cumin seeds, crushed or coarsely chopped
1 teaspoon dried oregano
½ teaspoon ground cinnamon
½ cup water
2 tablespoons tomato paste
2 tablespoons red-wine vinegar
2 cups diced onion
2 cups chopped seeded Cubanelle or Anaheim peppers
1 cup frozen corn kernels, thawed
½ cup pitted green olives, sliced
5 cloves garlic, minced
1 28-ounce can diced tomatoes
¼ teaspoon salt, or to taste
Freshly ground pepper to taste
Direction
In a large skillet, heat oil over medium-high heat. Put in bison (or beef) and sausage and cook for 5 to 6 minutes, using a wooden spoon to break the bison (or beef). If necessary, bring to a colander and drain to remove any extra fat, then bring back to the skillet. Put in cinnamon, oregano, cumin, and chili powder; cook while stirring over medium-high heat, until aromatic, 1 to 2 minutes. Mix in vinegar, tomato paste and water until blended.
Bring the meat mixture to a 5- to 6-quart slow cooker. Mix in garlic, olives, corn, peppers, and onion. Pour in tomatoes with their juice.
Cook with a cover on Low for 7 to 8 hours or on High for 4 hours. Stir the picadillo to blend and sprinkle with pepper and salt to season.
Nutrition Information
Calories: 310 calories;;Cholesterol: 70;Total Carbohydrate: 16
Sugar: 7;Protein: 28;Total Fat: 16
Fiber: 4
Saturated Fat: 4;Sodium: 535

844. Slow Cooker Sausage Apple Stuffing

Serving: 16 | Prep: 30mins | Cook: | Ready in:
Ingredients
3 tablespoons extra-virgin olive oil
1 large onion, chopped
2 cups chopped celery
8 ounces sweet Italian sausage, casing removed and crumbled
1¼ teaspoons poultry seasoning
½ teaspoon ground pepper
¼ teaspoon salt
1 pound stale whole-grain bread, cubed (about 8 cups; see Tip)
1 large Granny Smith apple, peeled and chopped
1 cup low-sodium chicken broth
Direction
Heat oil on medium heat in a large skillet. Put in onion and celery; cook and stir until softened for 10 minutes. Put in salt, pepper, poultry seasoning, and sausage; cook and stir until no longer pink for an additional 6 to 8 minutes.
Place to a 5- to 6-quart slow cooker. Put in broth, apple, and bread; stir to coat well. Cook, covered, on high for 2 hours.
Nutrition Information
Calories: 136 calories;
Saturated Fat: 1;Total Carbohydrate: 16
Sugar: 4;Protein: 7;Total Fat: 5;Sodium: 240
Fiber: 3;Cholesterol: 4

845. Slow Cooker Vegetarian Lasagna

Serving: 8 | Prep: | Cook: 30mins | Ready in:
Ingredients
1 large egg
1 15- to 16-ounce container part-skim ricotta
1 5-ounce package baby spinach, coarsely chopped
3 large or 4 small portobello mushroom caps, gills removed (see Tip), halved and thinly sliced
1 small zucchini, quartered lengthwise and thinly sliced
1 28-ounce can crushed tomatoes
1 28-ounce can diced tomatoes
3 cloves garlic, minced
Pinch of crushed red pepper (optional)
15 whole-wheat lasagna noodles (about 12 ounces), uncooked
3 cups shredded part-skim mozzarella, divided
Direction
In a big bowl, mix the spinach, egg, zucchini, ricotta and mushrooms together.
In a medium-sized bowl, mix the garlic, crushed red pepper (if desired) and diced and crushed tomatoes along with their juices together.
Use a good amount of cooking spray to grease a 6-quart or bigger slow cooker. Spread 1 1/2 cups of the tomato mixture evenly in the slow cooker and top it with 5 noodles, you may overlap the noodles a little bit and crack it to smaller pieces if need be to make sure that the tomato mixture is evenly-covered.
Scatter 1/2 of the ricotta-vegetable mixture evenly on top of the noodles and push it down firmly; put another even layer of 1 1/2 cups of the tomato mixture and top it off with 1 cup of mozzarella. Do the same layering process once more beginning with the noodles. Put a final layer of noodles on top and scatter the rest of the tomato mixture evenly over the noodles. Keep the remaining 1 cup of mozzarella in the fridge.
Cover the slow cooker and allow the mixture to cook for 2 hours on high setting or for 4 hours on low

setting. Switch the slow cooker off then top the lasagna with the chilled remaining mozzarella; cover the slow cooker and allow the cooked lasagna to rest for 10 minutes until the mozzarella cheese has melted.
Nutrition Information
Calories: 413 calories;Protein: 27;Cholesterol: 67;Total Carbohydrate: 49
Sugar: 9;Total Fat: 14
Saturated Fat: 8;Sodium: 665
Fiber: 7

846. Spanish Chicken Stew

Serving: 4 | Prep: 30mins | Cook: | Ready in:
Ingredients
1¼ pounds skinless, boneless chicken thighs, cut into 1- ½-inch pieces
12 ounces red potatoes, cut into ½-inch wedges
1 medium onion, thinly sliced
1 teaspoon minced garlic (2 cloves)
½ teaspoon dried thyme, crushed
¼ teaspoon salt
¼ teaspoon ground black pepper
1 (14.5 ounce) can no-salt-added diced tomatoes, undrained
1 medium red bell pepper, cut into ¼-inch strips
⅓ cup pimiento-stuffed olives, chopped
1 cup reduced sodium chicken broth
Direction
Mix together the black pepper, salt, thyme, garlic, onion, potato and chicken in a 3 1/2 or 4-quart slow cooker, then add broth and tomatoes.
Put cover and let it cook for 3 1/2 to 4 hours on high-heat setting or 7-8 hours on low-heat setting. Increase to high-heat setting if you're using low-heat setting. Mix in olives and sweet pepper. Put cover and let it cook for additional 30 minutes.
Nutrition Information
Calories: 297 calories;;Total Fat: 8
Saturated Fat: 2
Fiber: 4;Cholesterol: 113;Total Carbohydrate: 24
Sugar: 7;Sodium: 683;Protein: 32

847. Sweet And Sour Pork With Cabbage

Serving: 4 | Prep: 35mins | Cook: 5mins | Ready in:
Ingredients
1 large red sweet pepper, quartered and seeded
1 teaspoon water
1 (8 ounce) can pineapple chunks (juice pack)
2 tablespoons reduced-sodium soy sauce
1 tablespoon packed brown sugar or brown sugar substitute equivalent to 1 tablespoon brown sugar (see Tip)
1 tablespoon cornstarch
2 teaspoons grated fresh ginger
2 cloves garlic
2 teaspoons rice vinegar
4 teaspoons canola oil
1 medium green sweet pepper, seeded and cut into 1-inch pieces
1 (8 ounce) can bamboo shoots, drained
12 ounces boneless pork loin, bias-sliced across the grain into strips
4 cups shredded Napa cabbage
Direction
Put the red sweet pepper quarters, cut sides down, in the microwave-safe dish. Pour in water. Cover with the plastic wrap. Microwave for 4-5 mins on 100% power (high) until tender. Allow to stand until skin easily peels from the flesh, about 10 mins; peel and throw away the skin. Put red sweet pepper in the food processor; process, covered, until smooth. Drain the pineapple chunks, reserving 1/3 cup juice; put the pineapple chunks aside. Put rice vinegar, garlic, ginger, cornstarch, brown sugar, soy sauce and the reserved 1/3 cup of pineapple juice to red sweet pepper in food processor. Process, covered, until combined; put aside.
Heat a teaspoon of the oil in a large skillet over medium-high heat. Put in green sweet pepper; stir-fry until crisp-tender, about 2 mins. Put in bamboo shoots; stir-fry for half a minute. Remove the vegetables from pan. Put in the remaining 3 teaspoons oil to the pan. Put in the pork strips; stir-fry just until done, about 2-3 mins. Put in the red sweet pepper mixture; cook while stirring until bubbly and thickened, about half a minute. Cook while stirring for 2 mins longer. Mix in pineapple chunks and green sweet pepper mixture; heat through. Serve over the Napa cabbage.
Nutrition Information
Calories: 274 calories;
Sugar: 16
Saturated Fat: 2;Total Carbohydrate: 23;Sodium: 341
Fiber: 4;Cholesterol: 47;Protein: 22;Total Fat: 11

848. Tried And True Chili Mac

Serving: 8 | Prep: 25mins | Cook: | Ready in:
Ingredients
1½ pounds lean ground beef
1 large onion, chopped
3 cloves garlic, minced
1 (15 ounce) can chili beans in chili gravy
1 (14.5 ounce) can diced tomatoes and green chilies, undrained
1 cup lower-sodium beef broth
1 medium green sweet pepper, chopped
2 teaspoons chili powder
1 teaspoon ground cumin
8 ounces dried cavatappi or macaroni, cooked according to package directions
¼ cup shredded reduced-fat Cheddar cheese
Direction
Set a large skillet over medium heat and sauté onion, garlic and ground beef until brown and tender. Remove excess fat.
Mix cooked meat with undrained chili beans, undrained green chilies and tomatoes, broth, cumin, chili powder and sweet pepper in a 3 1/2- to 4-quart slow cooker.
Place cover and cook on low for 4-6 hours or on high for 2-3 hours. Mix in cooked pasta. Toss cooked pasta into the pot until well coated. Best served with grated cheese on top.
Nutrition Information
Calories: 343 calories;;Sodium: 510
Fiber: 5;Total Carbohydrate: 36;Cholesterol: 58
Sugar: 3;Protein: 26;Total Fat: 10
Saturated Fat: 4

849. Vegetarian Pinto Bean Sloppy Joes

Serving: 10 | Prep: | Cook: 30mins | Ready in:
Ingredients
2 tablespoons extra-virgin olive oil
2 medium carrots, sliced
1 large white onion, sliced
4 cloves garlic, minced
3 tablespoons chili powder

2 tablespoons balsamic vinegar
1 cup dry pinto beans, soaked (see Tip)
1 large red bell pepper, diced
1 8-ounce can no-salt-added tomato sauce
½ cup water
2 tablespoons reduced-sodium soy sauce or tamari
2 tablespoons tomato paste
4 cups very thinly sliced green cabbage
1 medium zucchini, chopped
1 cup corn, fresh or frozen (thawed)
3 tablespoons honey mustard
1 tablespoon brown sugar
1 teaspoon salt
10 whole-wheat hamburger buns

Direction
In a large skillet, heat oil over medium-high heat. Put in onion and carrots; cook and stir occasionally for 8 minutes, until beginning to brown. Mix in chili powder and garlic; cook while stirring for 15 seconds until aromatic. Take away from heat; mix in vinegar and scrape the browned bits up if any.
Spray a 6-quart slow cooker with cooking spray. For soaked beans, drain and rinse; bring to the slow cooker. Mix in tomato paste, soy sauce (or tamari), water, tomato sauce, and bell pepper to combine. Spread the carrot-onion mixture on top of the bean mixture, but don't mix the two together. (The layer on top prevents beans from drying out by keeping the beans submerged while cooking.) Cook with a cover on Low for 9 hours or High for 5 hours.
Mix in salt, brown sugar, honey mustard, corn, zucchini, and cabbage; cook for 30 minutes on High. Pour the mixture on buns and serve.

Nutrition Information
Calories: 281 calories;;Cholesterol: 0;Total Carbohydrate: 50;Protein: 11;Sodium: 721 Fiber: 11;Total Fat: 6
Saturated Fat: 1
Sugar: 13

850. Zesty Sloppy Joes

Serving: 8 | Prep: 20mins | Cook: | Ready in:
Ingredients
1½ pounds lean ground beef (see Tip)
1 cup onion, chopped
1 clove garlic, minced
1 (6 ounce) can vegetable juice
½ cup ketchup
½ cup water
2 tablespoons heat-stable sugar substitute
2 tablespoons canned jalapeño peppers, chopped (optional)
1 tablespoon mustard
2 teaspoons chili powder
1 teaspoon Worcestershire sauce
8 whole wheat hamburger buns, split and toasted
Shredded reduced-fat Cheddar cheese (optional)
Sweet pepper strips (optional)

Direction
Cook garlic, onion and ground beef in a big skillet until onion is soft and beef turns brown, then drain off fat.
In the meantime, mix together Worcestershire sauce, chili powder, mustard, jalapeno peppers (optional), sugar substitute, water, ketchup and vegetable juice in a 3 1/2- or 4-qt. slow cooker. Stir in the meat mixture.
Place a cover and cook on high heat setting about 3-4 hours or low heat setting for 6-8 hours. Scoop on bun halves with the meat mixture. If you want, use cheese to sprinkle over and serve along with sweet pepper strips.

Nutrition Information
Calories: 294 calories;;Cholesterol: 54;Total Carbohydrate: 29;Protein: 20
Saturated Fat: 4;Sodium: 500
Fiber: 2
Sugar: 10;Total Fat: 11

Chapter 11: Healthy Slow Cooker Recipes

851. A Crock Of Curried Pork Soup

Serving: 10 | Prep: 20mins | Cook: 8hours | Ready in:

Ingredients

1 teaspoon olive oil
4 zucchini, cut into 1/4-inch slices
1 head garlic, separated into cloves and sliced
1 (2 pound) pork roast
3 tablespoons curry powder, divided
salt and ground black pepper to taste
2 (10 ounce) cans diced tomatoes with green chile peppers
3 cubes vegetable bouillon
3/4 cup boiling water
2 tablespoons minced garlic
1 (15.5 ounce) can white beans, drained
1 (15 ounce) can garbanzo beans (chickpeas), drained
1/2 cup white rice

Direction

Coat the inside of the slow cooker's bottom with the olive oil. Lay the slices of garlic and slices of zucchini onto the olive oil layer; add the pork roast on top. Use pepper, salt, and 1 tbsp. of curry powder to season the roast.
Add the tomatoes along with the green chile peppers to the big measuring cup; mix in the bouillon cubes and the boiling water till becoming dissolve. Add the broth-tomato mixture to the slow cooker. Spread the minced garlic on the top of the roast.
Cook over Low heat roughly 6 hours or till the pork softens.
Move the pork roast into the dish and shred into bite-sized pieces with the fork. Add the shredded pork back to the slow cooker; put in the rest 2 tbsp. of the curry powder, rice, garbanzo beans, and white beans and mix.
Cook for 2 hours longer.

Nutrition Information

Calories: 230 calories;;Total Fat: 4.9;Sodium: 340;Total Carbohydrate: 30.1;Cholesterol: 32;Protein: 17.4

852. Amazing Apple Butter

Serving: 48 | Prep: 10mins | Cook: 10hours25mins | Ready in:

Ingredients

10 pounds apples, quartered
4 cups unsweetened apple juice
1 cup white sugar
1 tablespoon apple cider vinegar
1 1/2 teaspoons ground cinnamon
1/2 teaspoon ground cloves
1/2 teaspoon ground allspice
6 half-pint canning jars with lids and rings

Direction

Combine the apple juice and apples in a stockpot. Bring the mixture to a boil. Lower the heat and cook the mixture at a simmer for 20-30 minutes until the apples are mushy and soft.
Transfer the apples into the food mill. Process the mixture into a puree, discarding the peels and cores that remain in the mill. Pour the processed apples into the slow cooker.
Cook the mixture on high heat while the lid is off for overnight up to 24 hours until the volume reduces by half and the moisture has evaporated.
Stir the apple cider vinegar, allspice, sugar, cloves, and cinnamon through the apple puree.
Continue cooking the mixture on high heat for 2-6 more hours until the mixture will mound on a chilled plate without seeing any water that separates from the edges.
Sterilize the jars and their lids in boiling water for at least 5 minutes. Fill the hot and sterilized jars with the apple butter, filling them up to within 1/4-inch of the top. Use a knife or a thin spatula to run the insides of the jars until all the air bubbles have been removed. Use a moist paper towel to wipe the jars' rims until all food residues are removed. Top the jars with their lids and screw with rings.
Position the rack in the bottom of the large stockpot. Fill the stockpot halfway with water. Bring the water to a boil. Use a holder to lower the jars into the boiling water, making sure that the jars are arranged 2-inches apart. If necessary, add more boiling water until the level of the water reaches at least 1-inch above the tops of the jars. Once the water reaches into a rolling boil, cover the pot and process the jars for 5-10 minutes.
Remove the jars from the pot and transfer them onto the wood or cloth-covered surface, placing them a few inches apart. Let them cool. Press the top of the lid using your finger once they are cool to check if the seal is tight (the lid must not move up or down). Store the jars in a cool and dark area.

Nutrition Information

Calories: 75 calories;;Total Fat: 0.2;Sodium: 2;Total Carbohydrate: 19.7;Cholesterol: 0;Protein: 0.3

853. Amazing Pork Tenderloin In The Slow Cooker

Serving: 6 | Prep: 15mins | Cook: 4hours | Ready in:

Ingredients

1 (2 pound) pork tenderloin
1 (1 ounce) envelope dry onion soup mix
1 cup water
3/4 cup red wine
3 tablespoons minced garlic
3 tablespoons soy sauce
freshly ground black pepper to taste

Direction

In a slow cooker, arrange the pork tenderloin with the contents of the soup packet. Spread soy sauce, wine, and water over the top, flipping over the pork to cover. Carefully scatter garlic over the pork, retaining as much on top of the roast while cooking as possible. Scatter with pepper, then cook, covered, on low for 4 hours. Use with cooking liquid on the side as au jus.

Nutrition Information

Calories: 180 calories;;Cholesterol: 65;Protein: 24.5;Total Fat: 3.7;Sodium: 918;Total Carbohydrate: 5.8

854. Apple Tapioca Pudding

Serving: 6 | Prep: 15mins | Cook: 3hours | Ready in:

Ingredients

4 cups apples - peeled, cored and sliced
1/2 cup brown sugar
3/4 teaspoon ground cinnamon
1/2 teaspoon salt
2 tablespoons small pearl tapioca
1 lemon, juiced

1 cup boiling water
1/2 cup raisins (optional)
Direction
In a bowl, put tapioca, salt, cinnamon, brown sugar and apples, and toss till slices of apple are coated. Put mixture of apple in slow cooker. Add boiling water and lemon juice on apples.
Fix cooker to High and cook for 3 to 4 hours, to soften apples and thicken.
If wished, stir raisins in; serve while warm.
Nutrition Information
Calories: 137 calories;;Total Fat: 0.2;Sodium: 201;Total Carbohydrate: 36;Cholesterol: 0;Protein: 0.7

855. Ashley's African Peanut Soup
Serving: 20 | Prep: 30mins | Cook: 5hours | Ready in:
Ingredients
2 tablespoons olive oil
2 large skinless, boneless chicken breast halves
1 onion, chopped
2 red bell peppers, sliced
4 cloves garlic, minced
1 (28 ounce) can crushed tomatoes
2 sweet potatoes, peeled and cut into bite-size pieces
3 cups sliced carrots
4 cups chicken broth, or more as needed
1/2 teaspoon curry powder
1/2 teaspoon ground cumin
1/4 teaspoon chili powder
1/4 teaspoon cayenne pepper
1/4 teaspoon crushed red pepper flakes
1/4 teaspoon ground cinnamon
1/4 teaspoon ground black pepper
1 cup brown rice
1 cup crunchy peanut butter
Direction
In a skillet, heat olive oil on medium heat. Brown both sides of chicken breasts for about 5 minutes on each side. Put chicken breasts in a slow cooker. In the hot skillet, cook garlic, red bell peppers and onion for about 5 minutes until onions are translucent. Put cooked veggies in the slow cooker.
In the slow cooker, mix in black pepper, cinnamon, red pepper flakes, cayenne pepper, chili powder, cumin, curry powder, chicken broth, carrots, sweet potatoes and crushed tomatoes. Set cooker on high. Cook for 5-6 hours or cook for 10 hours on low. Mix in extra chicken broth if needed as you cook.
3 hours prior to serving, mix in brown rice. Mix peanut butter in at least 1 hour prior to serving. Shred the chicken meat. Serve hot.
Nutrition Information
Calories: 205 calories;;Cholesterol: 14;Protein: 10.8;Total Fat: 8.7;Sodium: 353;Total Carbohydrate: 22.3

856. Balsamic Pear, Chicken, And Asparagus
Serving: 4 | Prep: 20mins | Cook: 4hours | Ready in:
Ingredients
1 tablespoon vegetable oil
4 skinless, boneless chicken breast halves, cut into strips
1 onion, sliced thin
salt and ground black pepper to taste
2 ripe Bartlett pears, cored and sliced
1 pound fresh asparagus, trimmed
4 cloves garlic, minced
2 tablespoons balsamic vinegar
3 tablespoons apple juice
1 teaspoon dried rosemary
1 tablespoon grated fresh ginger
2 tablespoons dark brown sugar
Direction
In a skillet, heat the oil over medium heat. Cook the chicken for 3 to 5 minutes in the hot oil until totally browned; move to a slow cooker. Put the onion into the chicken and add salt and pepper to season. Arrange the asparagus and pears on top of the chicken mixture.
In a bowl, mix the sugar, ginger, rosemary, apple juice, balsamic vinegar and garlic, then pour over the asparagus. Use salt and pepper again to season.
Cook for 4 to 6 hours on Low.
Nutrition Information
Calories: 309 calories;;Cholesterol: 69;Protein: 29.1;Total Fat: 7.4;Sodium: 70;Total Carbohydrate: 33.5

857. Beer Chops I
Serving: 4 | Prep: 10mins | Cook: 8hours | Ready in:
Ingredients
1 onion, sliced
2 pork chops butterfly cut
1 (12 fluid ounce) can or bottle beer
2 cubes chicken bouillon
Direction
Lay onion slices on slow-cooker base. Slice butterfly chops in half and put over onions. Put in beer then put chicken bouillon squares. Put cover, cook 6-8 hours on low.
Nutrition Information
Calories: 112 calories;;Sodium: 591;Total Carbohydrate: 6.5;Cholesterol: 19;Protein: 7.9;Total Fat: 3.3

858. Better Slow Cooker Robust Chicken
Serving: 6 | Prep: 5mins | Cook: 8hours | Ready in:
Ingredients
1 1/2 pounds skinless, boneless chicken breast halves - cut into 1 inch strips
2 tablespoons bacon bits
1/4 cup chopped green olives
1 (14.5 ounce) can diced tomatoes, drained
1 (4.5 ounce) can sliced mushrooms, drained
1 (1.25 ounce) envelope dry chicken gravy mix
1/2 cup red wine
3 tablespoons Dijon mustard
1/4 cup balsamic vinegar
Direction
Mix vinegar, mustard, wine, gravy mix, mushrooms, tomatoes, olives, bacon bits, and chicken in a slow cooker. Combine together.
Put the lid on the slow cooker and cook for 6-8 hours on Low.
Nutrition Information
Calories: 198 calories;;Cholesterol: 62;Protein: 24.5;Total Fat: 4.7;Sodium: 946;Total Carbohydrate: 10.1

859. Bloody Mary Chicken
Serving: 4 | Prep: | Cook: | Ready in:
Ingredients
4 skinless, boneless chicken breast halves
1 (32 ounce) bottle bottled Bloody Mary mix
Direction

Rinse, skin, and discard the fat from chicken breasts and put in a slow cooker.
Pour over the chicken breasts with Bloody Mary mix, set the slow cooker to low and cook for 8 hours on low.
Nutrition Information
Calories: 181 calories;;Total Fat: 1.5;Sodium: 1163;Total Carbohydrate: 11;Cholesterol: 68;Protein: 29.3

860. Blueberry And Banana Steel Cut Oats

Serving: 4 | Prep: 10mins | Cook: 5hours | Ready in:
Ingredients
2 cups water
2 cups almond milk
2 cups blueberries
2 ripe bananas, mashed
1 cup steel-cut oats
2 tablespoons honey
2 teaspoons vanilla extract
1 teaspoon ground cinnamon
1/4 teaspoon salt
Direction
In the container of a slow cooker, stir salt, cinnamon, vanilla extract, honey, oats, bananas, blueberries, almond milk, and water together.
Cook on Low for 5-8 hours.
Nutrition Information
Calories: 315 calories;;Sodium: 231;Total Carbohydrate: 64.6;Cholesterol: 0;Protein: 6.8;Total Fat: 4.3

861. Blueberry And Chia Quinoa

Serving: 6 | Prep: 5mins | Cook: 6hours | Ready in:
Ingredients
4 cups soy milk
4 cups water
2 cups quinoa
2 cups blueberries
1/3 cup chia seeds
1/3 cup honey
Direction
In a slow cooker, stir in chia seeds, soy milk, water, honey, quinoa, and blueberries.
Cook for 6 to 8 hours on low setting.
Nutrition Information
Calories: 381 calories;;Total Fat: 6.4;Sodium: 91;Total Carbohydrate: 69.1;Cholesterol: 0;Protein: 13.7

862. Bone Broth

Serving: 8 | Prep: 10mins | Cook: 1Day30mins | Ready in:
Ingredients
cooking spray
1 (6 ounce) can tomato paste
2 pounds beef bones
6 cups cool water, or as needed
2 onions, thickly sliced
2 carrots
3 cloves garlic, crushed
2 bay leaves
Direction
Preheat the oven to 200º C (400º F). Use cooking spray to spray a roasting pan.
Next, spread the tomato paste on the beef bones and arrange in the prepared roasting pan.
Bake for about 30 minutes in the preheated oven, until the bones begin to brown.

Remove the bones to a slow cooker, add enough water to cover bones. Next, add bay leaves, garlic, carrots, and onions to the broth mixture.
Then cook on low setting for at least 24 hours.
Through a fine-mesh strainer, filter the broth into a container and chill.
Nutrition Information
Calories: 49 calories;;Total Carbohydrate: 11.4;Cholesterol: 0;Protein: 1.8;Total Fat: 0.2;Sodium: 186

863. CB's Black Eyed Peas

Serving: 10 | Prep: 15mins | Cook: 4hours10mins | Ready in:
Ingredients
4 slices bacon, chopped
1 pound dry black-eyed peas
6 cups water
1 onion, chopped
1 (14.5 ounce) can diced tomatoes, undrained
1 jalapeno pepper, finely chopped
1 clove garlic, minced
1 tablespoon chili powder
salt to taste
Direction
In a deep, big frying pan, put the bacon and let it cook for about 10 minutes on medium heat, mixing from time to time, until browned evenly.
In a slow cooker, put the chili powder, garlic, jalapeno pepper, tomatoes, onion, water and dried peas, then stir to blend. Mix in the bacon grease and bacon, then set the cooker on High. Let it cook for around 4hours until the peas become soft. Season salt to taste, then serve.
Nutrition Information
Calories: 168 calories;;Cholesterol: 4;Protein: 11.2;Total Fat: 2.5;Sodium: 181;Total Carbohydrate: 26.1

864. Chicken Tagine With Couscous

Serving: 6 | Prep: 20mins | Cook: 2hours30mins | Ready in:
Ingredients
1 3/4 pounds skinless, boneless chicken breast halves - cut into 1 inch pieces
2 large onions, thinly sliced
1/2 cup coarsely chopped dried apricots
1/3 cup raisins
1 1/4 cups low-sodium chicken broth
2 tablespoons tomato paste
2 tablespoons lemon juice
2 tablespoons all-purpose flour
1 1/2 teaspoons ground ginger
1 1/2 teaspoons ground cumin
1 teaspoon ground cinnamon
1/2 teaspoon black pepper
1/4 teaspoon curry powder (optional)
1/8 teaspoon cayenne pepper (optional)
1 cup couscous
1 cup boiling water
Direction
In a slow cooker, combine the apricots, raisins, onions, and chicken. Whisk the chicken broth, lemon juice, black pepper, cayenne, curry powder, flour, tomato paste, ginger, cinnamon, and cumin in a bowl. Pour this mixture into the cooker with chicken. Cover the cooker and set it on High setting. Cook for 2 1/2 hours. If you want to cook it on Low setting, cook it for 5 hours.

In a saucepan, place the couscous and mix in boiling water. Cover the pan and allow it to stand for 5 minutes until the water is absorbed completely and the couscous is tender. Use a fork to fluff the pasta. Scoop it into the plates and serve together with chicken tagine.
Nutrition Information
Calories: 340 calories;Protein: 32;Total Fat: 3.3;Sodium: 132;Total Carbohydrate: 45.7;Cholesterol: 69

865. Chicken Wild Rice Soup III

Serving: 6 | Prep: 20mins | Cook: 6hours | Ready in:
Ingredients
1 cup uncooked wild rice
3 cups diced, cooked chicken breast meat
2 tablespoons chicken bouillon granules
1 onion, chopped
5 cups water
4 potatoes, cubed
1 1/2 cups milk
2 tablespoons all-purpose flour
Direction
Bring water, onion, bouillon, chicken, and rice to a boil on a big saucepan over medium-high heat. Take out from heat and pour into a slow cooker. Mix in potatoes. Combine flour and milk and stir until smooth. Mix into soup mixture. Cook for 6 to 8 hours until the flavors are blended well and the potatoes and rice are soft.
Nutrition Information
Calories: 356 calories;;Total Fat: 6.8;Sodium: 114;Total Carbohydrate: 46.7;Cholesterol: 57;Protein: 26.8

866. Chicken And Corn Chili

Serving: 6 | Prep: 15mins | Cook: 12hours | Ready in:
Ingredients
4 skinless, boneless chicken breast halves
1 (16 ounce) jar salsa
2 teaspoons garlic powder
1 teaspoon ground cumin
1 teaspoon chili powder
salt to taste
ground black pepper to taste
1 (11 ounce) can Mexican-style corn
1 (15 ounce) can pinto beans
Direction
In the slow cooker, put salsa and chicken the evening prior you desire to eat this chili. Put with pepper, salt, chili powder, cumin and garlic powder. On Low setting, cook for 6 to 8 hours.
Before you desire to eat, approximately 3 to 4 hours, with 2 forks tear the chicken. Put the meat back to the pot and keep cooking.
Into the slow cooker, mix the pinto beans and corn. Allow to simmer till about to serve.
Nutrition Information
Calories: 188 calories;;Total Carbohydrate: 22.6;Cholesterol: 41;Protein: 20.4;Total Fat: 2.3;Sodium: 1012

867. Chicken And Fresh Tomato Slow Cooker Stew

Serving: 6 | Prep: 15mins | Cook: 7hours | Ready in:
Ingredients
5 potatoes, peeled and cubed
1 1/2 cups chopped fresh tomato
1 cup sliced carrot
1 onion, chopped
2 bay leaves
3 large skinless boneless chicken breast halves
2 (8 ounce) cans tomato sauce
1 (14.5 ounce) can chicken broth
1 1/2 teaspoons Italian seasoning
1/4 teaspoon red pepper flakes
water, as needed
Direction
In a slow cooker, mix together bay leaves, onion, carrot, tomato, and potatoes. Put chicken breasts on top of vegetables. In a bowl, mix Italian seasoning, chicken broth, and tomato sauce, spread on chicken breasts. If necessary, add in water to fully cover the chicken. Cook for 6 hours over low heat. Take out chicken breasts, cut into bite-size pieces then bring them back to the slow cooker. Keep cooking for another 1 to 2 hours until vegetables become tender.
Nutrition Information
Calories: 295 calories;;Total Fat: 2.8;Sodium: 467;Total Carbohydrate: 40.8;Cholesterol: 59;Protein: 27.4

868. Chicken With Sausage And Dried Fruit

Serving: 4 | Prep: 10mins | Cook: 9hours | Ready in:
Ingredients
4 skinless, boneless chicken breast halves
1 (6 inch) smoked turkey sausage link, sliced
1 green bell pepper, seeded and chopped
1 small onion, chopped
3 cloves garlic, minced
3/4 cup chopped dried apples
1/2 cup sweetened dried cranberries
1 tablespoon dried parsley
2 teaspoons dried chives
1 cup chicken stock
1 pinch salt and pepper to taste
Direction
In the bottom of a slow cooker, put chicken breasts. If you use frozen chicken, you don't need to thaw them. Lay cranberries, apples, garlic, onion, green pepper, and sausage over the chicken. Sprinkle chives and parsley over. Drizzle everything with chicken stock, and use pepper and salt to season. Put the lid on and cook for 8-9 hours on Low.
Nutrition Information
Calories: 297 calories;;Total Fat: 7;Sodium: 591;Total Carbohydrate: 27.2;Cholesterol: 93;Protein: 31.8

869. Cindy's Snappy Sensational Superfood Soup

Serving: 2 | Prep: 25mins | Cook: 8hours | Ready in:
Ingredients
3 yellow potatoes (such as Klondike Goldust®), cubed
1 (10 ounce) package frozen chopped spinach, thawed and drained
2 large carrots, chopped
2 turnips, diced
3 cloves garlic, minced
3/4 cup dry lentils
water, or amount to cover
Cindy's Magical Motorvatin' Spice Mix:
1/4 teaspoon chopped fresh basil
1 teaspoon chili powder
1/4 teaspoon ground cinnamon
1/4 teaspoon dried basil

1/4 teaspoon paprika
1/8 teaspoon ground turmeric
1/8 teaspoon cayenne pepper
1/8 teaspoon ground ginger
sea salt and ground black pepper to taste
Direction
In a slow cooker, combine lentils, garlic, turnips, carrots, spinach, and potatoes. Add enough water to cover the mixture.
Whisk black pepper, sea salt, ground ginger, cayenne pepper, turmeric, paprika, dried basil, cinnamon, chili powder, and fresh basil together in a mixing bowl; mix into the slow cooker.
Put the lid on the cooker and cook for 8 hours on High setting.
Nutrition Information
Calories: 518 calories;;Total Fat: 2.4;Sodium: 440;Total Carbohydrate: 99.8;Cholesterol: 0;Protein: 29.9

870. Clean Eating Refried Beans
Serving: 18 | Prep: 10mins | Cook: 8hours5mins | Ready in:
Ingredients
3 cups dried pinto beans
16 1/2 cups water, divided
3 tablespoons olive oil
1/2 teaspoon salt
1/4 teaspoon ground black pepper
Direction
In a slow cooker, add beans and 8 cups of water to cover, then soak beans for about 8-10 hours.
Drain and rinse beans and turn them back to slow cooker and pour in 8 cups of fresh water.
Cook beans on low heat about 8-10 hours, then drain.
In a skillet, mix together pepper, salt, olive oil, beans and 1/2 cup of water on medium heat, then mash beans to desired consistency.
Nutrition Information
Calories: 132 calories;;Cholesterol: 0;Protein: 6.9;Total Fat: 2.6;Sodium: 75;Total Carbohydrate: 20.1

871. Dee's Special Chicken
Serving: 4 | Prep: | Cook: | Ready in:
Ingredients
4 skinless, boneless chicken breast halves
salt and pepper to taste
1 teaspoon dried rosemary
1 teaspoon dried sage
1 teaspoon dried thyme
6 cloves garlic
1 (12 fluid ounce) can or bottle beer
2 sprigs fresh parsley, for garnish
Direction
Season chicken breasts with pepper and salt then broil till golden brown.
In a slow cooker, put the chicken along with beer, garlic, thyme, sage and rosemary. For 3 to 4 hours cook on high. Move the chicken breasts out then jazz it up with parsley, serve.
Nutrition Information
Calories: 182 calories;;Cholesterol: 68;Protein: 28.4;Total Fat: 1.7;Sodium: 89;Total Carbohydrate: 6

872. Deer Chop Hurry
Serving: 4 | Prep: 15mins | Cook: 6hours | Ready in:
Ingredients
2 pounds deer chops (venison)
1 cup ketchup
1/2 cup water
1 medium onion, chopped
1/2 cup packed brown sugar
1 (1 ounce) envelope dry onion soup mix
Direction
Thinly cut the deer chops then place them in a heavy skillet set on medium-high heat and brown them. Then place the meat in a slow cooker. Stir in dry onion soup mix, brown sugar, onion, water, and ketchup. Cook for 6 hours on low or until it is tender. Bake at 350°F for 1 hour if you want to cook it in a roaster.
Nutrition Information
Calories: 435 calories;;Sodium: 1353;Total Carbohydrate: 49.2;Cholesterol: 171;Protein: 48.2;Total Fat: 5.3

873. Easy Peasy Venison Stew
Serving: 8 | Prep: 30mins | Cook: 4hours15mins | Ready in:
Ingredients
2 pounds venison, cut into cubes
salt and pepper to taste
1 kiwi, peeled and sliced
1 1/2 cups red wine
1/4 cup all-purpose flour
extra-virgin olive oil
2 cloves garlic, minced
1 onion, cut into chunks
1 sprig rosemary leaves, minced
1 sprig thyme leaves, minced
balsamic vinegar
1/2 cup beef stock
5 potatoes, peeled and cubed
1 carrots, cut into 1/2 inch pieces
1 parsnips, cut into 1/2 inch pieces
1 (8 ounce) package sliced fresh mushrooms
Direction
Season venison with pepper and salt; put into bowl. Mix red wine and kiwi slices in till mixed evenly. Cover. Marinate overnight in the fridge.
Drain venison. Keep red wine marinade. Pick kiwi pieces out of venison. Put into red wine marinade. Squeeze as much marinade from venison as possible. In a big skillet/saucepan, heat olive oil on medium-high heat. Put floured venison cubes in hot oil. Cook for 5-10 minutes till browned on all sides. Put venison cubes into slow cooker. Mix thyme, rosemary, onion and garlic into skillet. Cook for 3 minutes till onion edges start to soften. Put the reserved red wine marinade and the balsamic vinegar in. Boil and cook for 5 minutes. Put onion mixture into the slow cooker. Mix mushrooms, parsnips, carrots, potatoes and beef stock in till mixed evenly. If needed, add water to just cover veggies.
Cover slow cooker; set to low. Cook for 4 hours till veggies are tender and venison pulls apart easily with a fork. Season with pepper and salt to taste; serve.
Nutrition Information
Calories: 345 calories;;Total Carbohydrate: 35.9;Cholesterol: 86;Protein: 28;Total Fat: 6.3;Sodium: 54

874. Easy Slow Cooker Thai Chicken With Basil
Serving: 8 | Prep: 15mins | Cook: 6hours | Ready in:
Ingredients

2 pounds skinless, boneless chicken breast, cubed
1 red bell pepper, cut into strips
1/4 cup soy sauce
2 tablespoons fish sauce
3 fresh red Thai chile peppers, minced
1 tablespoon freshly squeezed lime juice
1 tablespoon rice vinegar
1 tablespoon finely grated fresh ginger
1/2 cup chopped Thai basil, or to taste
1 pinch salt and freshly ground black pepper to taste
Direction
In a slow cooker, mix ginger, rice vinegar, lime juice, fish sauce, soy sauce, bell pepper and Thai chile, chicken.
Cook on low for about 5 1/2 hours until the chicken becomes tender. Place in basil and then cook for about 30 minutes longer until it's wilted into the sauce. Season with pepper and salt.
Nutrition Information
Calories: 127 calories;;Total Fat: 2.4;Sodium: 793;Total Carbohydrate: 2.2;Cholesterol: 59;Protein: 23

875. Easy And Quick Swiss Steak

Serving: 8 | Prep: 15mins | Cook: 8hours10mins | Ready in:
Ingredients
1 tablespoon vegetable oil
2 cups all-purpose flour
salt and pepper to taste
paprika to taste
2 pounds beef cube steaks
3 green bell pepper, sliced into rings
3 red bell pepper, sliced into rings
4 onions, sliced into rings
4 (14.5 ounce) cans crushed tomatoes
Direction
On medium heat, heat oil in a pan. Combine paprika, pepper, flour, and salt in a bowl; dredge steaks in the mixture. Brown each side of the steak in the pan; remove from heat.
Alternately layer steak, tomatoes, green bell pepper, onion, and red bell pepper in a slow cooker.
Cook on Low, covered, for 6-8 hours until the steaks are really tender.
Nutrition Information
Calories: 349 calories;;Total Fat: 8.7;Sodium: 305;Total Carbohydrate: 48.6;Cholesterol: 27;Protein: 21.6

876. Gluten Free Vegan Stock For The Slow Cooker

Serving: 8 | Prep: 25mins | Cook: 8hours | Ready in:
Ingredients
2 tablespoons olive oil
4 stalks celery, cut into 4-inch pieces
2 carrots, cut into large chunks
1 potato, cut into large chunks
1 onion, cut into 8 wedges
2 large outer leaves romaine lettuce
1/2 cup gluten-free beer
2 shallots, halved
1 fennel bulb, outer layers only
1/2 green bell pepper
1/8 apple
1/4 bunch flat-leaf parsley
10 whole black peppercorns
1 wedge lemon
1 (1 inch) piece ginger

2 tablespoons tamari (gluten-free soy sauce)
1 tablespoon vegan Worcestershire sauce (optional)
2 cloves garlic
1 bay leaf
8 cups water
Direction
Use olive oil to coat a slow cooker crock's bottom. In the slow cooker crock, place bay leaf, garlic, Worcestershire sauce, tamari, ginger, lemon, peppercorns, parsley, apple, bell pepper, fennel, shallots, beer, lettuce, onion, potato, carrots, and celery. Cover the ingredients with water.
Cook for 4 hours on High or 8-10 hours on Low.
Use a slotted spoon to remove any solid chunks from the liquid and discard.
Use a cheesecloth to line a colander, set over a large pot; use the cheesecloth to strain the broth.
Nutrition Information
Calories: 110 calories;;Total Fat: 3.7;Sodium: 330;Total Carbohydrate: 17.3;Cholesterol: 0;Protein: 2.8

877. Grandma's Slow Cooker Vegetarian Chili

Serving: 8 | Prep: 10mins | Cook: 2hours | Ready in:
Ingredients
1 (19 ounce) can black bean soup
1 (15 ounce) can kidney beans, rinsed and drained
1 (15 ounce) can garbanzo beans, rinsed and drained
1 (16 ounce) can vegetarian baked beans
1 (14.5 ounce) can chopped tomatoes in puree
1 (15 ounce) can whole kernel corn, drained
1 onion, chopped
1 green bell pepper, chopped
2 stalks celery, chopped
2 cloves garlic, chopped
1 tablespoon chili powder, or to taste
1 tablespoon dried parsley
1 tablespoon dried oregano
1 tablespoon dried basil
Direction
Mix together celery, bell pepper, onion, corn, tomatoes, baked beans, garbanzo beans, kidney beans and black bean soup in a slow cooker. Season with basil, oregano, parsley, chili powder and garlic. Cook on high setting for a minimum of 2 hours.
Nutrition Information
Calories: 260 calories;;Total Fat: 2;Sodium: 966;Total Carbohydrate: 52.6;Cholesterol: 1;Protein: 12.4

878. Greek Slow Cooker Chicken

Serving: 6 | Prep: 20mins | Cook: 4hours | Ready in:
Ingredients
1 (3 pound) whole chicken, skin removed
1 lemon, cut in half
6 cloves peeled garlic, or more to taste (divided)
6 red potatoes, sliced into 1-inch thick rounds
1 large onion, roughly chopped
1/4 cup white wine
1/4 cup olive oil
1 teaspoon chicken bouillon granules
1/4 cup boiling water
2 teaspoons dried oregano
salt and pepper to taste
Direction
Wash the inside and out of the chicken. Insert 3 garlic cloves and a lemon half in chicken cavity. Put the other lemon half aside.

Into a slow cooker crock, arrange the onions and sliced potatoes in layer. Scatter around the inside of cooker with the leftover three cloves of garlic then put chicken on vegetables. Add olive oil and wine. In boiling water, dissolve bouillon, and pour into the cooker.

Squeeze juice from the leftover half of lemon on top of chicken (drain out the seeds); scatter oregano over. Add black pepper and salt to season the chicken. Cook for 4-6 hours on High setting or for about 8-10 hours on Low setting with a cover. An inserted meat thermometer in the thickest portion of a thigh, without touching the bone, must register no less than 70 ° C or 160 ° F.

Nutrition Information
Calories: 471 calories;;Total Fat: 17.9;Sodium: 173;Total Carbohydrate: 39.8;Cholesterol: 96;Protein: 36.7

879. Ham And Chickpea Slow Cooker Soup

Serving: 6 | Prep: 20mins | Cook: 10hours | Ready in:
Ingredients
1 pound dry garbanzo beans
1 meaty ham bone
10 new potatoes, halved
5 carrots, chopped
1/2 cup frozen corn
ground black pepper to taste
Direction
In a big container, put the garbanzo beans and pour a couple of inches of cold water to cover, then allow it to stand for 8 hours to overnight.
On the next day, rinse the soaked beans and put them in a slow cooker; put the ham bone in the cooker and pour in enough water to cover the ham bone and beans by a couple of inches. Set the cooker to Low and let it cook for 8 hours.
Remove any foam from the surface of the soup and take out the ham bone. From the ham bone, strip as much meat as possible, then put the meat back into the slow cooker and get rid of the bone. Mix in the black pepper to taste, frozen corn, carrots and potatoes. Set the cooker on Low and let it cook for an hour, then increase the heat up to High and let it cook for another 1 hour (sums up to 10 hours of cooking time).
Nutrition Information
Calories: 427 calories;;Cholesterol: 0;Protein: 18.6;Total Fat: 4.9;Sodium: 63;Total Carbohydrate: 80.5

880. Healthier (but Still Awesome) Awesome Slow Cooker Pot Roast

Serving: 12 | Prep: 10mins | Cook: 8hours | Ready in:
Ingredients
2 (10.75 ounce) cans low-fat, low-sodium condensed cream of mushroom soup
1 large onion, chopped
3 pounds chuck roast
2 cups sliced carrots
1 pound small red potatoes
1/2 pound string beans
1/4 cup chopped parsley
Direction
In a slow cooker, combine the chuck roast, chopped onion and cream of mushroom soup together.
Let it cook for 3 to 4 hours on a high setting or 8 to 9 hours on low. Put the parsley, string beans, potatoes and carrots in about an hour and a half before the pot roast is done cooking.
Nutrition Information
Calories: 305 calories;;Cholesterol: 76;Protein: 24.1;Total Fat: 16.2;Sodium: 299;Total Carbohydrate: 14.7

881. Healthier Amazing Pork Tenderloin In The Slow Cooker

Serving: 6 | Prep: 15mins | Cook: 4hours | Ready in:
Ingredients
1 (2 pound) pork tenderloin
2 cups onion, sliced
1/2 cup water
3/4 cup red wine
3 tablespoons soy sauce
3 tablespoons minced garlic
freshly ground black pepper to taste
Direction
In a slow cooker, put the sliced onions and pork tenderloin. Drizzle soy sauce, wine and water over the top, flipping the pork to coat. Distribute the garlic over pork, leaving as much on top of the roast as possible. Dust with pepper. Cover and cook for 4 hours on low setting until the pork is slightly pink in the middle. An instant-read thermometer placed in the middle should register at least 63°C (145°F). Enjoy with cooking liquid on the side as au jus.
Nutrition Information
Calories: 179 calories;;Total Fat: 3.2;Sodium: 506;Total Carbohydrate: 6.4;Cholesterol: 65;Protein: 24.7

882. Healthier BBQ Pork For Sandwiches

Serving: 12 | Prep: 15mins | Cook: 4hours30mins | Ready in:
Ingredients
1 (14 ounce) can beef broth
3 pounds boneless pork ribs
1 cup shredded carrot
4 1/2 fluid ounces barbeque sauce
4 1/2 ounces mesquite sauce
Direction
In the slow cooker, pour the beef broth and add the pork ribs. Let it cook for about 4 hours on High, until the meat easily shreds. Take out the meat and use 2 forks to shred it.
Set an oven to preheat to 175°C (350°F). Move the shredded pork to a frying pan or Dutch oven and mix in the mesquite sauce, barbecue sauce and carrots. Let it bake in the preheated oven for about 30 minutes, until heated through.
Nutrition Information
Calories: 313 calories;;Cholesterol: 83;Protein: 30.3;Total Fat: 18.1;Sodium: 290;Total Carbohydrate: 5.1

883. Healthier Baked Slow Cooker Chicken

Serving: 6 | Prep: 25mins | Cook: 10hours | Ready in:
Ingredients
1 (2 to 3 pound) whole chicken
salt and ground black pepper to taste
1 teaspoon paprika
3 large carrots, split lengthwise and cut into 2-inch pieces
2 medium onions, quartered
2 tablespoons fresh chopped parsley
Direction

Wad a piece of aluminum foil into 3- to 4-in. ball, working in the same manner to make 3 pieces; arrange them on the bottom of a slow cooker. Rinse chicken under cold water, inside and out. Use paper towels to pat dry. Season paprika, pepper and salt on the chicken. Put the chicken into a slow cooker, on top of the crumbled aluminum foil.
Set the slow cooker on high for 1 hour; decrease to low for 4-5 hours. Add in vegetables; cook for around another 4-5 hours, or till the juices run clear and the chicken is not pink anymore. Sprinkle parsley over. Serve.
Nutrition Information
Calories: 216 calories;Protein: 18.3;Total Fat: 12.4;Sodium: 100;Total Carbohydrate: 7.2;Cholesterol: 51

884. Healthier Marie's Easy Slow Cooker Pot Roast

Serving: 8 | Prep: 20mins | Cook: 8hours | Ready in:
Ingredients
3 pounds chuck roast
salt and ground black pepper to taste
1 cup reduced-sodium beef stock
2 onions, chopped
2 pounds potatoes, peeled and cubed
3 carrots, chopped
1 stalk celery, chopped
1/4 cup chopped fresh parsley (optional)
Direction
Sprinkle salt and pepper into the chuck roast.
Use a big skillet and heat on medium high heat. Sear roast for about 4 minutes on each side until browned on all sides.
Put the roast into a slow cooker. Pour beef stock into the skillet. Let it boil while scraping browned bits from the bottom of the pan using wooden spoon. Add in broth and onions into the slow cooker. Cook with cover for 5 hours on Low. Add in potatoes, parsley, celery and carrots. Cook with cover for another 3 hours on low, until roast is tender and cooked through.
Nutrition Information
Calories: 350 calories;;Total Fat: 15.5;Sodium: 128;Total Carbohydrate: 25.4;Cholesterol: 79;Protein: 26.7

885. Healthier Slow Cooker Beef Stew I

Serving: 6 | Prep: 30mins | Cook: 10hours20mins | Ready in:
Ingredients
2 pounds beef stew meat, cut into 1 inch cubes
1/4 cup all-purpose flour
1/2 teaspoon salt
1/2 teaspoon ground black pepper
4 cloves garlic, minced
1 bay leaf
1 teaspoon paprika
1 teaspoon Worcestershire sauce
1 onion, chopped
1 1/2 cups reduced-sodium beef broth
3 potatoes, diced
4 carrots, sliced
1 stalk celery, chopped
3/4 pound butternut squash, peeled and cut into small chunks
1/2 head escarole, washed and torn into bite-sized pieces
Direction

In slow cooker, place beef. Mix in a small bowl pepper, flour, and salt together. Pour over meat and toss to coat. Stir in bay leaf, garlic, paprika, onion, Worcestershire sauce, beef broth, butternut squash, celery, carrots, and potatoes.
Cook while covered for 4 to 6 hours on High mode or for 10 to 12 hours on Low setting. Stir in escarole. Continue cooking while covered for 15 to 20 minutes until escarole is tender.
Nutrition Information
Calories: 468 calories;;Total Fat: 21.3;Sodium: 341;Total Carbohydrate: 39.1;Cholesterol: 83;Protein: 30.7

886. Healthier Slow Cooker Chicken Stroganoff

Serving: 4 | Prep: 10mins | Cook: 5hours30mins | Ready in:
Ingredients
1 tablespoon chopped carrot
1 tablespoon chopped parsley
1 tablespoon chopped onion
1 clove garlic
1/4 teaspoon lemon zest
1 teaspoon salt
1/4 teaspoon ground black pepper
4 skinless, boneless chicken breast halves - cubed
2 tablespoons butter
4 ounces Neufchatel cheese
8 ounces natural cream of chicken soup
1 cup frozen peas
Direction
In a food processor or a small blender, mix together the ground pepper, salt, lemon zest, garlic, onion, parsley and carrot and process until chopped finely, then move to a slow cooker. Add butter and chicken then mix. Let it cook for 5-6 hours on Low.
Stir in peas, chicken soup and Neufchatel cheese. Let it cook for about 30 minutes on High until heated through.
Nutrition Information
Calories: 330 calories;;Sodium: 1164;Total Carbohydrate: 6.9;Cholesterol: 108;Protein: 32.7;Total Fat: 16.9

887. Healthier Slow Cooker Chicken Taco Soup

Serving: 8 | Prep: 15mins | Cook: 7hours | Ready in:
Ingredients
1 onion, chopped
1 (16 ounce) can chili beans
1 (15 ounce) can black beans
1 (15 ounce) can whole kernel corn, drained
1 carrot, chopped
1 (8 ounce) can tomato sauce
2 (10 ounce) cans diced tomatoes with green chilies, undrained
1 (12 fluid ounce) can or bottle beer
1 1/2 tablespoons taco seasoning, reduced sodium
3 whole skinless, boneless chicken breasts
1/4 cup chopped fresh cilantro
1/2 cup shredded reduced-fat Cheddar cheese (optional)
1/4 cup light sour cream (optional)
2 ounces crushed baked tortilla chips (optional)
Direction
In a slow cooker, put the beer, diced tomatoes, tomato sauce, corn, chopped carrot, black beans, chili

beans and onion, then add taco seasoning and mix to combine. Lay the chicken breasts over the mixture, then press down a bit until just covered by the other ingredients. Put cover and allow it to cook for 5 hours on Low.
Take out the chicken breasts from the soup and let it cool long enough so it can be handled. Shred the chicken and mix it back into the soup. Keep on cooking for 2 hours on Low. Serve it with crushed tortilla chips, light sour cream, Cheddar cheese and cilantro.
Nutrition Information
Calories: 328 calories;;Cholesterol: 50;Protein: 28.8;Total Fat: 5.8;Sodium: 1275;Total Carbohydrate: 42.9

888. Healthier Slow Cooker Chicken And Dumplings

Serving: 8 | Prep: 10mins | Cook: 5hours35mins | Ready in:
Ingredients
4 skinless, boneless chicken breast halves
2 tablespoons butter
2 cups natural cream of chicken soup
1 onion, finely diced
3 carrots, sliced
10 ounces refrigerated reduced-fat biscuit dough, torn into pieces
1 cup frozen peas
Direction
In a slow cooker, put the onion, cream of chicken soup, butter and chicken. Put cover and let it cook for 5-6 hours on High. After 5 hours of cooking, stir in carrots.
In the slow cooker, put the torn biscuit dough for 30 minutes prior to serving. Let it cook for about 25 minutes until the dough is no longer raw in the middle. Lift the biscuits' edges and mix in the peas. Allow it to stand for about 10 minutes until it becomes warm, prior to serving.
Nutrition Information
Calories: 248 calories;;Total Fat: 7.1;Sodium: 758;Total Carbohydrate: 29.3;Cholesterol: 41;Protein: 16.2

889. Healthier Slow Cooker Chicken Tortilla Soup

Serving: 8 | Prep: 40mins | Cook: 3hours | Ready in:
Ingredients
1 pound boneless, skinless chicken breasts, cut into strips
1 (15 ounce) can whole peeled tomatoes, mashed
1 (10 ounce) can enchilada sauce
1 medium onion, chopped
2 banana peppers, chopped
2 cloves garlic, minced
2 cups water
1 (14.25 ounce) can reduced-sodium chicken broth
1 teaspoon cumin
1 teaspoon chili powder
1 teaspoon salt
1/4 teaspoon ground black pepper
1 bay leaf
1 (10 ounce) package frozen corn
1 tablespoon chopped cilantro
7 corn tortillas
vegetable cooking spray
Direction
In a slow cooker, put the garlic, banana peppers, onion, enchilada sauce, tomatoes and chicken. Pour in chicken broth and water. Put in bay leaf, ground pepper, salt, chili powder and cumin to season, then mix in cilantro and corn. Put cover on and let it cook for 3 to 4 hours on High, or 6-8 hours on Low.
Set an oven to preheat to 200°C (400°F).
Use cooking spray to coat both sides of the tortillas lightly. Slice the tortillas into strips, then spread on a baking tray.
Let them bake in the preheated oven for 10-15 minutes until they become crisp; sprinkle the tortilla strips on top of the soup.
Nutrition Information
Calories: 208 calories;;Sodium: 438;Total Carbohydrate: 23.7;Cholesterol: 43;Protein: 15.3;Total Fat: 6.8

890. Hearty Cabbage Rutabaga Slow Cooker Soup

Serving: 6 | Prep: 25mins | Cook: 5hours | Ready in:
Ingredients
1/4 large head cabbage, chopped
1/4 large rutabaga, diced
1 1/2 cups uncooked orzo pasta
1/2 large onion, finely chopped
1 whole head garlic, peeled and minced
3 tablespoons chopped fresh dill
6 cups water
2 cups vegetable broth
Direction
In a slow cooker, put vegetable broth, water, dill, garlic, orzo pasta, onion, rutabaga and cabbage. Cover cooker. Cook for 5-9 hours on low until soup is thick and veggies are tender.
Nutrition Information
Calories: 236 calories;;Sodium: 182;Total Carbohydrate: 48.9;Cholesterol: 1;Protein: 9;Total Fat: 1.1

891. Honey Wheat Bread IV

Serving: 12 | Prep: 30mins | Cook: 3hours | Ready in:
Ingredients
2 cups scalded milk
2 tablespoons vegetable oil
1/4 cup honey
3/4 teaspoon salt
1 (.25 ounce) package active dry yeast
3 cups whole wheat flour
1 cup all-purpose flour
Direction
In a small saucepan, heat the milk till bubbling, then take away from heat. Mix in the salt, honey and vegetable oil; allow to cool until lukewarm. Preheat a 3 and a half-quart or 5-quart slow cooker, then lightly grease the right baking dish.
In a large bowl, add the lukewarm milk mixture. Let the yeast dissolve in the milk. Mix in whole wheat flour and the all-purpose flour, 1 cup at a time. Thoroughly beat till the dough has pulled together. In the prepared baking dish, place the dough. Allow to rest for 5 minutes.
In a slow cooker, position the dish; cook while covered on high for 2 - 3 hours or till the loaf sounds hollow when tapped on the base. Cool on a wire rack, then serve.
Nutrition Information

Calories: 203 calories;;Total Fat: 3.8;Sodium: 164;Total Carbohydrate: 37.7;Cholesterol: 3;Protein: 6.8

892. Hunter's Roast

Serving: 8 | Prep: 15mins | Cook: 8hours | Ready in:
Ingredients
4 pounds venison rump roast
2 (12 fluid ounce) cans or bottles beer
1 (16 ounce) jar pepperoncini
Direction
Remove all gristle and fat from venison; put in slow cooker. Use enough beer to cover roast. Use pepperoncinis to cover.
Cover. Cook for 8 hours on low setting till meat falls apart and is tender.
Nutrition Information
Calories: 322 calories;Protein: 53;Total Fat: 5.8;Sodium: 1301;Total Carbohydrate: 5;Cholesterol: 193

893. Karen's Slow Cooker Pizza Chicken

Serving: 5 | Prep: 20mins | Cook: 8hours | Ready in:
Ingredients
4 skinless, boneless chicken breast halves - cut into bite size pieces
1 onion, chopped
1 green bell pepper, chopped
2 stalks celery, sliced
1 (10.75 ounce) can condensed tomato soup
1 (10.75 ounce) can condensed cream of mushroom soup
2 tablespoons tomato paste
1/2 cup water
1 tablespoon dried parsley
1 tablespoon dried oregano
1 tablespoon dried basil
1 bay leaf
salt and pepper to taste
Direction
Arrange celery, bell pepper, onion and chicken in a slow cooker. In a medium bowl, mix pepper, salt, oregano, parsley, water, tomato paste, cream of mushroom soup, basil and tomato soup. Blend well and transfer the mixture over chicken and vegetables in the slow cooker. Toss to coat and put in bay leaf.
Cook on low setting in 8 hours, until chicken and vegetables turn tender.
Nutrition Information
Calories: 226 calories;Protein: 25;Total Fat: 6;Sodium: 859;Total Carbohydrate: 18.7;Cholesterol: 55

894. Laura's Quick Slow Cooker Turkey Chili

Serving: 8 | Prep: 15mins | Cook: 4hours | Ready in:
Ingredients
1 tablespoon vegetable oil
1 pound ground turkey
2 (10.75 ounce) cans low sodium tomato soup
2 (15 ounce) cans kidney beans, drained
1 (15 ounce) can black beans, drained
1/2 medium onion, chopped
2 tablespoons chili powder
1 teaspoon red pepper flakes
1/2 tablespoon garlic powder
1/2 tablespoon ground cumin
1 pinch ground black pepper
1 pinch ground allspice
salt to taste
Direction
In a skillet, heat oil on moderate heat. Put turkey into the skillet and cook until browned evenly, then drain. Use cooking spray to coat the inside of a slow cooker, then stir in onion, black beans, kidney beans, tomato soup and turkey. Season with salt, allspice, black pepper, cumin, garlic powder, red pepper flakes, and chili powder.
Cover and cook on high for 4 hours or on low for about 8 hours.
Nutrition Information
Calories: 276 calories;;Cholesterol: 42;Protein: 21.2;Total Fat: 7.6;Sodium: 547;Total Carbohydrate: 32.8

895. Lorene's Slow Cooker Potato Soup

Serving: 10 | Prep: 15mins | Cook: 6hours | Ready in:
Ingredients
2 large onions, diced
4 stalks celery, chopped
4 pounds potatoes, diced
1 tablespoon dried dill weed
2 tablespoons olive oil
vegetable broth to cover
Direction
In a slow cooker, mix dill weed, potatoes, celery, and onions together; drizzle over the mixture with olive oil. In the slow cooker, add vegetable broth.
Cook for 6 hours on High, until the vegetables are soft.
Nutrition Information
Calories: 203 calories;;Total Fat: 3.3;Sodium: 394;Total Carbohydrate: 39.2;Cholesterol: 0;Protein: 5

896. Lower Sugar Spicy All Day Apple Butter

Serving: 32 | Prep: 20mins | Cook: 10hours | Ready in:
Ingredients
10 pounds apples - peeled, cored, and chopped
1/2 cup white sugar
4 teaspoons ground cinnamon
1 teaspoon ground cloves
1 teaspoon ground allspice
3/4 teaspoon ground nutmeg
1/4 teaspoon salt
1/4 cup sugar-free butter-flavored syrup
1/4 cup honey
1 tablespoon maple syrup
1 tablespoon Mexican vanilla extract
2 teaspoons lemon juice
1/2 teaspoon molasses
Direction
In a slow cooker, put apples. Dust with salt, nutmeg, allspice, cloves, cinnamon and sugar. Cover and cook for 2 hours on High.
Into the apple mixture, mix molasses, lemon juice, vanilla extract, maple syrup, honey, and butter-flavored syrup; mash apples using a fork or potato masher.
Lower heat to low, cover; keep cooking for 9 to 11 hours until thickened and dark brown, frequently stirring. Uncover and cook for another 1 to 2 hours.
Nutrition Information
Calories: 102 calories;;Total Carbohydrate: 26.8;Cholesterol: 0;Protein: 0.4;Total Fat: 0.3;Sodium: 25

897. Middle Eastern White Beans

Serving: 6 | Prep: | Cook: 6hours | Ready in:
Ingredients
1 1/2 cups dried white kidney beans, soaked overnight
3 tablespoons tomato paste
1 tablespoon red pimento sauce
3 cloves garlic, chopped
3 medium onions, chopped
1 tablespoon lemon juice
1 teaspoon ground cumin
2 tablespoons olive oil
salt and pepper to taste
1 (14.5 ounce) can beef broth
Direction
Mix pepper, salt, olive oil, lemon juice, cumin, onions, garlic, pimento sauce, tomato paste and beans in a slow cooker until the beans are coated. Add beef broth, followed by adequate water so that the beans are entirely submerged. Put a lid on and set it to high. Cook until the liquid thickens and the beans become tender, about 6 hours. There should be not much soup at all.
Nutrition Information
Calories: 229 calories;;Total Fat: 5.3;Sodium: 351;Total Carbohydrate: 36.5;Cholesterol: 0;Protein: 10.2

898. Momma OB's Chicken Chili
Serving: 8 | Prep: 15mins | Cook: 3hours | Ready in:
Ingredients
2 pounds skinless, boneless chicken breast meat - cubed
1/2 tablespoon olive oil
1 tablespoon Italian seasoning
2 (28 ounce) cans whole peeled tomatoes
1 (16 ounce) can chili beans, drained and rinsed
1 (15 ounce) can kidney beans, drained and rinsed
1 (1.25 ounce) package chili seasoning mix
1 (4 ounce) can diced green chile peppers
1 onion, minced
3 cloves garlic, minced
1/2 cup water
Direction
In a skillet, heat oil over medium heat then cook 1/2 of the Italian seasoning and chicken. Allow it to cook with frequent stirring until chicken is evenly brown and well-cooked.
In a slow cooker, mix water, onion, garlic, tomatoes, chile peppers, kidney beans, chili seasoning, chili beans and the rest of the Italian seasoning. Mix in juices and chicken.
Place cover and let it cook over high heat for 3 hours.
Nutrition Information
Calories: 281 calories;;Total Fat: 3.6;Sodium: 1300;Total Carbohydrate: 30.9;Cholesterol: 66;Protein: 34.8

899. Montigott
Serving: 16 | Prep: 30mins | Cook: 6hours | Ready in:
Ingredients
2 (10.75 ounce) cans condensed tomato soup
2 (15 ounce) cans tomato sauce
2 (6 ounce) cans tomato paste
1 pound turkey sweet Italian sausages, casings removed
1 pound turkey hot Italian sausages, casings removed
1 1/2 (16 ounce) packages mostaccioli pasta
1/2 cup milk
2 (16 ounce) packages shredded mozzarella cheese

Direction
In a slow cooker, put the tomato paste, tomato sauce, and tomato soup. Stir to blend. Crumble the sweet and hot Italian sausages into the mixture. Cook while stirring occasionally on low with a cover until the sauce is flavorful and the meat is cooked through, about 4-6 hours.
When the tomato sauce is nearly done, boil a big pot of lightly salted water. Add the mostaccoli pasta to the boiling water, cook for about 8-10 minutes, or until the pasta is soft. Drain and rinse.
Set the oven at 190°C (375°F). Spray the cooking spray onto an 8x8 in. baking dish and a 9x13 in. baking dish. Layer the noodles and the cheese in the prepared baking dishes to an even depth and end with the top layer of cheese. Drizzle a little milk on each layer of cheese except for the top one.
Bake in the preheated oven until cheese melts and turns a bit brown on top, about 15 minutes. Slice into wedges and put the sauce on top before serving.
Nutrition Information
Calories: 447 calories;;Total Fat: 16.6;Sodium: 1481;Total Carbohydrate: 44.4;Cholesterol: 80;Protein: 32.4

900. Moroccan Tagine
Serving: 6 | Prep: 15mins | Cook: 45mins | Ready in:
Ingredients
1 tablespoon olive oil
2 skinless, boneless chicken breast halves - cut into chunks
1/2 onion, chopped
3 cloves garlic, minced
1 small butternut squash, peeled and chopped
1 (15.5 ounce) can garbanzo beans, drained and rinsed
1 carrot, peeled and chopped
1 (14.5 ounce) can diced tomatoes with juice
1 (14 ounce) can vegetable broth
1 tablespoon sugar
1 tablespoon lemon juice
1 teaspoon salt
1 teaspoon ground coriander
1 dash cayenne pepper
Direction
In a big pan, heat the oil on medium heat and cook garlic, onion and chicken for about 15 minutes until it turns brown.
In the pan, stir in the lemon juice, sugar, broth, tomatoes with juice, carrot, garbanzo beans and squash. Sprinkle cayenne pepper, coriander and salt to season. Let the mixture boil and keep on cooking until the veggies are soft, or for 30 minutes.
Nutrition Information
Calories: 265 calories;;Total Carbohydrate: 44.7;Cholesterol: 20;Protein: 14.1;Total Fat: 4.3;Sodium: 878

901. Mushroom Lentil Barley Stew
Serving: 8 | Prep: 15mins | Cook: 12hours | Ready in:
Ingredients
2 quarts vegetable broth
2 cups sliced fresh button mushrooms
1 ounce dried shiitake mushrooms, torn into pieces
3/4 cup uncooked pearl barley
3/4 cup dry lentils
1/4 cup dried onion flakes
2 teaspoons minced garlic
2 teaspoons dried summer savory

3 bay leaves
1 teaspoon dried basil
2 teaspoons ground black pepper
salt to taste

Direction

In a slow cooker, combine together salt, pepper, basil, bay leaves, savory, garlic, onion flakes, lentils, barley, shiitake mushrooms, button mushrooms and the broth.

Cook with a cover for 10-12 hours on low heat or 4-6 hours on high heat. Discard the bay leaves. Serve.

Nutrition Information

Calories: 213 calories;;Total Fat: 1.2;Sodium: 466;Total Carbohydrate: 43.9;Cholesterol: 0;Protein: 8.4

902. NO YOLKS® Easy Slow Cooker Beef Noodle Stew

Serving: 4 | Prep: 10mins | Cook: 7hours | Ready in:

Ingredients

1 pound lean cubed stewing beef
1 onion, chopped
8 ounces whole or sliced button mushrooms
2 teaspoons minced garlic
1 teaspoon dried thyme leaves
1 teaspoon dried rosemary leaves
2 1/4 cups sodium-reduced beef broth, divided
1 (19 ounce) can diced tomatoes
2 tablespoons cornstarch
1 1/2 cups frozen diced mixed vegetables (such as carrots, green beans and peas), thawed
1/2 (12 ounce) package NO YOLKS® Dumplings

Direction

Into the crock of 4- or 5-qt. slow cooker, add rosemary, thyme, garlic, mushrooms, onion and beef. Mix in tomatoes and 2 cups of broth (about 500 mL). Set heat to Low and cook for 6 – 7.5 hours or maximum of 10 hours.

Turn heat to High. Mix the rest of the broth with cornstarch. Mix into slow cooker till well-combined; put in vegetables. Keep it covered and cook till thoroughly heated or for extra 20 - 30 minutes.

At the same time, based on the instructions on the package, prepare the noodles. Scoop hot stew on top of noodles to serve.

Nutrition Information

Calories: 449 calories;;Total Fat: 8.3;Sodium: 355;Total Carbohydrate: 56;Cholesterol: 60;Protein: 35.2

903. Old Fashioned Baked Beans

Serving: 10 | Prep: 15mins | Cook: 6hours20mins | Ready in:

Ingredients

10 cups water
2 cups dried navy beans
8 slices crisply cooked bacon, crumbled
1/2 cup chopped onion
1/2 cup packed brown sugar
1/4 cup molasses
1 teaspoon salt
3 cups water

Direction

Boil the navy beans and 10 cups of water in a big pot; let it cook at a boil for 2 minutes. Stir the salt, molasses, brown sugar, onion and bacon into the water.

Pour the mixture carefully into a slow cooker.

Let it cook for 4 hours on High, stirring from time to time.

Mix 3 cups of water into the mixture and keep on cooking for around 2 hours and 15 minutes more, until the beans become tender.

Nutrition Information

Calories: 242 calories;;Cholesterol: 8;Protein: 10.7;Total Fat: 3.7;Sodium: 417;Total Carbohydrate: 42.7

904. Paleo Chicken With Apple And Sweet Potato

Serving: 4 | Prep: 20mins | Cook: 8hours | Ready in:

Ingredients

1 pound skinless, boneless chicken breast halves
2 sweet potatoes, peeled and diced
1 cup unsweetened applesauce
1/2 cup chopped onion
1 tablespoon curry powder
2 cloves garlic, minced
2 teaspoons apple cider vinegar
1/2 teaspoon ground ginger
salt and ground black pepper to taste

Direction

In a resealable freezer bag, mix pepper with salt, ginger, apple cider vinegar, garlic, curry powder, onion applesauce, sweet potatoes and chicken; put in the freezer until ready to use.

Put the chicken blend in a slow cooker over Low heat; cover. Cook for about 8 hours until the chicken is soft.

Nutrition Information

Calories: 225 calories;;Sodium: 134;Total Carbohydrate: 23.5;Cholesterol: 65;Protein: 25.2;Total Fat: 3

905. Pinto Beans Muy Facil

Serving: 8 | Prep: 15mins | Cook: 4hours | Ready in:

Ingredients

1 pound dried pinto beans
1 onion, chopped
1 clove garlic, minced
2 jalapeno peppers, chopped
salt and ground black pepper to taste

Direction

Into a big bowl, put the pinto beans and submerge in few inches of water; immerse for at least 8 hours to 1 day. Let drain and wash prior to using.

In a slow cooker, put the jalapeno peppers, garlic, onion and soaked pinto beans; add sufficient water on mixture to submerge in few inches. Allow to cook for 4 to 6 hours on Medium-Low. Put black pepper and salt to season.

Nutrition Information

Calories: 194 calories;;Cholesterol: 0;Protein: 12;Total Fat: 0.9;Sodium: 2;Total Carbohydrate: 35.8

906. Pork Chops With Apples, Sweet Potatoes, And Sauerkraut

Serving: 4 | Prep: 15mins | Cook: 5hours | Ready in:

Ingredients

4 (1 inch thick) boneless pork chops
2 medium sweet potatoes, peeled and sliced 1/2 inch thick
1 medium onion, sliced
2 apples - peeled, cored and sliced
1 tablespoon brown sugar
1/2 teaspoon ground nutmeg
1/4 teaspoon salt
freshly ground black pepper to taste

1 (16 ounce) can sauerkraut, drained
Direction
Heat the skillet on medium-high heat and use the cooking spray to coat. Rapidly, brown pork chops on every side. Put aside.
Arrange the slices of the sweet potato in the bottom of a 3 - 4 qt. slow cooker. Use slices of the onion to cover, then slices of the apple. Scatter the salt, nutmeg and brown sugar on top of apples, and grind a small amount of the pepper. Add pork chops over the pile, and use the sauerkraut to cover. Keep covered, and cook over Low heat for roughly 5 hours. It could go 1 more hour without drying out though. Serve the veggies and pork along with the juice from slow cooker which is scooped over them.
Nutrition Information
Calories: 276 calories;;Total Fat: 5.6;Sodium: 968;Total Carbohydrate: 43.4;Cholesterol: 30;Protein: 14.6

907. Quick Chick!
Serving: 4 | Prep: 15mins | Cook: 6hours | Ready in:
Ingredients
3 boneless, skinless chicken breast halves
1 (12 ounce) jar turkey gravy
1/2 teaspoon paprika
1/2 teaspoon salt-free herb seasoning blend
1 teaspoon soy sauce
Direction
In a slow cooker, add the gravy and chicken. Spice with soy sauce, seasoning blend and paprika. Cook for 4 hours on High or for 6 - 8 hours on Medium. Shred chicken into pieces. Serve over potatoes, noodles or rice.
Nutrition Information
Calories: 135 calories;;Sodium: 530;Total Carbohydrate: 4.7;Cholesterol: 51;Protein: 22;Total Fat: 2.6

908. Refried Beans Without The Refry
Serving: 15 | Prep: 15mins | Cook: 8hours | Ready in:
Ingredients
1 onion, peeled and halved
3 cups dry pinto beans, rinsed
1/2 fresh jalapeno pepper, seeded and chopped
2 tablespoons minced garlic
5 teaspoons salt
1 3/4 teaspoons fresh ground black pepper
1/8 teaspoon ground cumin, optional
9 cups water
Direction
In a slow cooker, put cumin, pepper, salt, garlic, jalapeño, rinsed beans and onion. Put in water and mix to combine. Cook for 8 hours on High and put in more water if needed. The temperature is too high if more than 1 cup of water has evaporated while cooking.
Strain the beans when they are cooked but set aside the liquid. Use a potato masher to mash the beans. To attain desired consistency, put in more reserved water as needed while mashing.
Nutrition Information
Calories: 139 calories;Protein: 8.5;Total Fat: 0.5;Sodium: 785;Total Carbohydrate: 25.4;Cholesterol: 0

909. Savory Slow Cooker Squash And Apple Dish
Serving: 10 | Prep: 15mins | Cook: 4hours | Ready in:
Ingredients
1 (3 pound) butternut squash - peeled, seeded, and cubed
4 apples - peeled, cored and chopped
3/4 cup dried cranberries
1/2 white onion, diced (optional)
1 tablespoon ground cinnamon
1 1/2 teaspoons ground nutmeg
Direction
In a slow cooker, mix together nutmeg, cinnamon, onion, cranberries, apples and squash, then cook for 4 hours on High setting, until the squash is cooked through and softened. While cooking, stir the mixture from time to time.
Nutrition Information
Calories: 123 calories;;Total Fat: 0.4;Sodium: 6;Total Carbohydrate: 32.3;Cholesterol: 0;Protein: 1.6

910. Shrimp Jambalaya
Serving: 8 | Prep: 40mins | Cook: 9hours20mins | Ready in:
Ingredients
1 pound boneless, skinless chicken thighs, cut into 2-inch pieces
2 stalks celery, thinly sliced
1 medium green bell pepper, cut into 1 inch pieces
1 medium onion, chopped
2 cloves garlic, minced
1 (28 ounce) can crushed tomatoes, with liquid
1 tablespoon white sugar
1/2 teaspoon salt
1/2 teaspoon dried Italian seasoning
1/4 teaspoon cayenne pepper
1 bay leaf
1 cup uncooked orzo pasta
1 pound cooked shrimp, peeled and deveined
Direction
Mix chicken, green bell pepper, onion, garlic, celery, sugar, tomatoes with liquid, cayenne pepper, bay leaf, salt and Italian seasoning in a slow cooker; cover and cook on low heat for 7 to 9 hours.
Take out the bay leaf from the chicken mixture and stir in orzo. Increase heat to high and cook for 15 minutes until orzo is soft.
Mix in shrimps and cook for 2 minutes until shrimp is well heated.
Nutrition Information
Calories: 270 calories;;Sodium: 441;Total Carbohydrate: 30;Cholesterol: 145;Protein: 26.8;Total Fat: 5

911. Sleeper Heater Lentil Soup
Serving: 8 | Prep: 10mins | Cook: 4hours | Ready in:
Ingredients
3 cups brown lentils
1/4 cup chopped fresh parsley
1/4 cup curry paste
1 tablespoon grated fresh ginger root
2 tablespoons chopped fresh oregano
2 cloves garlic, chopped
1 tablespoon all-purpose flour
1 teaspoon paprika
Direction
In a 2.5-quart or 5-liter slow cooker, put the paprika, flour, garlic, oregano, ginger, curry paste, parsley and lentils, then mix until combined. Pour water to fill within 1/2-inch of the top. Put cover and let it cook for 4 hours on high or longer if possible.
Nutrition Information

Calories: 267 calories;;Total Fat: 0.9;Sodium: 149;Total Carbohydrate: 45.9;Cholesterol: 0;Protein: 18.9

912. Slow Cook 3 Bean Chili (Vegetarian And Gluten Free)

Serving: 12 | Prep: 20mins | Cook: 10hours | Ready in:
Ingredients
8 cups water
1 (16 ounce) package dry kidney beans
1 (15.25 ounce) can whole kernel corn, drained
1 (15 ounce) can crushed tomatoes
1 (8 ounce) package dry lentils
1 (8 ounce) package dry black beans
1 (6 ounce) can tomato paste
1/2 cup white sugar
2 tablespoons chili powder
1 tablespoon ground cumin
1 teaspoon paprika
2 tablespoons olive oil
3 onions, chopped
3 cloves garlic, minced
Direction
In a slow cooker, insert paprika, cumin, chilli powder, sugar, tomato paste, black beans, lentils, crushed tomatoes, corn, kidney beans and water. Stir. For the next 6 hours, leave it cooking on a high setting.
In a big skillet, pour the olive oil in and heat it up at moderate heat. Add garlic and onions, stirring and cooking them for around 5 minutes until the onion becomes transparent. Mix it into the chilli, stirring. At a low setting, proceed to cook chili for another 4 to 6 hours until the beans are entirely soft.
Nutrition Information
Calories: 390 calories;;Cholesterol: 0;Protein: 20.3;Total Fat: 4;Sodium: 293;Total Carbohydrate: 72.6

913. Slow Cooked Apple Peach Sauce

Serving: 12 | Prep: 10mins | Cook: 5hours | Ready in:
Ingredients
10 Macintosh apples, cored and chopped
4 fresh peaches, pitted and chopped
1 tablespoon ground cinnamon
Direction
Place fruit into a slow-cooker; dust with cinnamon. Set slow-cooker to high. Cover and cook on high for 3 hours, then set to low for 2 hours. Mix prior to serving.
Nutrition Information
Calories: 69 calories;;Sodium: 3;Total Carbohydrate: 18.3;Cholesterol: 0;Protein: 0.3;Total Fat: 0.2

914. Slow Cooked Baked Beans

Serving: 8 | Prep: 15mins | Cook: 11hours15mins | Ready in:
Ingredients
2 cups kidney beans
5 cups water
1 onion, chopped
1 1/2 teaspoons salt
4 ounces cured pork
1/4 cup molasses
4 tablespoons brown sugar
1 teaspoon dry mustard
1/4 cup ketchup
Direction
In a slow cooker, insert the pork, salt, onion, water and beans then cover it up. Set it to low and cook for 9 to 10 hours. After draining the beans, keep the liquid. Combine 1 cup of the bean liquid with ketchup, dry mustard, brown sugar and molasses. At a low setting, leave it cooking with a cover on for 1 hour.
Nutrition Information
Calories: 156 calories;;Sodium: 739;Total Carbohydrate: 28.1;Cholesterol: 6;Protein: 6.8;Total Fat: 2.3

915. Slow Cooker Apple Butter

Serving: 48 | Prep: 30mins | Cook: 22hours | Ready in:
Ingredients
12 pounds Golden Delicious apples - peeled, cored and sliced
1/2 cup apple cider vinegar
3 cups white sugar
1 cup brown sugar
1 tablespoon ground cinnamon
1/4 teaspoon ground cloves
1 teaspoon ground allspice
Direction
Combine the vinegar and apples in a large slow cooker. Cover it with its lid. Set the slow cooker on a high setting. Cook the mixture for 8 hours. Adjust the setting to low and cook it for 10 more hours.
Once the cooking is done, mix in clove, brown sugar, white sugar, allspice, and cinnamon. Cook the mixture for 4 more hours.
Nutrition Information
Calories: 116 calories;;Total Carbohydrate: 31.1;Cholesterol: 0;Protein: 0.4;Total Fat: 0;Sodium: 4

916. Slow Cooker Apple Cider Pot Roast

Serving: 4 | Prep: 15mins | Cook: 8hours5mins | Ready in:
Ingredients
8 cups apple cider
1 tablespoon brown sugar
1/2 teaspoon ground cloves
1/2 teaspoon whole cloves
1/2 teaspoon ground black pepper
1/2 teaspoon ground ginger
1/2 teaspoon ground cinnamon
1 (3 pound) bottom round roast
6 carrots, cut in half
6 potatoes, peeled and quartered
1/4 cup quick-mixing flour (such as Wondra®)
1 tablespoon dry brown gravy mix
salt and ground black pepper to taste
Direction
In a bowl, whisk cinnamon, ginger, pepper, whole cloves, ground cloves, brown sugar and apple cider together then empty the entire bowl into a plastic resealable bag. Insert the roast and coat with marinade. Squeeze the excess air out of the bag and seal it. Leave it marinating in the fridge for a minimum of 2 days up to 4 days.
In a slow cooker, mix the beef, marinade, potatoes and carrots together.
Place the roast in and adjust the setting to low. Leave the meat in the cooker for 8 hours until it is thoroughly cooked and tender.
Get 3 cups of cider broth from slow cooker and pour it into a pot. Stir quick-mixing flour into the cider broth and let it simmer for 5 minutes until gravy is thick. Mix pepper, salt and the brown gravy mix into the cider gravy.

On a platter, arrange the roast, potatoes and carrots nicely; then pour the cider gravy on top.
Nutrition Information
Calories: 867 calories;;Total Carbohydrate: 141.5;Cholesterol: 116;Protein: 51.1;Total Fat: 10.8;Sodium: 311

917. Slow Cooker Baked Beans

Serving: 12 | Prep: 1hours | Cook: 5hours | Ready in:
Ingredients
24 ounces dry white beans
1 pound ham hocks
1 onion, chopped
1/2 cup packed brown sugar
1/2 cup maple syrup
1 teaspoon salt
1 cup water
1/2 cup ketchup
2 tablespoons prepared mustard
Direction
Over high heat, add beans in a large pot and then cover with water. Heat to boil for ten minutes. Take away from the heat and allow to stand for one hour. Drain off water from the beans and then transfer them to a slow cooker. Add the onion, ham hocks, maple syrup, brown sugar, water and salt.
Combine thoroughly, cover the cooker and let cook for about 4 to 5 hours on high setting while stirring sometimes. During final hour of the cooking process, pour in the mustard and ketchup, take the ham out of hocks and get rid of the hocks. Combine thoroughly before serving.
Nutrition Information
Calories: 363 calories;;Total Fat: 8.6;Sodium: 368;Total Carbohydrate: 53.6;Cholesterol: 26;Protein: 19.4

918. Slow Cooker Baked Potatoes

Serving: 4 | Prep: 10mins | Cook: 4hours30mins | Ready in:
Ingredients
4 baking potatoes, well scrubbed
1 tablespoon extra virgin olive oil
kosher salt to taste
4 sheets aluminum foil
Direction
Use a fork to prick potatoes a few times and then rub the potatoes with olive oil. Drizzle salt on top and tightly wrap in foil. Transfer potatoes to a slow cooker, cover the cooker and then cook on Low for 7 1/2 to 8 hours or on High for 4 1/2 to 5 hours or until tender.
Nutrition Information
Calories: 254 calories;;Total Fat: 3.6;Sodium: 114;Total Carbohydrate: 51.2;Cholesterol: 0;Protein: 6.1

919. Slow Cooker Balsamic Chicken

Serving: 6 | Prep: 15mins | Cook: 4hours | Ready in:
Ingredients
2 tablespoons olive oil
4 skinless, boneless chicken breast halves, or more to taste
salt and ground black pepper to taste
1 onion, thinly sliced
4 cloves garlic
1 teaspoon dried oregano
1 teaspoon dried basil
1 teaspoon dried rosemary
1/2 teaspoon dried thyme
1/2 cup balsamic vinegar
2 (14.5 ounce) cans crushed tomatoes
Direction
Sprinkle olive oil into a slow cooker. Put chicken breasts atop oil and then season each breast with pepper and salt. Add on top of chicken breasts; thyme, rosemary, basil, oregano, onion slices, and garlic. Sprinkle balsamic vinegar atop seasoned breasts and top with tomatoes.
Let to cook in the slow cooker that is set to High for about 4 hours until the juices run clear and the chicken is no longer pink at the middle.
Nutrition Information
Calories: 200 calories;;Cholesterol: 43;Protein: 18.6;Total Fat: 6.8;Sodium: 223;Total Carbohydrate: 17.6

920. Slow Cooker Butternut Squash Soup

Serving: 8 | Prep: 25mins | Cook: 4hours10mins | Ready in:
Ingredients
2 large butternut squashes, seeded and sliced into rounds
4 carrots, peeled and cut into chunks
1 large yellow onion, quartered
8 cubes vegetable bouillon
1 white potato, peeled and cut into chunks
8 cups water
1 bay leaf
1 teaspoon garlic powder
1/2 teaspoon ground nutmeg
salt and ground black pepper to taste
Direction
Preheat the oven to 260 degrees C (500 degrees F). Use aluminum foil to line a baking sheet.
On the prepared baking sheet, spread onion, carrots, and squash into a single layer.
Bake for about 10 minutes in the preheated oven or until slightly browned. Cut rind from the squash and remove.
Put the bouillon cubes in a slow cooker. Add in potato, onions, carrots, and peeled squash pieces.
Pour water over vegetables and stir in black pepper, salt, nutmeg, garlic powder, and bay leaf.
Cook on high heat for 4 hours, stir one time. Remove the bay leaf.
Puree the soup with an immersion blender until smooth.
Nutrition Information
Calories: 194 calories;Protein: 4.4;Total Fat: 0.6;Sodium: 73;Total Carbohydrate: 49.1;Cholesterol: 0

921. Slow Cooker Calico Bean Soup

Serving: 9 | Prep: 5mins | Cook: 4hours | Ready in:
Ingredients
1 (16 ounce) package dried navy beans
1 meaty beef roast bone
2 (14.5 ounce) cans peeled and diced tomatoes
1 1/2 cups red wine
3 tablespoons dried minced onion flakes
1 tablespoon dried parsley
1 teaspoon paprika
1 tablespoon celery seed
2 bay leaves
1 teaspoon seasoned salt
1 tablespoon garlic powder
1 teaspoon white sugar

1/2 teaspoon ground black pepper
1 pinch crushed red pepper flakes
water to cover
Direction
Soak the beans overnight in water, rinse properly and drain.
In a slow cooker, mix the crushed red pepper flakes, ground black pepper, sugar, garlic powder, seasoned salt, bay leaves, celery seed, paprika, parsley, red wine, tomatoes, meat bones and soaked beans. Cover with enough water.
Cook on Low setting for about 3 - 4 hours, until beans become softened. Discard the bones then strip any meat from the bones and shred. Throw away the bones and transfer the meat back to the slow cooker. Let it heat through.
Nutrition Information
Calories: 234 calories;;Total Carbohydrate: 37.1;Cholesterol: 0;Protein: 12.4;Total Fat: 1;Sodium: 250

922. Slow Cooker Caribou Stew

Serving: 8 | Prep: 20mins | Cook: 8hours5mins | Ready in:
Ingredients
1/2 cup all-purpose flour
2 1/2 pounds moose meat, cut into cubes
1 tablespoon vegetable oil, or as needed
4 cups beef stock
3 large potatoes, peeled and cubed
4 carrots, cut into 1-inch pieces
4 stalks celery, cut into 1-inch pieces
1 large onion, chopped
1 (14 ounce) can diced tomatoes with juice
2 teaspoons dried oregano
2 teaspoons Worcestershire sauce
1 1/2 teaspoons dried thyme
1 teaspoon minced garlic
2 bay leaves
Direction
In a shallow bowl, put flour; coat meat by pressing it into flour and shake off excess flour.
In a large skillet, heat vegetable oil over medium heat; cook while stirring meat until all sides are brown, about 5 minutes. Put meat into a large slow cooker.
Pour beef stock over meat in slow cooker; put in bay leaves, garlic, thyme, Worcestershire sauce, oregano, diced tomatoes with juice, onion, celery, carrots, and potatoes. Mix mixture gently.
Cook for 8 hours on Low setting.
Nutrition Information
Calories: 327 calories;;Cholesterol: 69;Protein: 32.7;Total Fat: 3.5;Sodium: 243;Total Carbohydrate: 39.6

923. Slow Cooker Carrot Cake Steel Cut Oats

Serving: 16 | Prep: 10mins | Cook: 6hours | Ready in:
Ingredients
10 cups water
23 ounces unsweetened applesauce
2 cups steel cut oats
1 (10 ounce) bag shredded carrots
1 (8 ounce) can crushed pineapple, drained
1 cup raisins
1/3 cup granular no-calorie sucralose sweetener (such as Splenda®) (optional)
2 tablespoons ground cinnamon
1 tablespoon pumpkin pie spice
1 teaspoon salt (optional)
Direction
In a crock of a 7-quart or large slow cooker, add applesauce, carrots, raisins, oats, pineapple, cinnamon, pumpkin pie spice, sweetener, salt and water.
On low, cook for 6 hours.
Nutrition Information
Calories: 139 calories;;Sodium: 164;Total Carbohydrate: 30.1;Cholesterol: 0;Protein: 3.1;Total Fat: 1.4

924. Slow Cooker Chicken Creole

Serving: 4 | Prep: 10mins | Cook: 12hours | Ready in:
Ingredients
4 skinless, boneless chicken breast halves
salt and pepper to taste
Creole-style seasoning to taste
1 (14.5 ounce) can stewed tomatoes, with liquid
1 stalk celery, diced
1 green bell pepper, diced
3 cloves garlic, minced
1 onion, diced
1 (4 ounce) can mushrooms, drained
1 fresh jalapeno pepper, seeded and chopped
Direction
In a slow cooker, place chicken breasts. Sprinkle with Creole-style seasoning, pepper, and salt to season for taste. Mix in jalapeno pepper, mushroom, onion, garlic, bell pepper, celery, and tomatoes with liquid. Cook on High for 5 to 6 hours or on Low for 10 to 12 hours.
Nutrition Information
Calories: 189 calories;;Sodium: 431;Total Carbohydrate: 13.8;Cholesterol: 68;Protein: 29.6;Total Fat: 1.9

925. Slow Cooker Chicken Curry With Quinoa

Serving: 6 | Prep: 30mins | Cook: 4hours | Ready in:
Ingredients
1 1/2 pounds diced chicken breast meat
3/4 cup chopped onion
1 1/4 cups chopped celery
1 3/4 cups chopped Granny Smith apples
1 cup chicken broth
1/4 cup nonfat milk
1 tablespoon curry powder
1/4 teaspoon paprika
1/3 cup quinoa
Direction
In a slow cooker, put the paprika, curry powder, milk, chicken broth, apple, celery, onion and chicken, then mix until combined. Put on the cover and let it cook for 4-5 hours on Low. Mix in the quinoa during the last 35 minutes of cooking. Serve once the quinoa becomes tender.
Nutrition Information
Calories: 185 calories;Protein: 24.4;Total Fat: 3.1;Sodium: 75;Total Carbohydrate: 14.4;Cholesterol: 59

926. Slow Cooker Chicken Marrakesh

Serving: 8 | Prep: 25mins | Cook: 4hours | Ready in:
Ingredients
1 onion, sliced
2 cloves garlic, minced (optional)
2 large carrots, peeled and diced
2 large sweet potatoes, peeled and diced

1 (15 ounce) can garbanzo beans, drained and rinsed
2 pounds skinless, boneless chicken breast halves, cut into 2-inch pieces
1/2 teaspoon ground cumin
1/2 teaspoon ground turmeric
1/4 teaspoon ground cinnamon
1/2 teaspoon ground black pepper
1 teaspoon dried parsley
1 teaspoon salt
1 (14.5 ounce) can diced tomatoes

Direction

In a slow cooker, add the carrots, onion, garbanzo beans, garlic, chicken breast pieces, and sweet potatoes. Mix the black pepper, cumin, cinnamon, turmeric, salt, and parsley in a bowl; sprinkle over the vegetables and chicken. Pour in the tomatoes and stir to combine.
Cook while covered for about 4 to 5 hours on High setting until the sauce has thickened and the sweet potatoes are tender.

Nutrition Information

Calories: 290 calories;;Total Fat: 2;Sodium: 625;Total Carbohydrate: 36;Cholesterol: 66;Protein: 30.6

927. Slow Cooker Chicken Mole

Serving: 8 | Prep: 30mins | Cook: 9hours | Ready in:

Ingredients

1 cup chopped onion
1/3 cup golden raisins
1/3 cup currants
2 cloves garlic, minced
1 1/2 teaspoons ancho chile powder
2 tablespoons toasted sesame seeds
3/4 teaspoon ground cumin
3/4 teaspoon ground cinnamon
5 teaspoons cocoa powder
1/4 teaspoon hot pepper sauce, or to taste
1 (14.5 ounce) can diced tomatoes
1 cup tomato sauce
1 cup chicken broth
3 pounds skinless, boneless chicken breast halves
1/4 cup slivered almonds, for garnish

Direction

In a slow cooker, add chicken broth, tomato sauce, tomatoes, hot sauce, cocoa powder, cinnamon, cumin, sesame seeds, Chile powder, garlic, currants, raisins and onion, then stir to mix. Put in chicken breasts and stir to cover with sauce.
Cover and cook on Low 6 hours then raise heat to high and keep on cooking about 3 hours longer, until chicken is tender. Or cook on Low about 11-12 hours. Remove, shred and stir chicken back into the mole once it is tender, then serve with slivered almonds sprinkled over top.

Nutrition Information

Calories: 276 calories;;Total Fat: 6.7;Sodium: 320;Total Carbohydrate: 17.7;Cholesterol: 88;Protein: 36.1

928. Slow Cooker Chicken And Noodles

Serving: 6 | Prep: 30mins | Cook: 8hours | Ready in:

Ingredients

4 skinless, boneless chicken breast halves
6 cups water
1 onion, chopped
2 stalks celery, chopped (optional)
salt and pepper to taste
1 (12 ounce) package frozen egg noodles

Direction

In a slow cooker, arrange the onion, water, and chicken; use pepper and salt to taste. If desired, add in celery. Adjust the temperature to low and cook for 6-8 hours.
Once the chicken becomes tender, take away from the slow cooker; chop/tear into bite-sized pieces. In a small casserole dish, put aside to keep warm.
Increase the heat of the slow cooker to high and stir the frozen egg noodles. Cook until noodles become tender, bring the chicken pieces back into the broth. Change seasonings to taste as desired.

Nutrition Information

Calories: 311 calories;;Sodium: 81;Total Carbohydrate: 42;Cholesterol: 93;Protein: 26.4;Total Fat: 3.5

929. Slow Cooker Chocolate Banana Steel Cut Oats

Serving: 12 | Prep: 5mins | Cook: 6hours | Ready in:

Ingredients

cooking spray
10 cups water
2 cups steel-cut oats
2 pounds ripe bananas, mashed
1/2 cup unsweetened cocoa powder
1/3 cup granular no-calorie sucralose sweetener (such as Splenda®) (optional)

Direction

With cooking spray, lightly grease a 5qt or bigger slow cooker crock.
Stir sweetener, water, cocoa powder, mashed bananas, and oats in the slow cooker.
On Low setting, cook for six hours.

Nutrition Information

Calories: 180 calories;;Total Fat: 2.6;Sodium: 8;Total Carbohydrate: 36.9;Cholesterol: 0;Protein: 6

930. Slow Cooker Cider Applesauce (No Sugar Added)

Serving: 16 | Prep: 10mins | Cook: 4hours | Ready in:

Ingredients

5 pounds apples - peeled, cored, and thinly sliced
1 1/2 tablespoons ground cinnamon
1/2 teaspoon ground cloves
1/4 teaspoon ground nutmeg

Direction

Carefully arrange the apples in a layer in a slow cooker. Sprinkler the cloves, nutmeg and cinnamon over the apples.
Cook for 4 to 5 hours on high heat until the apples are soft. If a chunkier applesauce is desired, whisk the apples vigorously. If a smoother one is desired, use an immersion blender to make it into a puree.

Nutrition Information

Calories: 76 calories;;Cholesterol: 0;Protein: 0.4;Total Fat: 0.3;Sodium: 2;Total Carbohydrate: 20.2

931. Slow Cooker Cilantro Lime Chicken Tacos

Serving: 10 | Prep: 15mins | Cook: 5hours | Ready in:

Ingredients

3 sheets aluminum foil, rolled into balls
1 (5 pound) whole chicken
1 teaspoon seasoned salt (such as Pappy's Choice®), or more to taste
8 cloves garlic, or more to taste, crushed
8 limes, quartered
1/2 cup white wine
20 corn tortillas, warmed

1 bunch cilantro, chopped
Direction
In the bottom of a slow cooker crock, put aluminum foil balls.
Add seasoned salt to chicken for seasoning. Rub half of the garlic on the chicken's cavity's inside surfaces then leave them inside. Squeeze 8 lime quarters into cavity; drop in the cavity with the squeezed quarters. Put the chicken over the foil balls. Squeeze 8 more lime quarters atop the chicken's outside; drop squeezed lime quarters into the crock's bottom. Rub the leftover garlic atop the chicken's outside and place the garlic in the crock's bottom. Drizzle white wine into the crock.
Cook at Low for 5 to 6 hours, until the chicken meat breaks apart easily.
Transfer chicken to a chopping board. Separate meat from bones and thoroughly shred. Serve chicken on warmed tortillas with cilantro on top and lime wedge.
Nutrition Information
Calories: 358 calories;;Sodium: 216;Total Carbohydrate: 30.3;Cholesterol: 96;Protein: 35.6;Total Fat: 10.1

932. Slow Cooker Cinnamon Apple Steel Cut Oats

Serving: 10 | Prep: 15mins | Cook: 6hours | Ready in:
Ingredients
cooking spray
8 cups water
23 ounces unsweetened applesauce
1 1/2 cups steel cut oats
2 Granny Smith apples - peeled, cored, and diced
1/4 cup ground cinnamon, or to taste
1/3 cup granular no-calorie sucralose sweetener (such as Splenda®) (optional)
Direction
Lightly grease cooking spray on a 5-quart or larger slow cooker crock.
Mix sweetener, cinnamon, diced apple, oats, applesauce, and water in the greased slow cooker.
Cook on low for 6 hours.
Nutrition Information
Calories: 137 calories;;Total Fat: 1.6;Sodium: 8;Total Carbohydrate: 29.2;Cholesterol: 0;Protein: 3.3

933. Slow Cooker Garlic And Herb Pork Tenderloin

Serving: 4 | Prep: 10mins | Cook: 4hours15mins | Ready in:
Ingredients
1 garlic and herb pork tenderloin
6 large red potatoes
16 green beans, trimmed, or more to taste (optional)
1 cup water
salt and ground black pepper to taste
Direction
Preheat the outdoor grill to high heat, and slightly oil grate.
Grill the pork tenderloin for 2-3 minutes on each side till becoming seared on each side. Move the tenderloin into a slow cooker; put in the water, green beans and potatoes.
Cook the tenderloin in the slow cooker at Low setting for roughly 4 hours till the pork center is lightly pink. The instant-read thermometer inserted in middle should reach no less than 63 degrees C (145 degrees F). Use the ground black pepper and salt to season to taste.
Nutrition Information
Calories: 419 calories;;Sodium: 46;Total Carbohydrate: 89.6;Cholesterol: 12;Protein: 15.2;Total Fat: 1.5

934. Slow Cooker Ham And Beans

Serving: 8 | Prep: 10mins | Cook: 12hours | Ready in:
Ingredients
1 pound dried great Northern beans, soaked overnight
1/2 pound cooked ham, chopped
1/2 cup brown sugar
1 tablespoon onion powder
1 tablespoon dried parsley
1/2 teaspoon garlic salt
1/2 teaspoon black pepper
1/4 teaspoon cayenne pepper
water to cover
Direction
In a slow cooker, mix together the cayenne pepper, black pepper, garlic salt, parsley, onion powder, brown sugar, ham and beans. In the slow cooker, pour enough water to cover the mixture by approximately 2 inches. Set the slow cooker to low, then simmer for 12 hours, mixing from time to time.
Nutrition Information
Calories: 318 calories;;Cholesterol: 16;Protein: 17.8;Total Fat: 5.9;Sodium: 492;Total Carbohydrate: 49.8

935. Slow Cooker Homemade Beans

Serving: 12 | Prep: 20mins | Cook: 10hours | Ready in:
Ingredients
3 cups dry navy beans, soaked overnight or boiled for one hour
1 1/2 cups ketchup
1 1/2 cups water
1/4 cup molasses
1 large onion, chopped
1 tablespoon dry mustard
1 tablespoon salt
6 slices thick cut bacon, cut into 1 inch pieces
1 cup brown sugar
Direction
Drain beans, remove soaking liquid then put beans in a Slow Cooker.
Mix brown sugar, bacon, salt, mustard, onion, molasses, water, and ketchup into the beans until well combined.
Cover, allow to cook 8-10 hours on LOW setting, mixing from time to time if possible (if not, it's still ok).
Nutrition Information
Calories: 296 calories;;Sodium: 1312;Total Carbohydrate: 57;Cholesterol: 5;Protein: 12.4;Total Fat: 3

936. Slow Cooker Mediterranean Lentil Soup

Serving: 6 | Prep: 15mins | Cook: 6hours | Ready in:
Ingredients
18 ounces dry lentils
water to cover
1/2 cup olive oil
3 carrots, sliced
1 large red onion, grated
2 tablespoons tomato paste

2 cloves garlic cloves, peeled
2 teaspoons dried Greek oregano
2 bay leaves
salt and freshly ground black pepper to taste
Direction
Place lentils covered in water in a medium saucepan then boil; let it boil for 10 minutes then drain well. Put in the slow cooker.
Mix together pepper, salt, bay leaves, oregano, garlic, tomato paste, red onion, carrots and olive oil in a slow cooker; cover with 6-7 cups of water. Cook for 6-8 hours on low till lentils are soft.
Nutrition Information
Calories: 490 calories;;Total Fat: 19.1;Sodium: 101;Total Carbohydrate: 58.2;Cholesterol: 0;Protein: 22.9

937. Slow Cooker Mediterranean Stew

Serving: 10 | Prep: 30mins | Cook: 10hours | Ready in:
Ingredients
1 butternut squash - peeled, seeded, and cubed
2 cups cubed eggplant, with peel
2 cups cubed zucchini
1 (10 ounce) package frozen okra, thawed
1 (8 ounce) can tomato sauce
1 cup chopped onion
1 ripe tomato, chopped
1 carrot, sliced thin
1/2 cup vegetable broth
1/3 cup raisins
1 clove garlic, chopped
1/2 teaspoon ground cumin
1/2 teaspoon ground turmeric
1/4 teaspoon crushed red pepper
1/4 teaspoon ground cinnamon
1/4 teaspoon paprika
Direction
Mix garlic, raisins, broth, carrot, tomato, onion, tomato sauce, okra, zucchini, eggplant, and butternut squash together in a slow cooker. Use paprika, cinnamon, red pepper, turmeric, and cumin to season. Put the cover on and cook on Low until the vegetables are soft, about 8-10 hours.
Nutrition Information
Calories: 122 calories;;Sodium: 157;Total Carbohydrate: 30.5;Cholesterol: 0;Protein: 3.4;Total Fat: 0.5

938. Slow Cooker Mock Roast

Serving: 6 | Prep: 20mins | Cook: 8hours12mins | Ready in:
Ingredients
1 pound beef sirloin roast
1 pinch seasoned salt, or to taste
1 pinch ground black pepper, or to taste
1 teaspoon vegetable oil
3/4 cup chopped onion
1/4 cup chopped carrot
1/4 cup chopped celery
4 large potatoes, cubed
6 carrots, cut into bite-size pieces
2 teaspoons dried Italian herb seasoning
2 teaspoons dried parsley
1/4 teaspoon celery salt
1 (12 fluid ounce) can or bottle caffeinated citrus-flavored soda (such as Mountain Dew®)
4 1/2 teaspoons steak sauce (such as A1 Steak Sauce®)
Direction
To taste, sprinkle the beef with black pepper and seasoned salt. In a frying pan over medium heat, heat the vegetable oil; brown each side of the roast for about 3 minutes. Add the browned roast to a slow cooker, then sprinkle the celery, chopped carrot, and onion over the meat. Scatter the carrot pieces and potatoes over other ingredients, sprinkle on the celery salt, parsley, and Italian seasoning, then drizzle everything with the can of soda. Pour the steak sauce over.
Cook while covered on Low setting for 8 hours.
Nutrition Information
Calories: 348 calories;;Cholesterol: 26;Protein: 19.8;Total Fat: 3.9;Sodium: 269;Total Carbohydrate: 60.5

939. Slow Cooker Moroccan Chicken

Serving: 6 | Prep: 15mins | Cook: 5hours15mins | Ready in:
Ingredients
1 pound skinless, boneless chicken breast halves - cut into 2 inch pieces
4 cloves garlic, chopped
1 large onion, chopped
1 (28 ounce) can diced tomatoes
3 fresh peaches - peeled, pitted, and sliced
1 (15 ounce) can garbanzo beans, drained
1 cup chopped dried apricots
2 teaspoons ground cumin
1 teaspoon ground ginger
1 teaspoon cinnamon
1/2 teaspoon ground coriander
1/2 teaspoon cayenne pepper
2 cups chicken broth
1 tablespoon cornstarch
1 tablespoon water
3 tablespoons chopped fresh cilantro
1/3 cup slivered almonds, toasted
Direction
In the base of a slow cooker, position the chicken. Put in the cayenne pepper, coriander, cinnamon, ginger, cumin, dried apricots, garbanzo beans, peaches, tomatoes, onion, and garlic. Add the chicken broth.
Cook for 5 hours on Low.
Take the chicken out and keep warm. In a small bowl, mix the water and cornstarch together. Stir the cornstarch mixture into the slow cooker. Cook for around 15 minutes on High till the sauce has thickened. Move the chicken back to the slow cooker and let heat through. Before serving, top with almonds and fresh cilantro.
Nutrition Information
Calories: 284 calories;;Total Carbohydrate: 37.9;Cholesterol: 39;Protein: 20.7;Total Fat: 5.5;Sodium: 385

940. Slow Cooker Oats

Serving: 6 | Prep: 15mins | Cook: 6hours | Ready in:
Ingredients
1 cup steel cut oats
3 1/2 cups water
1 cup peeled and chopped apple
1/2 cup raisins
2 tablespoons butter
1 tablespoon ground cinnamon
2 tablespoons brown sugar
1 teaspoon vanilla extract
Direction

Put steel cut oats, brown sugar, water, apple, vanilla extract, raisins, cinnamon, and butter into a slow cooker. Mix to combine until sugar is dissolved. Cover cooker, switch to Low and let to cook for 8 hours (for softer texture) or 6 to 7 hours (for firm oats).
Nutrition Information
Calories: 208 calories;;Sodium: 35;Total Carbohydrate: 37.2;Cholesterol: 10;Protein: 3.9;Total Fat: 5.6

941. Slow Cooker Potato Soup

Serving: 8 | Prep: 10mins | Cook: 7hours40mins | Ready in:
Ingredients
8 pounds potatoes, peeled and cubed
1 small onion, chopped
2 tablespoons butter
2 cubes chicken bouillon
2 tablespoons dried parsley
6 cups water
2 cups milk
1/2 cup all-purpose flour
Direction
Put parsley, chicken bouillon cubes, butter, onion, potatoes, and water into a slow cooker. Cook for 6 to 8 hours on low setting.
Mix flour and milk together until smooth and stir into the soup at least 30 minutes before serving. Cook until the soup thickens, or for 30 minutes.
Nutrition Information
Calories: 443 calories;Protein: 10.2;Total Fat: 4.7;Sodium: 382;Total Carbohydrate: 91.9;Cholesterol: 13

942. Slow Cooker Pozole

Serving: 6 | Prep: 45mins | Cook: 7hours | Ready in:
Ingredients
1 dried chile negro (pasilla) soaked in boiling water for 30 minutes, and drained
2 (14.5 ounce) cans chicken broth
1 (14.5 ounce) can beef broth
3/4 pound pork tenderloin, cubed
3/4 pound skinless, boneless chicken breast halves - cut into 2 inch pieces
2 cups chopped onion
1 1/2 teaspoons crushed garlic
1 (4 ounce) can diced green chiles
1 (15 ounce) can white hominy, drained
1 (15 ounce) can yellow hominy, drained
1 bay leaf
2 teaspoons dried Mexican oregano
2 tablespoons ground cumin
Direction
Take out the stem from the rehydrated chile pepper. In the food processor or blender, mix with 1 can of the chicken broth, and process till becoming smooth. Add to the 5 - 6 qt. slow cooker.
Add in the rest can of the chicken broth, and put in the yellow and white hominy, green chilies, garlic, onion, chicken, pork, and beef broth. Use cumin, oregano and bay leaf to season. Keep covered, and cook over High heat for 4 - 5 hours, or over Low heat for 6 - 7 hours. Discard the bay leaf prior to serving.
Nutrition Information
Calories: 262 calories;;Sodium: 1365;Total Carbohydrate: 28.9;Cholesterol: 57;Protein: 24.6;Total Fat: 4.9

943. Slow Cooker Pumpkin Steel Cut Oats

Serving: 6 | Prep: 5mins | Cook: 6hours | Ready in:
Ingredients
cooking spray (such as Pam®)
6 cups water
1 (15 ounce) can pumpkin puree
1 1/2 cups steel-cut oats
1 cup brown sugar replacement (such as Splenda® Brown Sugar Blend)
2 tablespoons ground cinnamon
1 tablespoon pumpkin pie spice
Direction
Spray cooking spray over the crock of a slow cooker. In the prepared slow cooker, combine pumpkin pie spice, cinnamon, brown sugar replacement, oats, pumpkin puree, and water.
Cook for 6 hours on Low. Mix before eating.
Nutrition Information
Calories: 195 calories;;Total Fat: 2.9;Sodium: 198;Total Carbohydrate: 38.2;Cholesterol: 0;Protein: 5.9

944. Slow Cooker Ratatouille From RED GOLD®

Serving: 8 | Prep: 25mins | Cook: 5hours | Ready in:
Ingredients
1 medium onions, roughly chopped or quartered
2 garlic cloves, crushed
1 medium eggplant, skin on and diced
1 medium green bell pepper, diced
1 medium red bell pepper, diced
1 medium zucchini, diced
1 yellow summer squash, diced
1/4 cup extra-virgin olive oil
1 (6 ounce) can RED GOLD® Tomato Paste
1 (28 ounce) can RED GOLD® Crushed Tomatoes
1 teaspoon dried basil
1/2 teaspoon dried thyme
1/4 cup chopped fresh parsley
Salt and black pepper to taste
Direction
Place a 10-inch frying pan over medium heat for preheating. Drizzle with oil and when hot, quickly stir in the garlic and onions; keep cooking for 2 minutes. Mix in RED GOLD® Tomato Paste and stir to combine. Put in slow cooker.
Return the skillet to the heat. Heat oil and pour in summer squash, zucchini, red bell pepper, green bell pepper and eggplant. Cook until tender, 10-15 minutes. Pour into slow cooker.
Blend thyme, basil and RED GOLD® Crushed Tomatoes. Place the slow cooker on low heat and cook for about 5 hours.
Serve as an entrée or a side dish, sprinkle parsley on top. Ratatouille is perfectly cold and reheated the following day.
Nutrition Information
Calories: 164 calories;;Total Carbohydrate: 21.8;Cholesterol: 0;Protein: 4.7;Total Fat: 7.3;Sodium: 312

945. Slow Cooker Root Vegetable Tagine

Serving: 8 | Prep: 50mins | Cook: 9hours | Ready in:
Ingredients
1 pound parsnips, peeled and diced
1 pound turnips, peeled and diced
2 medium onions, chopped
1 pound carrots, peeled and diced

6 dried apricots, chopped
4 pitted prunes, chopped
1 teaspoon ground turmeric
1 teaspoon ground cumin
1/2 teaspoon ground ginger
1/2 teaspoon ground cinnamon
1/4 teaspoon ground cayenne pepper
1 tablespoon dried parsley
1 tablespoon dried cilantro
1 (14 ounce) can vegetable broth
Direction
Mix together prunes, apricots, carrots, onions, turnips and parsnips in a slow cooker. Season with cilantro, parsley, cayenne pepper, cinnamon, ginger, cumin and turmeric. Add vegetable broth.
Place on the cover, and let it cook on Low for 9 hours.
Nutrition Information
Calories: 131 calories;Protein: 2.8;Total Fat: 0.7;Sodium: 187;Total Carbohydrate: 31;Cholesterol: 0

946. Slow Cooker Root Veggie Winter Soup

Serving: 6 | Prep: 25mins | Cook: 5hours5mins | Ready in:
Ingredients
1 (32 ounce) carton low-sodium vegetable broth (such as Imagine™)
1 (10 ounce) can low-sodium chicken broth
1 1/4 cups water
1 teaspoon caraway seeds, divided
1/4 teaspoon dried cilantro, or more to taste
1 teaspoon dried tarragon
1/4 teaspoon coriander seeds
1 1/2 pounds colored carrots, peeled and sliced
1 pound parsnips, peeled and sliced
1 large rutabaga, peeled and cubed
1 large white onion, cut into large wedges
ground white pepper to taste
1 green onion, chopped
Direction
In a slow cooker on high setting, mix water, chicken broth, vegetable broth, dried cilantro and 1/2 tsp. caraway seeds.
In a spice grinder, pulse coriander seeds, tarragon and the remaining 1/2 tsp. caraway seeds until finely ground. Mix into slow cooker.
Mix in onion, rutabaga, parsnips and carrots. Cook on high setting until liquid boils up. Lower heat to low. Cook for 5 hours until veggies are tender when pricked with a fork.
Season using white pepper. Top with green onion.
Nutrition Information
Calories: 134 calories;;Total Fat: 0.7;Sodium: 197;Total Carbohydrate: 30.5;Cholesterol: 1;Protein: 3.6

947. Slow Cooker Rosemary And Red Pepper Chicken

Serving: 8 | Prep: 20mins | Cook: 7hours | Ready in:
Ingredients
1 small onion, thinly sliced
1 medium red bell pepper, seeded and thinly sliced
4 cloves garlic, minced
2 teaspoons dried rosemary
1/2 teaspoon dried oregano
8 ounces turkey Italian sausages, casings removed
8 (4 ounce) skinless, boneless chicken breast halves
1/4 teaspoon coarsely ground pepper
1/4 cup dry vermouth
1 1/2 tablespoons cornstarch
2 tablespoons cold water
salt to taste
1/4 cup chopped fresh parsley
Direction
Mix oregano, rosemary, garlic, bell pepper and onion in a 5 to 6 quarts slow cooker. Crumble over onion mixture with sausages. Rinse chicken then pat dry; organize in a single layer over sausage. Sprinkle with pepper. Pour in the vermouth. Cover and cook for 5 to 7 hours on Low setting, until chicken is soft and cooked through when pierced.
Move chicken to a warm, deep platter then cover to maintain warm.
Mix cold water with cornstarch in a small bowl. Mix into the cooking liquid in a slow cooker. Increase heat to High then cover. Cook for about 10 more minutes while mixing about 2 to 3 times until the sauce is thickened. Season with salt to taste. Spoon sauce over chicken, then dust with parsley.
Nutrition Information
Calories: 201 calories;;Total Fat: 4.4;Sodium: 457;Total Carbohydrate: 5;Cholesterol: 87;Protein: 32

948. Slow Cooker Southern Lima Beans And Ham

Serving: 8 | Prep: 15mins | Cook: 7hours | Ready in:
Ingredients
1 pound dried baby lima beans
2 quarts water
2 onions, coarsely chopped
1 meaty ham bone
1 cup leftover ham meat from bone, chopped
3 cups water, or as needed to cover
1 teaspoon Cajun seasoning
1/4 teaspoon freshly ground black pepper
1/4 teaspoon garlic salt, or to taste
1 pinch cayenne pepper
Direction
In a large bowl with 2 quarts of water, soak the lima beans for 8 hours or overnight. On the following day, let the lima beans drain, then move into a slow cooker along with ham, ham bone, and onions. Cover with 3 cups of water or more. Cover the cooker, adjust to High, then cook for 3 hours.
Fold in cayenne pepper, garlic salt, black pepper, and Cajun seasoning; adjust the cooker to Low, then cook for 4 more hours until the meat and beans are very soft.
Nutrition Information
Calories: 133 calories;;Total Carbohydrate: 17.8;Cholesterol: 9;Protein: 8.4;Total Fat: 3.4;Sodium: 346

949. Slow Cooker Spaghetti Sauce I

Serving: 10 | Prep: 10mins | Cook: 4hours | Ready in:
Ingredients
5 (29 ounce) cans tomato sauce
3 (6 ounce) cans tomato paste
3 cloves garlic, minced
1 onion, chopped
3 tablespoons dried rosemary
3 tablespoons dried oregano
3 tablespoons dried thyme
3 tablespoons dried parsley
1 bay leaf
1 pinch crushed red pepper flakes
Direction

In a large slow cooker, mix together red pepper, bay leaf, parsley, thyme, oregano, rosemary, onion, garlic, tomato paste and tomato sauce. Cook while stirring occasionally on high for 3-4 hours.
Nutrition Information
Calories: 157 calories;;Total Fat: 1.4;Sodium: 2534;Total Carbohydrate: 35.4;Cholesterol: 0;Protein: 8.2

950. Slow Cooker Spicy Black Eyed Peas

Serving: 10 | Prep: 30mins | Cook: 6hours | Ready in:
Ingredients
6 cups water
1 cube chicken bouillon
1 pound dried black-eyed peas, sorted and rinsed
1 onion, diced
2 cloves garlic, diced
1 red bell pepper, stemmed, seeded, and diced
1 jalapeno chile, seeded and minced
8 ounces diced ham
4 slices bacon, chopped
1/2 teaspoon cayenne pepper
1 1/2 teaspoons cumin
salt, to taste
1 teaspoon ground black pepper
Direction
In a slow cooker, pour the water then add the bouillon cube and mix until it dissolves. Mix together the pepper, salt, cumin, cayenne pepper, bacon, ham, jalapeno pepper, bell pepper, garlic, onion and black-eyed peas and mix to combine. Cover the slow cooker and let it cook for 6-8 hours on Low, until the beans become tender.
Nutrition Information
Calories: 199 calories;;Total Fat: 2.9;Sodium: 341;Total Carbohydrate: 30.2;Cholesterol: 10;Protein: 14.1

951. Slow Cooker Turkey Chili With Kidney Beans

Serving: 10 | Prep: 20mins | Cook: 4hours5mins | Ready in:
Ingredients
1 1/4 pounds ground turkey
2 onions, chopped
2 Anaheim chile peppers, chopped
2 (16 ounce) cans kidney beans, rinsed and drained
1 (16 ounce) can Mexican-style hot tomato sauce
1/4 cup chili powder
1/4 cup cornmeal
2 tablespoons minced garlic
1 tablespoon dried onion flakes
1 tablespoon unsweetened cocoa powder
1 tablespoon ground cumin
1 teaspoon ground black pepper
1 teaspoon white sugar
1 teaspoon dried parsley
1 teaspoon dried Mexican oregano
1 teaspoon beef base
1/2 teaspoon red pepper flakes
1/2 teaspoon ground coriander
1/2 cup water, or as desired
Direction
Heat a big skillet on moderate high heat. Cook and stir in the hot skillet the Anaheim chile peppers, onions and turkey for 5-7 minutes until crumbly and browned; drain and move the turkey mixture to a slow cooker.

Combine coriander, red pepper flakes, beef base, oregano, parsley, sugar, ground black pepper, cumin, cocoa power, onion flakes, garlic, cornmeal, chili powder, Mexican-style tomato sauce and kidney beans into turkey mixture. Put in enough water to get the preferred consistency.
Cook on high setting for about 4 hours or on low setting for about 8-10 hours.
Nutrition Information
Calories: 222 calories;;Cholesterol: 42;Protein: 17.8;Total Fat: 5.6;Sodium: 475;Total Carbohydrate: 27.1

952. Slow Cooker White Chicken Chili

Serving: 6 | Prep: | Cook: | Ready in:
Ingredients
PAM® Original No-Stick Cooking Spray
2 (15 ounce) cans Great Northern beans, undrained
1 pound boneless, skinless chicken thighs
1 (10 ounce) can RO*TEL Diced Tomatoes and Green Chilies, undrained
1 cup reduced sodium chicken broth
3/4 cup chopped yellow onion
1 1/2 teaspoons ground cumin
1 teaspoon dried oregano
Direction
Cover a 4-quart slow cooker with cooking spray. In slow cooker, put a can of beans; crush till smooth using a spoon or potato masher. Put another can of beans and the rest of the ingredients to slow cooker; mix to blend.
With cover, cook for 8 hours on Low or 4 hours on High. Gently part chicken into bite-size pieces.
Nutrition Information
Calories: 282 calories;;Total Fat: 5.7;Sodium: 261;Total Carbohydrate: 33.8;Cholesterol: 46;Protein: 24.4

953. Slow Cooked Habanero Chili

Serving: 10 | Prep: 20mins | Cook: 8hours | Ready in:
Ingredients
3 tablespoons olive oil
1 pound lean ground turkey
1 cup red bell pepper, chopped
3 cloves garlic, minced
1 (16 ounce) can kidney beans, rinsed and drained
1 (16 ounce) can black beans, rinsed and drained
1 cup rinsed and drained canned black-eyed peas
1 (15 ounce) can low sodium tomato sauce
1 dried habanero pepper, chopped
1 cup frozen corn kernels
1 tablespoon packed brown sugar
1 teaspoon Worcestershire sauce
1 tablespoon dried basil
1 teaspoon dried sage
salt to taste
Direction
In a big skillet, heat 1 tbsp. of olive oil on moderate high heat. Put in ground turkey and cook for 10 minutes until it is not pink anymore and browned evenly. Put the cooked meat into a slow cooker with a slotted spoon and drain off excess oil from the skillet.
Heat the remaining 2 tbsp. of olive oil in the same skillet on moderate high heat. Stir in garlic and red pepper; cook for 3 minutes until softened. Stir into the slow cooker with turkey.
Stir habanero pepper, tomato sauce, black-eyed peas, black beans and kidney beans into the turkey

mixture. Set the slow cooker on low and cook for 7 hours or on high for 3 hours.
Stir in sage, basil, Worcestershire sauce, brown sugar and corn one hour before cooking time is done. Keep on cooking the chili for the remaining hour. Season with salt to taste.
Nutrition Information
Calories: 240 calories;Protein: 16.6;Total Fat: 8.2;Sodium: 380;Total Carbohydrate: 27;Cholesterol: 33

954. Spiced Slow Cooker Applesauce

Serving: 8 | Prep: 10mins | Cook: 6hours30mins | Ready in:
Ingredients
8 apples - peeled, cored, and thinly sliced
1/2 cup water
3/4 cup packed brown sugar
1/2 teaspoon pumpkin pie spice
Direction
Put the apples in a slow cooker with water. Turn heat on Low. Cook for 6-8 hours. Add pumpkin pie spice and brown sugar, stirring occasionally. Cook for another half hour.
Nutrition Information
Calories: 150 calories;;Sodium: 8;Total Carbohydrate: 39.4;Cholesterol: 0;Protein: 0.4;Total Fat: 0.2

955. Spicy Chicken Thai Noodle Soup

Serving: 12 | Prep: 20mins | Cook: 8hours10mins | Ready in:
Ingredients
5 cups chicken broth
1 cup white wine
1 cup water
1 onion, chopped
3 green onions, chopped
3 cloves garlic, chopped
4 large carrots, cut into 1 inch pieces
4 large stalks celery, cut into 1 inch pieces
1/2 teaspoon salt
1 teaspoon ground black pepper
1 tablespoon curry powder
1/2 tablespoon dried sage
1/2 tablespoon poultry seasoning
1/2 tablespoon dried oregano
1 teaspoon ground cayenne pepper
2 tablespoons vegetable oil
3 skinless, boneless chicken breast halves - cut into 1 inch cubes
1 fresh red chile pepper, seeded and chopped
1/2 (12 ounce) package dried rice noodles
Direction
Mix chicken broth, poultry seasoning, wine, black pepper, water, oregano, onion, cayenne, green onion, carrots, salt, curry, garlic, sage, and celery in a slow cooker on low heat.
Over medium heat, cook the chicken in oil in a skillet until brown. Mix into the slow cooker.
Cook the soup for 5 hours on high or 8 hours on low. Mix in the red pepper about halfway through the cooking time. Mix in the noodles 15 minutes before serving.
Nutrition Information
Calories: 131 calories;;Total Fat: 3;Sodium: 155;Total Carbohydrate: 14.5;Cholesterol: 17;Protein: 7.9

956. Spicy Slow Cooker Black Bean Soup

Serving: 6 | Prep: 5mins | Cook: | Ready in:
Ingredients
1 pound dry black beans, soaked overnight
4 teaspoons diced jalapeno peppers
6 cups chicken broth
1/2 teaspoon garlic powder
1 tablespoon chili powder
1 teaspoon ground cumin
1 teaspoon cayenne pepper
3/4 teaspoon ground black pepper
1/2 teaspoon hot pepper sauce
Direction
Drain black beans; rinse.
Mix chicken broth, jalapenos and beans in a slow cooker; season using hot pepper sauce, pepper, cumin, cayenne, chili powder and garlic powder. Cook for 4 hours on high. Lower heat to low; cook till serving or for 2 hours.
Nutrition Information
Calories: 281 calories;;Sodium: 1012;Total Carbohydrate: 49.7;Cholesterol: 5;Protein: 17.7;Total Fat: 2

957. Spicy Turkey Chili

Serving: 8 | Prep: 10mins | Cook: 3hours | Ready in:
Ingredients
2 (5 ounce) cans turkey meat, drained
2 (15 ounce) cans kidney beans
2 (14.5 ounce) cans Italian-style stewed tomatoes
2 (1.25 ounce) packages chili seasoning mix
1 (4 ounce) can green chile peppers
1 (8 ounce) can tomato sauce
1 onion, diced
1 cup water
Direction
Mix turkey, tomato sauce, water, onion, chili peppers, beans, chili seasoning, and tomatoes in a slow cooker. Let it cook on Low setting for 3-4 hours. Serve it warm.
Nutrition Information
Calories: 213 calories;;Sodium: 1751;Total Carbohydrate: 30.8;Cholesterol: 23;Protein: 17;Total Fat: 3.7

958. Sweet And Simple Pork Roast

Serving: 8 | Prep: 10mins | Cook: 10hours | Ready in:
Ingredients
1 1/2 large sweet potatoes, peeled and cut into 1-inch chunks
2 cups baby carrots
1 sweet onion, cut into 1-inch chunks
3/4 cup white grape juice
1/2 cup unsweetened applesauce
1/4 cup water
1 (2 pound) pork roast
Direction
Whisk together the onion, carrots and sweet potatoes in the slow cooker. Whisk together the water, applesauce, and white grape juice in the bowl. Add half of the grape juice mixture on vegetables in the slow cooker. Add the pork roast over vegetables and add leftover grape juice mixture on top of pork. Cook over Low heat for 10 hours. Pour the accumulated juices on top of roast when serving.
Nutrition Information
Calories: 206 calories;;Total Carbohydrate: 26.2;Cholesterol: 40;Protein: 15;Total Fat: 4.5;Sodium: 98

959. Tunisian Slow Cooked Turkey Breast

Serving: 6 | Prep: 25mins | Cook: 3hours40mins | Ready in:
Ingredients
2 tablespoons all-purpose flour
1 teaspoon chipotle chili powder
1/2 teaspoon garlic powder
1/2 teaspoon ground cinnamon
1/2 teaspoon ground coriander
1/2 teaspoon salt
1/4 teaspoon ground black pepper
1 (4 pound) skinless, boneless turkey breast half
1 tablespoon olive oil
1 acorn squash, seeded and cut into quarters
3 large carrots, peeled and cut into 3 pieces
2 red onions, quartered
6 unpeeled garlic cloves
Direction
In a large resealable plastic bag, combine black pepper, salt, coriander, cinnamon, garlic powder, chipotle chili powder, and flour. Shake until thoroughly combined. Place in the turkey breast, seal, shake until turkey is evenly coated with the spice mix.
In a large skillet, heat oil over medium heat. Sear the seasoned turkey breast in the hot oil for 5 minutes per side until all sides are nicely browned, make sure that the meat will remain pink color inside.
In the bottom of a large slow cooker, place some garlic cloves, red onions, carrots, and acorn squash quarters. Top the vegetables with the browned turkey breast. Cover cooker.
Cook turkey breast for 3 1/2 to 4 hours on High or 7 to 8 hours on Low, until everything is tender.
Transfer turkey breast to a platter and set aside to cool for 10 minutes before slicing.
Peel garlic cloves and squash. Surround the turkey meat with the cooked vegetables. Spoon juices left in the slow cooker over turkey and vegetables. Serve.
Nutrition Information
Calories: 455 calories;;Cholesterol: 218;Protein: 81.1;Total Fat: 4.6;Sodium: 365;Total Carbohydrate: 19.2

960. Tykvenitsa Millet Breakfast Cereal

Serving: 6 | Prep: 15mins | Cook: 4hours | Ready in:
Ingredients
3 cups shredded pumpkin
2 cups water
2 cups rice milk
1 cup millet
1 tablespoon butter, or to taste
1 pinch salt to taste
Direction
Put millet, rice milk, water and pumpkin in a slow cooker and mix thoroughly.
Cook 4 to 5 hours on Low until creamy. Mix salt and butter into the cereal prior to serving.
Nutrition Information
Calories: 201 calories;;Sodium: 47;Total Carbohydrate: 36;Cholesterol: 5;Protein: 5.1;Total Fat: 4.1

961. Vegetarian Cassoulet

Serving: 8 | Prep: 20mins | Cook: 9hours | Ready in:
Ingredients
2 tablespoons olive oil
1 onion
2 carrots, peeled and diced
1 pound dry navy beans, soaked overnight
4 cups mushroom broth
1 cube vegetable bouillon
1 bay leaf
4 sprigs fresh parsley
1 sprig fresh rosemary
1 sprig fresh lemon thyme, chopped
1 sprig fresh savory
1 large potato, peeled and cubed
Direction
In a skillet, heat a little oil over medium heat. In oil, cook and stir carrots and onion until tender.
Combine bay leaf, bouillon, mushroom broth, onion, carrots, and beans in a slow cooker. Add water to cover ingredients if needed. Tie savory, thyme, rosemary, and parsley together, put into the pot. Choose Low setting, cook for 8 hours.
Mix in potato, keep cooking 1 more hour. Take away herbs then serve.
Nutrition Information
Calories: 279 calories;;Sodium: 141;Total Carbohydrate: 47.2;Cholesterol: 0;Protein: 15.3;Total Fat: 4.4

Chapter 12: Easy Slow Cooker Recipes

962. Bacon Cheese Breakfast Casserole
Serving: 8 | Prep: 35mins | Cook: | Ready in:
Ingredients
6 light multi-grain English muffins, cut into 1-inch pieces
Disposable slow cooker liner
Nonstick cooking spray
1 (12 ounce) package (18 slices) lower-sodium less-fat bacon, crisp-cooked, drained and coarsely chopped
½ medium zucchini, halved lengthwise and sliced (1 cup)
½ cup chopped onion (1 medium)
½ cup bottle roasted red sweet pepper, coarsely chopped
3 ounces Gouda cheese, shredded (¾ cup), divided
¼ cup finely shredded Parmesan cheese (about 1 ounce)
2 cups fat-free milk
1 cup refrigerated or frozen egg product, thawed if frozen
¼ teaspoon salt
¼ teaspoon black pepper
Direction
Preheat oven to 350°F. In a 15x10x1-inch baking pan, spread the English muffin pieces. Bake for 10 - 12 minutes or until dried. Take it out of the oven and let it cool. Meanwhile, use a disposable slow cooker liner to line the removable crockery liner of a 4-quart slow cooker; use cooking spray to coat; leave aside.
Toss the Parmesan, a half cup of the Gouda, roasted red pepper, onion, zucchini, bacon and bread cubes together in a very big bowl. Put the mixture in the prepared cooker. In the same bowl, whisk pepper, salt, egg product and milk together. In the cooker, spread egg mixture over the bread mixture. Use the back of a spoon to press lightly so the bread will be moistened completely.
In the slow cooker, arrange the crockery liner. Cook while covered on Low-heat setting for 3 to 3 and a half hours or till an instant-read thermometer reaches 200°F to 210°F when pinned into the middle of the casserole. To make sure of the even cooking, if possible, carefully rotate crockery liner 180° midway through cooking. Turn off the cooker. Take the crockery liner out of the cooker. Top with the leftover quarter cup of Gouda. Allow to rest for 30 minutes, then serve.
Nutrition Information
Calories: 222 calories;Protein: 17;Total Fat: 8
Saturated Fat: 3;Cholesterol: 23
Sugar: 5;Sodium: 565
Fiber: 7;Total Carbohydrate: 25

963. Barbecue Pulled Chicken
Serving: 8 | Prep: | Cook: 25mins | Ready in:
Ingredients
1 8-ounce can reduced-sodium tomato sauce
1 4-ounce can chopped green chiles, drained
3 tablespoons cider vinegar
2 tablespoons honey
1 tablespoon sweet or smoked paprika
1 tablespoon tomato paste
1 tablespoon Worcestershire sauce
2 teaspoons dry mustard
1 teaspoon ground chipotle chile
½ teaspoon salt
2½ pounds boneless, skinless chicken thighs, trimmed of fat
1 small onion, finely chopped
1 clove garlic, minced
Direction
In a 6-quart slow cooker, mix salt, ground chipotle, mustard, Worcestershire sauce, tomato paste, paprika, honey, vinegar, chiles and tomato sauce together until smooth. Add garlic, onion and chicken; stir to combine.
Put on the lid, then cook on low for approximately 5 hours till chicken can be pulled apart.
Move the chicken to a cutting board, then use a fork to shred. Move the chicken back to the sauce, thoroughly stir, then serve.
Nutrition Information
Calories: 214 calories;Protein: 25;Total Fat: 8;Sodium: 321
Fiber: 1;Cholesterol: 130
Sugar: 6
Saturated Fat: 2;Total Carbohydrate: 9

964. Beef And Red Bean Chili
Serving: 6 | Prep: 1hours10mins | Cook: | Ready in:
Ingredients
1 cup dry red beans or dry kidney beans
1 tablespoon olive oil
2 pounds boneless beef chuck, cut into 1-inch cubes
1 large onion, coarsely chopped
1 (14 ounce) can beef broth
1 to 2 chipotle chile peppers in adobo sauce, finely chopped, plus 2 tsp. adobo sauce
2 teaspoons dried oregano, crushed
1 teaspoon ground cumin
½ teaspoon salt
1 (14.5 ounce) can diced tomatoes with mild green chiles
1 (15 ounce) can tomato sauce
¼ cup snipped fresh cilantro
1 medium red sweet pepper, chopped
Direction
Rinse out the beans and place them into a Dutch oven or big saucepan, then add in water enough to cover them. Allow the beans to boil then drop the heat down. Simmer the beans without a cover for 10 minutes. Take off the heat and keep covered for an hour.
In a big frypan, heat up the oil upon medium-high heat, then cook onion and half the beef until they brown a bit over medium-high heat. Move into a 3 1/2 or 4 quart crockery cooker. Do this again with what's left of the beef. Add in tomato sauce, tomatoes (not drained), salt, cumin, oregano, adobo sauce, chipotle peppers, and broth, stirring to blend. Strain out and rinse beans and stir in the cooker.
Cook while covered on a low setting for around 10-12 hours or on high setting for around 5-6 hours. Spoon the chili into bowls or mugs and top with sweet pepper and cilantro.
Nutrition Information
Calories: 288 calories;;Total Fat: 7;Sodium: 702
Fiber: 6;Protein: 31
Saturated Fat: 2;Cholesterol: 67;Total Carbohydrate: 24
Sugar: 5

965. Buffalo Chicken Salads

Serving: 6 | Prep: 15mins | Cook: | Ready in:
Ingredients
1½ pounds skinless, boneless chicken breast halves
½ cup Wing Time® Buffalo chicken sauce or reduced-sodium Buffalo sauce
4 teaspoons cider vinegar
1 teaspoon Worcestershire sauce
1 teaspoon paprika
⅓ cup light mayonnaise
2 tablespoons fat-free milk
2 tablespoons crumbled blue cheese
2 romaine hearts, chopped
1 cup whole grain croutons
½ cup very thinly sliced red onion
Direction
Place chicken in a 2-quarts slow cooker. Mix together Worcestershire sauce, 2 teaspoons of vinegar and Buffalo sauce in a small bowl; pour over chicken.
Dust with paprika. Cover and cook for 3 to 4 hours on low-heat setting.
Mix the leftover 2 teaspoons of vinegar with milk and light mayonnaise together in a small bowl at serving time; mix in blue cheese. While chicken is still in the slow cooker, pull meat into bite-sized pieces using two forks.
Split the romaine among 6 dishes. Spoon sauce and chicken over lettuce. Pour with blue cheese dressing then add red onion slices and croutons on top.
Nutrition Information
Calories: 274 calories;;Cholesterol: 79;Total Carbohydrate: 11
Sugar: 2;Protein: 27;Total Fat: 13
Saturated Fat: 2;Sodium: 396
Fiber: 2

966. Cheese Fondue With Fennel Tomatoes

Serving: 12 | Prep: | Cook: 30mins | Ready in:
Ingredients
1½ tablespoons extra-virgin olive oil
2 cups diced fennel
1 cup diced onion
1 (14 ounce) can no-salt-added diced tomatoes, drained well
¼ teaspoon salt
Freshly ground pepper to taste
10 ounces Emmentaler or Swiss cheese, shredded (3½ cups)
6 ounces Comté or Gruyère cheese, shredded (2 cups)
2 tablespoons all-purpose flour, plus more as needed
1 teaspoon fennel seeds, gently crushed
¼ teaspoon cayenne pepper
1¼ cups light, fruity white wine, such as dry Riesling
Direction
Pour very hot water in a fondue pot or a small slow cooker until full; set it aside to warm.
On medium heat, heat oil in a big pan. Cook and stir often onion and fennel for 8-10 minutes until translucent; add pepper, salt and tomatoes. Cook for 2-4 minutes while occasionally mixing until any liquid evaporates. Take off from the heat.
In a medium bowl, mix cayenne fennel seeds, flour and both cheeses together.
On medium heat, heat wine in a medium heavy-bottomed pot until hot yet not boiling. Add a handful of cheese mixture at a time, mix well until melted after each addition. Take off from the heat then mix in the vegetable mixture.
Drain the fondue pot or the slow cooker then dry. Transfer the fondue then keep it warm on a warm setting or on low heat to serve. Mix in 1-2 tsp. of flour if it begins to separate.
Nutrition Information
Calories: 202 calories;;Total Fat: 13
Saturated Fat: 7
Fiber: 1
Sugar: 2;Protein: 11;Sodium: 175;Cholesterol: 37;Total Carbohydrate: 6

967. Chile, Cheese, And Scrambled Egg Grits

Serving: 8 | Prep: 10mins | Cook: | Ready in:
Ingredients
Nonstick cooking spray
4½ cups reduced-sodium chicken broth or reduced-sodium vegetable broth
1 cup yellow or white grits
½ teaspoon to 1 teaspoon ground cumin
½ teaspoon salt
¾ cup shredded reduced-fat Cheddar cheese
1 (4 ounce) can diced green chile peppers, undrained
2 cloves garlic, minced
4 eggs
1 pinch salt
Direction
In a 3 1/2- or 4-quart slow cooker, line a disposable slow cooker liner. Spray liner with cooking spray. Combine garlic, diced green chile peppers with liquid, cheese, half teaspoon salt, cumin, grits, chicken or vegetable broth in a large bowl. Bring mixture to the prepared cooker.
Cook with a cover for 7 to 9 hours on low-heat setting or for 3 1/2 to 4 1/2 hours on high-heat setting, mixing once halfway through cooking. Turn the cooker off.
In a small bowl, beat eggs with 1 pinch salt; pour over grits. Allow to sit with a cover, for 30 minutes before serving, mixing twice.
Nutrition Information
Calories: 159 calories;
Fiber: 1;Cholesterol: 104;Total Carbohydrate: 15;Total Fat: 6
Saturated Fat: 3;Sodium: 611
Sugar: 1;Protein: 9

968. Creamy Chicken Noodle Soup

Serving: 8 | Prep: 25mins | Cook: | Ready in:
Ingredients
1 (32 fluid ounce) container reduced-sodium chicken broth
3 cups water
2½ cups chopped cooked chicken (about 12 ounces)
3 medium carrots, sliced (1½ cups)
3 stalks celery, sliced (1½ cups)
1½ cups sliced fresh mushrooms (4 ounces)
¼ cup chopped onion
1½ teaspoons dried thyme, crushed
¾ teaspoon garlic-pepper seasoning
3 ounces reduced-fat cream cheese (Neufchâtel), cut up
2 cups dried egg noodles
Direction
Mix together the garlic-pepper seasoning, thyme, onion, mushrooms, celery, carrots, chicken, water and broth in a 5 to 6-quart slow cooker.

Put cover and let it cook for 3-4 hours on high-heat setting or 6-8 hours on low-heat setting.
Increase to high-heat setting if you are using low-heat setting. Mix in the cream cheese until blended. Mix in uncooked noodles. Put cover and let it cook for an additional 20-30 minutes or just until the noodles become tender.

Nutrition Information
Calories: 170 calories;;Sodium: 381
Sugar: 3;Protein: 17;Total Fat: 6
Saturated Fat: 2
Fiber: 2;Cholesterol: 54;Total Carbohydrate: 12

969. Easy Chicken Enchiladas

Serving: 6 | Prep: 20mins | Cook: 30mins | Ready in:
Ingredients
1 (8 ounce) package cream cheese
1 cup salsa
2 cups chopped cooked chicken breast meat
1 (15.5 ounce) can pinto beans, drained
6 (6 inch) flour tortillas
2 cups shredded Colby-Jack cheese

Direction
Preheat an oven to 175 degrees C (350 degrees F). Coat a 9x13 inch baking dish lightly with grease.
Over medium heat, mix salsa and cream cheese in a small saucepan. Cook while stirring until melted and blended well. Mix in pinto beans and chicken. Fill the tortillas with the mixture, roll and transfer to the prepared baking dish. Add cheese all over the top. Cover using aluminum foil.
Bake for about 30 minutes or until heated through. Garnish with toppings you love like sour cream or tomatoes and lettuce.

Nutrition Information
Calories: 565 calories;;Sodium: 1166;Total Carbohydrate: 32.8;Cholesterol: 120;Protein: 32.6;Total Fat: 34.1

970. Eggplant Chickpea Stew

Serving: 8 | Prep: | Cook: 45mins | Ready in:
Ingredients
1 ounce dried porcini mushrooms
3 cups hot water
2 large eggplants (about 1½ pounds each)
3 tablespoons extra-virgin olive oil, divided
2 large onions, thinly sliced
6 cloves garlic, minced
2 teaspoons dried oregano, crumbled
1 small (1-inch) cinnamon stick
1 teaspoon salt
1 teaspoon freshly ground pepper
1 bay leaf
1 cup dried chickpeas, rinsed and soaked overnight (for a quick-soak method, see Tip) and drained
1 28-ounce can tomatoes (see Note), drained and coarsely chopped
¼ cup finely chopped fresh parsley

Direction
Set an oven to preheat to 400 degrees F.
In a bowl, mix together the hot water and dried mushrooms. Mix well and allow it to stand for 30 minutes. Strain it through a paper towel-lined sieve and put the liquid aside. Chop the mushrooms finely.
In the meantime, skin the eggplants, if preferred, and slice it in half lengthwise. Brush 2 tbsp. of oil generously on the cut sides. Put it on a rimmed baking tray, cut side down and let it roast for about 25 minutes until it becomes tender. Allow it to stand until it is cool enough to touch. Slice it into 1-inch cubes and move to a 4-quart or bigger slow cooker.
In the meantime, in a big frying pan, heat the leftover 1 tbsp. of oil on medium heat, then add onions and let it cook for 3-6 minutes, stirring often, until it becomes soft. Add chopped mushrooms, bay leaf, pepper, salt, cinnamon stick, oregano and garlic and let it cook and stir for a minute. Add chickpeas and reserved mushroom soaking liquid, then boil. Let it cook for 5 minutes, stirring from time to time. Move to the slow cooker and mix to blend with the eggplant.
Put a cover and let it cook for 7-8 hours on Low or around 4 hours on High, until the chickpeas become very tender. Take out the bay leaf and cinnamon stick. Mix in parsley and tomatoes.
Variation: Turn the 3 cups of remaining stew into the Chickpea and Eggplant Baked Pasta. Set an oven to preheat to 350 degrees F. Use cooking spray to coat an 8-inch square or a similar 2-quart baking dish. Boil a big pot of water. Cook the 8-oz. of whole-wheat fusilli following the package instructions, then drain and wash. In a small bowl, mix together the 1 tbsp. extra-virgin olive oil and 1/2 cup course dry whole-wheat breadcrumbs. In a big bowl, toss the pasta with 2 tbsp. lemon juice, 1/4 cup chopped fresh mint or basil, 1 cup crumbled feta cheese and 3 cups of stew. Spread the mixture in the prepped baking dish and put the breadcrumb mixture on top. Let it bake for about 30 minutes until the topping turns crispy and golden. Sprinkle with 1/4 cup of chopped fresh mint or basil on top.
Note: To make your own breadcrumbs, cut the crusts from the whole-wheat bread. Tear the bread into pieces and process it in a food processor until it forms coarse crumbs. Spread it on a baking tray and let it bake for around 10-15 minutes at 250 degrees F, until it becomes dry. One bread slice makes approximately 1/3 cup dry breadcrumbs. For store-bought coarse dry breadcrumbs we like Ian's brand, labeled "Panko breadcrumbs." Find them at well-stocked supermarkets.

Nutrition Information
Calories: 220 calories;;Cholesterol: 0;Total Carbohydrate: 33
Sugar: 11;Total Fat: 7
Saturated Fat: 1;Sodium: 392
Fiber: 11;Protein: 9

971. Ethiopian Spiced Chicken Stew

Serving: 8 | Prep: | Cook: 40mins | Ready in:
Ingredients
1½ cups red lentils
2½ pounds boneless, skinless chicken thighs, trimmed
1 tablespoon butter
2 teaspoons extra-virgin olive oil
4 cups chopped red onions
5 cloves garlic, finely chopped
1 tablespoon minced fresh ginger
5 tablespoons berbere spice blend (see Tip)
½ cup dry red wine
1 14-ounce can diced tomatoes
2 cups reduced-sodium chicken broth

Direction
In a medium bowl, wash lentils in cold water until the water runs clear; drain and distribute in a slow

cooker of 5 to 6-quarts in an even layer. Put the chicken over the lentils.
Heat butter and oil over medium - high heat in a big skillet. Put in onions and cook when the butter has melted, mixing often, for 4 to 6 minutes, until tender and translucent. Put in ginger and garlic and cook for 1 to 2 minutes, mixing often, until fragrant. Put in berbere and cook, whisking, for 2 to 4 minutes, until very fragrant. Mix in wine, scraping the onion mixture from the bottom of the pan, and mix in the tomatoes with their juice.
Put in the onion mixture to the slow cooker over the chicken, and pour in broth.
Cover and cook on high for 5 hours or on low for 7 to 8 hours, until the chicken is falling-apart soft. Mix the stew to blend.
Nutrition Information
Calories: 430 calories;
Saturated Fat: 4;Sodium: 666;Protein: 38;Total Fat: 14;Total Carbohydrate: 35
Sugar: 5
Fiber: 7;Cholesterol: 98

972. Fennel Pork Stew
Serving: 8 | Prep: | Cook: 20mins | Ready in:
Ingredients
8 cups thinly sliced fennel (2-3 medium bulbs), plus ¼ cup chopped fronds
1 medium onion, halved and thinly sliced
2½ pounds pork shoulder or Boston butt, trimmed of excess fat and cut into 2-inch chunks
1½ teaspoons kosher salt, divided
1½ teaspoons freshly ground pepper, divided
2 tablespoons extra-virgin olive oil, divided
¾ cup dry white wine, such as Sauvignon Blanc
4 cloves garlic, minced
1 tablespoon finely chopped fresh rosemary
2 teaspoons finely chopped fresh oregano
1 28-ounce can whole tomatoes, drained
Direction
Spread onion and fennel evenly in a 5-6-qt. slow cooker. Refrigerate, covered, the fennel fronds.
Add three-fourths teaspoon each of pepper and salt onto the pork. In a Dutch oven or a large skillet, bring 1 tablespoon of oil to medium-high heat. Put in about 1/2 of pork and brown for 4-5 minutes. Remove to the slow cooker. Do the same process with leftover pork and oil. Pour wine into the pan, scraping up browned bits; take off the heat.
Season pork with three-fourths teaspoon each of leftover pepper and salt, oregano, rosemary and garlic. Add on drained tomatoes and wine from the skillet.
Cook, covered over low heat for 7-8 hours or over high heat for 5 hours. Blend stew well until incorporated; add use reserved fronds to decorate.
Nutrition Information
Calories: 249 calories;;Sodium: 303;Total Carbohydrate: 9
Sugar: 4;Protein: 20;Total Fat: 13
Saturated Fat: 4
Fiber: 3;Cholesterol: 70

973. Fireside Beef Stew
Serving: 6 | Prep: 20mins | Cook: | Ready in:
Ingredients
1½ pounds boneless beef chuck pot roast
1 pound butternut squash, peeled, seeded and cut into 1-inch pieces
2 small onions, cut into wedges
2 cloves garlic, minced
1 (14 ounce) can reduced-sodium beef broth
1 (8 ounce) can tomato sauce
2 tablespoons Worcestershire sauce
1 teaspoon dry mustard
¼ teaspoon ground black pepper
⅛ teaspoon ground allspice
2 tablespoons cold water
4 teaspoons cornstarch
1 (9 ounce) package frozen Italian green beans
Direction
Cut out the fat from the meat. Divide meat into 1-inch chunks. Add it into a 3 1/2 to 4 1/2-quart slow cooker. Add garlic, onions, and squash. Mix in allspice, pepper, dry mustard, Worcestershire sauce, tomato sauce and beef broth
Let cook while covered for 8 to 10 hours at low-heat mode or 4 to 5 hours at high-heat mode.
At low-heat mode, turn to high-heat mode. Mix cornstarch with cold water in a small bowl. Mix the green beans and cornstarch mixture into the cooker.
Let cook while covered for 15 more minutes or until thickened.
Nutrition Information
Calories: 207 calories;;Total Fat: 4
Saturated Fat: 1;Sodium: 440;Total Carbohydrate: 15;Protein: 27
Fiber: 3;Cholesterol: 67
Sugar: 5

974. Flemish Beef Stew
Serving: 8 | Prep: | Cook: 45mins | Ready in:
Ingredients
4 teaspoons canola oil, divided
2 pounds bottom round, trimmed of fat and cut into 1-inch cubes
¾ pound sliced cremini, or white button mushrooms
3 tablespoons all-purpose flour
2 cups brown ale, or dark beer
4 large carrots, peeled and cut into 1-inch pieces
1 large onion, chopped
1 clove garlic, minced
1½ tablespoons Dijon mustard
1 teaspoon caraway seeds
¾ teaspoon salt
½ teaspoon freshly ground pepper
1 bay leaf
Direction
Heat 2 teaspoons of oil over medium heat in a big skillet. Put in half the beef; brown on all sides, flipping frequently, for 5 minutes. Move to a slow cooker (6 quarts in size). Drain any fat from the pan. Put in the leftover 2 teaspoons oil and brown the rest of the beef. Move to the slow cooker.
Set the skillet back to medium heat; put in mushrooms and cook, mixing often, for 5 to 7 minutes until the liquid is given off and evaporates to a glaze. Dust the flour over the mushrooms; cook for 10 seconds undisturbed, then mix and cook for another 30 seconds. Drizzle in ale (or beer); boil and stir constantly for about 3 minutes to decrease foaming until bubbling and thickened. Move the mushroom blend to the slow cooker.
Put the bay leaf, pepper, salt, caraway seeds, mustard, garlic, onion and carrots in the slow cooker. Toss to mix.

Cover and cook on low for about 8 hours until the beef is very soft. Remove the bay leaf prior to serving.
Nutrition Information
Calories: 301 calories;;Sodium: 361
Fiber: 2;Cholesterol: 81;Total Carbohydrate: 17;Total Fat: 10
Saturated Fat: 3
Sugar: 5;Protein: 31

975. Fork Tender Pot Roast

Serving: 8 | Prep: 25mins | Cook: | Ready in:
Ingredients
1 2½ to 3-pound boneless beef chuck pot roast
1 tablespoon olive oil
1 cup coarsely chopped carrot (2 medium)
2 stalks celery, cut into 1-inch pieces
1 cup coarsely chopped onion (1 large)
1 clove garlic, minced
1 bay leaf
¾ cup lower-sodium beef broth
¼ cup dry red wine
2 tablespoons quick-cooking tapioca, crushed
1 tablespoon dried Italian seasoning, crushed
1 tablespoon tomato paste
1 teaspoon garlic powder
¾ teaspoon ground black pepper
½ teaspoon dry mustard
½ teaspoon paprika
⅛ teaspoon salt
4 cups mashed potatoes (optional)
Direction
Brown meat in hot oil over medium - high heat on all sides in a big skillet. Take away from heat and put aside.
Mix bay leaf, garlic, onion, celery and carrot in a 3 1/2 or 4-quarts slow cooker (see Tip). Put meat on top. Mix salt, paprika, dry mustard, pepper, garlic powder, tomato paste, Italian seasoning, tapioca, wine and broth in a medium bowl. Drizzle over meat in cooker.
Cover and cook for 10 to 12 hours on low-heat setting or for 5 to 6 hours on high-heat setting. Move meat to a serving dish for serving. Use a slotted spoon to remove vegetables. Remove and discard bay leaf. Skim fat from the leftover sauce; pour sauce over vegetables and meat. Serve with mashed potatoes if desired.
Nutrition Information
Calories: 241 calories;;Cholesterol: 62;Total Carbohydrate: 7
Sugar: 2;Protein: 32;Total Fat: 8;Sodium: 204
Fiber: 1
Saturated Fat: 2

976. Greek Chicken Vegetable Ragout

Serving: 6 | Prep: | Cook: 40mins | Ready in:
Ingredients
1 pound carrots, cut into 1¼-inch pieces, or 3 cups baby carrots
1 pound (3-4 medium) yellow-fleshed potatoes, such as Yukon Gold, peeled and cut lengthwise into 1¼-inch-wide wedges
2 pounds boneless, skinless chicken thighs, trimmed
1 14-ounce can reduced-sodium chicken broth
⅓ cup dry white wine
4 cloves garlic, minced
¾ teaspoon salt
1 15-ounce can artichoke hearts, rinsed and quartered if large
1 large egg
2 large egg yolks
⅓ cup lemon juice
⅓ cup chopped fresh dill
Freshly ground pepper to taste
Direction
Spread up the sides and over the bottom of a big or 4-quart slow cooker with potatoes and carrots. Top the vegetables with chicken. In a medium-sized saucepan, boil salt, garlic, wine, or broth over medium-high heat. Add to the vegetables and chicken. Put a cover on and cook on low for 4-4 1/2 hours or on high for 2 1/2-3 hours, until the vegetables are soft and chicken has thoroughly cooked.
In the slow cooker, put artichokes. Put a cover on and cook for 5 minutes on high. In the meantime, in a medium-sized bowl, stir together lemon juice, egg yolks, and egg.
With a slotted spoon, move the vegetables and chicken to a serving bowl. Put a cover on and keep warm. Pour approximately 1/2 cup of the cooking liquid into the egg mixture. Stir until smooth. Stir the egg mixture into the slow cooker with the left cooking liquid. Put a cover on and cook for 15-20 minutes, until thickened a bit and an instant-read thermometer display 160°F when you insert it into the sauce, stirring 2-3 times. Mix in pepper and dill. Add the sauce to the vegetables and chicken and enjoy.
Nutrition Information
Calories: 326 calories;
Fiber: 5;Total Carbohydrate: 28
Sugar: 5;Protein: 29;Total Fat: 10
Saturated Fat: 3;Sodium: 778;Cholesterol: 214

977. Pasta With Marinara Sauce

Serving: 8 | Prep: 20mins | Cook: | Ready in:
Ingredients
1 (28 ounce) can whole Italian-style tomatoes, cut up and undrained
4 medium carrots, coarsely chopped (2 cups)
3 stalks celery, sliced (1½ cups)
1 large onion, chopped (1 cup)
2 small green bell peppers, chopped (1 cup)
1 (6 ounce) can no-salt-added tomato paste
½ cup water
2 teaspoons sugar (optional)
2 teaspoons dried Italian seasoning, crushed
3 cloves garlic, minced
½ teaspoon salt
¼ teaspoon black pepper
1 bay leaf
4 cups hot cooked whole-grain spaghetti (8 ounces dried)
1 ounce Parmesan cheese, shaved into shards
Fresh herb sprigs (optional)
Direction
Combine bay leaf, tomatoes, black pepper, carrots, salt, celery, garlic, onion, Italian seasoning, bell peppers, sugar if using, water, and tomato paste in a 3 1/2 or 4-qt slow cooker.
Cook for 8-10hrs on low or 4-5hrs on high while covered.
Remove the bay leaf. Serve sauce on top of hot cooked pasta with sprinkled Parmesan on top. Top with herb sprigs to garnish if desired.
Nutrition Information
Calories: 188 calories;;Sodium: 401

Fiber: 6;Cholesterol: 2;Total Carbohydrate: 35;Protein: 9;Total Fat: 2
Sugar: 10
Saturated Fat: 1

978. Pulled Pork With Caramelized Onions

Serving: 8 | Prep: | Cook: 1hours | Ready in:
Ingredients
1 tablespoon extra-virgin olive oil
3 large onions, thinly sliced
⅓ cup raw cane sugar, such as Demerara or turbinado (see Notes)
4 cloves garlic, minced
1 teaspoon dried oregano
1 teaspoon freshly ground pepper
½ teaspoon salt
⅓ cup cider vinegar
1 cup chili sauce, such as Heinz
1½-3 teaspoons minced chipotle chile in adobo sauce (see Notes)
3 pounds boneless pork shoulder or blade (butt) roast, trimmed
Direction
On medium-high heat, heat oil in a big pan. Cook onions in hot oil for 3-6mins while occasionally stirring until they start to soften; put in sugar. Cook for another 6-8mins while occasionally stirring until the onions are golden brown. Add salt, garlic, pepper, and oregano; cook and stir for a minute. Pour in vinegar then boil. Cook for 30secs to 1min until the liquid mostly evaporates. Take off heat; mix in chipotle and chili sauce to taste.
Put pork in a four-quart or bigger slow cooker; pour in sauce to cover. Cover then cook on High for 4hrs or on Low for 8hrs until the meat is almost falling apart. Shred the pork with 2 forks on a cutting board; mix back into the pot with sauce.
For the variation, use three cups of leftover pulled pork into Pulled-Pork Torta. Preheat the oven to 375 degrees F. Use cooking spray to grease a 9-in round baking pan or deep-dish pie pan. Warm three cups of finely shredded Pulled Pork and Caramelized Onions with sauce. Drain one can of 14oz. diced tomatoes with no-added-salt, set the juice aside. In a bowl, mix with a quarter cup diced Spanish-style chorizo or pepperoni; stir well. Slather about half a cup mixture on the bottom of the prepared pan to cover it. Add one 8-in flour tortilla on top (preferable whole-wheat). Spread 1/3 of the remaining mixture on top of the tortilla then put another tortilla on top. Repeat two more times, ending with the 4th tortilla on top. Pour in the reserved tomato juice on top then use foil to cover; bake for 20mins. Discard the foil then top with 3/4 cup shredded Monterey Jack cheese; bake for another 20mins until the torta bubbles and the cheese melts. Cool for 10mins. Serve with a quarter cup each of chopped fresh cilantro and finely chopped scallions on top, if desired.
The Spanish-style chorizo can be found with other cured sausages in supermarkets. It is a fully-cooked and seasoned smoked pork sausage.
Nutrition Information
Calories: 355 calories;;Cholesterol: 90
Sugar: 14;Protein: 25;Total Fat: 18
Saturated Fat: 6
Fiber: 3;Total Carbohydrate: 20;Sodium: 664

979. Sausage And Sweet Pepper Hash

Serving: 10 | Prep: 5mins | Cook: | Ready in:
Ingredients
¾ (12 ounce) package cooked smoked chicken sausage, quartered lengthwise and cut into ½-inch pieces
1 teaspoon olive oil
1½ cups sliced sweet onion
Nonstick cooking spray
1½ pounds new potatoes, cut into ½-inch pieces
2 teaspoons snipped fresh thyme or ½ teaspoon dried thyme, crushed
½ teaspoon black Pepper
¼ cup reduced-sodium chicken broth
2 cups chopped green, red, and/or yellow sweet peppers
½ cup shredded Swiss cheese (2 ounces) (optional)
2 teaspoons snipped fresh tarragon or parsley
Direction
On medium heat, cook sausage in a big non-stick pan for 5 mins until brown; take the sausage out of the pa. On medium-low heat, heat oil in the same pan. Cook and stir onion for 5 mins until the onion is tender and begins to turn brown.
Grease using cooking spray or place a disposable liner at the base of a 3 1/2 or 4qt slow cooker. Mix black pepper, sausage, thyme, onion, and potatoes together in the prepared slow cooker; pour in broth. Set on low heat and cook, covered, for 5-6hrs or cook for 2 1/2-3 hours on high heat. Mix in sweet peppers; add cheese if desired.
If set on low heat, adjust the cooker to high heat mode. Cook for another 15 mins while covered. Serve using a slotted spoon; add tarragon on top.
Nutrition Information
Calories: 116 calories;;Cholesterol: 18;Sodium: 172
Saturated Fat: 1
Fiber: 2;Total Carbohydrate: 18
Sugar: 5;Protein: 6;Total Fat: 3

980. Slow Cooked Beans

Serving: 6 | Prep: | Cook: 10mins | Ready in:
Ingredients
1 pound dried beans, such as cannellini beans, black beans, kidney beans, black-eyed peas, great northern beans or pinto beans
1 onion, chopped
4 cloves garlic, minced
6 sprigs fresh thyme, or 1 teaspoon dried
1 bay leaf
5 cups boiling water
½ teaspoon salt
Direction
Soak beans for 6 hours or overnight in cold water enough to cover them by 2-inches. (Use the quick-soak technique as an alternative: Put beans in a large pot covered with enough water by 2 inches. Bring to a boil over high heat. Take it away from heat and allow it to stand for 1 hour).
Strain the beans and transfer them to a slow cooker. Add bay leaf, thyme, garlic, and onion. Add in boiling water. Cook for 2 to 3 1/2 hours on high, covered, until the beans are tender. Mix in salt and cook for 15 more minutes, covered.
Nutrition Information
Calories: 253 calories;
Saturated Fat: 0;Sodium: 201
Fiber: 19
Sugar: 1;Protein: 15;Total Fat: 1;Cholesterol: 0;Total Carbohydrate: 48

981. Slow Cooked Brisket In Onion Gravy

Serving: 14 | Prep: | Cook: 1hours | Ready in:
Ingredients
5 pounds flat-cut beef brisket (see Note), trimmed
2 tablespoons extra-virgin olive oil, divided
4 large onions, thinly sliced
6 cloves garlic, minced
1 teaspoon dried thyme
1 teaspoon coarsely ground pepper
1 6-ounce can tomato paste
2 cups reduced-sodium beef broth
1 teaspoon salt
2 tablespoons butter, softened
2 tablespoons all-purpose flour
1 tablespoon Worcestershire sauce
Direction
Slice the brisket into 2 or 3 pieces small enough to fit in a Dutch oven; pat dry. In the Dutch oven, heat 1 tablespoon of oil over medium - high heat. Lower the heat to medium; brown the brisket, one at a time, for 2 minutes each side, putting in an extra tablespoon oil if needed to avoid sticking. Move the brisket to a slow cooker (5 quarts or bigger).
Put in the leftover 1 tablespoon of oil. Put in onions; cook for 3 to 6 minutes, mixing occasionally, until soft. Put in pepper, thyme and garlic and cook for a minute, mixing. Whisk in tomato paste. Put in salt and beef broth; boil.
Place the onion blend to the slow cooker. Cover and cook on high for 4 to 5 hours or on low for 8 to 10 hours until the brisket reaches the desired tenderness.
Place the brisket to a cutting board, then cut or shred. Put in a serving plate; cover to keep warm. Move gravy to a saucepan. Boil over medium-high heat; rapidly boil for 5 minutes to decrease slightly.
In the meantime, in a small bowl, stir flour and butter until creamy and smooth. Lower the heat once the gravy has reduced to keep a simmer. Mix in the Worcestershire sauce. Stir half of the butter blend into the gravy, then return to a simmer. Cook, mixing, for 1 to 3 minutes until it thickens slightly. If the gravy doesn't thicken enough (it should have a cream soup texture), put in the remaining butter blend and repeat. Do not overcook. Enjoy the brisket with the gravy.
Variation: To create Brisket Sloppy Joes, use 2 cups gravy and 3 cups remaining brisket. Heat 1 tablespoon extra-virgin olive oil over medium heat in a big saucepan. Put in 1 seeded and minced jalapeno pepper (optional) and 1 seeded and diced green bell pepper; cook for 3 to 4 minutes, mixing occasionally, until soft. Put in 1?4 teaspoon salt, 2 teaspoons of chili powder and 1 drained 14-ounce can diced tomatoes and cook for a minute, mixing. Put in 2 tablespoons brown sugar, 2 tablespoons molasses, 2 cups Onion Gravy and 3 cups chopped Slow-Cooked Brisket; mix well. Cover and simmer to meld flavors for 10 minutes. Serve on onion or warm whole-wheat buns.
Nutrition Information
Calories: 248 calories;
Fiber: 1;Cholesterol: 92;Total Carbohydrate: 8;Protein: 30;Total Fat: 10
Saturated Fat: 4;Sodium: 386
Sugar: 4

982. Slow Cooker Beef Stroganoff

Serving: 6 | Prep: 30mins | Cook: | Ready in:
Ingredients
1½ pounds beef stew meat
2 teaspoons vegetable oil
2 cups sliced fresh mushrooms
1 medium onion, chopped (½ cup)
2 cloves garlic, minced
½ teaspoon dried oregano, crushed
½ teaspoon salt
¼ teaspoon dried thyme, crushed
¼ teaspoon black pepper
1 bay leaf
1 (14.5 ounce) can lower-sodium beef broth
⅓ cup dry sherry or lower-sodium beef broth
1 (8 ounce) carton light sour cream
2 tablespoons cornstarch
2 cups hot cooked noodles
Snipped fresh parsley (optional)
Direction
Cut fat off from the beef. Slice beef into 1-inch pieces. Cook half of the beef at a time in hot oil in a large frying pan over medium heat until brown. Skim the fat.
In a 3 and a half-quart or 4-quart slow cooker, place bay leaf, pepper, thyme, salt, oregano, garlic, onion, and mushrooms. Put in beef. Put sherry and broth over.
Cook while covered for 8 - 10 hours on low-heat setting or for 4 - 5 hours on high-heat setting. Throw away the bay leaf.
Switch to high-heat setting if using low-heat. Blend cornstarch and sour cream in a medium bowl. Slowly stir in about 1 cup of the hot cooking liquid together. Blend the sour cream mixture into the cooker. Cook while covered for around 30 more minutes or until thickened. Serve over hot cooked noodles. Top each serving with parsley if you like.
Nutrition Information
Calories: 257 calories;
Saturated Fat: 5;Sodium: 312
Sugar: 4;Total Fat: 10
Fiber: 2;Cholesterol: 74;Total Carbohydrate: 14;Protein: 26

983. Slow Cooker Beef Tacos With Rhubarb Salsa

Serving: 8 | Prep: 45mins | Cook: | Ready in:
Ingredients
2 tablespoons chili powder
1 tablespoon dried oregano
1 tablespoon ground cumin
½ teaspoon garlic powder
1½ teaspoons salt, divided
3 pounds beef chuck, trimmed and cut into 1-inch cubes
1 tablespoon avocado oil or grapeseed oil
1 large onion, halved and sliced
1 cup low-sodium beef broth
3 tablespoons tomato paste
1 cup chopped fresh rhubarb
1 teaspoon white sugar
½ cup chopped yellow bell pepper
1-2 jalapeños, seeded if desired, finely chopped
¼ cup finely chopped red onion
¼ cup chopped fresh cilantro
1 tablespoon lime juice
16 corn tortillas
Lime wedges for serving

Direction
In a small bowl, combine 1 1/4 teaspoons salt, garlic powder, cumin, oregano and chili powder. Sprinkle two tablespoons mixture on the beef.
In a large frying pan, heat oil over medium-high heat. Put in the beef and cook for 5-6 mins total or until it is browned on all sides, stirring occasionally. Put onion slices in a slow cooker (about 5- to 6-quart). Put in beef. Stir tomato paste and broth into remaining spice mixture and transfer over beef. Cook, covered, on low for 8 hours or on high for 4 hours. Use 2 forks to shred beef. Whisk back into the liquid.
In the meantime, in a medium bowl, toss sugar and rhubarb together. Allow to sit 10 mins. Put in remaining 1/4 teaspoon of salt, cilantro, lime juice, red onion, jalapeño to taste and bell pepper; mix to combine.
Serve the beef with lime wedges, the rhubarb salsa and tortillas.
Nutrition Information
Calories: 359 calories;;Total Fat: 11
Fiber: 5;Protein: 37
Saturated Fat: 3;Sodium: 675;Cholesterol: 100;Total Carbohydrate: 29
Sugar: 3

984. Slow Cooker Chicken Tortilla Soup

Serving: 8 | Prep: 30mins | Cook: 8hours | Ready in:
Ingredients
1 pound shredded, cooked chicken
1 (15 ounce) can whole peeled tomatoes, mashed
1 (10 ounce) can enchilada sauce
1 medium onion, chopped
1 (4 ounce) can chopped green chile peppers
2 cloves garlic, minced
2 cups water
1 (14.5 ounce) can chicken broth
1 teaspoon cumin
1 teaspoon chili powder
1 teaspoon salt
1/4 teaspoon black pepper
1 bay leaf
1 (10 ounce) package frozen corn
1 tablespoon chopped cilantro
7 corn tortillas
vegetable oil
Direction
Put tomatoes, green chiles, garlic, enchilada sauce, onion, and chicken in a slow cooker.
Pour in the chicken broth and water and season it with chili powder, pepper, cumin, bay leaf, and salt. Mix in cilantro and corn. Cover it up and let it cook for 6-8 hours on low setting or 3-4 hours on high setting.
Heat up an oven to 400 degrees Fahrenheit or 200 degrees Celsius.
Brush both of the tortilla sides with oil lightly. Cut them up into strips and then place them on the baking sheet.
Bake them in the heated oven until they're crisp or for about 10-15 minutes. Serve it by placing the tortilla strips over the soup.
Nutrition Information
Calories: 262 calories;;Total Fat: 10.8;Sodium: 893;Total Carbohydrate: 24.7;Cholesterol: 45;Protein: 18

985. Slow Cooker Garlic Mashed Potatoes

Serving: 16 | Prep: 15mins | Cook: | Ready in:
Ingredients
4 pounds Yukon Gold potatoes, diced (½ inch)
¾ cup finely chopped shallots
3 large cloves garlic, peeled
½ cup water
1½ cups buttermilk, at room temperature
¼ cup unsalted butter, melted
1¼ teaspoons salt
½ teaspoon ground pepper
Direction
In a 5 to 6-quart slow cooker, mix together the water, garlic, shallots and potatoes. Let it cook on High for 4 hours. Turn off the slow cooker, then add pepper, salt, butter and buttermilk and mash until blended and nearly smooth.
Nutrition Information
Calories: 133 calories;
Sugar: 1;Total Fat: 3;Sodium: 227;Total Carbohydrate: 23;Protein: 3
Saturated Fat: 2
Fiber: 2;Cholesterol: 9

986. Slow Cooker Lamb Stew With Artichokes White Beans

Serving: 6 | Prep: | Cook: 30mins | Ready in:
Ingredients
1 cup dry small white beans or navy beans, soaked (see Tip)
2 pounds boneless leg of lamb, trimmed and cubed (1-inch)
4 cups reduced-sodium beef broth
8 shallots, ends trimmed and peeled, but left whole
4 cloves garlic, sliced
8 cups chopped escarole
1 15-ounce can artichokes, drained and quartered
Zest and juice of 1 lemon
½ teaspoon pepper
¼ teaspoon salt
¼ cup chopped fresh dill
Direction
Drain the soaked beans and combine them with garlic, shallots, broth, and lamb in a 5-6 quart slow cooker. Cook on a high setting for 4 hours or on a low setting for 8 hours.
Add salt, pepper, lemon juice, lemon zest, artichokes, and escarole to the slow cooker. Cook while covered on high setting until the escarole wilts, around 10 minutes. Serve with a sprinkle of dill.
Nutrition Information
Calories: 373 calories;;Total Fat: 7
Sugar: 3;Total Carbohydrate: 37;Protein: 40
Saturated Fat: 3;Sodium: 747
Fiber: 9;Cholesterol: 91

987. Slow Cooker Moroccan Lentil Soup

Serving: 12 | Prep: | Cook: 30mins | Ready in:
Ingredients
2 cups chopped onions
2 cups chopped carrots
4 cloves garlic, minced
2 teaspoons extra-virgin olive oil
1 teaspoon ground cumin
1 teaspoon ground coriander
1 teaspoon ground turmeric
¼ teaspoon ground cinnamon
¼ teaspoon ground pepper
6 cups vegetable broth or reduced-sodium chicken broth

2 cups water
3 cups chopped cauliflower
1¾ cups lentils
1 28-ounce can diced tomatoes
2 tablespoons tomato paste
4 cups chopped fresh spinach or one 10-ounce package frozen chopped spinach, thawed
½ cup chopped fresh cilantro
2 tablespoons lemon juice
Direction
In a 5-6-quart slow cooker, mix together pepper, cinnamon, turmeric, coriander, cumin, oil, garlic, carrots, and onions. Add tomato paste, tomatoes, lentils, cauliflower, water, and broth and toss until thoroughly blended.
Put the lid on and cook on Low for 8-10 hours or on High for 4-5 hours until the lentils are soft.
Mix in spinach during the last 30 minutes of cooking.
Mix in lemon juice and cilantro right before serving.
Nutrition Information
Calories: 153 calories;
Saturated Fat: 0;Sodium: 200
Sugar: 7;Total Fat: 2
Fiber: 10;Cholesterol: 0;Total Carbohydrate: 28;Protein: 9

988. Slow Cooker Pasta E Fagioli Soup Freezer Pack

Serving: 6 | Prep: 15mins | Cook: | Ready in:
Ingredients
2 cups chopped onions
1 cup chopped carrots
1 cup chopped celery
1 pound cooked Meal-Prep Sheet-Pan Chicken Thighs (see associated recipe), diced
4 cups cooked whole-wheat rotini pasta
6 cups reduced-sodium chicken broth
4 teaspoons dried Italian seasoning
¼ teaspoon salt
1 (15 ounce) can no-salt-added white beans, rinsed
4 cups baby spinach (half of a 5-ounce box)
4 tablespoons chopped fresh basil, divided (optional)
2 tablespoons best-quality extra-virgin olive oil
½ cup grated Parmigiano-Reggiano cheese
Direction
In a resealable large plastic bag, place celery, onions, and carrots. Add the cooked chicken and pasta in another bag. Ensure that bags are properly sealed and store in the freezer for a maximum of five days. Transfer the bags to the refrigerator and thaw overnight.
In a large slow cooker, drop the vegetable mixture adding the broth, salt and Italian seasoning. Cover the pot with a lid and leave it for 7 1/4 hours on low, to cook.
Gently drop thawed chicken and pasta with spinach, beans and 2 tablespoon of basil. Let it cook for another 45 minutes.
Add spinach, beans, 2 tablespoons basil, if using, and the defrosted chicken and pasta. Cook for 45 minutes more. Scoop a good amount of soup into a bowl adding in some cheese and a tiny drizzle of olive oil. If desired, top with two tablespoons of basil.
Nutrition Information
Calories: 457 calories;;Total Fat: 18;Cholesterol: 72
Sugar: 4;Protein: 34
Saturated Fat: 4;Sodium: 653
Fiber: 8;Total Carbohydrate: 42

989. Slow Cooker Shredded Beef Tacos With Pico De Gallo

Serving: 8 | Prep: 45mins | Cook: | Ready in:
Ingredients
Tacos
3 tablespoons chili powder
1 tablespoon dried oregano
1 tablespoon ground cumin
¼ teaspoon salt
½ teaspoon cayenne pepper
½ teaspoon garlic powder
3 pounds beef chuck, trimmed and cut into 1-inch cubes
1 tablespoon extra-virgin olive oil
1 large onion, halved and sliced
1 cup low-sodium beef broth
3 tablespoons tomato paste
16 corn tortillas
Lime wedges for serving
Pico de Gallo
¾ cup diced tomato (about 1 medium)
½ cup chopped fresh cilantro
¼ cup finely diced red onion
1 jalapeño pepper, seeded if desired, finely diced
1 tablespoon lime juice
¼ teaspoon salt
Direction
Preparing the beef: In a small bowl, mix together the garlic powder, cayenne, salt, cumin, oregano and chili powder, then sprinkle 2 tablespoons of the mixture on the beef.
In a big frying pan, heat the oil on medium-high heat, then add the beef and let it cook for 5 to 6 minutes in total, stirring from time to time, until all sides turn brown.
In a 5 to 6-quart slow cooker, put the onion, then add the beef. Whisk together the leftover spice mixture, tomato paste and broth and pour it on top of the beef. Let it cook for 8 hours on Low or 4 hours on High. Use 2 forks to shred the beef and mix it back into the liquid.
Preparing the pico de gallo: In a medium bowl, mix together the salt, lime juice, jalapeño, red onion, cilantro and tomato.
Serve the beef with lime wedges, pico de gallo and tortillas.
Nutrition Information
Calories: 521 calories;;Total Fat: 17
Fiber: 6;Total Carbohydrate: 28
Sugar: 3;Protein: 64
Saturated Fat: 5;Sodium: 409;Cholesterol: 177

990. Slow Cooker Southwestern Bean Soup

Serving: 6 | Prep: 20mins | Cook: | Ready in:
Ingredients
1 tablespoon extra-virgin olive oil
1 large onion, diced
1 large stalk celery, diced
1 large carrot, diced
2 cups water
4 cups reduced-sodium chicken broth, "no-chicken" broth or vegetable broth (32-ounce carton)
½ cup pearl barley
⅓ cup dried black beans
⅓ cup dried great northern beans
⅓ cup dried kidney beans

1 tablespoon chili powder
1 teaspoon ground cumin
½ teaspoon dried oregano
¾ teaspoon salt
Direction
In a 5- to 6-quart slow cooker, mix oil, barley, celery, carrot, water, broth, barley, kidney beans, black beans, great northern beans, cumin, chili powder, oregano and salt. For 7 to 8 hours on low or about 4 hours on high, cover and cook beans until tender.
Nutrition Information
Calories: 196 calories;;Sodium: 402
Fiber: 8
Sugar: 3;Protein: 10;Total Fat: 4
Saturated Fat: 1;Cholesterol: 0;Total Carbohydrate: 32

991. Slow Cooker Sweet Potato Casserole With Marshmallows

Serving: 12 | Prep: 20mins | Cook: | Ready in:
Ingredients
3 pounds sweet potatoes, peeled and diced (½ inch)
2 tablespoons light brown sugar
3 tablespoons melted butter
1 teaspoon vanilla extract
1 teaspoon salt
½ teaspoon ground pepper
½ teaspoon ground cinnamon
¼ teaspoon ground nutmeg
½ cup mini marshmallows
½ cup toasted chopped pecans
Direction
In a 5-6 qt. slow cooker, mix nutmeg, cinnamon, pepper, salt, vanilla, butter, brown sugar and sweet potatoes together; stir to coat. Cook for 3 hours on High.
Move to a serving dish; top with marshmallows and pecans. The heat from the sweet potatoes will melt the marshmallows slightly.
Nutrition Information
Calories: 159 calories;;Total Fat: 6;Sodium: 227;Total Carbohydrate: 25;Cholesterol: 8
Sugar: 10;Protein: 2
Saturated Fat: 2
Fiber: 3

992. Slow Cooker Turkish Lamb Vegetable Stew

Serving: 8 | Prep: | Cook: 20mins | Ready in:
Ingredients
1½ pounds lean boneless leg of lamb, trimmed and cut into 1¼-inch pieces
1¼ teaspoons salt, divided
1½ tablespoons extra-virgin olive oil, divided
2 large onions, thinly sliced
4 cloves garlic, minced
½ teaspoon dried oregano
Freshly ground pepper, to taste
1 large all-purpose potato, preferably Yukon Gold, peeled and cut into ⅜-inch-thick slices
½ pound green beans, trimmed
1 small eggplant, cut into ⅜-inch-thick slices
1 medium zucchini, cut into ⅜-inch-thick slices
6 bay leaves
1 14-ounce can diced tomatoes
3 tablespoons chopped fresh parsley
Direction
Use 1/4 teaspoon of pepper and salt to season the lamb. In a big, heavy frying pan, heat 1/2 tablespoon of oil over medium-high heat. Put in 1/2 of the lamb and sear for 2-4 minutes until fully browned, flipping. Move to a 4-qt. slow cooker. Add the other 1/2 tablespoon of oil to the frying pan and brow the leftover lamb. Add to the slow cooker.
Add the leftover 1/2 tablespoon of oil to the frying pan and lower the heat to medium. Add onions and cook for 3-5 minutes until tender, mixing. Add oregano and garlic; cook for another 1 minute, mixing. Add tomatoes and simmer, using a fork or potato masher to mash. Take away from heat and put 1/2 of the mixture on the lamb.
In the pot, put 1 layer of potatoes, use 1/4 teaspoon of pepper and salt to season. Add green beans, and then zucchini and eggplant, use 1/4 teaspoon of pepper and salt to season each layer. Spread over the vegetables with the leftover of the onion-tomato mixture. Put bay leaves on top.
Put a cover on and cook for 4 hours on high, until the vegetables and lamb are completely soft. Remove the bay leaves. Enjoy hot, use parsley to garnish.
Nutrition Information
Calories: 190 calories;;Total Carbohydrate: 15;Protein: 16;Total Fat: 8;Sodium: 466
Fiber: 5;Cholesterol: 43
Sugar: 6
Saturated Fat: 2

993. Slow Cooker Vegetable Soup

Serving: 8 | Prep: 35mins | Cook: | Ready in:
Ingredients
1 medium onion, chopped
2 medium carrots, chopped
2 stalks celery, chopped
12 ounces fresh green beans, cut into ½-inch pieces
4 cups chopped kale
2 medium zucchini, chopped
4 Roma tomatoes, seeded and chopped
2 cloves garlic, minced
2 (15 ounce) cans no-salt-added cannellini or other white beans, rinsed
4 cups low-sodium chicken broth or low-sodium vegetable broth
2 teaspoons salt
½ teaspoon ground pepper
2 teaspoons red-wine vinegar
8 teaspoons prepared pesto
Direction
In a big or 6 quart slow cooker, mix the pepper, salt, broth, white beans, garlic, tomatoes, zucchini, kale, green beans, celery, carrots and onion. Cook for 6 hours on Low or 4 hours on High.
Add in vinegar and put 1 teaspoon of pesto on top of each soup serving.
Nutrition Information
Calories: 174 calories;;Sodium: 733
Fiber: 8;Total Carbohydrate: 26;Protein: 10;Total Fat: 4
Saturated Fat: 1;Cholesterol: 0
Sugar: 5

994. Slow Cooker Yankee Bean Pot

Serving: 8 | Prep: | Cook: 20mins | Ready in:
Ingredients
1 pound dried navy or great northern beans
1 teaspoon canola oil
2 medium onions, chopped

4 ounces Canadian-style bacon, diced (¾ cup)
6 cloves garlic, minced
1 teaspoon dried thyme leaves
Pinch of crushed red pepper
¼ cup pure maple syrup, or molasses
¼ cup ketchup
2 tablespoons Worcestershire sauce
1 tablespoon dry mustard
½ pound smoked ham hock, pork neck bones or turkey wings (optional)
3 cups boiling water
2 bay leaves
1-2 tablespoons cider vinegar
Hot sauce, such as Tabasco, to taste
¼ teaspoon salt
Freshly ground pepper, to taste
Direction
In a large bowl, arrange beans and pour in cold water to cover. Allow to soak for minimum of 8 hours to overnight (You can add 2 quarts of water and beans to a large pot. Bring to a boil. Boil for 2 minutes. Take away from the heat and allow to stand for an hour). Drain the beans and wash. Arrange in a slow cooker.
In a large non-stick skillet, heat the oil over medium-high heat. Put in bacon and onions; cook and regularly stir for 5 minutes until they turn light golden and become soft. Put in the crushed red pepper, thyme, and garlic; cook and stir for 1 more minute. Place over the beans.
Place mustard, Worcestershire, ketchup, molasses or maple syrup over the beans; then stir to blend. Bury the turkey wings, neck bones, or ham hock into the beans if using. Pour in the boiling water and add bay leaves on top.
Put on a cover and cook on low for 11 hours or on high for 4 1/4 hours, until beans become tender. Remove bones and bay leaves. Flavor with pepper, salt, hot sauce, and vinegar. Then serve it hot.
Nutrition Information
Calories: 272 calories;;Cholesterol: 7;Protein: 16
Sugar: 12;Total Fat: 2
Saturated Fat: 0;Sodium: 306
Fiber: 9;Total Carbohydrate: 48

995. Southwestern Three Bean Barley Soup

Serving: 6 | Prep: | Cook: 30mins | Ready in:
Ingredients
1 tablespoon extra-virgin olive oil
1 large onion, diced
1 large stalk celery, diced
1 large carrot, diced
9 cups water
4 cups (32-ounce carton) reduced-sodium chicken broth, "no-chicken" broth or vegetable broth
½ cup pearl barley
⅓ cup dried black beans
⅓ cup dried great northern beans
⅓ cup dried kidney beans
1 tablespoon chili powder
1 teaspoon ground cumin
½ teaspoon dried oregano
¾ teaspoon salt
Direction
Heat oil inside a Dutch oven on medium heat. Add carrot, celery and onion; cook for 5 minutes till soft, occasionally mixing. Add oregano, cumin, chili powder, kidney beans, great northern beans, black beans, barley, broth and water; let it lively simmer on high heat. Lower the heat to maintain simmering; cook for 1 3/4-2 1/2 hours till beans are tender, occasionally mixing, if needed or desired, add 1/2 cup more water at a time. Season with salt.
Slow-cooker option: Instead of 9 cups, use 2 cups of water; mix together all ingredients inside a 5-6-qt. slow cooker then cover and cook for 7-8 hours on low or 4 hours on high till the beans are tender.
Nutrition Information
Calories: 205 calories;
Saturated Fat: 1;Cholesterol: 0;Total Carbohydrate: 36;Protein: 9;Total Fat: 3;Sodium: 454
Fiber: 11
Sugar: 3

996. Spanish Potato Omelet

Serving: 6 | Prep: 15mins | Cook: 45mins | Ready in:
Ingredients
1/2 cup olive oil
1/2 pound potatoes, thinly sliced
salt and pepper to taste
1 large onion, thinly sliced
4 eggs
salt and pepper to taste
2 tomatoes - peeled, seeded, and coarsely chopped
2 green onions, chopped
Direction
Heat olive oil in a big skillet or frying pan set over medium-high temperature. Lightly season potatoes with salt and pepper then fry until crisp and golden brown.
When the potatoes become golden, add in the onions. Cook and stir until onions start to brown and soften. In another bowl, place eggs and sprinkle with salt and pepper to taste. Whisk eggs then pour it into the pan, stirring gently to blend well. Turn heat down to low and continue cooking until eggs start to brown on the bottom.
Using a spatula, loosen the bottom of the omelet. Cover pan with a big plate, turned upside down, and carefully flip the omelet out onto it. Slip the omelet back into the pan with the uncooked side down. Continue to cook until eggs are done. Serve warm with tomato and green onion as garnish.
Nutrition Information
Calories: 252 calories;;Total Fat: 21.5;Sodium: 54;Total Carbohydrate: 10.7;Cholesterol: 124;Protein: 5.4

997. Sweet Ginger Root Vegetables

Serving: 8 | Prep: 15mins | Cook: | Ready in:
Ingredients
2¾ pounds red and/or golden beets, trimmed, peeled, and cut into ¾-inch wedges
12 ounces carrots, peeled and cut into 3-inch pieces (halve any thick pieces) (4 medium)
2 teaspoons grated fresh ginger
½ cup pomegranate juice
¼ teaspoon salt
1 tablespoon cornstarch
1 tablespoon water
¼ cup sugar
Direction
Combine the salt, pomegranate juice, ginger, carrots and beets in a 3 1/2 or 4-quart slow cooker.
Cover and cook the mixture on low-heat setting for 6 hours or on high-heat setting for 3 hours. Turn to high-heat setting when using a low-heat setting. Mix

cold water and cornstarch together and stir the mixture into the beet mixture together with the sugar or sugar substitute. Cover the slow cooker and cook for 20 more minutes, until bubbly and thick.

Nutrition Information
Calories: 122 calories;
Fiber: 6;Total Carbohydrate: 28
Sugar: 21;Protein: 3;Sodium: 225

998. Tangy Cherry Barbecue Sausage

Serving: 36 | Prep: 15mins | Cook: | Ready in:
Ingredients
2 medium onions, finely chopped (1 cup)
⅔ cup cherry preserves
¼ cup no-salt-added tomato paste
¼ cup cider vinegar
1 teaspoon ground chipotle chile pepper
2 pounds cooked light smoked Polish sausage or smoked turkey sausage, cut into 72 slices (about ½-inch thick)
Direction
Mix together the chipotle chile pepper, vinegar, tomato paste, cherry preserves and onions in a 2-qt. slow cooker, add sausage slices and toss to combine. Cover and cook for 4 hours on low heat setting, then serve it right away. Or keep it warm for up to 1 hour on low heat setting, stirring occasionally, serve with toothpicks.

Nutrition Information
Calories: 60 calories;
Sugar: 3;Sodium: 227;Cholesterol: 16;Total Carbohydrate: 5;Total Fat: 1
Saturated Fat: 0
Fiber: 0;Protein: 4

999. Vegetable And Pasta Soup

Serving: 6 | Prep: 20mins | Cook: | Ready in:
Ingredients
1 (15 ounce) can cannellini (white kidney) beans, rinsed and drained
1 (8 ounce) package fresh button mushrooms, quartered
1 cup frozen whole kernel corn
1 cup chopped onion
1 cup finely chopped carrots
1 cup coarsely chopped zucchini
2 cloves garlic, minced
6 cups unsalted vegetable or chicken stock
1 (6 ounce) can no-salt-added tomato paste
2 teaspoons dried Italian seasoning, crushed
½ teaspoon salt
1 (9 ounce) package frozen Italian green beans
½ cup dried multigrain rotini or elbow pasta
2 tablespoons snipped fresh parsley
2 tablespoons finely shredded Parmesan cheese
Direction
Combine garlic, zucchini, carrots, onion, corn, mushrooms, and cannellini beans in a 3 1/2 to 5 quart slow cooker. Stir in salt, Italian seasoning, tomato paste, and stock.
Cook while covered on low setting for 7-8 hours or on high setting for 3 1/2-4 hours. If using a low setting, turn the heat up to high. Stir in the pasta and frozen beans, then cook, covered, for 45 more minutes.
Stir in parsley before serving and sprinkle with cheese.

Nutrition Information
Calories: 213 calories;;Total Carbohydrate: 42
Sugar: 13;Protein: 10;Sodium: 598
Fiber: 8
Saturated Fat: 0;Cholesterol: 1;Total Fat: 1

1000. Veggies, Turkey, And Pasta

Serving: 8 | Prep: 40mins | Cook: | Ready in:
Ingredients
1 pound turkey breast tenderloin, cut into ¾-inch cubes
2 teaspoons olive oil
2 (14.5 ounce) cans no-salt-added diced tomatoes, undrained
1 (10.75 ounce) can reduced-fat and reduced-sodium condensed cream of mushroom soup
4 medium carrots, sliced (2 cups)
3 stalks celery, sliced (1½ cups)
3 medium onions, chopped (1½ cups)
4 cloves garlic, minced
2 teaspoons dried Italian seasoning, crushed
½ teaspoon salt
¼ teaspoon black pepper
8 ounces dried multigrain penne pasta (2¾ cups dried)
¼ cup finely shredded Parmesan cheese (1 ounce)
Direction
Cook turkey in hot oil in a 12-inch skillet until all sides are lightly browned.
Stir soup and tomatoes together in a 4- to 5-quart slow cooker. Stir in pepper, salt, Italian seasoning, garlic, onions, celery, carrots and browned turkey. Cook with a cover for 7-8 hours on low-heat setting or 3 1/2-4 hours on high-heat setting.
In the meantime, cook penne pasta as directed on the package; drain. Stir penne gently into the cooker.
Serve in shallow bowls and top cheese over each serving.

Nutrition Information
Calories: 260 calories;;Total Carbohydrate: 36
Sugar: 7;Protein: 20
Fiber: 4;Cholesterol: 38;Total Fat: 4
Saturated Fat: 1;Sodium: 440

1001. Wine Tomato Braised Chicken

Serving: 10 | Prep: | Cook: 45mins | Ready in:
Ingredients
4 slices bacon
1 large onion, thinly sliced
4 cloves garlic, minced
1 teaspoon dried thyme
1 teaspoon fennel seeds
1 teaspoon freshly ground pepper
1 bay leaf
1 cup dry white wine (see Tip)
1 28-ounce can whole tomatoes, with juice, coarsely chopped
1 teaspoon salt
10 bone-in chicken thighs (about 3¾ pounds), skin removed, trimmed
¼ cup finely chopped fresh parsley
Direction
Cook the bacon on medium heat in the big skillet for roughly 4 minutes or till becoming crisp. Move to the paper towels to let drain. Break up into crumbles once cooled.
Drain off all except 2 tbsp. of the fat from the pan. Put in the onion and cook on medium heat, mixing, for 3-6 minutes or till becoming tender. Put in the bay leaf, pepper, fennel seeds, thyme and garlic and cook, mixing, for 60 seconds. Pour in the wine, boil and boil

for 2 minutes, scraping up any of the browned bits. Put in the tomatoes along with their juice and salt; whisk them well.

Add the chicken thighs into the 4-qt. (or bigger) slow cooker. Drizzle the bacon on top of chicken. Add tomato mixture on top of chicken. Keep covered and cooked roughly for 6 hours over Low heat or roughly 3 hours over High heat or till chicken softens very much. Discard the bay leaf. Sprinkle with the parsley then serve.

Variation: Turn 2 cups each of the remaining chicken and sauce into the Braised Chicken Gumbo. Heat 1 tbsp. of the extra-virgin olive oil on medium heat in the big sauce pan. Put in 1 diced medium red/green bell pepper and 2 tbsp. of the all-purpose flour and cook, whisking, for roughly 2 minutes or till flour turns golden brown and pepper starts to become tender. Put in 1/8-1/4 tsp. of the cayenne pepper, three quarters cup of the instant brown rice (see the Tip), 1 cup of the sliced okra (which can be fresh/frozen, thawed), 2 cups of the reduced-sodium chicken broth, 2 cups of the sauce, and 2 cups of the shredded chicken. Boil. Lower the heat and let simmer for roughly 10 minutes or till okra softens and flavors are melded.

Tip: Mix in 1 cup of any remaining cooked rice instead if you use the not-instant rice. Otherwise, if you have the time, put in half cup of the quicker-cooking whole-grain rice, like Kalijira rice/Bhutanese red rice, and the extra 1.25 cups of the chicken broth prior to putting in okra. Cook for roughly 25 minutes (or following the direction on package) or till rice nearly softens then put in okra and let simmer till it softens.

Nutrition Information
Calories: 240 calories;
Saturated Fat: 3;Sodium: 395;Total Carbohydrate: 5
Sugar: 2;Protein: 24;Total Fat: 12
Fiber: 2;Cholesterol: 84

www.ingramcontent.com/pod-product-compliance
Lightning Source LLC
Chambersburg PA
CBHW081106080526
44587CB00021B/3475